PCAT
PHARMACY COLLEGE
ADMISSION TEST

Related Titles

Becoming a Healthcare Professional

Health Occupations Entrance Exams

Pharmacy Technician Exam

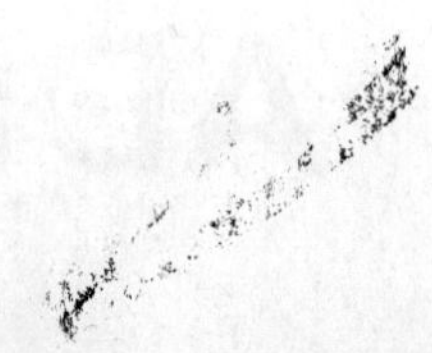

PCAT PHARMACY COLLEGE ADMISSION TEST

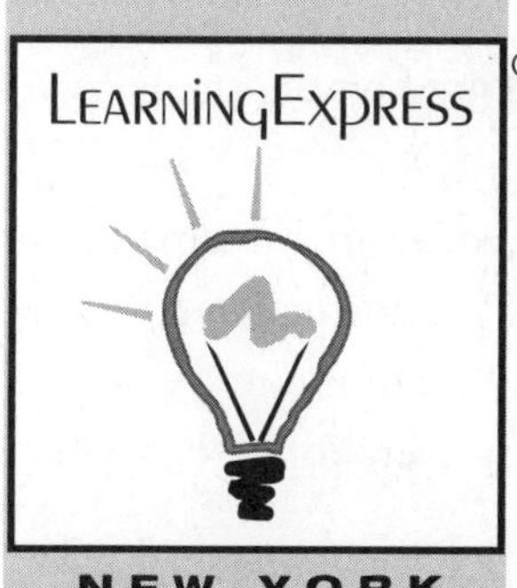

NEW YORK

Published in the United States by LearningExpress, LLC, New York.

Library of Congress Cataloging-in-Publication Data:
PCAT : pharmacy college admission test.—1st ed.
p. ; cm.
Pharmacy college admission test
ISBN-13: 978-1-57685-787-8
ISBN-10: 1-57685-787-5
1. Pharmacy colleges—United States—Entrance examinations—Study guides. 2. Pharmacy—Examinations, questions, etc. I. LearningExpress (Organization). II. Title: Pharmacy college admission test. [DNLM: 1. College Admission Test—Examination Questions. 2. Pharmacy—Examination Questions. 3. Schools, Pharmacy—Examination Questions. 4. Test Taking Skills—Examination Questions. QV 18.2]
RS105.P36 2011
615'.1076—dc22

2011006975

Printed in the United States of America

9 8 7 6 5 4 3 2 1

ISBN 978-1-57685-787-8

For more information or to place an order, contact LearningExpress at:
2 Rector Street
26th Floor
New York, NY 10006

Or visit us at:
www.learnatest.com

CONTENTS

CONTRIBUTORS

Glen Brizius (Chemistry)

Glen Brizius has a Ph.D. in Organic Chemistry from the University of South Carolina, where he graduated with honors. Glen is a synthetic chemist and a scientific innovator with expertise developing chemical solutions for polymers, textiles, perfumes and fragrances, and manufacturing and natural products industries. He is a recipient of a number of prestigious fellowships and awards including a National Research Council (NRC) Fellowship and is a sought-after speaker at numerous events and organizations, guest researcher at NASA, and a member of the research faculty at Georgia Tech. Glen's areas of expertise include: TEM; SEM; NMR; IR; MS; GC; HPLC; GPC; UV-Vis; Fluorescence Spectroscopy/Quantum Yield Determination; DSC; TGA; CD; Polarizing Microscopy; LED Fabrication, and Electrochemistry.

Ann Cohen (Writing and Reading Comprehension)

Ann Cohen is a freelance writer/editor based in New York City. A graduate of the University of Pennsylvania, she has spent 20 years in the non-profit sector, 10 of them as director of development and communications for a medical research institute. Ms. Cohen is a co-author of *The Complete Idiot's Guide to Dangerous Diseases and Epidemics* and served as editorial consultant on *Timebomb*, a book about multi-drug resistant tuberculosis in Russia. She has also contributed to a number of test preparation books including those for NCLEX-RN, Advanced Placement Study in English Language, English Composition, U.S. Government and Politics, U.S. History and World History, and the MAT.

Allison Dunne (Verbal Ability)
Allison Dunne is a National Public Radio member station writer, reporter, and producer who covers science and other topical issues. Most recently she has worked on a series of science and technology pieces funded by a National Science Foundation grant. In addition to being an independent reporter/producer, Allison has been a news bureau chief and reporter for a public radio station. She has also been a news anchor and co-host on commercial radio in New York. Her work has been broadcast on public and commercial radio stations across the country. Allison graduated with honors with a BS in Journalism from Boston University.

Michael Hough (Biology)
Michael Hough is a graduate of the State University of New York College of Environmental Science and Forestry (SUNY ESF), where he earned his M.S. degree in Plant Ecology. He is currently an adjunct professor at the State University of New York College at Cortland and has taught classes in General Biology, Zoology, Botany, and Environmental Science.

Jeffrey Linson (Chemistry)
Jeffrey Linson has a degree in chemistry from Yale University. He is currently an information technology project manager specializing in web technologies, e-commerce, retail, and accounting and reporting systems. He is an experienced test preparation tutor and has worked as a consultant with major multinational companies, including International Paper, Pfizer—Warner-Lambert, Pepsi International, Pepsi—North America, and the former Sea-Land Services division of CSX. Jeffrey is a member of the Project Management Institute (PMI).

Phillip Montgomery (Chemistry)
Phillip Montgomery is a general chemistry student and teaching assistant in organic chemistry, an Undergraduate Research Scholar at the University of North Carolina, Asheville, and a member of the American Chemical Society. Phillip's areas of interest are inorganic synthesis and catalysis, especially green catalysis involving chromium centered complexes.

Louiza Patsis (Chemistry)
Louiza Patsis received a Bachelor of Arts in Chemistry and an M.S. in biomedical journalism from New York University. She is a Ph.D. candidate and is currently working on her dissertation in the NYU Palmer School of Information Science Doctoral Program on the topic of telemedicine. Louiza has many years of experience in continuing medical education, pharmaceutical advertising, and publishing and, in her day-to-day consulting business, works closely with physicians, PharmDs, the Food and Drug Administration, and the National Drug Authority. Her areas of interest include: biochemistry, genetics, oncology, virology, and toxicology, among others. She is a member of the American Association for the Advancement of Science, National Writers Union, National Association of Science Writers, American Medical Writers Association, National Academy of Science, American Women in Science, and Landmark Education. She is also the author of *The Boy in a Wheelchair, Life, Work and Play: Poems and Short Stories*, and two editions of *Pocket Guide to Fitness.*

Robin Pickering (Biology)

Robin Pickering has a Bachelor of Arts from the University of Kentucky–Lexington, and has completed pre-pharmacy course work in Biology, Microbiology, Anatomy & Physiology, Biochemistry, Chemistry, Organic Chemistry, and Physics. Robin is also the author of numerous certification test preparation books.

Michael Sapko (Chemistry)

Michael Sapko is an M.D. with a Ph.D. in Neuroscience from the University of Maryland. He has received numerous awards including the National Research Service Award from the National Institute of Neurological Diseases and Stroke and the American Society for Neurochemistry Young Investigator Educational Enhancement Award. He is the author of several peer-reviewed articles in such prestigious publications as the International Archives of Medicine, the Journal of Neurochemistry, and Experimental Neurology, among others. He is currently a freelance medical/science writer and has written test preparation materials for the MCAT, NCLEX, USMLE, and Praxis exams along with a variety of other projects.

Michael Solomon (Quantitative Ability)

Michael Solomon, CISSP, PMP, CISM, GSEC, holds an M.S. in Mathematics and Computer Science from Emory University, a Bachelor of Science in Computer Science from Kennesaw State University, and is currently pursuing a Ph.D. in Computer Science and Informatics at Emory University. He is a full-time security speaker, consultant, and author, and a former college instructor who specializes in development and assessment security topics. Previously, he was an instructor in the Kennesaw State University's Computer Science and Information Sciences (CSIS) department, where he taught courses on software project management, C++ programming, computer organization and architecture, and data communications. As an IT professional and consultant, he has worked on projects for more than 100 major companies and organizations. He has also contributed to various security certification books and has authored an e-learning course as well.

Shan Siddiqi (Chemistry)

Shan Siddiqi is a freelance writer and a current medical student at the University of Sydney in Australia. He earned his undergraduate degree from the University of Missouri with a major in chemistry (medicinal) and minors in medical physics, radioenvironmental sciences, and biology. His research background centers around projects in medicinal chemistry and clinical pharmacology, often in combination with molecular biology and microbiology. Combined with his undergraduate training in chemistry, his background in clinical pharmacology and his graduate medical training help to create a solid foundation for producing PCAT preparation materials.

Ann Marie Souzzi (Chemistry)

Anne Marie Souzzi, a graduate of Columbia University and the University of Illinois at Urbana–Champaign, has been an Adjunct Professor at Cornell University, The University of California at Berkeley, The University of Illinois at Urbana–Champaign, Niagara University, The State University of NY at Buffalo SUNY, and St. John's University among others. She has taught college-level Physics, Chemistry, Organic Chemistry, Anatomy and Physiology, Biology, Biological Organic Chemistry, Biochemistry, Pharmacokinetics, and Medicinal Chemistry, as well as other science and math subjects. She has written numerous papers and has contributed to many test preparation guides on subjects as diverse as the MCAT, AP Statistics, NCLEX, and the GRE. She is currently a second-year medical student.

Sean Thomas (Quantitative Ability)

Sean Thomas is a Ph.D. candidate in Mathematics with a specialization in arithmetic hyperbolic 3-manifolds and additional education in Computer Science at Emory University. His areas of study include Fuchsian Groups, Algebraic Number Theory, and Arithmetic Hyperbolic 3-Manifolds. He is a graduate instructor in Probability and Statistics as well as Calculus I and II. He is a graduate of Rollins College, where he tutored students in Precalculus, Calculus I/II/III, Linear Algebra, Discrete Mathematics, and Abstract Mathematics.

PCAT
PHARMACY COLLEGE ADMISSION TEST

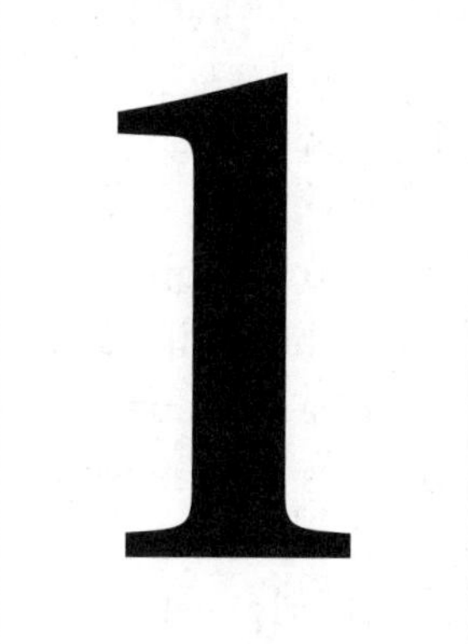

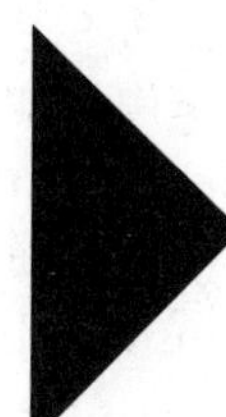

CHAPTER 1 THE PROFESSION

If you ask people on the street what they think of when they hear the word *pharmacist*, the odds are they will tell you a pharmacist is the person behind the counter at the local drugstore who wears a white coat and dispenses medications. They would probably also tell you that they have a high level of respect for pharmacists, a profession consistently identified as among the most trusted in the United States.

If you're considering pharmacy as a career, you probably already know that working as a neighborhood pharmacist is only one of a number of career paths for those with a pharmacy degree. With that in mind, this chapter includes an overview of the profession, including a brief history, information on the profession's future prospects, working environment, typical salaries/benefits, and career opportunities, as well as useful information on educational requirements, postgraduate training, and Internet resources.

Background and History of the Profession

The profession of pharmacist arose in the United States in response to the importation of drugs and medications from Europe. In Colonial times, there were no regulations or legal standards for medications and no labeling requirements. People purchased medications from doctors, at general stores, or from wholesalers and importers.

The first pharmacy college opened in Philadelphia in 1821, and by midcentury, special expertise and education were required to prepare medications. The American Pharmacists Association (the APhA) pushed for standards, including labeling and ingredient lists, when it was first organized in 1852.

It may surprise you to learn that until the mid-1900s, the majority of doctor's offices included dispensaries (facilities for compounding and preparing medications) and patients did not need prescriptions to buy drugs. Medication labeling laws were not passed until 1938. This began to create the distinction between over-the-counter medications and prescription medications. In 1952, a law was passed designating the Food and Drug Administration (FDA) as the arbiter of whether a medication could be offered over-the-counter or as a prescription only.

As the number of prescription medications have increased and become more complex, so too have the qualifications necessary to become a pharmacist. Today, pharmacists must complete four years of study and complete a PharmD degree from a school approved by the Accreditation Council for Pharmacy Education (ACPE). Graduates must then pass specific exams to become licensed to practice in the United States. All states require the North American Pharmacist Licensure Exam (NAPLEX) and a specified number of hours of experience in a practice setting (which can be met while in school). Forty-four states also require pharmacists to pass the Multistate Pharmacy Jurisprudence Examination (MPJE), which tests pharmacists' knowledge of pharmacy law.

Future Prospects of the Profession

According to the *Occupational Outlook Handbook, 2010–2011 Edition* (United States Department of Labor's Bureau of Labor Statistics), the employment of pharmacists is expected to grow by 17% through 2018, higher than average compared to other professions. A shortfall of around 160,000 pharmacists is predicted by 2020, according to the findings of a conference sponsored by the Pharmacy Manpower Project, Inc. Demand for pharmacists is being spurred by the "graying" of the population, as the increasing number of middle-aged and elderly seek medical attention, including prescription drugs.

The drive to expand healthcare, including prescription drug coverage, is also expected to impact the demand for pharmacists. According to the *Occupational Outlook Handbook*, employers in many parts of the country report difficulty finding and retaining sufficient numbers of pharmacists, and there are currently anywhere from 7,000 to 10,000 unfilled positions in the United States at any given time.

Career Opportunities

It may surprise you to learn just how varied the career opportunities for a pharmacist are. For instance, you can work for a company that owns and operates drugstores (according to the Bureau of Labor Statistics, about 65% of pharmacists work in a retail environment). Your career path might consist of starting in a store, and then possibly progressing to a regional, divisional, or corporate position, if your interests lie in that direction. Some pharmacists even open their own pharmacy. Many pharmacists find fulfillment by spending their entire careers working day-to-day directly with consumers. There's a lot more to these in-store positions than knowing about the composition and properties of medications and dispensing them. These pharmacists also act as health educators, checking patients' medications lists to watch for side effects and interactions for patients taking multiple drugs, and teaching patients how to take their drugs properly and safely. Just think about how many times you have asked your own local pharmacist for recommendations or help.

Pharmacists may also work in hospitals, nursing homes, or other extended care facilities. In such cases, they usually begin working in a hospital pharmacy and progress to being in charge of one or a group of hospital pharmacies overseeing things like medication procurement and distribution. According to the Bureau of Labor Statistics, about 22% of pharmacists work in a hospital setting.

Positions are also available at pharmaceutical companies in research and development, or marketing, sales, and administration. And of course there's the possibility of teaching at a pharmacy school or doing research at a university.

Working Environment

The day-to-day environment in which pharmacists work tends to be clean, well-lighted, and well-ventilated. Pharmacists may be required to wear gloves, masks, or other personal protective equipment (PPE) if they are working with dangerous drugs or need to maintain a sterile environment. Pharmacists typically spend much of the day on their feet. According to the Bureau of Labor Statistics, most pharmacists work about 40 hours a week, although about 20% work part-time. Depending on the type of employment, some night, weekend, and holiday hours may be required.

Salary and Benefits

Pharmacist jobs pay fairly well, and many have good benefits, too. According to the Bureau of Labor Statistics and the website Payscale.com, the mean salary for pharmacists in 2009 was $106,630, and the range was from $60,000 to $124,000. Around 83% of those positions offered medical benefits, 67% offered dental benefits, and 51% offered vision benefits.

Education

In order to be a practicing pharmacist in the United States, you must earn a PharmD degree from an accredited school of pharmacy. The ACPE or the APhA are the best resources to go to for up-to-date information on accredited schools. For some specific career paths, especially those involving research, it's necessary to get a graduate degree or a PhD.

Before Applying to Pharmacy School

Each pharmacy school has its own specific requirements with respect to the course work you must complete before applying for its pharmacy program. However, you typically will be required to complete two years of specific undergraduate prepharmacy study before being admitted to a PharmD program. This requirement means taking courses in natural sciences like biology (some schools may also require anatomy, physiology, and microbiology); chemistry (general and organic); physics; as well as statistics, precalculus, and calculus. You must also take the Pharmacy College Admission Test (PCAT™) for admission to most programs.

Applying to Pharmacy School

The Pharmacy College Application Service (PharmCAS) provides a centralized application service that allows you to use one application to apply to multiple PharmD programs. PharmCAS accepts applications beginning in July for admission to pharmacy school in the fall of the following calendar year. To complete the PharmCAS application, you will need an official academic transcript, your PCAT scores, and reference letters. Visit the PharmCAS website (www.pharmcas.org) for more information. Not all pharmacy schools participate in the PharmCAS, so make sure to check the application procedures for each school to which you intend to apply.

What You'll Learn in Pharmacy School

During your four years of pharmacy school, you will take courses that help you learn about all aspects of drug therapy. You will also learn how to communicate information about drugs and overall care with patients and healthcare providers. In addition you will learn professional ethics, public health, and business management. Pharmacy college students also work with licensed pharmacists in practice settings as part of the required training in order to become licensed.

Training

In addition to educational and licensing requirements previously mentioned, some pharmacy school graduates gain additional training through residency programs or fellowships (which typically last one or two years). Pharmacy residencies are postgraduate training programs that usually require the completion of a research project. This additional training is often mandatory if you want to work in a clinical setting. Pharmacy fellowships are more specific and individualized. They are designed to prepare you to work in a specialized area of pharmacy, like a research laboratory.

For those of you who may want to own your own pharmacy, it may make sense for you to take business classes or even consider getting a master's degree in business administration (MBA). You may also find that an advanced degree in public administration or public health may lead to expanded career opportunities.

Resources

There are a number of resources available online that you can consult for further information about a career as a pharmacist. The American Association of Colleges of Pharmacy (www.aacp.org) is the national organization representing pharmacy education in the United States. The Student Center page on its website provides links to a pharmacy school locator, pharmacy career information, and information for current student pharmacists about pharmacy residency and internship opportunities. At the National Association of Boards of Pharmacy website, www.nabp.net, you can find links to the various state Boards of Pharmacy throughout the United States, as well as in Canada and New Zealand. It also provides information about the NAPLEX and the MPJE, and much more. The Pharmacy Choice site (www.pharmacychoice.com) is another very valuable resource. It is a Web portal that provides links to a plethora of information, including news and information about pharmacy careers and education.

There are many career paths and opportunities for students who complete pharmacy school. The rest of this book will help you prepare for the PCAT so that you can get a good score, be accepted into pharmacy school, and start down the road to your career as a licensed pharmacist.

CHAPTER 2

THE PCAT EXAM

You've bought this book to prepare for the PCAT™, or Pharmacy College Admission Test. One of the most important ways to begin that preparation is to become familiar with the process of registering for the exam, the subjects the exam covers, the number of sections and times for each section, and the exam format. This chapter will help you get started. Note: Information in this chapter is current as of the date of publication. For the most recent information, refer to the official PCAT website, www.pcatweb.info.

Overview of the PCAT

The PCAT exam is a test for students who want to go to pharmacy school. Scores are submitted to pharmacy colleges as part of the application process. The objective of the test is to assess specific skill sets among applicants and to use the scores to determine which students are best qualified and show the most aptitude for a career in pharmacy.

The test takes four hours and is offered four times a year, on a Saturday in January, June, August, and October, at around 200 locations throughout the United States and Puerto Rico, with additional locations in Canada and Qatar. It has seven sections (five multiple choice and two writing) with a short break midway through the exam. Each multiple-choice section has 48 questions. Subjects covered include biology, chemistry, quantitative ability, reading comprehension, verbal ability, and essay writing.

In October 2010, the first candidates were selected randomly to take a computer-based test (CBT) version of the PCAT. Beginning in July 2011, all students will take the CBT version. The CBT version of the PCAT is exactly the same as the paper-and-pencil version—the order of questions is the same, the scoring is the same, and the reporting is the same.

Registering for the Exam

You can register to take the test online by going to the PCAT website, www.pcatweb.info. Fill out the forms carefully and be sure to check for spelling or typos. Enter your name and address exactly as they appear on the two pieces of identification you will be using to secure admission to the Test Center on test day. If you don't have access to online registration, you can call 1-800-622-3231 to request the paper registration form.

The registration fee is $150, and you can pay by credit card. This fee includes a personal score report that will be sent to you, and three score reports to be sent to three pharmacy schools of your choice. You should indicate which schools you want to receive these reports at the time of registration. If you want your scores to be sent to more than three schools, you may request additional scoring reports at a cost of $20 each. Paper registration costs an additional $50. There is a $49 charge for late registration.

Seating at Test Centers is on a first come, first served basis, so register as early as you can. Be sure to choose a date that leaves enough time for your scores to be sent to the schools you're applying to before their deadlines.

Within two days of registering online (one week for paper registration) you will get an email notice that tells you how to access your Registration Confirmation, which verifies that your registration is complete. Make sure all of the information is accurate or you may have trouble getting in to the Test Center on test day. If changes have to be made, they must be made by the late registration deadline.

About a week before the test date, you will get another email telling you how to access and print your Admission Ticket from your "My Profile" page on the PCAT website. You will need Microsoft Internet Explorer to print the ticket. That ticket will give you the exact location of the Test Center, and the time you are to be there. Verify that all of the information is correct. If it's not, it's up to you to contact PSE Customer Relations at 1-800-622-3231. You must have your Admission Ticket with you in order to get into the Test Center.

Your personal score report will be sent to the address you list when you register for the test. Changes of address can be made up until the late registration date.

If you need to cancel your registration, you may be able to receive a partial refund if your request is received before the registration cancellation deadline, which you can find on the PCAT website.

When and How Often Should You Take the Test?

As noted previously, the PCAT is offered four times a year, in January, June, August, and October. Since most schools don't penalize applicants for taking the test more than once, we recommend you take it in June or August of the year before you intend to start pharmacy school. That way you have time to take the test again in October if you need to, and submit that score to the schools you choose. Each pharmacy school has specific admission requirements, so if you are thinking about taking the test more than once, check the websites or catalogs from the schools you're interested in to make sure that they allow you to submit multiple PCAT scores. Note, however, that without special permission from Pearson you may only take the PCAT up to five times.

What to Expect at the Test Center

You must bring the Admission Ticket to get into the Test Center. Along with your Admission Ticket, bring two forms of valid identification. One must have a photograph of you and your signature (driver's license, passport, or other government-issued identification card). Valid secondary forms of identification include credit cards, library cards, or a utility bill (if your name and address are exactly the same as they are on your Admission Ticket). Bring several sharpened No. 2 pencils with erasers.

Do not bring food, beverages, books, papers, highlighters, rulers, notes, earplugs, calculators, pagers, PDAs, cell phones, recording devices, cameras, headphones, or any other electronic devices or reference materials. You may not wear a baseball cap or any hat with a brim into the testing room, unless worn for a religious or medical reason that has been preapproved by Pearson.

During the test, purses and backpacks will be stored in a designated area provided by the Test Center. If you need access to any of your personal belongings during one of the breaks, you must get permission from the Test Center staff.

Remember, you won't be able to get into the Test Center if you don't have a valid Admission Ticket and two forms of identification that match the information on that Admission Ticket. You will also be denied admission if you show up late either before the test starts or after the break. These policies are strictly enforced, so keep your eye on the time!

During the Test

You must follow all of the instructions and rules that the Test Center staff explains to you. If you have any questions, ask them before the test starts, because there are no questions allowed after you begin.

There will be one rest break halfway through the test. As mentioned previously, if you need to leave the test room during the break, you have to get permission from the examiner, and someone will be with you while you're outside of the testing room.

On the back of your PCAT answer booklet, there is an Acknowledgment statement that you are required to sign, and a bubble you have to fill in that indicates you have read and signed the statement ***or your test will not be scored, your scores will not be reported to you or to any recipient schools, and your fees will not be refunded.***

No Score Option

Before the test begins, the examiner will tell you how to request the No Score Option. Choosing this option means that scores will not be reported to you or to the schools you requested. You can't change your mind, and you can't get your money back, but the schools you're applying to won't know that you took the test, so if you know you've had a bad day, it might make sense to choose this option and take the test again at a later date.

Outline of the Exam

The PCAT covers the following topics:

- **Writing:** Conventions of Language and Problem Solving
- **Verbal Ability:** Analogies and Sentence Completion
- **Biology:** General Biology, Microbiology, Anatomy, and Physiology
- **Chemistry:** General Chemistry and Organic Chemistry
- **Reading Comprehension:** Comprehension, Analysis, and Evaluation
- **Quantitative Ability:** Basic Math, Algebra, Probability and Statistics, Precalculus, and Calculus

Each multiple-choice question has four possible answers. Some include diagrams or illustrations. The two essays test more than whether you can use correct grammar and spell words correctly. They are used to see whether you can communicate clearly, persuasively, and logically on paper. Essay topics include general health and science, and political, social, or cultural issues. You will have 30 minutes to write each essay.

The test uses the following format and order:

- **Writing:** 30 minutes, first essay that asks you to address a problem related to a general health, science, social, cultural, or political issue
- **Verbal Ability:** 30 minutes, 48 multiple-choice questions focusing on nonscientific vocabulary in the form of analogies (60%) and sentence completion (40%) questions
- **Biology:** 30 minutes, 48 multiple-choice questions on general biology (60%), microbiology (20%), and human anatomy and physiology (20%)
- **Chemistry:** 30 minutes, 48 multiple-choice questions on general chemistry (60%) and organic chemistry (40%)
- Short break after the first four sections
- **Writing:** 30 minutes, second essay that asks you to address a problem related to a general health, science, social, cultural, or political issue
- **Reading Comprehension:** 50 minutes, 6 passages, 48 multiple-choice questions that test you on your comprehension (30%), evaluation (30%), and analysis (40%) of passages on scientific topics
- **Quantitative Ability:** 40 minutes, 48 multiple-choice questions on basic math (15%), algebra (20%), probability and statistics (20%), precalculus (23%), and calculus (22%)

You may work only on each section in order, and may not go back to any earlier sections once you have completed them. Of the 48 questions in each of the five multiple-choice sections, 40 count toward your score and eight are experimental. One of the two writing sections is also experimental. Since you won't know which questions or sections are scored and which are experimental, it's important to do your best on all parts of the test. You should start by answering the questions that are easiest for you, but because there is no penalty for guessing, watch the clock as you work so that you are sure to have time to answer every multiple-choice question. (See Chapter 3, "The LearningExpress Test Preparation System," for tips and strategies on how to maximize your PCAT score.)

Scoring

Each of the five multiple-choice sections of the PCAT is given a score between 200 and 600 based on the number of questions you answer correctly. You will also receive a percentage ranking for each section, which compares your performance against the results of others taking the test.

Essays are scored separately on a scale from zero (incomplete) to 5 (outstanding).

They are judged on conventions of language—grammar, spelling, and composition—as well as on your ability to construct a logical argument. A score of 5 represents superior capability, 3 is adequate, and a zero means an incomplete answer to the essay question (see Chapter 4, "Writing," for more information). Your writing score will be a number only; there is no percentile ranking reported for the PCAT essays.

Approximately six weeks after the test, you will receive your scores in the mail, and official transcripts will be sent to the institutions to which you requested your scores be reported. The score report you receive will show scaled scores and percentiles for each of the five multiple-choice subtests and a composite score for the full test. Writing subtest scores are scored based on a specific rubric and reported separately. Your scores are kept on record for five years.

Pharmacy School Admissions Requirements

Just as with those who take the SAT and ACT to gain admission into undergraduate schools, pharmacy schools consider PCAT test results in combination with grades (high school and undergraduate), references, and personal interviews. Admission requirements vary by school, though most expect you to have completed specific course work in biology, chemistry, math, and English prior to admission. You should check the websites of the schools you're interested in to be sure you've completed all the relevant course work and met any other special requirements. Remember, your PCAT scores are only part of the equation, but by studying and preparing, you can ensure that they will be a strong part of your application.

CHAPTER 3

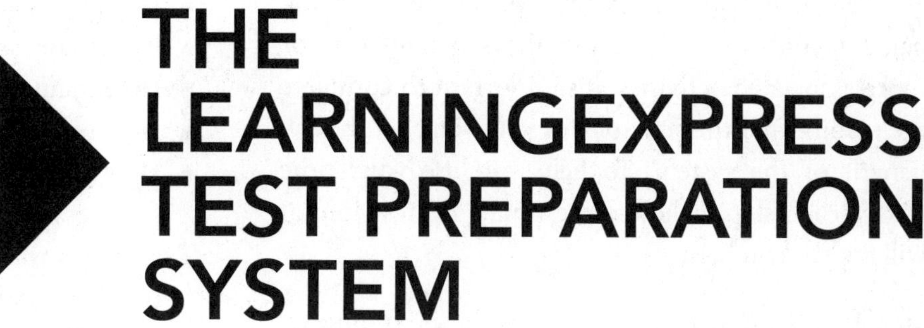

THE LEARNINGEXPRESS TEST PREPARATION SYSTEM

It takes significant preparation to score well on any written exam, and the PCAT is no exception. The LearningExpress Test Preparation System, which was developed by leading test experts exclusively for LearningExpress, guides you through the preparation process and helps you develop the skills and the attitude you need to be your best on test day.

The LearningExpress Test Preparation System addresses typical obstacles that stand in the way of successful test taking:

- Being unfamiliar with the exam format
- Being paralyzed by test anxiety
- Leaving your preparation to the last minute or not preparing at all
- Not mastering vital test-taking skills like how to pace yourself through the exam, how to use the process of elimination, and how to make educated guesses
- Not being in tip-top mental and physical shape

The LearningExpress Test Preparation System gives you *control.* Our nine easy-to-follow steps, put you in charge of your preparation and your performance on the PCAT. After completing this chapter, you will know what you need to do to get a high score.

Each of the nine steps reviewed on the following pages includes reading about the step and one or more associated activities. It's important to complete the reading and the activities, or you won't get the full benefit of the system. To help you use your time wisely, each step includes an estimate of how long it will take to complete.

Step 1.	Get information	30 minutes
Step 2.	Conquer test anxiety	20 minutes
Step 3.	Make a plan	50 minutes
Step 4.	Learn to manage your time	10 minutes
Step 5.	Learn to use the process of elimination	20 minutes
Step 6.	Guessing on the PCAT	20 minutes
Step 7.	Reach your peak performance zone	10 minutes
Step 8.	Get your act together	10 minutes
Step 9.	Do it!	10 minutes
Total		**3 hours**

We estimate that working through the entire system will take you approximately three hours. It's perfectly okay if you work at a faster or slower pace. It's up to you to decide whether you should set aside a whole afternoon or evening to work through the Learning-Express Test Preparation System in one sitting, or break it up and do just one or two steps a day for the next several days.

Step 1: Get Information

Time to complete: 30 minutes
Activity: Read the Introduction to this book.

The first step in the LearningExpress Test Preparation System is to determine everything you can about the type of information you will be expected to know as well as how your knowledge will be assessed.

What You Should Find Out

Knowing the details will help you study efficiently and help you feel a sense of control. Here's a list of things you might want to find out:

- What skills are tested?
- How many sections are on the exam?
- How many questions are in each section?
- How much time is allotted for each section?
- How is the exam scored, and is there a penalty for guessing/wrong answers?
- Can you write in the exam booklet, or will you be given scratch paper?

You will find answers to these questions in Chapters 1 and 2 of this book and on the PCAT website located at: www.pcatweb.info.

Step 2: Conquer Test Anxiety

Time to complete: 20 minutes
Activity: Take the Test Anxiety Quiz.

Now that you know what's on the test, the next step is to address one of the biggest obstacles to success: *test anxiety.* Test anxiety may not only impair your performance on the exam itself, but it can also keep you from preparing properly. In Step 2, you will learn stress management techniques that will help you succeed on your exam. Practicing these techniques as you work through the activities in this book will help them become second nature to you by exam day.

Combating Test Anxiety

A little test anxiety is a good thing. Everyone gets nervous before a big exam—and if that nervousness motivates you to prepare thoroughly, so much the better. Many athletes report pregame jitters, which they are able to harness to help them perform at their peak. Stop here and answer the questions on the Test Anxiety Quiz to determine your level of test anxiety.

TEST STRESS QUIZ

You need to worry about test anxiety only if it is extreme enough to impair your performance. The following questionnaire will provide a diagnosis of your level of test anxiety. In the blank before each statement, write the number that most accurately describes your experience.

0 = Never
1 = Once or twice
2 = Sometimes
3 = Often

______ I have gotten so nervous before an exam that I put down the books and did not study for it.
______ I have experienced disabling physical symptoms such as vomiting and severe headaches because I was nervous about an exam.
______ I have simply not shown up for an exam because I was afraid to take it.
______ I have experienced dizziness and disorientation while taking an exam.
______ I have had trouble filling in the little circles because my hands were shaking too hard.
______ I have failed an exam because I was too nervous to complete it.
______ **Total: Add up the numbers in the blanks above.**

Your Test Stress Score

Here are the steps you should take, depending on your score. If you scored:

- **Below 3:** Your level of test anxiety is nothing to worry about; it is probably just enough to give you that little extra edge.
- **Between 3 and 6:** Your test anxiety may be enough to impair your performance, and you should practice the stress management techniques in this section to try to bring your test anxiety down to manageable levels.
- **Above 6:** Your level of test anxiety is a serious concern. In addition to practicing the stress management techniques listed in this section, you may want to seek additional, personal help. Call your local high school or community college and ask for the academic counselor. Tell the counselor that you have a level of test anxiety that sometimes keeps you from being able to take the exam. The counselor may be willing to help you or may suggest someone else you should talk to.

Stress Management before the Exam

If you feel your level of anxiety is getting the best of you in the weeks before the exam, here are things you can do to bring the level down:

- **Prepare.** There's nothing like knowing what to expect to put you in control of test anxiety. That's why you're reading this book. Use it faithfully, and you will be ready on test day.
- **Practice self-confidence.** A positive attitude is a great way to combat test anxiety. Stand in front of the mirror and say to your reflection, "I'm prepared. I'm confident. I'm going to ace this exam. I know I can do it." Say it into a recorder, and play it back once a day. If you hear it often enough, and you use the LearningExpress method to study for the PCAT, it will be true.
- **Fight negative messages.** Every time someone talks to you about how hard the exam is or how it's difficult to get a high score, think about your self-confidence messages. If the someone with the negative messages is you—telling yourself you don't do well on exams, that you just can't do this—don't listen. Turn on your recorder and listen to your self-confidence messages.

- **Visualize.** Visualizing success can help make it happen—and it reminds you of why you're doing all this work in preparing for the exam. Imagine yourself in your first day of classes or beginning the first day of your dream job.
- **Exercise.** Physical activity helps calm your body and focus your mind. Besides, being in good physical shape can actually help you do well on the exam. Go for a run, lift weights, go swimming—and exercise regularly.

Stress Management on Test Day

There are several ways you can bring down your level of test stress and anxiety on test day. They'll work best if you practice them in the weeks before the exam, so you know which ones work best for you.

- **Breathe deeply.** Take a deep breath in while you count to five. Hold it for a count of one, and then let it out on a count of five. Repeat several times.
- **Move your body.** Try rolling your head in a circle. Rotate your shoulders. Shake your hands from the wrist.
- **Visualize again.** Think of the place where you are most relaxed: lying on the beach in the sun, walking through the park, or wherever relaxes you. Now, close your eyes and imagine you're actually there. If you practice in advance, you will find that you need only a few seconds of this exercise to experience a significant increase in your sense of relaxation and well-being.

When anxiety threatens to overwhelm you *during* the test, there are still things you can do to manage your stress level:

- **Repeat your self-confidence messages.** You should have them memorized by now. Say them quietly to yourself, and believe them!
- **Visualize one more time.** This time, visualize yourself moving smoothly and quickly through the exam, answering every question correctly, writing a well-organized essay, and finishing just before time is up. Like most visualization techniques, this one works best if you've practiced it ahead of time.
- **Find an easy question.** Skim over the questions on Part I until you find an easy question, and then answer it. Getting even one question answered correctly gets you into the test-taking groove.
- **Take a mental break.** Everyone loses concentration once in a while during a long exam. It's normal, so you shouldn't worry about it. Instead, accept what has happened. Say to yourself, "Hey, I lost it there for a minute. My brain is taking a break." Put down your pencil, close your eyes, and do some deep breathing for a few seconds. Then go back to work.

Try these techniques ahead of time and see if they work for you!

Step 3: Make a Plan

Time to complete: 50 minutes
Activity: Construct a study plan.

There is no substitute for careful preparation and practice over time. So the most important thing you can do to better prepare yourself for your exam is to create a study plan or schedule and then follow it. This will help you avoid cramming at the last minute, which is an ineffective study technique that will only add to your anxiety.

On the following pages, you will find four examples of study schedules based on the amount of time you have before the PCAT exam. If you're the kind of person who needs deadlines and assignments to motivate you for a project, here they are. If you're the kind of person who doesn't like to follow other people's plans, you can use the suggested schedules to construct your own.

Once you make your plan, make a commitment to follow it. Set aside at least 20 minutes every day for studying and practice. This will do more good than two hours crammed into a Saturday. If you have months before the test, you're lucky. Don't put off your studying until the week before. Start now. Even ten minutes a weekday, with half an hour or more on weekends, can make a big difference in your score.

Schedule A: The Leisure Plan

This schedule gives you at least six months to sharpen your skills and prepare for the PCAT. The more prep time you give yourself, the more relaxed you'll feel.

- **Test day minus six months:** Read Chapters 2, 4, and 5 ("The PCAT Exam," "Writing," and "Verbal Ability"). Start going to the library once every two weeks to read books or information about successful writing strategies. Find other people who are preparing for the exam, and form a study group.
- **Test day minus five months:** Read Chapters 6 and 7 ("Biology" and "Chemistry") and work through the exercises.
- **Test day minus four months:** Read Chapter 8 ("Reading Comprehension") and work through the exercises. You're still continuing with your reading, aren't you?
- **Test day minus three months:** read Chapter 9 ("Quantitative Ability") and work through the exercises.
- **Test day minus two months:** Use your scores from the chapter exercises to help you decide where to concentrate your efforts this month. Go back to the relevant chapters and reread the information. Continue working with your study group.
- **Test day minus one month:** Review the end of chapter quizzes.
- **Test day minus one week:** Take and review the practice test. See how much you've learned in the past months. Concentrate on what you've done well, and decide not to let any areas where you still feel uncertain bother you.
- **Day before test:** Relax. Do something unrelated to the PCAT. Eat a good meal and go to bed at your usual time.

Schedule B: The Just-Enough-Time Plan

If you have three to six months before the test, that should be enough time to prepare. This schedule assumes four months; stretch it out or compress it if you have more or less time.

- **Test day minus four months:** Read Chapters 4, 5, and 8 ("Writing," "Verbal Ability," "Reading Comprehension") and work through the exercises. Start going to the library once every two weeks to read books or information about successful writing strategies.
- **Test day minus three months:** Read Chapters 6 and 7 ("Biology" and "Chemistry") and work through the exercises.
- **Test day minus two months:** Read Chapter 9 ("Quantitative Ability") and work through the exercises. You're still continuing with your reading, aren't you?
- **Test day minus one month:** Take the practice test. Use your score to help you decide where to concentrate your efforts this month. Go back to the relevant chapters and reread the information, or get the help of a friend or teacher.
- **Test day minus one week:** Review Chapters 4 to 9 one last time, and take the online practice test. See how much you've learned in the past months. Concentrate on what you've done well, and decide not to let any areas where you still feel uncertain bother you.

- **Day before test:** Relax. Do something unrelated to the PCAT. Eat a good meal and go to bed at your usual time.

Schedule C: More Study in Less Time

If you have one to three months before the test, you still have enough time for some concentrated study that will help you improve your score. This schedule is built around a two-month time frame. If you have only one month, spend an extra couple of hours a week to get all these steps in. If you have three months, take some of the steps from Schedule B and fit them in.

- **Test day minus eight weeks:** Read Chapters 4, 5, and 8 ("Writing," "Verbal Ability," and "Reading Comprehension"). Work through the exercises in these chapters. Review areas you're weakest in.
- **Test day minus six weeks:** Read Chapters 6 and 7 ("Biology" and "Chemistry") and work through the exercises.
- **Test day minus four weeks:** Read Chapter 9 ("Quantitative Ability") and work through the exercises.
- **Test day minus two weeks:** Take the practice exam. Then, score it and read the answer explanations until you're sure you understand them. Review the areas where your score is lowest.
- **Test day minus one week:** Take the online practice exam. Then review both exams, concentrating on the areas where a little work can help the most.
- **Day before test:** Relax. Do something unrelated to the PCAT. Eat a good meal and go to bed at your usual time.

Schedule D: The Cram Plan

If you have three weeks or less before the test, you really have your work cut out for you. Carve half an hour out of your day, every day, for studying. This schedule assumes you have the whole three weeks to prepare; if you have less time, you will have to compress the schedule accordingly.

- **Test day minus three weeks:** Take the practice test at the end of this book, and review the correct answers and the explanations. Work through the exercises in the chapters. Review areas you're weakest in.
- **Test day minus two weeks:** Read the material in Chapters 4 to 9 and work through the exercises.
- **Test day minus one week:** Evaluate your performance on the chapter quizzes. Review the parts of the chapters that explain the skills you found the hardest. Get a friend or teacher to help you with the sections in which you had the most difficulty.
- **Test day minus two days:** Take the online practice exam. Review your results. Make sure you understand the answer explanations. Review the sample essay outline in Chapter 4.
- **Day before test:** Relax. Do something unrelated to the PCAT. Eat a good meal and go to bed at your usual time.

Step 4: Learn to Manage Your Time

Time to complete: 10 minutes to read, many hours of practice
Activities: Practice these strategies as you take the sample exams.

Steps 4, 5, and 6 of the LearningExpress Test Preparation System put you in charge of your PCAT experience by showing you test-taking strategies that work. Practice these strategies as you take the sample quizzes and practice exams in this book. Then you will be ready to use them on test day.

First, you will take control of your time on the PCAT. Start by understanding the format of the test.

The seven sections of the test are always given in the same order:

- **Section 1: Written Essay**, 30 minutes
- **Section 2: Verbal Ability**, 30 minutes, 48 multiple-choice questions
- **Section 3: Biology**, 30 minutes, 48 multiple-choice questions
- **Section 4: Chemistry**, 30 minutes, 48 multiple-choice questions.
- **Section 5: Written Essay**, 30 minutes
- **Section 6: Reading Comprehension**, 50 minutes, 48 multiple-choice questions
- **Section 7: Quantitative Ability**, 40 minutes, 48 multiple-choice questions

You will want to practice using your time wisely on the practice tests and chapter quizzes, while trying to avoid making mistakes at the same time as working quickly.

- **Listen carefully to directions.** By the time you get to the test, you should know how it works. But listen carefully in case something has changed.
- **Pace yourself.** Glance at your watch every few minutes and compare the time to how far you've gotten in the section. Leave some extra time for review, so that when one-quarter of the time has elapsed, you should be more than a quarter of the way through the section, and so on. If you're falling behind, pick up the pace.
- **Keep moving.** Don't spend too much time on one question. If you don't know the answer, skip the question and move on. Circle the number of the question in your test booklet and come back to it later.
- **Keep track of your place on the answer sheet.** If you skip a question, make sure you skip on the answer sheet, too. Check yourself every five to ten questions to make sure the question number and the answer sheet number match.
- **Don't rush.** You should keep moving; but rushing won't help. Try to keep calm and work methodically and quickly.

Step 5: Learn to Use the Process of Elimination

Time to complete: 20 minutes
Activity: Complete the worksheet on Using the Process of Elimination.

After time management, the next most important tool for taking control of your test is using the process of elimination wisely. It's standard test-taking wisdom that you should always read all the answer choices before choosing your answer. This helps you find the right answer by eliminating wrong answer choices. And, sure enough, this standard wisdom applies to the PCAT. Let's say you're facing a question that goes like this:

9. **Sentence 6:** I would like to be considered for the assistant manager position in your company my previous work experience is a good match for the job requirements posted.

Which correction should be made to sentence 6?

a. Insert *Although* before *I.*
b. Insert a question mark after *company.*
c. Insert a semicolon and *However* before *my.*
d. Insert a period after *company* and capitalize *my.*
e. No corrections are necessary.

If you happen to know that sentence 6 is a run-on sentence and you know how to correct it, you don't need to use the process of elimination. But let's assume that, like some people, you don't. So, you look at the answer choices. *Although* sure doesn't sound like a good choice, because it would change the meaning of the sentence. So, you eliminate choice **a**—and now you have only four answer choices to deal with. Mark an X next to choice **a** so you never have to read it again. Move on to the other answer choices.

If you know that the first part of the sentence does not ask a question, you can eliminate answer **b** as a possible answer. Make an X beside it. Choice **c**, inserting a semicolon, could create a pause in an otherwise long sentence, but inserting the word *However* might not be correct. If you're not sure whether this answer is correct, put a question mark beside it, meaning "well, maybe."

Answer choice **d** would separate a very long sentence into two shorter sentences, and it would not change the meaning. It could work, so put a check mark beside it meaning "good answer—I might use this one." Answer choice **e** means that the sentence is fine like it is and doesn't need any changes. The sentence could make sense as it is, but it is definitely long. Is this the best way to write the sentence? If you're not sure, put a question mark beside answer choice **e**.

Now, your question looks like this:

Which correction should be made to sentence 6?

X a. Insert *Although* before *I.*
X b. Insert a question mark after *company.*
? c. Insert a semicolon and *However* before *my.*
✓ d. Insert a period after *company* and capitalize *my.*
? e. No corrections are necessary.

You've got just one check mark, for a *good answer*. If you're pressed for time, you should simply mark choice **d** on your answer sheet. If you've got the time to be extra careful, you could compare your check mark answer to your question mark answers to make sure that it's better. (It is: Sentence 6 is a run-on, and should be separated into two shorter, complete sentences.)

It's good to have a system for marking good, bad, and maybe answers. We recommend using this one:

X = bad
✓ = good
? = maybe

If you don't like these marks, devise your own system. Just make sure you do it long before exam day—while you're working through the quizzes and practice test in this book—so you won't have to worry about it during the exam.

Even when you think you're absolutely clueless about a question, you can use the process of elimination to get rid of one answer choice. By doing so, you're better prepared to make an educated guess, as you will see in Step 6. More often, the process of elimination allows you to get down to only two possible right answers. Then you're in a strong position to guess, which you should do since guessing is not penalized on the PCAT. And sometimes, even though you don't know the right answer, you find it simply by getting rid of the wrong ones, as you did in this example.

Try using your powers of elimination on the questions that follow. The answer explanations show one possible way you might use the process to arrive at the right answer.

USING THE PROCESS OF ELIMINATION

Use the process of elimination to answer the following questions.

1. Ilsa is as old as Meghan will be in five years. The difference between Ed's age and Meghan's age is twice the difference between Ilsa's age and Meghan's age. Ed is 29. How old is Ilsa?
   a. 4
   b. 10
   c. 19
   d. 24

2. "All drivers of commercial vehicles must carry a valid commercial driver's license whenever operating a commercial vehicle." According to this sentence, which of the following people need NOT carry a commercial driver's license?
   a. a truck driver idling his engine while waiting to be directed to a loading dock
   b. a bus operator backing her bus out of the way of another bus in the bus lot
   c. a taxi driver driving his personal car to the grocery store
   d. a limousine driver taking the limousine to her home after dropping off her last passenger of the evening

3. Smoking tobacco has been linked to
   a. increased risk of stroke and heart attack.
   b. all forms of respiratory disease.
   c. increasing mortality rates over the past ten years.
   d. juvenile delinquency.

4. Which of the following words is spelled correctly?
   a. incorrigible
   b. outragous
   c. domestickated
   d. understandible

Answers

Here are the answers, as well as some suggestions as to how you might have used the process of elimination to find them.

1. d. You should have eliminated choice **a** immediately. Ilsa cannot be 4 years old if Meghan is going to be Ilsa's age in five years. The best way to eliminate other answer choices is to try plugging them into the information given in the problem. For instance, for choice **b**, if Ilsa is 10, then Meghan must be 5. The difference in their ages is 5 years. The difference between Ed's age, 29, and Meghan's age, 5, is 24. Is 24 two times 5? No. Then choice **b** is wrong. You could eliminate choice **c** in the same way and be left with choice **d**.

2. c. Note the word *not* in the question, and go through the answers one by one. Is the truck driver in choice **a** *operating a commercial vehicle*? Yes, idling counts as "operating," so he needs to have a commercial driver's license. Likewise, the bus operator in choice **b** is operating a commercial vehicle; the question does not say the operator has to be on the street. The limo driver in choice **d** is operating a commercial vehicle, even if it does not have a passenger in it. However, the cabbie in choice **c** is not operating a commercial vehicle, but his own private car.

USING THE PROCESS OF ELIMINATION (*continued*)

3. a. You could eliminate choice **b** simply because of the presence of the word *all.* Such absolutes hardly ever appear in correct answer choices. Choice **c** looks attractive until you think a little about what you know—are there not fewer people smoking these days, rather than more? So how could smoking be responsible for a higher mortality rate? (If you did not know that *mortality rate* means the rate at which people die, you might keep this choice as a possibility, but you would still be able to eliminate two answers and have only two to choose from.) Choice **d** is plain silly, so you could eliminate that one, too. Now you are left with the correct choice, **a**.

4. a. How you used the process of elimination here depends on which words you recognized as being spelled incorrectly. If you knew that the correct spellings were *outrageous, domesticated*, and *understandable,* then you were home free. You probably knew that at least one of those words was spelled wrong.

Step 6: Guessing on the PCAT

Time to complete: 20 minutes
Activity: Complete the worksheet on Your Guessing Ability.

Armed with the process of elimination, you're ready to make educated guesses. Since there is no guessing penalty, you should be sure to answer every multiple-choice question on the test.

YOUR GUESSING ABILITY

The following are ten really hard questions. You are not supposed to know the answers. Rather, this is an assessment of your ability to guess when you don't have a clue. Read each question carefully, just as if you did expect to answer it. If you have any knowledge at all about the subject of the question, use that knowledge to help you eliminate wrong answer choices.

ANSWER GRID

1.	ⓐ	ⓑ	ⓒ	ⓓ	**5.**	ⓐ	ⓑ	ⓒ	ⓓ	**9.**	ⓐ	ⓑ	ⓒ	ⓓ
2.	ⓐ	ⓑ	ⓒ	ⓓ	**6.**	ⓐ	ⓑ	ⓒ	ⓓ	**10.**	ⓐ	ⓑ	ⓒ	ⓓ
3.	ⓐ	ⓑ	ⓒ	ⓓ	**7.**	ⓐ	ⓑ	ⓒ	ⓓ					
4.	ⓐ	ⓑ	ⓒ	ⓓ	**8.**	ⓐ	ⓑ	ⓒ	ⓓ					

1. September 7 is Independence Day in
- **a.** India.
- **b.** Costa Rica.
- **c.** Brazil.
- **d.** Australia.

2. Which of the following is the formula for determining the momentum of an object?
- **a.** $p = mv$
- **b.** $F = ma$
- **c.** $P = IV$
- **d.** $E = mc^2$

3. Because of the expansion of the universe, the stars and other celestial bodies are all moving away from each other. This phenomenon is known as
- **a.** Newton's first law.
- **b.** the big bang.
- **c.** gravitational collapse.
- **d.** Hubble flow.

4. American author Gertrude Stein was born in
- **a.** 1713.
- **b.** 1830.
- **c.** 1874.
- **d.** 1901.

5. Which of the following is NOT one of the Five Classics attributed to Confucius?
- **a.** *I Ching*
- **b.** *Book of Holiness*
- **c.** *Spring and Autumn Annals*
- **d.** *Book of History*

6. The religious and philosophical doctrine that holds that the universe is constantly in a struggle between good and evil is known as
- **a.** Pelagianism.
- **b.** Manichaeanism.
- **c.** neo-Hegelianism.
- **d.** Epicureanism.

7. The third chief justice of the U.S. Supreme Court was
- **a.** John Blair.
- **b.** William Cushing.
- **c.** James Wilson.
- **d.** John Jay.

8. Which of the following is the poisonous portion of a daffodil?
  a. the bulb
  b. the leaves
  c. the stem
  d. the flowers

9. The winner of the Masters golf tournament in 1953 was
  a. Sam Snead.
  b. Cary Middlecoff.
  c. Arnold Palmer.
  d. Ben Hogan.

10. The state with the highest per capita personal income in 1980 was
  a. Alaska.
  b. Connecticut.
  c. New York.
  d. Texas.

Answers

Check your answers against the following correct answer choices.

1. c.
2. a.
3. d.
4. c.
5. b.
6. b.
7. b.
8. a.
9. d.
10. a.

How Did You Do?

You may have simply gotten lucky and actually known the answer to one or two questions. In addition, your guessing was more successful if you were able to use the process of elimination on any of the questions. Maybe you didn't know who the third chief justice was (question 7), but you knew that John Jay was the first. In that case, you would have eliminated choice **d** and, therefore, improved your odds of guessing correctly from one in four to one in three.

According to probability, you should get $2\frac{1}{2}$ answers correct, so getting either two or three right would be average. If you got four or more right, you may be a really terrific guesser. If you got one or none right, you may need to work on your guessing skills. Keep in mind, though, that this is only a small sample. You should continue to keep track of your guessing ability as you work through the sample questions in this book. Circle the numbers of questions you guess on as you make your guess; or, if you don't have time while you take the practice exams, go back afterward and try to remember which questions you guessed at.

Remember, on an exam with four answer choices, your chances of getting a right answer is one in four. So keep a separate "guessing" score for each exam. How many questions did you guess on? How many did you get right? If the number you got right is at least one-fourth of the number of questions you guessed on, you are at least an average guesser, maybe better—and you should always go ahead and guess on a real exam. If the number you got right is significantly lower than one-fourth of the number you guessed on, you would, frankly, be safe in guessing anyway, but maybe you would feel more comfortable if you guessed only selectively, when you can eliminate a wrong answer or at least have a good feeling about one of the answer choices.

Step 7: Reach Your Peak Performance Zone

Time to complete: 10 minutes to read; weeks to complete!
Activity: Complete the Physical Preparation Checklist.

To get ready for a challenge like a big test, you have to take control of your physical, as well as your mental, state. Exercise, proper diet, and rest will ensure that your body works with, rather than against, your mind during your preparation and on test day.

Exercise

If you don't already have a regular exercise program going, the time while you're preparing for an exam is an excellent time to start one. And if you're already keeping fit—or trying to get that way—don't let the pressure of preparing for an exam fool you into quitting. Exercise helps reduce stress by pumping good-feeling hormones called *endorphins* into your system. It also increases the oxygen supply throughout your body, including your brain, so you will be at peak performance on exam day.

A half hour of vigorous activity—enough to break a sweat—every day should be your aim. If you're really pressed for time, every other day is acceptable. Choose an activity you like and get out there and do it. Jogging with a friend always makes the time go faster, as does running with an iPod.

Diet

A balanced diet will help you achieve peak performance. Limit your caffeine and junk food intake. Eat plenty of fruits and vegetables, along with proteins and carbohydrates. Foods that are high in lecithin (an amino acid), such as fish and beans, are especially good brain foods. The night before the test, you might carbo-load the way athletes do before a contest.

Rest

You probably know how much sleep you need every night to be at your best, even if you don't always get it. Make sure you do get that much sleep, though, for at least a week before the exam.

If you're not a morning person and your test will be given in the morning, you should reset your internal clock so that your body doesn't think you're taking an exam at 3 A.M. You have to start this process well before the day of the test. The way it works is to get up half an hour earlier each morning and go to bed half an hour earlier that same night. Don't try it the other way around; you will just toss and turn if you go to bed early without having gotten up early. The next morning, get up another half an hour earlier, and so on. How long you will have to do this depends on how late you're used to getting up. Use the Physical Preparation Checklist to make sure you're in tip-top form.

PHYSICAL PREPARATION CHECKLIST

For the week before the test, write down what physical exercise you engaged in and for how long and what you ate for each meal. Remember, you are trying for at least half an hour of exercise every other day (preferably every day) and a balanced diet that is light on junk food.

Exam minus 7 days

Exercise: ______________ for _____ minutes

Breakfast: ______________________________

Lunch: ______________________________

Dinner: ______________________________

Snacks: ______________________________

Exam minus 6 days

Exercise: ______________ for _____ minutes

Breakfast: ______________________________

Lunch: ______________________________

Dinner: ______________________________

Snacks: ______________________________

Exam minus 5 days

Exercise: ______________ for _____ minutes

Breakfast: ______________________________

Lunch: ______________________________

Dinner: ______________________________

Snacks: ______________________________

Exam minus 4 days

Exercise: ______________ for _____ minutes

Breakfast: ______________________________

Lunch: ______________________________

Dinner: ______________________________

Snacks: ______________________________

Exam minus 3 days

Exercise: ______________ for _____ minutes

Breakfast: ______________________________

Lunch: ______________________________

Dinner: ______________________________

Snacks: ______________________________

Exam minus 2 days

Exercise: ______________ for _____ minutes

Breakfast: ______________________________

Lunch: ______________________________

Dinner: ______________________________

Snacks: ______________________________

Exam minus 1 day

Exercise: ______________ for _____ minutes

Breakfast: ______________________________

Lunch: ______________________________

Dinner: ______________________________

Snacks: ______________________________

Step 8: Get Your Act Together

Time to complete: 10 minutes to read; time to complete will vary.
Activity: Complete the Final Preparations worksheet.

You're in control of your mind and body; you're in charge of test anxiety, your preparation, and your test-taking strategies. Now, it's time to take charge of external factors, like the testing site and the materials you need to take the test.

Find Out Where the Exam Is and Make a Trial Run

Make sure you know exactly when and where your test is being held. Do you know how to get to the exam site? Do you know how long it will take to get there? If not, make a trial run, preferably on the same day of the week at the same time of day. On the Final Preparations worksheet, make note of the amount of time it will take you to get to the test site. Plan on arriving 10 to 15 minutes early so you can get the lay of the land, use the bathroom, and calm down. Then figure out how early you will have to get up that morning, and make sure you get up that early every day for a week before the test.

Gather Your Materials

The night before the exam, lay out the clothes you will wear and the materials you have to bring with you to the test. Plan on dressing in layers; you won't have any control over the temperature of the examination room. Have a sweater or jacket you can take off if it's warm. Use the checklist on the Final Preparations worksheet to help you pull together what you will need.

Don't Skip Breakfast

Even if you don't usually eat breakfast, do so on the morning of the test. A cup of coffee or can of soda doesn't count. Don't eat doughnuts or other sweet foods, either. A sugar high will leave you with a sugar low in the middle of the test. A mix of proteins and carbohydrates is best. Cereal with milk and just a little sugar or eggs with toast will do your body a world of good.

Step 9: Do It!

Time to complete: 10 minutes, plus test-taking time.
Activity: Ace the PCAT!

Fast-forward to test day. You're ready. You made a study plan and followed through. You practiced your test-taking strategies while working through this book. You're in control of your physical, mental, and emotional state. You know when and where to show up and what to bring with you. In other words, you're well prepared!

When you're done with the test, you will have earned a reward. Plan ahead for an after-test celebration. Call up your friends and suggest a party, look forward to a nice dinner with your family, or pick out a movie to see—whatever your heart desires.

And then go into the test, full of confidence, armed with test-taking strategies you've practiced until they're second nature. You're in control of yourself, your environment, and your performance on the exam. You're ready to succeed. So do it. And look forward to your future as someone who has scored well on the PCAT!

FINAL PREPARATIONS

Getting to the Exam Site

Location of exam site: ____________________

Date: ____________________

Departure time: ____________________

Do I know how to get to the exam site? Yes ____ No ____ (If no, make a trial run.)

Time it will take to get to exam site ____________________

Things to Lay Out the Night Before

Clothes I will wear ______

Sweater/jacket ______

Watch ______

Photo ID ______

Four #2 pencils ______

Other Things to Bring/Remember

____________________ ____________________

____________________ ____________________

____________________ ____________________

____________________ ____________________

____________________ ____________________

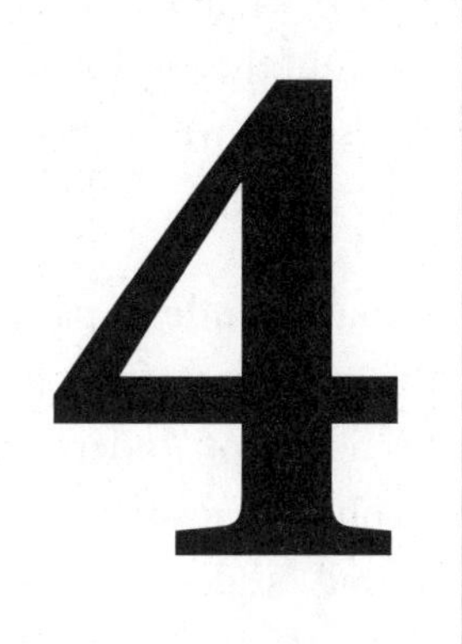

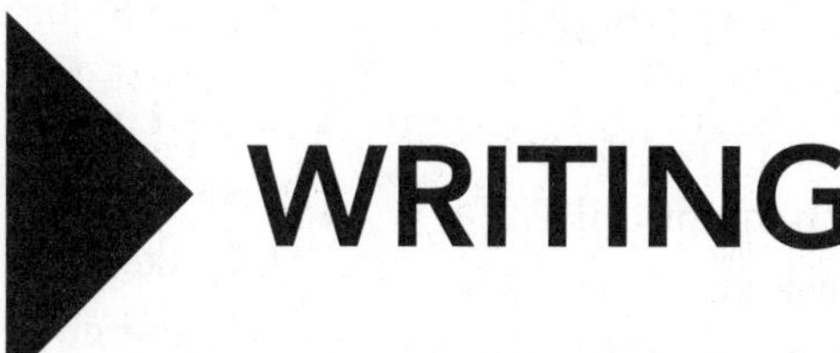

CHAPTER 4 WRITING

Getting a good score on the writing portion of the PCAT takes more than just being able to use correct grammar, spelling, and punctuation. It's also about your ability to make a logical argument in writing.

You will have to write two essays on the PCAT. One is scored, and one is experimental, but since you won't know which is which it's important to do a good job on both essays. The essays present a topic and ask you to write about a possible solution. The subjects will cover general health, science, politics, and culture. Your score will reflect whether you are able to present a clear and logical argument. It will not reflect whether your solution is correct.

The best essays that will receive the highest scores will include a proposed solution, three examples of how that solution might work, an evaluation of an alternative solution, and a conclusion. They will also be presented clearly, logically, and precisely, and be grammatically correct.

PCAT Essay Scoring Explained

You will receive two scores for your PCAT essay: one for Conventions of Language, and one for Problem Solving. The scores use a scale of zero to 5. A zero represents an incomplete essay. A 5 is one that is considered outstanding. A 3 represents an adequate, or acceptable, essay.

Your Conventions of Language score is based on grammar, spelling, mechanics, and punctuation. The second score is Problem Solving, which addresses your ability to propose a solution to the problem in the essay prompt, and whether you present a logical argument that supports your proposed solution. Your solution should be organized into distinct parts—an introduction, an explanation, examples, counterexamples or alternative solutions, and a conclusion.

The following sections review the PCAT scoring rubric. They will help you figure out what you need to focus on as you study, read, and write practice essays.

Conventions of Language

This portion of your score is related to the mechanics of your writing:

- 5.0—Superior
  A superior essay is one in which the writer spells correctly, uses excellent grammar, knows the rules of punctuation, and shows some sophistication in terms of sentence structure and mechanics. This includes things such as varying the length of your sentences and using compound and complex sentences correctly.

- 4.0—Efficient
  An efficient essay is one in which the writer makes a few mistakes in sentence formation, usage, or mechanics, but the errors do not negatively impact the flow and meaning of the answer.

- 3.0—Adequate
  An adequate essay is one in which the writer makes several spelling, grammar, and usage mistakes, but overall the writer applies the conventions of language fairly well. Errors may interfere with the flow of the essay, but the essay's meaning is still apparent, and the essay is well structured.

- 2.0—Limited
  A limited essay is one that includes a pattern of mistakes that affect the meaning of the answer, and therefore indicates a lack of understanding of how to structure a cohesive response. Grammar, spelling, punctuation, and usage mistakes are significant enough to affect the quality and clarity of the response.

- 1.0—Weak
  In a weak essay, the writer shows limited ability to apply the conventions of language, with frequent and serious spelling, grammar, punctuation, and structural mistakes. The response is difficult to follow and understand.

- 0—Invalid
  An invalid essay is one in which the Writing section of the answer booklet has been left blank, or the essay is written in a foreign language or is illegible.

Problem Solving

Your Problem Solving score is related to your ability to present a logical, convincing, and well-structured argument in writing.

- 5.0—Superior
  In a superior essay, the writer develops a powerful, sophisticated, logical, organized argument, and communicates that argument effectively. The writer's proposed solution is clear and detailed, using facts and specific examples. The writer also discusses and evaluates an alternative solution or solutions.

- 4.0—Efficient
  An efficient essay makes a persuasive argument that is well composed, but may include a small amount of questionable reasoning or minor lapses in logic. The solution relates to the problem and includes specific examples. Multiple possible solutions, or one or more alternative solutions are mentioned, with some attempt at evaluation.

- 3.0—Adequate
  An adequate response uses important principles of effective composition and clearly discusses the problem and solution, but is too general to be convincing. This essay lacks the detailed, in-depth examples of higher-scoring responses. The writing is logical, but loosely organized and may include digressions or unnecessary information and repetition, which weaken the argument.

- 2.0—Limited
  A limited essay does not properly address the problem, and does not provide clearly stated solutions. Examples are limited, incomplete, or irrelevant. The essay is not well organized, and the loose structure of ideas weakens the flow and argument.

- 1.0—Weak
  A weak response is one in which the solution does not clearly relate to the problem presented, or it is unconvincing. Contradictory information may be present, along with digressions and redundancies or repetition. Chaotic organization may make it hard to follow the logic of the response.

- 0—Invalid
  An invalid essay is one in which the writer has either left the Writing section of the answer booklet blank or has written in a foreign language, written illegibly, written in a way that indicates an inability or refusal to attempt a response, or written on a topic other than the one assigned.

Writing a Good Essay

Even if writing isn't your strong suit, practice and preparation can help you get a good score on your PCAT essay. One of the most important things you can do is understand how you should spend the 30 minutes you will have to write each essay. If you are tempted to read the prompt and start writing immediately, don't do it! A few minutes of outlining can mean the difference between scoring a 2 and scoring a 5!

Understand What's Being Asked

The first thing you should do is read the prompt, which will be something like this: "Discuss a solution to the problem of the United States' dependence on foreign oil." Make sure you focus your thinking on the specific issue you're being asked to write about. In this example, while it might be relevant to mention the impact of oil on the environment, that shouldn't be the focus of your answer, because the prompt is asking you about dependence on foreign oil, not to evaluate whether Americans are using too much oil or energy.

Outline

It is still not time to start writing your essay yet. Once you have focused on exactly what you're being asked to write about, you should spend a few minutes writing an outline. Then you can take that outline and use it as the framework for writing your essay. This should take you no more than five minutes.

Your outline should have five parts:

1. Introduction
2. Proposed solution
3. Three or four elements of that solution
4. Alternative solution and evaluation
5. Conclusion

Using the example mentioned earlier, your outline might look like this:

> Introduction: Dependence on foreign oil adds to deficit, slows economic growth, and supports unstable governments.
>
> Solution: A comprehensive program of public/private investment to support the development of alternative sources of fuel and energy.
>
> Elements of solution: Tax breaks for research and development of alternative energy, public/private partnerships to encourage the development of alternative energy sources, tax incentives for carmakers producing fuel-efficient cars and hybrids, and tax breaks for consumers who buy those cars.
>
> Alternative solution: Wind turbines, which require large open spaces to operate, may be unsightly to neighbors, and may also kill birds who fly into them.
>
> Conclusion: A combined public/private partnership that develops a comprehensive program could have a significant impact on consumption of foreign oil, and simultaneously be good for the environment.

See pages 33–35 to read the essay that was written based on this outline.

Write Your Essay

After writing your outline, take the next 20 minutes to write your essay. Be clear and concise. Remember to use at least three examples to back up your thesis. Your introductory paragraph should give a brief overview of the problem/issue and present your solution. The next three paragraphs should include your explanation and examples. The last paragraph should draw a conclusion.

Proofread!

While you are writing your essay, keep an eye on the clock. Make sure you leave five minutes at the end so you can proofread your work. This is when you make sure your argument is logical and well constructed; make sure you've used at least three examples; check for clarity; and check spelling, grammar, punctuation, and sentence structure.

Other Strategies to Help Increase Your Essay Score

There are additional things you can do to help improve your PCAT essay scores. Write practice essays, review grammar and punctuation rules, and read examples of well-structured solutions to problems, which you can find in newspapers and magazines, especially on the opinion pages.

Grammar and Punctuation

Many people, especially those who have focused their studies on science, have not studied English writing skills since they were in high school. But even if that is not your situation, make sure you review spelling, grammar, and punctuation rules. Getting them right is a great way to increase your score. A brief overview follows, but it's probably worth doing a full review using a textbook if you have one handy.

Sentence Structure

Make sure you write complete and correct sentences. Each sentence contains a subject, about which something is said, and a verb, which says something about the subject. Together they make up a clause. Every sentence must have at least one clause.

The subject and verb must match, or agree in person and in number. If the subject of a sentence is singular, the verb must also be singular. Examples: **I** (a singular subject) **am** (a singular verb that agrees with the singular subject) going to the store. **My husband and my daughter** (a plural subject) **are** (a plural verb that agrees with the plural subject) going to the store. Make sure that your verbs are also in the correct tense (past, present, or future) to appropriately reflect the specific time at which the event being described in the sentence occurs.

Be sure to avoid sentence fragments and run-on sentences. A sentence should express one and only one complete thought. It may have several parts, or clauses, but each part must contribute to a unified idea. If you are using a lot of commas, take time when you proofread your essay to make sure you aren't stringing together words that should be separated into multiple sentences. Keep the rule of one complete thought in mind when you write your essays and when you proofread them.

As you develop your solution to the problem presented on the PCAT essay, you should also make sure that you describe the solution using the active voice. That means writing sentences where the subject directly performs the action. Active: **BP found oil** after drilling in the Gulf of Mexico. Passive: **Oil was found** after drilling in the Gulf of Mexico.

Punctuation

Use commas to separate items in a series when there are more than two items. You should also use commas to separate descriptive words, or adjectives, before nouns, and to set off interpolative phrases or clauses. Also use commas after introductory phrases.

Semicolons may be used to separate independent clauses, and should be used between independent clauses connected by words such as therefore, nevertheless, and moreover. Use a colon to signal that what follows is a list, definition, explanation, or restatement of what has gone before.

You should probably avoid the use of contractions such as *don't* or *isn't* on your PCAT essay, as they are signs of informality. In other words, use apostrophes only to indicate the possessive form of a noun.

Writing Style

The style that works best for the PCAT essays is direct and precise. This means using concrete examples where you can, and replacing bulky wording with fewer words that are more exact. To do this effectively, use the active voice, use clear language instead of vague language, use the words you need, and don't add extra words because you think they make you sound knowledgeable. The PCAT essays are relatively short, so be sure to avoid redundancy—do not repeat yourself. Stay away from clichés and jargon, and use an appropriate degree of formality. Finally, avoid sexist or biased language.

Another helpful hint is to read articles in newspapers and magazines ahead of time. Many of them are written using a similar structure to what you're asked to do in your PCAT essay. Opinion pieces and editorials will be particularly helpful. The point is not so much whether you agree with them; instead it's whether you can recognize the structure of a good argument and apply that structure to your essays.

Practice writing good essays, and time yourself when you do it. Make sure you take the first five minutes to prepare an outline, write for 20 minutes, and leave five minutes at the end for proofreading. Look at the two scoring rubrics at the beginning of this chapter and try to score your own work.

Commonly Misspelled and Misused Words

There are words that can be easily, and incorrectly, spelled or interchanged. As you do your grammar review, you should pay close attention to them so that you don't make careless mistakes that will cost you points on your PCAT essays. The following are a few examples.

Make sure that you know the difference between **there**, **their**, and **they're**. *There* is a place. The word *their* shows belonging or possession. (Their shoes were at the front door.) And *they're* is a contraction for *they are*. Since your PCAT essay should be written in a formal style, you should stay away from using contractions such as *they're*.

It's also important for you to remember the difference between **its** and **it's**. *It's* is a contraction, short for *it is*. Once again, stay away from using *it's* in your PCAT essay, because it is too informal. Like the word *their* in the preceding paragraph, the word *its* shows belonging or possession.

You can use the following to remember the difference between **principal** and **principle**. The *principal* of your school can be your pal. The kind of "principle," or rule, you might discuss in your PCAT essay ends in *-le*.

Here are just a few words that are often misspelled:

dependent (*-ent*, not *-ant*)
gauge (*-au*, not *-ua*)
judgment (not judgement)
license (not lisence)
maintenance (*-ance* at end, not *-ence*)
occasion/occasionally (two *c*'s, one *s*)
occurrence (*-ence*, not *-ance*)
receive (*-eive*, not *-ieve*)

It makes sense to study words like these so you walk into the test confident that you will not lose points for spelling mistakes.

Effective and Ineffective Essay Writing

Writing an effective essay for the PCAT involves two separate aspects. The first is doing your best to make sure your spelling, grammar, mechanics, and usage are correct. If you feel confident in your ability to do well on this aspect of the essay, which is one of your two scores, you don't have to spend a lot of time reviewing rules and spelling. However, if these areas are weaknesses for you, don't despair. Instead, prepare. Study grammar and usage rules, review commonly misspelled words, and practice, practice, practice. The time you spend reviewing can have a direct impact on your Conventions of Language score.

The second part is about making a logical argument. You need to think through your answer, outline it carefully, and before you start writing, review your outline. Make sure you've included an introduction, a proposed solution, three elements of that solution, an alternative solution and a sentence or two about whether it might work, and a conclusion. Then use your outline to structure your essay.

Paragraphs

As a rule, the paragraphs of your PCAT essay should be three sentences or more. You can make an exception for a conclusion, though it's best to include at least two sentences.

Writing a Good Paragraph

A paragraph is a piece of writing that consists of several sentences. A paragraph should always have complete, correct, and concise sentences. As well, it should be easy to read and well organized. The paragraph itself should focus on one subject, theme, or central idea. Each paragraph should have its own main idea, and the sentences in it should support or be related to that main idea.

A paragraph contains several elements. Some paragraphs will have only one main point, whereas others will have two or three. In your PCAT essay, make sure your first and last paragraphs have clear concluding sentences. Some of your paragraphs in the middle of the essay, where you go through your proposed solution to the stated problem, may end with openings for transitions as you move from one element of your solution to the next.

- Topic sentence: tells the reader what the paragraph is about and gets the reader interested
- First main point: proves, backs up, or explains the topic sentence

- Second main point: Backs up or provides a reason for the first main point
- Third main point: can help prove the topic sentence or back up first or second main point
- Conclusion: sums up the ideas in the paragraph and may complete the topic or may provide a transition to the next paragraph

Here's an example that follows this format:

> One part of the solution would be for the federal government to provide a series of incentives, including tax breaks, for companies pursuing research and development of alternative energy solutions. In our current economy, some of those incentives could be focused on providing tax breaks to companies that hire new employees. In addition, incentives could be offered to companies that can move their research processes along quickly and bring products to the marketplace within specific time frames.

The topic sentence lets the reader know right away that this paragraph is about one part of the solution of the U.S. dependence on foreign oil. The main idea is providing incentives to companies that pursue research and development of alternative energy solutions. The second main idea is that by providing incentives, we can support companies that hire new employees. The third main idea is that incentives could help products reach the marketplace faster. As this paragraph is in the middle of an essay, it does not draw a conclusion. Instead, by making it clear in the first sentence that it addresses one part of the proposed solution, it allows the essay writer to transition smoothly to the next part of the solution in the following paragraph.

Good Conclusion

The following is the concluding paragraph of a sample essay responding to a prompt about the problem of U.S. dependence on foreign oil. The whole essay, a good response, is one you will review later in this chapter:

> The implementation of a comprehensive program of public and private investment could have a significant impact on the United States' dependence on foreign oil. In addition, it would be good for the environment. A solution such as this one, with multiple positive outcomes, is one that our country can and should pursue.

This conclusion reviews the proposed solution, a comprehensive program of public and private investment, discusses its potential impact, and closes by saying it is a solution that should be pursued.

Weak Conclusion

A weak conclusion to the same essay follows.

> In conclusion, the United States is too dependant on foreign oil, and must implement solutions that will have an effect on the problem.

This conclusion has a few problems. The word *dependant* is misspelled. It should be *dependent*, with an *e*. In addition, it is only one sentence long, and it does not restate any specific solutions or elements of solutions to the problem. Instead it merely restates that there is a problem that needs solutions.

Sample Essays

Essay 1

Prompt: Discuss a solution to the problem of the United States' dependence on foreign oil.

Good Response

The United States' dependence on oil as fuel, and in particular on oil that is purchased from foreign countries, contributes to the U.S. deficit, slows our economic growth, and provides indirect support for unstable and dangerous foreign governments. Developing and implementing a comprehensive program to reduce our dependence on foreign oil that combines public and private efforts and investment is the best way to deal with this significant problem.

One part of a solution would be for the federal government to provide a series of incentives, including tax breaks to companies pursuing research and development of alternative energy solutions. In our current economy, some of those incentives could be focused on providing tax breaks to companies that hire new employees. In addition, incentives could be offered to companies that can move their research processes along quickly and bring products to the marketplace within specific time frames.

Public/private partnerships to increase the use of alternative energy also make sense. The federal government could raise revenue for these investments by increasing the federal gas tax. This would have a two-pronged effect because it could also decrease consumption. Additional incentives could be provided for carmakers that increase gas mileage and make and sell more hybrid cars, as well as tax breaks for consumers who buy the cars.

Although wind power has been put forth as part of the solution to this problem, there are some challenges with the low-technology methods used to harness it. Wind farms require hundreds of tall turbines that take up a significant amount of space, produce loud noise, and may be harmful to birds and other wildlife. Today they are not a viable large-scale solution.

The implementation of a comprehensive program of public and private investment could have a significant impact on the United States' dependence on foreign oil. In addition, it would be good for the environment. A solution such as this one, with multiple positive outcomes, is one that our country can and should pursue.

Analysis of Response

This response is good because it meets the standards of the Conventions of Language score: correct spelling, correct grammar, proper sentence structure, and proper mechanics and organization. The five paragraphs are well laid out and create the structure for a good Problem Solving score. In terms of the Problem Solving score, this essay develops a sophisticated and logical argument, communicates that argument effectively via the use of specific examples, presents and evaluates an alternative solution, and sums up the argument clearly in the concluding paragraph.

Weak Response

The United State is too dependant on foreign oil and this is bad for the country. It's a problem and we need to come up with a way to fix it.

One solution is to increase the tax that the government could charge people when they fill there cars up with gas. Then this money could be used to help pay for companies' to make cars that get better gas mileage.

Another solution is to look into other types of energy for people to use for power for there homes, cars, and other appliances, two examples are solar and wind power.

If we do these things, we can help to solve the problem of our over dependance on foreign oil.

Analysis of Response

Although this response does lay out a logical argument, it is filled with spelling, grammatical, and mechanical/structural mistakes.

The introductory paragraph repeats the prompt, states that a solution is needed, and does not state what that solution might be. When you write the introductory paragraph of your essay, be sure to do more than just restate the problem.

The second paragraph does include a solution, but the writer uses the incorrect word *there* (place) when *their* (possessive) is correct. And the word *companies* in the second sentence is not possessive, so there should be no apostrophe.

In the third paragraph, the writer again uses *there* incorrectly. The proper word, again, is *their*. Further, the sentence is a run-on. It should have a period after *appliances*. The second sentence should read: Two examples of alternative energy sources are solar power and wind power.

The concluding paragraph once again includes misspelling of the word *dependence*, has an extra space (*overdependence*), and restates the problem without summing up the proposed conclusion.

The paragraphs are also short, and they do not provide enough detail. There is no counterexample, an element that is not necessary to receive a decent score of 3, but that is important to include in order to score a 5. These mistakes are significant enough not only to lead to a low Conventions of Language score, but to impact the Problem Solving score as well.

Essay 2

Prompt: Discuss a solution to the problem of inadequate science education in U.S. high schools.

Good Response

The United States has fallen to 21st in the world in science education. This impacts our country's future competitiveness economically and technologically because many twenty-first-century jobs and twenty-first-century challenges will involve science and technology. It is vital that we implement new teaching methods to engage students in science before they reach the high school level, and that we continue to nurture and encourage their interest while they are in high school.

The first part of this solution requires rethinking the way science is taught at the elementary and secondary school levels. One of the best ways to engage students is to have students actively participate in learning: science teachers should, as often as possible, have their students conduct actual experiments, preferably working in groups. This type of active learning and engagement will be more effective than sitting in the classroom listening to a teacher talk, or watching a video. If possible, integrating the use of computers into the experiments will also help students become comfortable with computers as teaching tools.

Implementing this more active approach will be most effective if students work in teams, not only because they will learn from one another and inspire one another, but also because there are studies that show project-based learning helps to boost creativity. In addition, the team approach enables teachers to follow what the students are doing more easily than if experiments were conducted individually, and it decreases the cost of materials.

Another important element of this solution is to incorporate student participation in science competitions and after-school programs offered by schools and nonprofit organizations around the country. If high school science teachers encourage their students to enter competitions and become involved in extracurricular programs, the students can choose the specific areas that interest them, and they can work with others who have similar interests and help to inspire each other. In many instances, these programs include interaction with mentors who work in scientific fields. This is one of the best ways to get students engaged—to have adults talk to students about the adults' own work and how they learned to do it. If such mentor programs are not available, science teachers should try to get scientists to come into classrooms and talk to students.

Finally, some organizations offer summer internships or special science programs for high school students. Science teachers should encourage their students to apply to such programs. The teachers should also help the students with their applications, since that will be a helpful way for them to judge a student's true level of interest.

The alternative, to do in the classroom exactly what we are doing now, is likely to lead to further declines that this country can ill afford. We need to excite and entice today's students into the worlds of science. We should try to relate those sciences to students' everyday interests in order to spur their curiosity.

If we are able to inspire students by making science come alive for them long before they get to high school, if we offer as many hands-on opportunities as possible, and if we encourage students to interact with mentors and scientists, we have an opportunity to have a major positive impact on this significant gap in our current educational system.

Analysis of Response

As with the essay about foreign oil dependence, this essay would receive a high score because it is well structured in terms of Conventions of Language, and it presents a clear, logical argument, including an alternative solution and brief evaluation.

In the first paragraph, the writer makes a broad, general statement that illustrates the depth of the problem, and then develops the solution using strong language for paragraph transitions that shows a sophisticated command of language and argument.

The writer presents three elements of a solution, which address the way science is taught from the perspective of teachers and students, and adds two additional pieces involving the use of mentors and integration of after-school programs, which make the argument stronger.

In this case, the alternative solution is to continue with the same policies, procedures, and teaching methods that have helped to cause the problem. Although it is a simple, short paragraph, it is a mechanical and grammatical device to draw attention to the weakness of the current situation, so it is effective and will receive a good score.

The conclusion sums up the argument and ends by stating that if the elements of the solution were put in place, the system would improve.

Weak Response

The United States is not doing well in science education. Our students are not learning science, and that means they are not going to be enough scientists in the future. If we don't try to make changes, this will be an ongoing problem.

One way to solve the problem of bad science education is high school is to hire better science teachers who will be able to do a better job teaching their students the things they have to learn about science.

Another way to solve the problem of bad science education is to make the work more interesting for students so that they don't lose interest in science because they are bored or don't understand the work.

Another way to solve the problem of bad science education is to have scientists and other people who work in scientific fields come into classrooms and talk to students about what they do. This could help some students want to be scientists because they like what they here or think the work would be interesting.

One thing we know, is if we keep dong what we are doing, the situation won't improve.

But if we can help students get more interested in science, and keep them interested, we can have an impact on this serious problem. And then we will have students ready to be scientists in the future.

Analysis of Response

This is not a bad essay, but it is not as strong as the first example. Its weaknesses include repetition at the start of paragraphs two, three, and four; repetition of other words and phrases; the use of *they* where *there* would be correct; the use of the contraction *don't* instead of *do not* (remember, this is formal writing, and contractions should be avoided); and a bare-bones argument that does not include any information about how changes would be made.

In other words, this essay is similar to the strong one in some ways, so take some time to compare the two and you will be able to see the differences, which will help you approach your PCAT essays prepared to write a strong response.

Essay 3

Prompt: Discuss a solution to the problem of childhood obesity.

Good Response

Over the past 25 years, rates of childhood obesity in the United States have skyrocketed, leading to a variety of health problems among young people, including an increase in the incidence of diabetes. It is important that we work to slow this trend, not only because of its health implications for young people now, but because of the impact obesity will have on their health throughout their lifetimes.

The best way to combat childhood obesity is through a combination of healthy eating and exercise. While it is difficult to control a child's eating habits at home, schools can play a part by offering healthy food choices, and by teaching students about the importance of eating only healthy food. This can include materials that students can take home and share with their families.

These days, school budgets are stretched thin, and as a result, many schools do not offer physical education for students. This puts many students at risk. A possible solution is for the federal government, through a collaboration of the Department of Education and the Department of Health and Human Services, to have a two-step campaign. The first would be education regarding the importance of exercise for children, and the second would be to restore funding that would support physical education for students in school. Each state has published standards for physical education for elementary school, junior high school, and high school students. Starting by requiring states to provide classes where students have a chance to meet those standards makes good sense. Linking these standards to good health outcomes for students will help to make the case for funding.

Participation on sports teams can be beneficial as well, so parents should encourage students to join teams, or to participate in after-school programs in districts where there are no school-sponsored sports teams. If neither of those options is available, families should be encouraged to participate in outdoor activities together—even if it is just taking a half-hour walk a few days a week.

Although a good argument can be made for government policies such as adding calorie counts to fast-food restaurant menus, and they are a positive step, such education is only the first step in changing behavior. Public health agencies in towns, cities, states, and at the federal level need to provide easily accessible information on healthy and affordable alternatives. Fast-food restaurants have already begun offering lower-calorie, healthier entrees, and they should be encouraged to continue that practice, although it is not possible to require them to do so.

Although childhood obesity is a problem that will take years to solve, a combination of education, advocacy, and exercise as described here will begin to help reverse this dangerous and troubling trend.

Analysis of Response

Like the other good responses in this chapter, the introduction to this essay provides specific examples to illustrate why the problem presented is one that needs to be solved. The proposed solution has multiple elements that intertwine to address the problem through more than one channel—a sophisticated response.

Because grammar, spelling, mechanics, and usage are correct, this essay would also receive a high score for Conventions of Language.

Weak Response

The rate of childhood obesity in the United States is high, and this leads to health problems for people when they are young and as they grow up. It is important to address this problem so that our society can be healthier.

The first step is for children to eat better. Parents and schools should provide healthy meals and healthy snacks. It's better to cook dinner at home than it is to go out to a fast-food restaurant for dinner where the food is high in calories and not very healthy.

Children also need to get exercise at least a few days a week in gym class at school, after school, or at home. Parents can help here by getting outside with their kids and playing catch or going for a walk. Or students can join sports teams after school so that they get exercise.

If children eat better and exercise more, we will begin to address the serious problem of childhood obesity.

Analysis of Response

While there are some good elements in this response, it is too simple to receive a high score. The grammar and mechanics are satisfactory, but the sentences and paragraph structure are very simple. The essay needs more details.

For example, it may be correct to say that children should eat healthier, but it is important to add additional details because children often are not the ones making their eating decisions. Schools and parents have to become involved by offering healthy choices—the good essay includes that information while this weaker essay does not. The same is true for the paragraph about exercise. Even if you don't know that many schools no longer provide physical education, like the writer of the first essay says, if you think about the problem that is presented to you, it will be possible for you to indicate that you know where certain solutions are not as simple as they sound. If you acknowledge that, your essay will be stronger.

As with Essay 2, it makes sense for you to read the strong response and the analysis, and then read this response and analysis. The comparison will help you to write a stronger PCAT essay.

Essay 4

Prompt: Discuss a solution to the problem of illiteracy in the United States.

Good Response

The ability to read is fundamental to functioning effectively in today's complex world. Unfortunately, with holes in our educational system, there are students who are passed from grade to grade even though their reading skills are not up to the proper standard. This leads to illiteracy issues for children and for adults as well.

An obvious solution is to stop passing students from one grade to the next unless they are able to show through classroom work and through their performance on standardized tests that their reading skills are appropriate for their grade level. This is more complicated than it sounds because of the lack of funding for education that is a consequence of growing state and local budget deficits. While it is a challenge, this is a key point for intervention to solve the problem, so it is worth government reexamination of resources at all levels so that tutors and special classes can be provided to help those who are not learning to read.

Reinforcement should also happen at home. For students whose parents do not know how to read or do not speak English as their first language, additional resources such as reading programs at local public libraries can provide some of the additional reinforcement these young students need. In addition, libraries can be used as the home for adult literacy programs—sponsored by local governments and nonprofit organizations. Collaborations with nonprofit organizations make particularly good sense here because they will know how to get around the stigma some adults feel regarding admitting that they don't know how to read.

While some would say that extending the school year through the summer would help students improve their literacy skills, this is likely to be even more expensive than developing specific tutoring programs during the school year because it would involve not only paying teachers, but also all of the associated costs of keeping schools open when they would typically be closed.

By providing extra tutoring, creating after-school programs using libraries, and helping parents learn to read, our society can begin to improve literacy rates. This improvement will have benefits for people of all ages.

Analysis of Response

As you should be starting to see by the time you review this example, this essay is strong because it has a good introductory paragraph, provides specific examples that would address the problem of illiteracy, includes solutions to address illiteracy both among children and among adults, includes a counterexample and analysis, and has a strong conclusion.

It is also structurally, grammatically, and mechanically correct, and free of spelling errors.

Weak Response

If people don't learn to read, they will have problems in their lives. They may not be able to pay their bills, do their taxes, or help teach their children to read.

Schools need to do a better job teaching students to read. They should spend more hours in school. They should take more tests to tell if they're learning. Teachers should make students read out loud to the class. Parents need to read to they're children too.

Without reading, it's hard to get through life, so it's important for children to learn to read.

Analysis of Response

It is easy to tell that this is a very poorly written essay. There are mechanical mistakes and spelling mistakes, and the essay is too short. The Conventions of Language score for this example would be a 1 or possibly even a zero.

On the Problem Solving front, there aren't enough examples, and there is no logical argument presented. It is not enough to say that "schools need to do a better job teaching students to read." That is the starting point, whereas in a PCAT essay you have to attempt to indicate how something like teaching reading might be done more effectively than it is being done now. Compare this with the good response to the same prompt and you will see the difference.

Summing It Up

As you write practice essays, remember to come back to these examples so that you can check the structure of your essays. Since you will receive two separate scores for each essay—a Conventions of Language score and a Problem Solving score—be sure to spend some time looking at the quality of your answers from both perspectives.

Conventions of Language

Did you write an essay that is grammatically and mechanically correct? Do all of your subjects and verbs agree in number and use the proper tense? Did you check your spelling? Do your paragraphs have topic sentences and main ideas to back up the topics? Did you vary your sentence structure?

Problem Solving

Have you presented a logical argument with an introductory statement of your proposed solution to the stated problem? Did you include two or three paragraphs with examples that further explain your solution? Did you remember to include a counterexample and short explanation of why it might not be the right solution, or might not be a good short-term solution? Did you write a clear conclusion that summarizes your answer without repeating the exact same words you used in your introduction?

If you can answer yes to all, or at least most, of these questions, then the quality of your practice essays is high and you should be ready to get good scores on this portion of your PCAT.

It All Comes Back to Reading

Even if you feel like you write well and are fully prepared to ace your PCAT essays, you should still read as much as you can. Focus on finding articles or essays that are written in order to argue a position. They will be the best guides for you on how to create a logical argument for your PCAT essay. Opinion pages in the newspaper and on the Internet are likely to be your best sources for this kind of writing.

CHAPTER

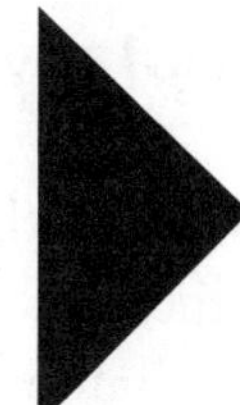

VERBAL ABILITY

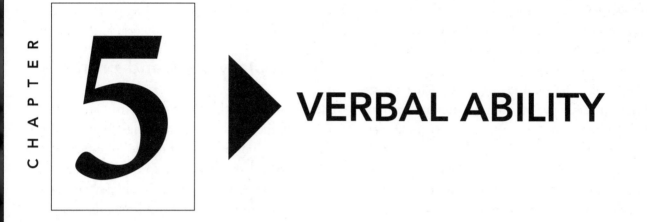

The Verbal Ability portion of the PCAT contains 48 questions, 60% of which are analogies, and 40% of which are sentence completion exercises. You may be wondering why you need to demonstrate verbal ability as part of your proficiency to be accepted into a pharmacy college, especially when the vocabulary used in the Verbal Ability section is essentially nonscientific, and when you are being tested to a much greater extent on biology, chemistry, and mathematics. Being able to communicate effectively is important for success not only in any graduate-level school, but in almost every profession; and to communicate effectively includes possession of a broad vocabulary and the ability to infer meanings from hard-to-understand words and sentences. A successful pharmacy student will not only excel at math and science, but also speak and write competently and be able to resort to a power of deduction and the ability to make connections among words.

You will learn how to seek the correct answers for analogies and sentence completions later in this section. First, it is important to lay the groundwork to help you with vocabulary, as vocabulary and the ability to figure out what certain words mean will guide you toward the correct answers for analogies and sentence completions. While a broad knowledge of vocabulary certainly will pay off on this test, it is the ability to choose words based on the context of a sentence or, in the case of an analogy, based on the relationship among words, that will enable you to do well on the Verbal Ability section.

You have a lot of studying ahead. Chances are you will not memorize an entire dictionary or hundreds of words. Yet committing to learning new words every day will go a long way toward helping you on the Verbal Ability section of the PCAT. In your everyday reading or listening, whenever you come across or hear a word you do not know, jot down the word and look up its definition as soon as possible. About an hour or two later, see if you can remember the definition. The next day, test yourself on that word again. Keep a running list of these words. You will likely read or hear unfamiliar words, or words whose meaning escapes you, not only through reading, but via all sorts of media, from radio programs to text or video on websites.

Vocabulary Lists and Prompts

The following are the common prefixes and suffixes, and their more common meanings. If you do not know the definition of any of the examples of the prefixes or suffixes, then head for the dictionary, online or on the bookshelf. This should get you started on your own mini-dictionary. Learning the following should put you on the right course for helping to decipher words with which you are unfamiliar.

VOCABULARY PROMPTS—COMMON PREFIXES

PREFIXES	MEANING	EXAMPLES
a-,	to, toward	aloft, around
a-, an-	not, without	apolitical, asymmetrical; anarchy, annihilate
ab-, abs-	away from	abnormal, abject; absent, abstain
ante-	before	antebellum, antecedent
anti-	against	antioxidant, antithesis
auto-	self	autograph, autonomous
bene-	good	benefactor, benevolent
bi-	two	bicentennial, binary
circum-	around	circumspect, circumvent
co-	with	coexist, coincide
contra-	against	contradict, contravene
de-	reverse, away from, down	decompress, devolve
dis-	not	disquiet, distasteful

VOCABULARY PROMPTS—COMMON PREFIXES *(continued)*		
PREFIXES	**MEANING**	**EXAMPLES**
dys-	bad	dysfunction, dyspeptic
ecto-	outside	ectoplasm
en-, em-	put into, bring about	engage, entrust; empower, embolden
endo-	inside	endodontics
ex-	out	except, expunge
extra-	beyond	extracurricular, extraordinary
hydr-, hydro-	water	hydrology
hyper-	over, excessively	hyperbole
hypo-	under	hypochondria
in-	in	inculcate, induct
in-, im-	not	inexplicable, involuntary; impervious, immodest
inter-	between, among	intervene, interdisciplinary
intra-	within, between	intramuscular, intramural
intro-	into, within	introduce, introspective
macro-	large	macroeconomics, macroscopic
mal-	bad	malevolent, malfunction
micro-	small	microcosm, microelectronics
mis-	bad(ly), wrong(ly)	mislead, misunderstand
mono-	one, single	monoculture, monolithic
multi-	many	multinational, multiplex
neo-	new	neonatal, neophyte
non-	not	nonfiction, nonrefundable
omni-	all	omnipotent, omniscient
over-	above, excessive(ly)	overcast, overlay; overexpose, overwrought
pan-	all	panacea, panoply
peri-	around	peripatetic, peripheral
poly-	many	polygraph, polymorphous
post-	after	postpone, postscript

(continued)

VOCABULARY PROMPTS—COMMON PREFIXES *(continued)*		
PREFIXES	**MEANING**	**EXAMPLES**
pre-	before	preclude, preoccupy
pro-	before	procede, propel
pro-	in favor of	proponent
proto-	first	prototype
pseudo-	fake	pseudonym
re-	again, back	rebound, repatriate, restore
retro-	backward(s)	retroactive, retrograde
semi-	half	semiannual, semicircle
semi-	partly	semiconscious, semisweet
sub-	below, under	subway, subterranean; subjugation, submissive
super-	above, over	superlative, superimpose
syn-, sym-	together, at the same time	synchronize, symmetrical
tele-	far	telephonic, telescope
trans-	across	transgress, transmission
tri-	three	tricycle, tripod
un-	not	unknown, unsightly
uni-	one	unidirectional, uniform

VOCABULARY PROMPTS—COMMON SUFFIXES		
SUFFIXES	**MEANING**	**EXAMPLES**
-able, -ible (adjective)	able, capable	capable, tenable; susceptible, sensible
-acy, -cy (noun)	state of, quality of	democracy, legitimacy, advocacy, normalcy
-al (noun)	action, result of action	reversal, transmittal
-al (adjective)	pertaining to	conventional, mercurial
-ance, -ence (noun)	state of, quality of	acceptance, defiance; eminence, resurgence
-ancy, -ency (noun)	act of, state of	expectancy; dependency, clemency, complacency
-ant, -ent (noun)	one who, that which	accountant, miscreant, dependent, resident; contaminant, repellant, consistent, evanescent

VOCABULARY PROMPTS—COMMON SUFFIXES *(continued)*		
SUFFIXES	**MEANING**	**EXAMPLES**
-ate (noun)	state	estate, magnate
-ate (verb)	cause to be	capitulate, formulate
-dom (noun)	place, state of being	kingdom, martyrdom
-en (noun)	made of	golden, wooden
-en (verb)	become, cause to become	embolden, hearten
-er, -or (noun)	one who; that which	complainer, producer, counselor, professor; forerunner, modifier, indicator, simulator
-esque (adjective)	reminiscent of	grotesque, picturesque
-ful (adjective)	marked by	fanciful, merciful
-ic, -ical (adjective)	pertaining to, having the quality of	phantasmic, magical, apologetic, critical
-ify, -fy (verb)	to make, to become	mollify, specify; liquefy, stupefy
-ion (noun)	condition, action, act of	accumulation, contemplation
-ious, -ous (adjective)	characterized by	perspicacious, vicarious; glamorous, momentous
-ish (adjective)	having the quality of	cartoonish, nightmarish
-ism (noun)	doctrine, belief	patriotism, solipsism
-ist (noun)	one who	biochemist, egoist
-ity, -ty (noun)	having the quality of, state of	affordability, credibility; gritty, lefty
-ive (adjective)	having the nature of	creative, explosive
-less (adjective)	without	harmless, powerless
-ment (noun)	condition of	assessment, nourishment
-ness (noun)	condition, state of being	acuteness, dampness
-ology (noun)	science or study of	ornithology, pathology, epidemiology
-ory (noun)	place for, serves for; marked by	conservatory, dormitory; exploratory, satisfactory
-sion, -tion (noun)	condition of, action of	affiliation, modification
-y (adjective)	marked by, somewhat	lousy, spiny

Now that you are more equipped to decipher unfamiliar words, it is time to explore sentence completion exercises.

Sentence Completion Exercises

There are two types of sentence completion exercises in the PCAT Verbal Ability section. One leaves out a single word for the test taker to choose, and the second type omits two words. These sentences can be referred to as one-blank and two-blank exercises. For both types, it is a good idea to come up with your own word(s) for the blank(s), or even word sense, before reading the multiple-choice answers. Then, in the case of a one-blank sentence completion, look among the answer choices for a synonym. If you see one and it makes as much sense as your word, then it probably is the correct choice. In addition, pay attention to the tone of the sentence, its logical flow, and grammar. If an answer choice has the correct meaning for the blank but is not the correct part of speech, then it is not the correct answer.

If you are unable to pick out a synonym among the choices, you should return to the sentence and starting looking for clues. These clues are words such as: *but, however, not, moreover, in addition, more, most, few, less, yet, since, although*, and *even though*; and the list continues. For example:

> He walked out of the building _____, even though he said he was in a hurry.
>
> **a.** irritated
> **b.** quickly
> **c.** slowly
> **d.** abruptly

The clue phrase here is *even though*, letting you know you are looking for an answer that would mean the opposite to *in a hurry*. The only choice that makes sense is **c**, slowly.

For two-blank sentence completions, be sure both words in an answer choice fit. If one word fits perfectly but the second word only sort of fits, eliminate that answer choice and select another.

> When it seemed that nothing could _____ a crushing defeat to the home team, the opponents committed a _____ that handed over an unexpected victory.
>
> **a.** invite . . . play
> **b.** prevent . . . mistake
> **c.** create . . . mystery
> **d.** deliver . . . misstep

There are a few clues in this sentence: *nothing* and *unexpected*. The correct answer is choice **b**, prevent . . . mistake. Answer choice **a** is incorrect because *invite* does not make sense given how the sentence flows logically, even though the second word choice, *play*, does fit. Similarly, choice **d** is incorrect; one word fits and the other does not. In this case, although the second word choice, *misstep*, works, *deliver* does not. A word like *deliver* would work if the sentence used *victory* in place of *crushing defeat*, and *unexpected defeat* instead of *unexpected victory*. Neither words in choice **c** make sense, so **c** is incorrect.

Analogies

Your scientific and logical mathematical thinking will be useful in decoding analogies. Just as you look for the relationship between, say, two compounds or two medicinal interactions, you will look for the relationship between two word sets. Simply put, analogies are word relationships. Rather than considering the interaction between two pharmaceuticals, you are considering the interaction between words. On the test, you will be given the first word pair, along with the first word of a second word pair. Your job is to find the second word for the second word pair based on the relationship, or bond, of the first word pair. Consider this plugging in the unknown variable, like in algebra. For example:

CARPET : FLOOR :: CURTAIN :

a. lamp
b. paisley
c. couch
d. window

Approach this analogy by forming a sentence based on the relationship of the first word pair. A carpet covers a floor as a curtain covers a window. Therefore, choice **d**, window, is the correct choice. None of the others fit the sentence as logically.

When constructing your analogy relationship sentence, it may sometimes make sense to word the sentence starting with the second word of the given pair, especially if you are having difficulty forming a sentence bridging word one to word two. How would you phrase the following analogy starting with *milk*?

REFRIGERATOR : MILK :: FREEZER : ICE CREAM

____

____

The sentence could read: Milk is kept in the refrigerator just as ice cream is kept in the freezer.

Now, phrase the same analogy starting with *refrigerator.*

____

____

The sentence could read: A refrigerator houses milk just as a freezer houses ice cream.

It is important to pay attention to parts of speech. If the first word of the word pair is a noun, the first word of the second pair will be a noun. If the second word of the first pair is an adjective, the second word of the second pair must be an adjective. Thus, the test taker would choose an adjective from among the answer choices. The first word pair may contain different parts of speech (for example a verb and a noun), but the second pair has to match in the same order. For example:

SIT : CHAIR :: DRIVE : CAR

(VERB : NOUN :: VERB : NOUN)

In fact, the PCAT may ask the test taker to complete a grammatical analogy, such as:

FOUND : FIND :: SLEPT :

a. sleeping
b. pillow
c. sleep
d. sleepy

The first word pair contains two verbs, the first in the past tense, and the second in the present tense. Therefore, the second word pair must mirror the first pair in parts of speech, and, in the case of a verb, in the verb tense as well. In this example, the answer must be a verb in the present tense, given that *find* is in the present tense. The correct answer is choice **c**, sleep.

There are many more types of analogies. The following examples and explanations describe the more common types, and include those types likely to be on the PCAT.

This next analogy demonstrates a cause-and-effect relationship.

BACTERIA : INFECTION :: SPARKS : FIRE
Bacteria can lead to/cause infection. Sparks can lead to/cause a fire.

Here is an example of an analogy containing antonyms:

CAUTIOUS : RECKLESS :: INEXCUSABLE : FORGIVABLE

An analogy of synonyms is:

BEGIN : COMMENCE :: RUIN : DESTROY

Another type of analogy is one in which the first two words are similar in meaning, but one word has a different level of intensity, carrying the meaning to a different degree. For example:

BIG : ENORMOUS :: SMALL : MICROSCOPIC
Enormous is extremely big, whereas microscopic is extremely small.

Analogies that exhibit part-to-whole relationships are another common type. For example:

PAGES : BOOK :: SHINGLES : ROOF

This could read: A book contains pages just as a roof contains shingles. Another way to interpret this analogy is: Many pages make up a book. Many shingles make up a roof. Simply stated, pages are part of a book and shingles are part of a roof.

Here is a variation on the part-to-whole analogy, where the relationship is such that, in the word pair, one word is a type of the other word, such as:

BIOLOGIST : SCIENTIST :: ELM : TREE
A biologist is a type of scientist, and an elm is a type of tree.

Workers and their professions, or hobbyists and their activities, constitute another analogy category. These types of analogies can be about workers and their tools (CHEMIST : BEAKER :: ACCOUNTANT : CALCULATOR); tools and their functions (KNIFE : CUT :: PEN : WRITE); and other related associations, such as where workers perform their jobs (PROFESSOR : COLLEGE :: ARTIST : STUDIO). There are, of course, variations of these types of analogies.

Again, the aforementioned analogy types are just some of the more common ones found on the PCAT.

Take care not to make relationship sentences too long, or complicated, when figuring out analogies. The test questions are not intended to prompt intricate and circuitous trains of thought. Rather, the test taker is expected to figure out the word relationships in a direct manner.

Drawing a Blank

There could be an analogy or sentence completion for which you simply cannot figure out the meanings of the viable answer choices. You realize you will have to guess. You still have a last resort here, not terribly scientific, but something to consider. Suppose you have a one-blank sentence completion, and, given the context, you are able to eliminate two of the answer choices, but you cannot decide between the remaining ones. You have already applied your prefix/suffix knowledge and come up clueless. Now could be the time to apply a simplistic, though sometimes workable, solution. On an educated hunch, decide whether the word sounds positive or negative. Then, having assessed the type of word for which the sentence calls, plug in your choice.

Of course, this is something to use infrequently and only in a sentence completion for which you truly have no idea. For analogies, given that the answer is all about the word relationship, you would have to make the positive/negative word guess based on that relationship.

Practice Questions

Sentence Completions

1. Punishment alone will never _____ in putting an end to crime.
a. languish
b. succeed
c. resolve
d. portend

2. He was very easily approached, being naturally the most _____ man in the room.
a. pugnacious
b. sheepish
c. imperious
d. affable

3. His _____ temperament was disclosed in the deep color of his cheeks.
a. sanguine
b. plaintive
c. wistful
d. despairing

4. Leaving a life of bare essentials and meagerness, he found all the luxury and _____ money could provide in his new surroundings.
a. eagerness
b. sparseness
c. indulgences
d. extravagant

5. The crew seemed to have been overcome by the same _____ influence that had subdued Mother Nature, for they all lay about the deck sleeping or dozing.
a. prosaic
b. somnolent
c. indolent
d. obtuse

6. Many people imagine that all the evils _____ society spring from want, but this is only _____ true.
a. plaguing . . . entirely
b. ridiculing . . . practically
c. belying . . . exceptionally
d. afflicting . . . partially

7. Young and _____ animals are more prone to attacks of _____ diseases than are old and mature animals.
a. mature . . . invasive
b. immature . . . infectious
c. ill . . . benign
d. aged . . . genetic

8. In spite of exhibiting _____ and respect, the king, who was fast becoming intoxicated with success and corrupted by outside influences, gradually cooled in his _____ toward the philosopher Aristotle.
a. friendship . . . attachment
b. compunction . . . repentance
c. amity . . . detachment
d. bemusement . . . enmity

9. Objects to be _____ with the compound microscope are usually examined by transmitted light, and must be _____ enough to allow the light to pass through.
a. scrutinized . . . opaque
b. viewed . . . transcendent
c. studied . . . transparent
d. dissected . . . pellucid

10. They would overhear conversations and speculate on many things. Thinking they were doomed, they would return from their posts _____ and _____.
   a. dauntless . . . confounded
   b. languid . . . discouraged
   c. indefatigable . . . heartened
   d. phlegmatic . . . encouraged

Analogies

1. PARADE : STREET :: BARBECUE : _______
   a. kitchen
   b. matches
   c. patio
   d. grill

2. PIXEL : IMAGE :: FIBER : _______
   a. design
   b. rug
   c. thread
   d. lies

3. CHIROPRACTOR : ALIGNMENT :: NUTRITIONIST : _______
   a. diet
   b. doctors
   c. exercise
   d. fasting

4. ANGRY : INDIGNANT :: IMPERTINENT : _______
   a. indelible
   b. relevant
   c. officious
   d. irate

5. SPATULA : UTENSIL :: FUNGUS : _______
   a. mushroom
   b. botany
   c. spore
   d. organism

6. ABACUS : CALCULATOR :: CANDLE : _______
   a. lamp
   b. flame
   c. wick
   d. incinerator

7. GROUPER : FISH :: FLEA : _______
   a. beagle
   b. insect
   c. tick
   d. pesticide

8. JOYOUS : EXUBERANT :: ATTENTIVE : _______
   a. oblivious
   b. cognizant
   c. contemplative
   d. obsequious

9. DESPONDENT : HOPEFUL :: UNAPOLOGETIC : _______
   a. contrite
   b. despairing
   c. impenitent
   d. hopeless

10. ETNA : ITALY :: ST. HELENS : _______
   a. mountain
   b. Sicily
   c. United States
   d. Europe

11. ECOLOGY : BIOLOGY :: PERSONAL FINANCE : _______
   a. mathematics
   b. microeconomics
   c. market research
   d. retirement

12. POMEGRANATE : SEEDS :: BROCCOLI : _______

- **a.** vegetable
- **b.** florets
- **c.** stalk
- **d.** recipes

13. COMPOSURE : EQUANIMITY :: BELLIGERENCE : _______

- **a.** truculence
- **b.** peacefulness
- **c.** pugnacious
- **d.** patience

14. CROCODILE : HERPETOLOGY :: ORCA : _______

- **a.** ornithology
- **b.** hydrology
- **c.** dolphin
- **d.** cetology

15. NIGHTMARES : STRESS :: HEADACHES : _______

- **a.** migraine
- **b.** aspirin
- **c.** dehydration
- **d.** anatomy

Answers and Explanations

Sentence Completions

1. b. Clue words in this sentence are *alone* and *never*, indicating punishment can accomplish something toward ending crime, but cannot do it alone. Answer choice **a** is wrong because *languish* means to suffer neglect or hardship, which does not make sense here. Both **c** and **d** are wrong not only because of their meanings, but because they are not to be followed by the preposition *in*, which does appear in the sentence. One may *resolve* problems. However, it is incorrect to say one may *resolve in* problems. Similarly, one may *portend* disaster. However, it is incorrect to say one may *portend in* disaster. *Portend* means to give as an omen of, warning of, or to forecast, signify.

2. d. The clue here is *easily approached.* A person embodying answer choices **a**, **b**, or **c** would not be easily approached, as *pugnacious* is to be combative in nature; *sheepish* means meek or timid; and *imperious* signifies being arrogantly domineering. Therefore, the only logical choice is *affable*, meaning approachable, characterized by ease and friendliness.

3. a. The answer must describe a temperament that might cause one's cheeks to possess a deep color. The correct answer, choice **a**, *sanguine*, fits because sanguine means both relating to blood, as well as, in the context of disposition, having a ruddy complexion and temperament thought to be characteristic of a person having blood as the dominant bodily humor. None of the remaining answers works. This sentence completion is a straight vocabulary test: **b**, *plaintive*, means melancholy; **c**, *wistful*, means having a sad yearning; and **d**, *despairing*, is synonymous with hopeless. Thus, none of these types of temperaments would be apparent in the color of one's cheeks.

4. c. Because the sentence is about a person leaving behind *bare essentials and meagerness*, the answer will be an antonym for either *bare essentials* or *meagerness*, and be synonymous with the person's new finding of *luxury*. Answer choice **a** makes no sense, and **b** is a synonym for *meagerness*, which is incorrect. At first glance, **d** makes sense, as it is somewhat synonymous with *luxury*, but it is the wrong part of speech. *Extravagant*, an adjective, would have to be presented as a noun, *extravagance*, to be correct.

5. b. The words *same* and *subdued* are useful clues in this sentence. You are looking for a word that would describe a type of influence that would bring about *sleeping or dozing*, and *somnolent*, meaning sleepy or drowsy, is the correct choice. Choice **a**, *prosaic*, means factual or dull; **c**, *indolent*, can be defined as lazy; and **d**, *obtuse*, can mean stupid, or difficult to comprehend.

6. d. While the first word of answer choice **a** is a good fit, the second word is not. Pay attention to the sentence clues for the second word choice: *but* and *only*. Neither word in answer choice **b** fits logically. As for answer choice **c**, it is a stretch, but one could argue that the first word works. *Belie* means to misrepresent, contradict. However, the second word, *exceptionally*, makes no sense. Again, look at the word *only* preceding the second blank. This leaves answer choice **d** as the only appropriate and logical choice.

7. b. The clue in this sentence is *old and mature*, at the end of the sentence. Given *old* and *mature* are similar words to describe one category of animals, you are looking for a word that can be paired with *young* to describe a different category. *Young* is the opposite of *old*, so look for a word that is the opposite of *mature*. This knocks out answer choices **a** and **d**, because, even though the second words in both choices fit, the first words do not. Answer choice **c** is incorrect because *ill* is not an antonym for *mature*, and *benign* is illogical, given that one would not be *prone to attacks* of a *benign* nature.

8. **a.** The beginning of the sentence, *In spite of,* is a strong clue as to what word should fill the second blank. The phrase lets you know the king will be cooling in something positive, in a feeling that could tie in with *respect.* When approaching the sentence this way, choice **a** is the only clear choice in terms of the second word. You need to make sure the first word in choice **a** also is a good fit. When you read the whole sentence, it is likely you will plug in a word that would go well with *respect,* but not necessarily be a synonym. Here, *friendship* works well, so answer choice **a** is indeed a good fit. In answer choice **c**, *amity*, which means friendship, also works, though the second word choice, *detachment*, does not, thus eliminating choice **c**. Answer choices **b** and **d** test your vocabulary, though neither choices fit. In choice **b**, *compunction* can be defined as anxiety arising from a sense of guilt. In choice **d**, *bemusement* is bewilderment, confusion, and *enmity* is a feeling of hostility, or animosity.

9. **c.** The first word choice has to be an action enabled by a microscope. For this, answer choices **a**, **b**, and **c** all work. The second blank must contain a word that has to do with allowing light to pass through, as the end of the sentence indicates. This knocks out *transcendent*, in choice **b**, which makes no sense in the context, and *opaque* in choice **a**, which does not work, either, as *opaque* means blocking the passage of light. For the second blank, both answer choices **c** and **d** are appropriate, as *transparent* signifies capable of transmitting light, or clear. *Pellucid* is a synonym for transparent. However, the first word in choice **d** does not logically fit, leaving **c** as the correct answer.

10. **b.** Though the sentence blanks are separated by just one word, there is a very helpful clue: *Thinking they were doomed.* You also learn in the sentence that the people who were thinking they were doomed were also at work, as they were returning from their posts. Therefore, they could be tired. Certainly, the answer will contain words that a doomed person would likely feel. The first words of answer choices **b** and **d** make sense. In **b**, *languid* means weak and listless; and in **d**, *phlegmatic* means sluggish or apathetic. However, only answer choice **b** makes sense when it comes to the second word. The first word of answer choice **c**, *indefatigable*, is incorrect, as it signifies the opposite of what a doomed person would likely feel. *Indefatigable* means tireless. The second word in choice **c** also is illogical. In answer choice **a**, *dauntless* means tireless, which does not make sense given the context, even though the second word, *confounded*, meaning confused, could fit, though it is not the best choice. Moreover, given that *dauntless* is illogical, you can eliminate answer choice **a**.

Analogies

1. **c.** This analogy relates an activity to where the activity takes place. A parade takes place in the street as a barbecue takes place on a patio. While a barbecue conceivably, though dangerously, could take place in a *kitchen* **a**, a barbeque is more commonly and logically known to take place outdoors, outside a dwelling, like on a *patio* **c**, lawn, or deck. Answer choices **b**, *matches*, and **d**, *grill*, make no sense, though they are words associated with barbecues.

2. b. This is a part-to-whole analogy. Several pixels make up an image just as several fibers make up a rug. Remember to keep your relationship sentences simple. Answer choice **c**, *thread*, is incorrect because it is similar to a fiber, and the first two words, *pixel* and *image*, are not synonyms. Answer choice **a**, *design*, does not follow the logic of the first word pair, and **d** is there to throw off any test taker who misreads *fiber* as *fibber*.

3. a. This analogy concerns workers and their functions, in a sense. You could construct a sentence like: A chiropractor is concerned with/concentrates on a person's alignment. A nutritionist is concerned with/concentrates on a person's diet **a**. In this case, answer choices **b** and **d**, *doctors* and *fasting*, respectively, have no place in the word relationship. Answer choice **c** may have given you pause, as a *nutritionist* may be concerned with exercise, but a nutritionist is concerned with a person's diet first and foremost. Though not among these answer choices, a *trainer* would be a more appropriate choice to pair with *exercise*.

4. c. The word relationship in this analogy is based on synonyms. *Angry* is a synonym for *indignant* as *impertinent* is a synonym for *officious*. Answer choice **b**, *relevant*, is an antonym for *impertinent*, and answer choice **d**, *irate*, is a synonym for the words in the first word pair, but not for *impertinent*. Answer choice **a**, *indelible*, which means unforgettable or lasting, is out of place here.

5. d. This is an analogy where one word in the pair is a type of the second word. Here, a spatula is a type of utensil just as a fungus is type of organism. Answer choice **a**, *mushroom*, does not work because it is the second word of the pair. Given the first word pair relationship, *mushroom* would have to precede *fungus* for the analogy to work, as a mushroom is a type of fungus; a fungus is not a type of mushroom. Remember, you cannot flip the order of the second word pair in your relationship sentence. The sentence you devise for the given word pair must read in the same order as the second word pair. Answer choice **b**, *botany*, is illogical, and answer choice **c**, *spore*, does not work. Several spores make up a fungus, but this is not a part-to-whole analogy, or else the first word pair would have a sentence such as: *Several spatulas make up a utensil*, which is neither logical nor true.

6. a. The relationship in this analogy describes an object that came before, or was a precursor to, the second object for the same use. An abacus preceded the calculator to figure out calculations, whereas the candle preceded the lamp to give light. Answer choices **b** and **c**, *flame* and *wick*, are related to a candle, but are not precursors to a candle. One that burns to ashes is the meaning of **d**, *incinerator*, so answer choice **d** is incorrect because candles are generally used to give light, not burn something to ashes. Moreover, the candle is not considered a precursor to an incinerator.

7. b. A grouper is a type of fish just as a flea is a type of insect. While a flea may be found on the type of dog that is a *beagle* **a**, a flea is not a type of beagle. A *tick*, answer choice **c**, is a type of insect, as a flea is; and answer choice **d**, *pesticide*, is not logical. A pesticide may be used to exterminate a flea, but this analogy is not one of function or act.

8. **d.** This is an analogy where the relationship of the word pair is one of degree. In this case, the second word of the word pair has a higher level of intensity in meaning; that is, it takes the first word to a more extreme degree. It may be easier to construct a sentence starting with the second word of the given pair. *Exuberant* is being extremely *joyous*. So you are looking for a word that is similar to *attentive*, but means extremely so. Answer choice **d**, *obsequious*, means overly attentive to a fault, fawning, and is the only logical choice. Answer choice **a**, *oblivious*, is the opposite of attentive. Answer choice **b**, *cognizant*, is related to *attentive*, but not to a different degree. Answer choice **c**, *contemplative*, makes no sense. The constructed sentence could read: To be exuberant is to be extremely joyous while to be obsequious is to be extremely attentive.

9. **a.** This analogy contains antonyms. *Despondent* is the opposite of *hopeful*, whereas *unapologetic* is the opposite of *contrite*. Answer choice **b**, *despairing*, is a synonym for the first word of the given pair, *despondent*, but is not an antonym for *unapologetic*; and answer choice **c**, *impenitent*, is a synonym for *unapologetic*, not an antonym. Answer choice **d**, *hopeless*, is an antonym for *hopeful*, which is the second word of the first pair; it would have to mean the opposite of the first word of the second pair, *unapologetic*, to be correct.

10. **c.** Geography is the key to this analogy. Mount Etna is a volcano in Italy, whereas Mount St. Helens is a volcano in the United States. Answer choice **a**, *mountain*, is a related word to volcano, but has no bearing on the word relationship at hand, so is incorrect. *Sicily* (**b**) does not fit because *St. Helens* is not in *Sicily*, plus the analogy sets up a country as the second word, and *Sicily* is part of Italy, not a separate country. Answer choice **d** is incorrect because, again, *St. Helens* is in the United States, but also it is wrong because *Europe* is too broad a region for the analogy.

11. **b.** This word relationship involves subsets. *Ecology* is a subset, or branch, of *biology*, just as *personal finance* is a subset, or branch, of *microeconomics*. While one might rely on *mathematics* or *market research* (answer choices **a** and **c**, respectively) in personal finance, neither *mathematics* nor *market research* is considered a branch of personal finance, so **a** and **c** are incorrect. Answer choice **d** is wrong, as *retirement* has nothing to do with *personal finance* given the word relationship.

12. **b.** This is a part-to-whole analogy. One way to phrase the relationship here is: A pomegranate contains many seeds just as broccoli contains many florets. This relationship rules out answer choice **a**, *vegetable*, because while broccoli is a type of vegetable, broccoli does not contain vegetables. Answer choice **c**, *stalk*, also is incorrect because it is singular, not plural. Answer choice **d**, *recipes*, does not fit the word relationship, as broccoli cannot contain recipes.

13. a. This analogy is one of synonyms, and tests both vocabulary as well as parts of speech. *Composure* is similar to *equanimity*, just as *belligerence* is similar to *truculence*. Composure and equanimity signify even-temperedness, even under stress. Truculence and belligerence indicate a state of aggressiveness, ferociousness. Notice that all four words in this analogy are nouns, so while **c**, *pugnacious*, carries a meaning similar to belligerence, *pugnacious* is an adjective; it would have to appear in its noun form, *pugnacity*, to be the correct answer. Answer choice **d**, *patience*, though a noun, is not the opposite of belligerence, and answer choice **b**, *peacefulness*, could be an antonym for belligerence, not a synonym.

14. d. Knowing the *-ologies* will help in selecting the correct answer, but if you do not know the meanings of all the words ending in *-ology*, then try to figure out the rest of the word. The correct answer choice is **d**, because *cetology* is the study of whales, and an *orca* is a type of whale. This mirrors the relationship of the first word pair, as a *crocodile* is a type of reptile, and *herpetology* is the study of reptiles. If you did not know *cetology* is the study of whales but you know *-ology* is the study of some science, you might figure out Cetacea has to do with the order of marine mammals containing whales. If you were clueless about *cetology*, perhaps you were able to rule out a more common *-ology*: choice **a**, *ornithology*, which is the study of birds. Answer choice **b**, *hydrology*, is incorrect because it means the study of water (*hydr-*, *hydro-* is water), and while whales certainly live in the water, *hydrology* is not the study of whales in water. While a *dolphin* is also a mammal that lives in the water, the relationship to *orca* does not follow the relationship of the first word pair, so **c** is incorrect. Another way to interpret this analogy is: A crocodile is a type of reptile studied in herpetology, whereas an orca is a type of whale studied in cetology.

15. c. This analogy concentrates on possible symptoms. The relationship can be read as: Nightmares can be symptomatic of stress just as headaches can be symptomatic of dehydration. Answer choice **a**, *migraine*, is incorrect because *migraine* is a type of headache, not a symptom of one. Answer choice **b**, *aspirin*, does not work because aspirin can be a cure for headaches, not a possible symptom. *Anatomy* (**d**) has no relationship whatsoever to any of the given words. If you were unable to construct a sentence similar to the one in this explanation, then try building a bridge starting with the second word of the first word pair: Stress can lead to nightmares just as dehydration can lead to headaches. Remember, sometimes constructing the relationship sentence starting with the second word of the given pair can help to uncover the relationship.

CHAPTER

6 BIOLOGY

The Biology section of the PCAT contains 48 multiple-choice questions, covering general biology, microbiology, and human anatomy and physiology.

General Biology

Sixty percent of the questions (about 28 or 29 questions) on the biology section of the PCAT exam will be on general biology topics.

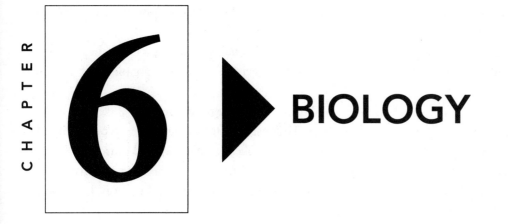

Unity and Diversity of Life

Biologists use the contrasting terms *unity* and *diversity* to describe life. *Unity* is used because all life forms, no matter how simple or complex, perform the same processes, have the same cellular mechanisms, and contain genetic material. *Biological diversity*, or *biodiversity*, in contrast, describes the vast variety of living organisms and the ecosystems different groups of organisms form.

Biological Organization

Biological organization has both internal and external components. Internally, organization begins at the chemical level where the least amount of energy is expended. Smaller organizational levels require less energy, while bigger, more complex organizational levels require more energy. Externally, organisms are organized according to how they interact with the environment. The hierarchy of organization runs from the least complex to the most complex, from the smallest energy requirement to the largest. As complexity increases, so does the energy needed to maintain the organizational level.

The following outlines biological organization from the lowest to the highest energy levels.

Chemical Organization

- **Subatomic particles:** The subatomic particles are protons, electrons, and neutrons.
- **Atoms:** There are 117 elements, which are the building blocks of all matter, both living and nonliving. The smallest indivisible unit of an element is the atom.
- **Molecules:** Atoms of the same or different elements form covalent chemical bonds to create molecules. Compounds contain at least two different elements. Therefore, all compounds are molecules, but molecules with only one type of atom are not compounds.

Cellular Organization

- **Organelle:** Molecules make up organelles, each of which has a specific task in the eukaryotic cell. All organelles must work in unison to keep the cell alive. Only eukaryotic cells have organelles.
- **Cell:** Life begins here. Each cell has all of the characteristics of a living organism.

Multicellular Organization

- **Tissues:** The four basic tissue types are epithelial, connective, nervous, and muscle.
- **Organs:** The tissues combine to form organs such as the heart, lungs, skin, liver, kidneys, and spleen.
- **Organ systems:** The organs combine to form the organ systems: integumentary, skeletal, muscular, cardiovascular, lymphatic, nervous, immune, respiratory, digestive, urinary, endocrine, reproductive, and the special senses.
- **Organism/species:** Breeding begins at this level. An organism is an individual of one particular type.

Ecological Organization

- **Population:** A population is a group of organisms. All organisms are of the same species.
- **Community:** A community is all of the organisms living in a particular area. Each group is one population. It consists of all of the populations of different species living in the same area.
- **Ecosystem:** An ecosystem includes the community of organisms living in a particular area, the nonliving environment (e.g., the air, water, sun, soil, and topography), and the interactions between the community and the nonliving environment.
- **Biosphere:** The biosphere is the entire planet Earth and all of its communities.

PROCESSES COMMON TO ALL LIFE FORMS

The following are processes common to all life forms:

Metabolism. Metabolism is the most important driving force behind life. It consists of catabolic reactions, which break down large macromolecules, releasing energy, and anabolic reactions, which build up complex molecules and require energy inputs.

Nutrient uptake. All life forms must have the ability to ingest nutrients so that catabolic reactions can take place. Carbon-hydrogen bonds are broken to release energy to the organism. The raw materials and energy, usually in the form of ATP (adenosine triphosphate) can then be used in anabolic reactions to synthesize the proteins needed for cell growth and differentiation.

Elimination. Waste products from metabolic reactions must be excreted through the surfaces of cells, as gases through pores or the stomata of plants, or in higher-level organisms through urination, defecation, and expiration. Plants also store waste products in the vacuoles of cells. These waste products are not excreted but remain in the vacuole until the cell dies.

Control mechanisms. All cellular metabolic processes require enzymes. Enzymes control the rates of reactions or *catalyze* reactions. Organisms must be able to regulate reactions so that they can control cell chemistry. Positive catalysts speed reactions, while negative catalysts, or *inhibitors*, slow reactions. These biological regulators can produce three possible outcomes. The reaction can be turned on, it can be turned off, or it can keep going. Since these processes operate to offset disrupting changes, they tend to keep things constant, are stabilizing, and attempt to maintain homeostasis. *Homeostasis* refers to the processes by which metabolic equilibrium is actively maintained.

Maintaining, initiating, or shutting down reactions is controlled by feedback mechanisms. The most common feedback mechanism is referred to as *negative feedback*. The final product often shuts down the reaction or diminishes the effect of the input. Negative feedback mechanisms operate based on a set point, and are often compared to a thermostat. The swing between the set point and the abnormal is very small. If the factor being regulated is still within a certain range of the set point, the response is to do nothing or maintain the reaction. If it is outside of this range, the response is to turn the reaction on. When the set point is reached, the reaction is shut down. In other words, between a turn-on point in the abnormal range and the set point, which is the turn-off point, the reaction is maintained. *Positive feedback* is when a variable is altered even more in the same direction. A chain of events is initiated to intensify the reaction, resulting in massive changes and sometimes explosive outcomes. This is why positive feedback mechanisms are much less common. The levels of the product of a reaction go way up, far out of a normal range, and then decrease commensurately. The classic example is the hormone oxytocin during childbirth. Contractions cause the release of oxytocin, which stimulates more contractions, which stimulates the release of more oxytocin, resulting in contractions that escalate in frequency and intensity. The cycle stops at delivery and the oxytocin levels return to normal.

Response to stimuli. All life forms must have some type of sensory device to perform data collection and some method by which that data is interpreted and appropriate responses are generated. Feedback mechanism systems also apply to responses to stimuli. Examples of stimuli that invoke a response include changes in the color, intensity, or direction of light; changes in temperature, pressure, and sound; and changes in the chemical composition of the surrounding soil, air, or water. Certain one-celled organisms retreat from bright light, cells in the retina respond to light, and plant stems grow toward the light. Plant roots grow toward a water source, and animals search out water in response to thirst. The Venus flytrap responds to touch by folding its leaves inward to capture insect prey. Animals search out food in response to hunger and flee predators in response to a threat.

(continued)

PROCESSES COMMON TO ALL LIFE FORMS (*continued*)

Reproduction. All life forms must have the ability to make more of themselves. There are two kinds of reproduction: asexual and sexual. The directions for reproduction come from the genes. A *gene* is a set of directions for how to make proteins. Genes are composed of *deoxyribonucleic acid* (*DNA*). *Chromosomes* are a conglomeration of genes, each of which contains the DNA directions. The order or sequence of four nitrogenous bases in DNA, adenine (A), guanine (G), cytosine (C), and thymine (T), establish the protein to be produced. In both forms of reproduction the DNA must be duplicated. At the cellular level, the DNA must be duplicated and passed on.

In asexual reproduction, first the DNA duplicates an exact copy, and then the cell splits in half. Every generation is the same as those before. In sexual reproduction, which occurs at the organism level, there must be sharing of genetic material between organisms. The DNA in the next generation is mixed. Therefore, specialized cells called *gametes* are required to house one-half of the genetic makeup for the next generation. The female gamete is the egg (ova), and the male gamete is the sperm. When the sperm penetrates the egg, fertilization occurs and a *zygote* is formed. The resulting organism is not a clone of its parent, but rather has half of its genes from the male parent and the other half from the female parent.

Adaptation. All organisms can trace their ancestry to one common ancestor. However, individual organisms within a group exhibit changes in the DNA. Natural genetic variations within a population of organisms may result in traits that benefit some individuals and disadvantage others. Beneficial DNA changes enhance survival and reproduction, whereas detrimental changes diminish the chances of survival and reproduction. This is the basis of the process of *natural selection* in which certain traits become more (or less) prevalent in a population. New novel proteins arise due to *mutations* in the DNA. The order of the four nitrogenous bases is changed in various ways so that different proteins are produced.

Sometimes mutations result in superior environmental adaptation. However, environments change over time. Thus, a trait that could be advantageous in a particular environment can become disadvantageous as the environment changes. Other times, mutations, such as cancer and sickle-cell anemia, result in traits that are immediately harmful to the organism. Mutated genes are passed down to future generations, resulting in a gradual change in the population over time. Natural selection is one of the important methods by which *evolution* occurs within a population of organisms.

Genetic recombination can also result in new and different proteins being produced that generate new traits. A DNA or RNA (ribonucleic acid) molecule is broken and joined to a different DNA or RNA molecule. Gene transfer between species, or *horizontal gene transfer*, which is now thought to be the foremost type of genetic transfer for single-celled organisms, is another way in which evolution occurs.

Systematics

The diversity of life can be demonstrated by the nearly two million species of organisms that have been documented to date. Each year, biologists identify approximately 15,000 additional species. To catalog this vast collection of diverse organisms and their evolutionary relationships, *systematic biology*, or *systematics*, is used. Systematics provides a framework by which organisms are named, described, collected, classified, and identified according to their evolutionary relationships and environmental adaptations. Evolutionary or phylogenic trees are used to show the relationships between organisms and the amount of evolution that has taken place. The *biogeography* or geographical distribution of populations of organisms is also documented.

Taxonomy

Taxonomy specifically deals with three of the metrics of systematics: naming, describing, and classifying organisms. Traditionally, organisms were grouped and classified based on similarities that arose along the evolutionary path. This was a constantly changing process as theoretical constructs were revised and data reinterpreted. Recently, bacteria have been identified and classifications have been updated according to DNA analysis. Paul Hebert, an evolutionary biologist at the University of Guelph, Ontario, and his colleagues have developed a method called *DNA bar-coding* to identify species based on a gene in the mitochondrial DNA. DNA found in the mitochondria, rather than the cell nucleus, is far more prone to mutations. Therefore, differentiating between closely related species is simplified.

Binomial Nomenclature

DNA bar-coding may eventually upend the system developed by Carolus Linnaeus in the mid-eighteenth century, which has endured with modifications to the present day. Linnaeus developed a hierarchical system based on the structural similarities among groups. The bottom of the hierarchy is the most specific, assigning a genus and a specific epithet to individual species. This system is referred to as *binomial nomenclature*, because it uses a two-part name. Latin words ensure that the name is universally recognized across language barriers. For example, the genus for maple trees is *Acer*. The red maple is therefore classified as *Acer rubrum*, and the silver maple as *Acer saccharinum*. Color is one of the descriptive specific epithets used to distinguish between species of the same genus. Shape or form, the discoverer's name, and the location of origin are other methods for assigning specific epithets. The genus is capitalized, the specific epithet is generally in lowercase, and both parts of the name are either italicized or underlined. Closely related species, such as all maple trees, are grouped in the same genus.

Taxonomic Categories

The next level in the hierarchy, family, includes genera that are closely related. For example, the pine family, Pinaceae, comprises ten commonly accepted genera, including: *Abies* (firs), *Cedrus* (cedars), *Larix* (larches), *Picea* (spruces), *Pinus* (pines), and *Tsuga* (hemlocks). Above the family category is the order. Orders include closely related families. Next are classes, which include related orders. Related orders are grouped into phyla. At the top of the hierarchy are kingdoms and domains. The term **taxon** refers to a structured grouping of organisms at any level in the hierarchy. For example, the phylum Magnoliophyta (flowering plants) is a taxon that includes the two classes Liliopsida (monocots) and Magnoliopsida (dicots).

The levels of taxonomic classification are as follows:

- domain
- kingdom
- phylum
- class
- order
- family
- genus
- specific epithet or specific name

Domains and Kingdoms

Beginning with Aristotle circa 350 B.C., two kingdoms were defined: Plantae and Animalia. The advent of microscopy changed this. First a third kingdom, Protista, was incorporated to accommodate bacteria and other microorganisms. Next, the distinction was made between Prokaryotes (before nucleus) and Eukaryotes (true nucleus), although no new kingdoms were added. Prokaryotes do not have a cell nucleus, nor do they have membrane-bound cell organelles. Eukaryotes have both a membrane-bound nucleus and membrane-bound organelles.

Next, a five-kingdom system was devised based on cell structure and methods of nutrient uptake. Specifically, fungi were removed from the kingdom Plantae and put into their own kingdom, and the prokaryotes were put into their own kingdom. Finally, RNA analysis revealed that there are two evolutionarily different groups of bacteria: eubacteria and archaebacteria. The most commonly used classification system today includes three domains with six embedded biological kingdoms.

DOMAIN	KINGDOMS			
Eubacteria	Eubacteria			
Archaea	Archaeabacteria			
Eukarya: four kingdoms	Protista	Fungi	Plantae	Animalia

Kingdom Characteristics

The various kingdoms each have their own characteristics, as follows:

Eubacteria

The Eubacteria kingdom contains small, simple, single-celled prokaryotes. They have peptidoglycan (a mucoprotein) in their cell walls. Most are decomposers, some are photosynthetic autotrophs, and some are parasitic and pathogenic.

Archaeabacteria

Members of the kingdom Archaeabacteria are also single-celled prokaryotes, but they can do more advanced protein synthesis. Many are bacteria that are able to live in extreme conditions such as extreme alkalinity (alkaliphiles) or acidity (acidophiles). There are halophiles, which live in high salinity; thermophiles, which live in high temperatures; and methanogens, which live in low-oxygen environments and produce methane gas as a by-product. One key structural difference is that those Archae that do have cell walls contain no peptidoglycan, unlike the Eubacteria. Most Archaebacteria have cell walls, but the genera *Thermoplasma* and *Ferroplasma* do not. Methanobacteria have pseudopeptidoglycan in their cell walls.

Protista

Members of the Eukarya domain in the Protista kingdom are single-celled or simple multicellular eukaryotic organisms. The Protista kingdom has traditionally been used to group what are known to be unrelated organisms that do not fit into the other kingdoms. There are three informal groups: protozoa, algae, and slime and water molds. Protozoa are typically motile and are known as the animal-like protists. Protozoa do not have a cell wall. Their outer surface is composed largely of proteins and is called a *pellicle.*

Algae are important producers and an important oxygen source in marine and freshwater ecosystems. Some green algae are multicellular autotrophs. Since they are photosynthetic, some classification systems put them in the kingdom Plantae. The cell walls of algae vary, though most have cellulose alone or in combination with other substances. The euglenoids lack a cell wall and have a proteinaceous pellicle like the protozoans. The cell walls of golden-brown algae and diatoms are composed of cellulose and pectic substances to form a type of hemicellulose. The diatoms have silica deposits in the hemicellulose, making their cell walls firm and resilient. The yellow-green algae have similar cell walls, with some species also containing silica deposits. Green algae have cell walls composed mostly of cellulose and some hemicellulose, and some green algae have calcium carbonate deposits. Red algae and brown algae have polysaccharides in addition to cellulose.

Slime and water molds do not have chitin in their cell walls. This is one of the defining characteristics of the Fungi kingdom, which is why the slime and water molds are included in the Protista kingdom instead. Water molds (Oomycetes) have cell walls composed of cellulose compounds and glycan. They also display DNA sequences that are far more similar to diatoms and golden and brown algae than they are to fungi. Slime molds are divided into two categories: cellular slime molds and plasmodial, or acellular, slime molds. Both have complex life cycles. During the feeding stage, plasmodial slime molds become a multinucleate mass of cytoplasm with no cell walls, called a plasmodium. During the feeding stage, cellular slime molds are individual cells with a cell wall.

Fungi

Members of the Eukarya domain in the Fungi kingdom are unicellular and multicellular heterotrophs. They are decomposers that accomplish nutrient uptake via absorption. They do not perform photosynthesis. Some are parasitic and pathogenic. Their cell walls are made of chitin. The Fungi kingdom includes yeasts, molds, and mushrooms.

Plantae

Members of the Eukarya domain in the Plantae kingdom are multicellular autotrophs. They are the photosynthetic green plants. Their cell walls are composed of cellulose. They have multicellular reproductive organs. Some classification systems put green algae in the plant kingdom, rather than in the kingdom Protista. One feature that sets plants apart from the multicellular photosynthetic green algae is that they produce a multicellular embryo inside an archegonium. Plants are the primary producers for all living organisms on land and an essential oxygen source for the atmosphere.

Animalia

Members of the Eukarya domain in the Animalia kingdom are multicellular heterotrophs. They ingest food and commonly exhibit tissue differentiation and complex organ systems. Most use muscle contractions to move. Their responses to stimuli are controlled by nervous tissue. They are consumers and can be herbivores, carnivores, omnivores, or detritus feeders.

Ecological Classifications

Ecological classifications are as follows:

Autotrophs

Autotrophs are self-feeders or producers. They are capable of synthesizing their own organic substances from inorganic compounds. Autotrophs produce their own sugars, lipids, and amino acids using carbon dioxide as a source of carbon, and ammonia or nitrates as a source of nitrogen. Plants, algae, and photosynthetic bacteria are producers because they can make their own food via photosynthesis. Chemosynthetic bacteria are also autotrophs and the primary producers in hydrothermal vent communities on ocean floors.

Heterotrophs

Heterotrophs are consumers, which must ingest food. They obtain their energy from carbohydrates and other organic material. All animals and most bacteria and fungi are heterotrophic, as are most protozoans.

Decomposers

Decomposers are bacteria and fungi, which begin digestion externally using enzymes. They then absorb the partially broken-down materials from dead plants and animals and the waste of other organisms. Decomposers are very important for any ecosystem, ensuring that the producers (for example, plants) get their essential nutrients and that dead matter and waste do not accumulate. They return nutrients to the soil by breaking down multicellular complexes.

Herbivores

Herbivores are animal consumers that eat only plants. They are the **primary consumers**. Herbivores can fully digest grains and plants that do not produce fruit.

Carnivores

Carnivores are animal consumers that eat only meat. They eat the primary consumers and thus are referred to as **secondary consumers**. Carnivores generally eat herbivores, but may also eat omnivores and rarely other carnivores. Carnivores that eat other carnivores are referred to as **tertiary consumers**.

Omnivores
Omnivores are animal consumers that eat either plants or other animals. Most omnivores eat both herbivores and other omnivores. Some are **scavengers**, which eat the entirety of dead animals and plants. Many omnivores also consume the eggs of other animals. Omnivores cannot digest some of the substances in grains and non-fruit-bearing plants, unlike herbivores.

Detritus Feeders (Detritivores)
Detritivores are animal consumers such as earthworms, shrimp, dung beetles, and blue crabs. They ingest dead or decaying organisms (mostly plants) and fecal material. Most detritivorous animals eat both the detritus and the communities of microorganisms that colonize and decompose the dead organic matter. Detrivores directly ingest dead and decomposing organic matter, whereas decomposers secrete enzymes to digest organic matter and then absorb the molecules.

Phylogeny
Phylogenetics is the science of phylogeny, the evolutionary path of a group of organisms from a common ancestor. It is one of the components of systematics, which includes classification and taxonomy. Systematics seeks to establish the phylogeny for a group of organisms. Phylogeny, therefore, is based on hypotheses, which are in turn based on the available data regarding the molecular, structural, developmental, and behavioral similarities between species. These similarities are used to group organisms into a chronological pattern that outlines the relationships among them.

Homologous Structures
Homology refers to the existence of the same structure in two or more species that originated in a common ancestor. They do not necessarily share the same function. For example, the forelimbs of all four-limbed vertebrates have a humerus, radius, ulna, carpals, metacarpals, and phalanges. However, humans use their forearms for picking up and holding objects and other prehensile tasks, while other vertebrates use the same bone structures for different types of locomotion. Birds and bats use the same bone structure to fly. Cats and dogs use the same structures to walk, run, and jump. Fish and whales use the same structures to swim. All amphibians, reptiles, birds, and mammals—the vertebrates know as tetrapods (four limbs)—evolved from an ancestor with a three-part limb. This structure, called the pentadactyl limb, consists of an upper limb with one bone, a lower limb with two bones, and a hand or foot with five digits. These **homologous** structures with a common evolutionary origin that evolved into different variations over time are an example of **divergent evolution**. The related species evolved in different ways, so they developed different traits for the same structure.

Homoplasy
A trait that appears to be homologous, but upon closer examination is revealed to have been independently acquired due to environmental factors rather than due to a common ancestor, displays homoplasy. If a biological trait or function is similar in two groups of organisms, but it was not inherited from a common ancestor, **convergent evolution** has occurred. The trait or function is an environmental adaptation that both species converged upon despite having different heredity. Thus it is an **analogous** trait, rather than homologous trait. One example is the development of eyes in squids and octopi (cephalopods) and in mammals. The evolution of cephalopods and mammals diverged around 500 million years ago when the evolution of the phylum Chordata split into the subphyla Vertebrata and Invertebrata, yet cephalopods and mammals both developed an advanced camera eye.

Conversely, if two species have a common ancestor and a common environment but are geographically separated and independently evolve analogous traits, **parallel evolution** has occurred. The classic example is the marsupial fauna of Australia and the placental mammals of Afro-Eurasia and the Americas. The two lineages are descendants of a common ancestor, which followed independent evolutionary pathways following the breakup of ancient land masses. Within these isolated populations some very similar body forms evolved. For example, morphologically (i.e., in form and structure), the pouched marsupial mouse of Australia and the harvest mouse of Europe and Asia are strikingly similar, as are the marsupial mole and the common mole.

HOMOPLASY			
TERMINOLOGY	TRAIT	ANCESTOR	ENVIRONMENT
homoplasy; convergent evolution	analogous	different; not closely related	similar
homoplasy; parallel evolution	analogous	same; closely related	similar; geographically separated

Plesiomorphic Characters

Systematists regard organisms with many homologous structures as closely related. The distinctions between homology and homoplasy, however, are not always easy to see. To begin creating taxonomic relationships, systematists look at the traits of the highest level of the hierarchy they are studying to determine which traits existed in the ancestral species that are still seen in all of the descendant groups. These traits are referred to as the *shared ancestral characters* or **plesiomorphic** characters.

Synapomorphic Characters

If two or more taxa share characteristics that are found in their most recent common ancestor, it is referred to as *shared derived characters*, or **synapomorphic** characters. Depending on how broad or narrow the taxon being looked at is, the same trait may be classified as plesiomorphic or synapomorphic. In a broad structured group, the trait may be derived, whereas in a narrower taxon it is an ancestral trait. The key is to find shared characters that can help to establish branch points in the taxonomic tree.

Molecular Systematics

Some species are so alike that their phenotypes (observable traits) are nearly indistinguishable. In these cases, molecular biology is used to compare the nucleotide sequences in the DNA and RNA and the amino acid sequences in the proteins. The more subunit sequences that correspond, the more closely related two species are. Furthermore, certain DNA nucleotide sequences can be examined for the number of differences, and the result may indicate the amount of time that has passed since two groups branched from a common ancestor. These stretches of DNA can therefore serve as a **molecular clock**. These molecular clock sequences exhibit a more or less consistent rate of change in the number of mutations that arise over a specific period of time. Thus, if we estimate that a gene that codes for a specific protein exhibits nitrogenous base changes at the rate of one per 50 million years, and two species are found to differ by four bases, then we can estimate that the species diverged from a common ancestor 200 million years ago.

Ribosomal RNA can likewise be used to construct or reconstruct evolutionary histories (phylogenies). It was differences in ribosomal RNA that led to the splitting of the prokaryotes into the two domains, Archaea and Eubacteria. Ribosomal RNA in the prokaryotes is found in three sizes: 5S, 16S, and 23S. The S refers to a sedimentation coefficient called the **Svedberg unit**. Heavier structures have higher sedimentation coefficients. The base pairs in the 5S and 16S sizes were analyzed to determine that the Archaea are actually more closely related to the Eukarya than they are to Eubacteria. Mitochondrial DNA sequences have been used to determine that dogs are more closely related to wolves than they are to jackals and coyotes. Whereas no more than 12 base differences were found between dogs and wolves, at least 20 were found between dogs and both coyotes and jackals.

Taxonomic Groupings

Systematists have devised three taxonomic groupings. A single organism and all of its descendants is called a **monophyletic taxon**. Monophyletic taxa are referred to as **natural groups** because they represent all close relatives in an evolutionary tree. They are also referred to as **clades**. A single organism and some, but not all, of its descendants are called a **paraphyletic taxon**. Both shared derived characters (synapomorphic characters) and shared ancestral characters (plesiomorphic characters) are used when a paraphyletic taxon is established. For example, the class Reptilia is a paraphyletic taxon because it does not include all of the descendants of the ancestral reptile Diapsida, which would include the class Aves (birds). The class Aves has been assigned to a class of equal ranking. Classic systematists consider the class Reptilia to stand on its own because the included organisms do not exhibit the derived characters found in birds, including feathers.

Unlike the other kingdoms, the kingdom Protista is not a monophyletic taxon. It has traditionally been used to group what are known to be unrelated organisms that do not fit into the other kingdoms. Systematists have recently made various attempts to group the paraphyletic protists into monophyletic taxa based on genetics, biochemistry, and ultrastructure. A grouping considered to be invalid by systematists because it includes no recent common ancestor for several evolutionary lines is called a **polyphyletic taxon**. Homoplasies that arose due to convergent evolution likely caused biologists to construct these taxa in the past, but true evolutionary relationships do not support their continued existence.

Cell Biology

This section reviews information with respect to cell biology that you should be familiar with for the PCAT exam.

Cell Theory

The cell theory states that all organisms are composed of at least one cell, that the cell is the smallest entity that exhibits all of the characteristics of living things, and that all cells came from a preexisting cell. That is, every cell had to have an ancestor, and every cell can perform all of the processes common to all life forms: metabolism, nutrient uptake, elimination, biochemical control mechanisms, response to stimuli, and genetic adaptation. The six components of the cell theory are:

1. All living organisms are composed of similar units of organization called cells.
2. The cell is the smallest structural and functional unit of all living organisms.
3. Some organisms are unicellular, while others are multicellular.
4. All cells arise from preexisting cells. Cells cannot spontaneously come into being. There is no spontaneous generation.
5. Cells contain hereditary information and can reproduce. The hereditary information is passed on during cell division.
6. In organisms of similar species, the cells have largely the same chemical composition.

The hole in the cell theory that might one day cause it to be revised is that we do not know how the first cell came into being. How did macromolecules assemble into cells? Furthermore, mitochondria and chloroplasts reproduce independently from the rest of the cell and contain their own genetic material. The endosymbiotic theory (discussed later) provides an explanation for the origin of these organelles.

Cell Size

Cells must remain small because as a cell becomes larger, the surface area-to-volume ratio decreases. Less and less surface is available to exchange the materials needed by and produced by the increasing internal volume. In other words, the available pathways to get nutrients from the outside and eliminate waste (toxins) from the cell do not increase enough to handle the increased volume of nutrients needed by and waste produced by the increased size of the cell. The result is that as a cell gets bigger there comes a time when its surface area is insufficient to meet the demands of the cell's volume and the cell stops growing.

Prokaryotic Cells

Prokaryotic cells are small and simple, with few structures. The only membrane, or phospholipid structure, is the cell membrane. They contain no internal membrane-bound organelles. They do not have a nucleus. Prokaryotic cells are members of the domains Eubacteria and Archaea. The disadvantage of having no membrane-bound organelles is that prokaryotic cells cannot compartmentalize. The cell and the genetic material must be able to coexist as a whole. No functions can be monitored or differentiated. This necessarily dictates that prokaryotic cells must remain small and simple.

STRUCTURES OF THE PROKARYOTIC CELL

- **Cell wall:** In the watery environments in which prokaryotic cells exist, a cell wall that is rigid in structure is crucial in order to give the cell shape and protect it from the watery environs. The cell wall is constructed with a mucoprotein called peptidoglycan. This combination of cross-linked peptides and glycogen is stiffened by the carbohydrate layers connected by amino acids.
- **Plasma membrane:** The cell membrane, or plasma membrane, is a semipermeable phospholipid bilayer. It allows free passage of certain materials and selects others for import or export. It performs many of the functions allocated to the organelles in eukaryotes.
- **Protoplasm:** The protoplasm comprises all of the internal parts of the cell—that is, everything surrounded by the plasma membrane. The watery part of the protoplasm is called the **cytosol**.
- **Nucleoid:** Prokaryotic cells have a single circular chromosome, or circular DNA molecule. It is not enclosed in a membrane. It contains the genes that code for the proteins needed by the cell. The survival of the cell depends on the existence of genetic material to instruct the cell how to build the proteins needed for life.
- **Ribosome:** The ribosomes are the site of protein synthesis. They are small complexes of RNA. Prokaryote ribosomes disassemble into two subunits with densities of 50S and 30S (Svedberg units). The two subunits fit together and work in unison to translate messenger RNA (mRNA) into a polypeptide chain to synthesize a protein. The smaller 30S subunit is composed of a 23S ribosomal RNA (rRNA) subunit, a 5S rRNA subunit, and 34 proteins. The larger 50S ribosomal subunit is composed of a 16S rRNA subunit and 21 proteins. The two subunits combine during protein synthesis to form a complete 70S ribosome. The Svedberg units for each ribosomal subunit cannot be added together to calculate the Svedberg unit for the ribosome because sedimentation rate does not scale linearly with the mass or volume of the particle.
- **Flagella:** The function of flagella is movement. Only some prokaryotes have flagella. They provide mobility to the cell. In order to accomplish this, the flagella must be flexible, or able to change its shape. The only macromolecule that can change shape is protein. The protein flagella are made of is called flagellin. The flagellin forms a hollow tube with a hook at the end. The N and C termini of the protein form the inside of the helical tube and allow it to polymerize into a filament. In contrast, eukaryotic cells have flagella constructed with microtubules assembled from dimmers of the globular protein tubulin.

Eukaryotic Cells

Eukaryotic cells are relatively large compared to prokaryotic cells. They are far more complex and contain membrane-bound organelles and a membrane-bound nucleus to house the genetic material. This design serves to concentrate molecules where they are needed, increasing cell efficiency markedly. Many cell processes can proceed simultaneously. Reactive compounds can be kept safely segregated away from other parts of the cell where they could inflict harm.

STRUCTURES OF THE EUKARYOTIC CELL

- **Cell wall:** A cell wall is found in members of the kingdoms Plantae and Fungi and some protists such as diatoms. The function of the cell wall is to provide rigidity, strength, support, and shape. It is generally rectangular and constant in shape. The cell walls of plants are made of cellulose. The cell walls of fungi are made of chitin.
- **Plasma membrane:** The eukaryotic cell membrane, or plasma membrane, is also a semipermeable phospholipid bilayer. Animal cells do not have a cell wall. Therefore, their outer boundary is the plasma membrane. This allows them to have flexibility of shape and ensures that no two are alike. Eukaryotic animal cells therefore do not display the uniformity of eukaryotic plant and fungi cells with their rigid cell walls. The cell membrane is embedded with proteins that perform most of the cell functions. Glycoproteins and glycolipids (proteins and lipids with short carbohydrate chains) are attached on the extracellular side of the membrane. The function of the plasma membrane is to allow molecules and ions to enter and leave the cell as necessary. Thus, the plasma membrane organizes the biochemistry of the cell. The embedded proteins perform transportation, communication, adhesion, and recognition functions.

  Channel proteins form pores for the facilitated transport of small molecules and ions across the cell membrane. The pores formed by channel proteins are often gated, or regulated. **Carrier proteins** transport attached molecules and ions via facilitated diffusion and active transport. **Recognition proteins** identify a particular cell type. They also function in self versus foreign identification. Most cell recognition proteins are glycoproteins. The carbohydrate chains are different in different species. Different types of cells in a single organism also have different carbohydrate chains. Glycolipids may also take part in cell recognition.

  Receptor proteins are the adhesion and communication proteins. They bind specific molecules such as hormones and cytokines. They act as the communication office for the cell, allowing it to interact with other cells. The specificity of receptor proteins allows the cell to respond to the outside environment in many different ways. When a molecule binds to the cell, it instigates a change inside the cell. This process is called **signal transduction**. Insulin receptors are one example of a receptor protein. The binding of insulin to a cell prompts the cell to send glucose transport proteins to the plasma membrane for export.
- **Protoplasm and cytoplasm:** Everything inside the cell membrane is classified as the protoplasm. The portion of the protoplasm outside the nucleus is the cytoplasm. The cytoplasm is a mixture of macromolecules, monosaccharide, polysaccharides, amino acids, proteins, lipids, ions, and water. The **cytosol** is the soluble portion of the cytoplasm. The protoplasm inside the nucleus is the **nucleoplasm**.
- **Nucleus:** The nucleus is notable for three main characteristics: DNA, a double membrane, and pores. The genes are stored on the chromosomes in the nucleus. The genes are organized into chromosomes to allow cell division to take place. The nucleus organizes the uncoiling of DNA to replicate key genes. It is also

responsible for transporting regulatory factors and gene products via the nuclear pores, and for the production of the messages (messenger ribonucleic acid or mRNA) that code for proteins. Finally, the nucleus is where the ribosomes are produced (in the nucleolus).

- **Nucleolus:** The nucleolus is a discrete, highly active DNA region of the nucleus. It is always active and densely stained. It is such a distinct area of the nucleus that it is sometimes called a suborganelle, though it is not surrounded by a membrane. Composed of protein and RNA, it is usually associated with a specific chromosomal site. It is involved in ribosomal RNA (rRNA) synthesis and the formation of ribosomes. The ribosomes then move out of the nucleus to positions on the rough endoplasmic reticulum (RER) to perform their work in protein synthesis.
- **Centriole:** Centrioles are cylindrical structures located near the nucleus in eukaryotic animal cells. Most plant and fungi cells do not contain centrioles. A centriole consists of a ring of nine evenly spaced bundles of three microtubules each. A few deviations display nine bundles of two or nine bundles of only one microtubule each. The microtubule bundles are arranged in a layout referred to as 9 + 0 because nine microtubule bundles are arranged in a circle and none in the center. Centrioles play a role in the formation of cilia and flagella. A pair of centrioles forms a **centrosome**. The centrosome is also referred to as the microtubule organizing center (MTOC). During animal cell division, the mitotic spindle forms between centrioles. They produce the microtubules that form the spindle fibers, which separate the chromosomes during cell division. During animal cell division, the centrosome divides and the centrioles replicate to create two new centrosomes, each with its own pair of centrioles. The two centrosomes move to opposite ends of the nucleus, and from each centrosome, microtubules grow into a spindle that is responsible for separating the replicated chromosomes into the two daughter cells.
- **Ribosome:** Ribosomes are composed of ribosomal RNA (rRNA) and protein and consist of two subunits that are joined together during translation. They are found both on the RER and free in the cytoplasm. Eukaryotic ribosomes are larger than prokaryotic ribosomes. The two subunits are 40S and 60S. The complete ribosome is 80S. The 60S subunit consists of a 5S rRNA, a 28S rRNA, a 5.8S rRNA, and approximately 49 proteins. The 40S subunit consists of an 18S rRNA and approximately 33 proteins. They are the site of protein synthesis. They receive and translate genetic instructions for the formation of specific proteins or polypeptides.
- **Endoplasmic reticulum:** The endoplasmic reticulum (ER) is a complex composed of parallel membranous tubules and flattened sacs surrounding the nucleus. It is a series of internal channels formed by invaginations of the cell membrane. It connects the nuclear membrane with the pores in the plasma membrane. This helps the cell to get more surface area for a better exchange rate. In other words, it puts the nucleus in greater contact with the cell environment. There are two kinds of ER: smooth and rough. The smooth ER (SER) provides a surface area for lipid synthesis, particularly phospholipids and steroids. It also metabolizes carbohydrates and steroids and controls calcium concentration. The SER makes a pathway for transporting molecules within the cell. Molecules are placed into transition vesicles (transfer molecules produced in the rough ER) and sent to the Golgi apparatus and other parts of the cell. The SER also provides a storage area for molecules synthesized by the cell. The rough ER (RER) is so named because ribosomes are attached to its outer surface. The RER produces and modifies newly formed proteins, manufactures new membrane, and performs roles in the transport of these proteins and membrane to other locations within the cell.

(continued)

- **Golgi complex:** The Golgi complex is composed of constituents called **cisternae**. Cisternae are flat disks. These flat disks are stacked in piles that range from three to 20 high. They are surrounded by a complex network of tubules and vesicles. The Golgi complex is the packaging center for storage, distribution, and excretion. Many Golgi apparati are found in kidney cells. They are responsible for sorting proteins and lipids received from the RER and the SER. They also modify certain proteins and glycoproteins and fold polypeptides to create proteins. These molecules are sorted and packaged into vacuoles and vesicles for storage, for transport to other parts of the cell, or for secretion.
- **Mitochondria:** The mitochondria are rod-shaped structures in the cytoplasm surrounded by two membranes. The exterior of the organelle is defined by the outer membrane. The inner membrane folds in on itself multiple times, providing a large surface area for chemical reactions. The folds are called **cristae**. Mitochondria have their own DNA and ribosomes and replicate to create new mitochondria. Mitochondria function during cellular respiration to produce adenosine triphosphate (ATP), the energy supply molecule for life processes. This is why they are often referred to as the powerhouses of the cell.
- **Vesicles and vacuoles:** Vesicles are single-phospholipid membrane-bound storage and transport containers. They are small and numerous in the cell. Due to their semipermeable membrane, vesicles can have an internal environment that differs from the exterior environment in the cytosol. They function to organize cellular substances to keep the cell environment safe. In addition to transport and storage, they are involved in metabolism and can function as enzyme storage compartments and as chemical reaction chambers. Vacuoles are a type of vesicle that contains mostly water. Vacuoles in plant cells are large, and there is only one or a few in a cell. For example, amoebas have a food vacuole that contains any food item that the amoeba has recently consumed. Plant cells have a central vacuole that contains water and substances such as amino acids, sugars, and other compounds that the plant needs. Some waste products are also stored in the central vacuole. In addition, because it is filled with water it provides turgor pressure to support the cell, providing it with rigidity and structure. The central vacuole is one of the reasons plant leaves stand upright. This push from turgor pressure is noticeably absent when a house plant is in need of water. The central vacuole also holds toxins that cannot be excreted. Water-soluble pigments that lend color to leaves, flowers, and fruit are also commonly stored in the central vacuole.
- **Lysosomes and peroxisomes:** Lysosomes are a type of membrane-bound vesicle. They are referred to as a suicide sac or destruction vacuole because they contain digestive enzymes to break down macromolecules. They are synthesized by the endoplasmic reticulum and the Golgi complex and can break down nucleic acids, proteins, and polysaccharides. They take in and break down older nonfunctioning or sick cells and organelles so that the products can be reused to make new organelles. Peroxisomes are also membrane-bound organelles. They also contain enzymes that catalyze a variety of metabolic reactions. Examples include the detoxification of harmful substances such as alcohol and hydrogen peroxide. In cellular respiration, the final acceptor in the electron transport chain is an oxygen atom. Oxygen readily accepts the electrons, which then combine with protons (H^+) to form water. Occasionally, oxygen reacts with other substances in the electron transport chain and only one electron is transferred, creating the reduced O_2^- called superoxide. This must be converted to hydrogen peroxide (by the enzyme superoxide dismutase) and then the H_2O_2 must be converted to water (by the enzyme catalase). Both O_2^- and H_2O_2 can react with DNA or proteins to disrupt cell functions and cause cell death.

- **Cytoskeleton:** The cytoskeleton is composed of microfilaments, intermediate filaments, and microtubules. Microfilaments are made of the protein **actin**. Their solid, rodlike construction provides cellular support. Their flexibility enables them to also perform tasks associated with movement of both the cell and the organelles, engulfing material in the extracellular environment (phagocytosis), and cell division. Intermediate filaments are composed of polypeptide chains. Their sturdy construction bolsters the cytoskeleton and supports cell shape. Microtubules are composed of the protein **tubulin**. They form hollow tubes which also provide structural support for the cell. They are also flexible and function in movement tasks such as cell and organelle movement and cell division. Centrioles, cilia, and flagella all contain microtubules. Eukaryotic animal cells, which do not have a rigid cell wall, require the support of the cytoskeleton to stabilize their shape. Cell movements, for example the crawling movement of white blood cells and amoebas or the contraction of muscle cells, depend on cytoskeletal filaments. In both mitosis and meiosis, the cytoskeleton organizes and controls the movement of the chromosomes during cell division. It also functions in the constriction of animal cells during cytokinesis.
- **Flagella and cilia:** Flagella in eukaryotes and cilia are both composed of tubulin, a globular protein. Tubulin dimmers are assembled into microtubes. The microtubules are arranged in what is referred to as a 9 + 2 layout in which nine microtubules are bundled in a circular arrangement with two in the middle. A basal body, which is constructed in the 9 + 0 layout of a centriole, anchors the flagella or cilia into a membrane. Flagella and cilia both serve movement functions. The tubules expand and contract, for example, to propel a euglena through the water or a sperm cell through the seminal fluid. Ciliated epithelia cells in the trachea use air currents to push out dirt, dust, and debris. Ciliated cells in the fallopian tubes pull the egg along to the uterus.
- **Chloroplasts:** Eukaryotic plant cells contain chloroplasts. They are enclosed in a double membrane just as mitochondria are. The *stroma* comprises the portion inside the inner membrane. The stroma is filled with fluid in between infoldings of the thylakoid membrane, which forms disklike sacs called *thylakoids*. The thylakoid membrane encloses the fluid-filled thylakoid interior space called the *thylakoid compartment* or *lumen*. The light-independent (dark) reactions of photosynthesis occur in the stroma where photosynthetic enzymes are stored. The stroma also contains a number of genes that contain the complete instructions for construction of the chloroplast, but not for all of its functions. The light-dependent reactions of photosynthesis take place on the thylakoid membrane, where chlorophyll and other photosynthetic pigments are stored. Sometimes the thylakoids form a stack called a **grana**. Between the inner membrane and the outer membrane is a section simply referred to as the intermembrane space. The outer membrane is permeable. The function of the chloroplasts is photosynthesis. The goal is to create glucose, the carbon-hydrogen bonds that cells need to function. This requires the pigment chlorophyll. The general reaction for photosynthesis is: Sunlight + CO_2 + $H_2O \rightarrow C_6H_{12}O_6$ + O_2. Although there are some photosynthetic bacteria, they do not have chloroplasts. Prokaryotes have no membrane-bound organelles. However, photosynthetic bacteria do have thylakoid membranes.

Similarities and Differences between Prokaryotic and Eukaryotic Cells

The following table highlights the similarities and differences between prokaryotic and eukaryotic cells.

PROKARYOTIC CELL VERSUS EUKARYOTIC CELL		
TRAIT	**PROKARYOTIC CELL**	**EUKARYOTIC CELL**
cell size	relatively smaller	relatively larger
plasma membrane	present; boundary with environment	present—boundary with environment
cytoplasm	present; fluid contents needed for chemical reactions	present—fluid contents needed for chemical reactions
DNA	present; genetic information in single circular DNA strand	present—genetic information in genes organized on chromosomes in the nucleus
ribosomes	present; workbench for protein assembly; relatively smaller; subunits with densities of 50S and 30S; complete 70S ribosome	present—workbench for protein assembly; relatively larger; subunits with densities 60S and 40S; complete 80S ribosome
membrane-bound organelles	none	present
nucleus	none; have nucleoid; 1 circular chromosome not enclosed in a membrane	present
cell wall	mostly present; key component is peptidoglycan; mycoplasma bacteria lack cell walls; most archaebacteria have cell walls; thermoplasma and ferroplasma do not; methanobacteria have pseudopeptidoglycan	present in plant and fungi cells; plants cellulose; fungi chitin; some protists have cell walls; some algae (euglenoids) have no cell wall; most algae have cell walls composed of cellulose alone or in combination with hemicellulose, silica, calcium carbonate, or polysaccharides; water molds have cell walls composed of cellulose compounds and glycan
flagella	sometimes present; made of flagellin (protein)	sometimes present: composed of microtubules made of tubulin (protein)
centrioles	none	present only in animal cells
chloroplasts	none	present only in plant cells
central vacuole	none	present only in plant cells

Similarities and Differences between Eukaryotic Plant Cells and Eukaryotic Animal Cells

The following table highlights the similarities and differences between eukaryotic plant cells and eukaryotic animal cells.

EUKARYOTIC PLANT CELL VERSUS EUKARYOTIC ANIMAL CELL		
TRAIT	**EUKARYOTIC PLANT CELL**	**EUKARYOTIC ANIMAL CELL**
cell wall	present	none
chloroplasts	present	none
central vacuole	present	none; both plant and animal cells contain vacuoles, but a central vacuole that dominates the cell is found only in plant cells.

Cell Junctions

In multicellular eukaryotes, cells are joined together in various ways depending on the function necessary for that cell type or location. One way that animal cells are joined is with a *spot desmosome* or *anchoring junction*. Spot desmosomes hold cells together and anchor the internal intermediate filaments. They are extensions of the cytoskeleton. Proteins go out to the membrane and congregate like a button to hold cells together. However, they are not leakproof. They are found in cells that need to stretch—for example, in the skin and bladder.

A second way that animal cells are joined is with a *tight* or *occluding junction*. Occluding junctions form bands around a cell where they are joined in localized spots to adjacent cells. The bands form a complex that increases in efficiency with each additional band. No chemicals can be transferred at these points—for example, the blood-brain barrier. None of the spaces are wide enough to allow passage. They form a leakproof barrier.

A third way that animal cells are joined is by *gap* or *communication junctions*. They form regions in the cell membrane where communication takes place. Cells on opposite sides of the junction deposit special proteins in the plasma membrane that form channels to transport both nutrient molecules and electrical currents between the connected cells. They allow for the rapid movement of both materials and messages between cells; for example, in cardiac cells they can be used to send signals for contraction.

Plant cells are joined together by *plasmodesmata*, which are similar to gap junctions. Plasmodesmata are delicate strands of cytoplasm that extend through the cell membrane and the cell wall to interconnect cells to form a transportation system. Plants need to rapidly move the glucose made in the leaves to the rest of the plant. They must also move water quickly. Osmosis would be much too slow. These extensions form the transportation system of the plant.

Endosymbiotic Theory

The endosymbiotic theory posits that prokaryotic microbes are the precursors of some eukaryotic organelles. Cells, possibly resembling amoebas, developed nuclei when a piece of the plasma membrane pinched off and enveloped the chromosomes. These primitive pre-eukaryotes then phagocytized, or engulfed, prokaryotic cells with which they formed symbiotic relationships. Engulfing aerobic bacteria similar to the *Rickettsia* led to the development of the mitochondria. Ingesting photosynthetic cyanobacteria led to the development of chloroplasts. Over numerous generations, the rudimentary chloroplast-like structure stopped developing a cell wall and discarded DNA that was not useful to the host cell.

Data that support the endosymbiotic theory include the fact that cells that develop without mitochondria and chloroplasts cannot manufacture them after the fact. Genes that encode for these two organelles do not contain a full set of instructions for all of the proteins from which they are constructed. They are similar in size to prokaryotic cells. These two organelles also contain a single circular gene with many similarities to the DNA molecule found in bacteria and few similarities to the genes in the cell nucleus. They can also produce their own proteins, and the methods they use to do so are similar to the ways in which bacterial cells produce proteins. In eukaryotic cells, the first amino acid in the transcript is methionine. In prokaryotic cells, the first amino acid is a modified methionine called fMet. Chloroplasts and mitochondria display fMet. Mitochondria and chloroplasts also have their own ribosomes that have 30S and 50S subunits like prokaryotes, not 40S and 60S like eukaryotes. *Giardia* and *Trichomonas*, early eukaryotic microbes, have a nuclear membrane, but do not have mitochondria.

Fluid-Mosaic Model

The construction of the plasma membrane is often referred to as the fluid-mosaic model. The membrane is mosaic-like because the framework of the phospholipid bilayer is mixed with integral membrane proteins that span the entire thickness of a lipid bilayer and it is also embedded with macromolecules of proteins, glycoproteins, and glycolipids. The membrane is fluid, allowing these protein, lipid, and phospholipid molecules to move laterally within its hydrophobic core. The way in which the phospholipid molecules combine to form the membrane creates a double layer that separates the aqueous cytoplasm from the aqueous extracellular fluid (ECF) surrounding the cell. The phosphate group is the polar, hydrophilic head facing on each side of the bilayer toward a watery mixture. The two fatty acids are the nonpolar, hydrophobic tails. The two nonpolar tails face one another together in bilayer. This hydrophobic core of the two nonpolar fatty acids acts as an electrical insulator allowing diffusion of small hydrophobic solutes across the membrane, but inhibiting the diffusion of charged and hydrophilic or water-soluble molecules.

Plasma Membrane Construction

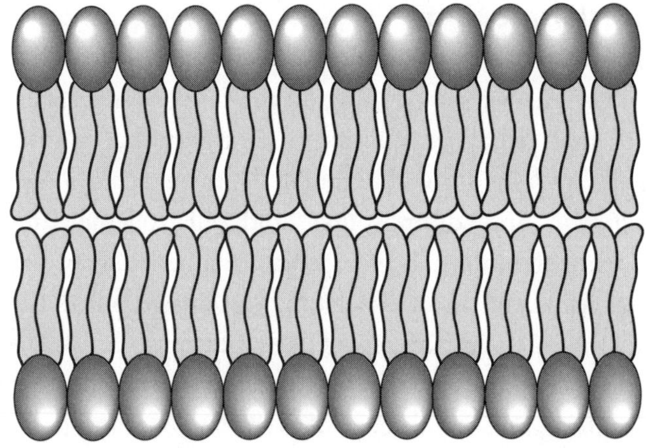

The various protein molecules within the hydrophobic membrane core create conduits for the entry and exit of both charged and hydrophilic molecules. By controlling the proteins that are produced, cells control membrane permeability and thus cell chemistry. The proteins are the key to the membrane's ability to be selectively permeable. The glycoproteins and glycolipids, which extend out to the exterior of the cell, are the marker antigens that determine cell uniqueness. They allow the cell to determine if an adjacent cell is the same or a foreign cell, thus providing recognition between cells. These proteins form the differences between membranes. Cholesterol, an additional component of the mosaic in animal cells, is added to stiffen the membrane and removed to make it more fluid.

Mixture Terminology

You should be familiar with the following mixture terminology:

- **Solution:** When two substances are mixed together, the substance of the greater amount is called the **solvent**. The substance that is mixed with the solvent is called the **solute**. Water is the most common solvent. Solutions with water as the solvent are called aqueous solutions. In a solution, the solute disappears. Even with a microscope, you cannot tell where the solute ends and the water begins. The solute molecules completely dissolve in the water so that you cannot see any solute particles. The two become one. The solution is **homogeneous** (the composition is uniform) and transparent, and no individual flecks can be seen.
- **Suspension:** In a suspension, the solute particles do not dissolve in the solvent. You can see solute particles. It is **heterogeneous** and opaque and you cannot see through it—for example, blood. In heterogeneous mixtures of two substances, there are two phases present (solid, liquid, or gas); thus the two substances are distinct and easily identified.
- **Colloid:** A colloid is halfway between a solution and a suspension. The solute is partially dissolved in the solvent. It is homogeneous and translucent. Light goes through, but you cannot see through it—for example, fog or smog. To force a colloid to become a suspension, you can use heat. The saying "The fog burned off" is in fact valid. It is forced into solution by the heating of the environment.

Movement of Molecules across the Plasma Membrane

The interior of the plasma membrane is a hydrophobic environment created by its phospholipid molecule construction. The head of each phospholipid molecule is a negatively charged hydrophilic phosphate group. The two tails are two highly hydrophobic hydrocarbon chains (two fatty acids).

Phospholipid

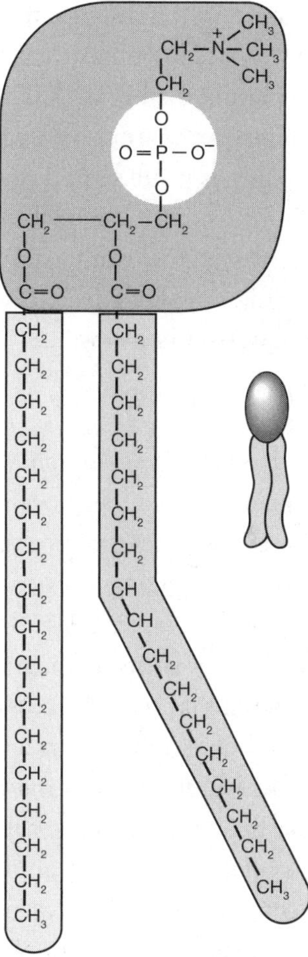

The two fatty acid tails of each phospholipid molecules point toward one another in the interior of the membrane, making it a hydrophobic environment. The negatively charged phosphate groups face out into the hydrophilic environments both intracellularly and extracellularly. Whether a molecule can diffuse through the plasma membrane, and the rate at which it can do so, depends on its ability to cross the hydrophobic interior. Therefore, nonpolar, hydrophobic molecules such as hydrocarbons, oxygen (O_2), and carbon dioxide (CO_2) can dissolve in the membrane and cross with ease. However, hydrophilic molecules such as ions and polar molecules cannot pass. Very small polar molecules that are not charged can pass through. Thus water (H_2O) is small enough to pass between the lipids in the interior of the membrane. Because most of the distance molecules would have to move across the membrane is nonpolar or hydrophobic, the plasma membrane's phospholipid bilayer is a natural barrier to most molecules important to living things such as proteins and sugars, as well as sodium, potassium, calcium, and chloride ions. Thus, after a cell goes through the trouble of making a sugar or protein, it will not just dissolve out of the cell into the surrounding water and be lost.

Diffusion

Diffusion is a type of *passive transport*, which means that the movement of molecules does not require an input of energy. Diffusion describes a gradual change in concentration with or along a concentration gradient. The concentration gradient describes the relative concentration of solutes within an area that can either include a membrane that must be crossed or not include such a membrane. When there are no intervening factors, solutes will move from the area of greater concentration to the area of lesser concentration. This movement of solutes from high concentration to low concentration continues until the area, or the two sides of a membrane, reach equilibrium. At equilibrium, molecular movement does not stop, but rather there is no more *net movement* of solute molecules. Across the plasma membrane, the molecules that enter and leave balance one another out. The cell has no control over the process of diffusion, although across the plasma membrane particles must be small enough to fit through pore openings in the phospholipid bilayer. Diffusion is dictated by the concentration gradient. The two most important molecules that move across the plasma membrane via diffusion are carbon dioxide (CO_2) and oxygen (O_2). Diffusion is how cells become oxygenated and how carbon dioxide is expelled.

Some of the factors that affect the rate of diffusion are:

- **Mass of the particles**: The heavier the particles, the slower the diffusion rate. For example, hydrogen gas diffuses more quickly than carbon dioxide gas.
- **Temperature**: The higher the temperature, the faster the diffusion rate.
- **Concentration gradient**: The greater the difference in the concentration gradient, the faster the diffusion rate. For example, solute will diffuse more rapidly across a semipermeable membrane when the gradient is two molar to one-tenth molar (2M:0.1M) rather than two-tenths molar to one-tenth molar (0.2M:0.1M).
- **State of the solute**: The gaseous state will diffuse faster than the liquid state, which will diffuse faster than the solid state.

Osmosis

Osmosis is another form of passive transport. It is the diffusion of water across a membrane. This means that there is a solution on each side of the membrane. To determine the net movement of water that will occur, tonicity is measured. *Tonicity* refers to the osmotic pressure of the two solutions on either side of the semipermeable membrane. Solutes in the solutions exert osmotic pressure when they cannot cross the membrane. Solutes that can freely cross via diffusion do not exert osmotic pressure on the membrane. Thus, osmosis occurs when there are solutes that are impermeable on either side of the membrane. Therefore, you must compare the strength of the two solutions. Which one has more impermeable solutes?

Water will always move to the hypertonic solution. *Hypertonic* refers to the more highly concentrated solution—that is, the solution with more solutes and less water. *Hypotonic* refers to the less concentrated solution—that is, the solution with less solutes and more water. Water will always move from where there is more water to where there is less water to establish equilibrium. *Isotonic* refers to the state in which there is an equal amount of solutes on each side of the membrane. At isotonicity, there will be no more net movement of water across the membrane.

When describing tonicity, it is important to understand that the terms describe relative concentrations. Thus, if there is a higher concentration of impermeable solutes outside a cell, the cell is described as being hypotonic to its environment. The cell has less solutes. Conversely, the environment is hypertonic to the cell. There are more impermeable solutes extracellularly. In cases in which the environment is hypertonic to the cell, dire consequences can occur. Water must leave the cell in order for equilibrium to be established on either side of the membrane. When water exits a eukaryotic animal cell, the cell shrinks, taking on a scallop-edged shape in a process called **crenation**. In eukaryotic plant cells, the plasma membrane separates from the inflexible cell wall but remains joined by the gap-junction-like plasmodesmata. Recall that the plasmodesmata form the transportation system for both glucose and water for the plant. This means that not only does the cell become distorted in shape, but the transportation channels are crimped and blocked as well. In a process called **plasmolysis**, the rigid cell wall remains intact, but the central vacuole significantly decreases in size as H_2O flows out of the cell and the cytoplasm collapses.

When the environment is hypotonic to the cell, the opposite occurs. Water enters the cell from the exterior where there are less solutes and more water. Remember, water moves to where there is less water, in this case, to the interior of the cell. Eukaryotic animal cells will swell up until they lyse or burst. This process is called **osmotic lysis** or **cytolysis**. Eukaryotic plant cells are protected from cytolysis by the rigid cell wall. They become turgid, or swollen and distended, but they do not lyse.

Facilitated Transport

Facilitated transport is a form of passive transport with the concentration gradient. No energy is required. Certain proteins in the cell membrane act as channels (channel proteins) or as transporters (carrier proteins), allowing specific ions or proteins to enter and leave the cell.

Facilitated transport follows the principles of natural diffusion. The solutes move from where there are more solutes to where there are less solutes. Whether the ions or proteins enter or exit depends primarily on the concentration of each solute on either side of the membrane, but also on the size of the channel. Channel proteins are responsible for rapid water transport. The channel and carrier proteins responsible for allowing water-soluble substances such as small polar molecules and ions to cross the phospholipid bilayer with no energy cost are also referred to as **passive transport proteins**.

Active Transport

In the pump systems of active transport, the opposite of natural diffusion occurs. Energy in the form of adenosine triphosphate (ATP) is required in order to transport molecules and ions against the concentration gradient. These substances must be moved from an area, either intracellularly or extracellularly, where there are less solutes to an area where there are more solutes. Carrier or transport proteins are needed. Interactions with ATP change the shape of these proteins so that specific ions, for example, Na^+, K^+, Ca^{+2}, and H^+, can be pumped across the membrane.

If uncharged solutes are small enough, they can move down their concentration gradients directly across the lipid bilayer by simple diffusion. Examples of such solutes are ethanol, carbon dioxide, and oxygen. Most solutes, however, can cross the membrane only if there is a membrane transport protein (a carrier protein or channel protein) to transfer them.

Passive transport, in the same direction as a concentration gradient, occurs spontaneously, whereas active transport against a concentration gradient requires an input of energy. Only carrier proteins can carry out active transport, but both carrier proteins and channel proteins can carry out passive transport.

Bulk Transport

The movement of large macromolecules or large quantities of material across the plasma membrane is accomplished by bulk transport methods. **Endocytosis** describes the ingestion of large amounts of materials. The cell and plasma membrane surround and engulf matter in the extracellular fluid (ECF) that surrounds the cell. Part of the cell membrane folds back on itself to create a pocket. The plasma membrane surrounding the desired items fuses to create a vesicle called an **endosome**.

Two special classifications of endocytosis are phagocytosis and pinocytosis. **Phagocytosis** is referred to as cell eating. It is when large particles such as bacterial cells are ingested. The endosome created from this process is given a special name due to its size: a **phagosome**. Not all cells perform phagocytosis. Amoebas are phagocytes, as are neutrophils and macrophages, which function in the immune response to foreign matter. Neutrophils and macrophages engulf bacteria. Phagosomes eventually fuse with lysosomes, which contain the enzymes needed to break down the bacteria and destroy them. **Pinocytosis** is referred to as cell drinking. This process occurs when liquid or small droplets of broken-down or dissolved matter are ingested. In contrast to phagocytosis, pinocytosis occurs in almost all cells and it is a continuous process rather than a specialized function that occurs on an as-needed basis. Small pinocytic vesicles also fuse with lysosomes for enzymatic digestion via hydrolysis. Pinocytosis allows cells to test the surrounding ECF to see what molecules and ions are there and to uptake those that the cell is lacking.

Exocytosis works in the opposite direction and serves several important functions. Vesicles from the cell interior move to the cell membrane, where they fuse with it. This replaces the lost plasma membrane used to create the endosome. Exocytic vesicles also expel the unneeded components from the ECF brought in by endosomes; other waste products, including toxins; and proteins, including enzymes. Exocytosis is also used to expel hormones, neurotransmitters, and antibodies via secretion into the ECF. Finally, when the endosome is created, some of the integral membrane proteins are turned inward. During exocytosis when the vesicle fuses with the plasma membrane, it turns inside out so that the integral membrane proteins are once more properly exposed to the extracellular fluid.

Exocytic vesicles are sometimes endosomes that return to the plasma membrane to empty their contents back out into the ECF. The Golgi apparatus and ER also manufacture and package exocytic vesicles for cell export. Endosomes are also pinched off and fused with lysosomes to create exocytic vesicles. Lysosomes themselves can be exocytic vesicles, carrying new pieces of membrane to patch holes in the plasma membrane. Secretory cells, such as exocrine cells in the pancreas, manufacture a lot of enzymes. These proteins must be released as needed for digestive processes to occur in other organs. They are amassed in secretory granules formed by the Golgi apparatus and transported to the cell membrane for expulsion.

Enzymes

An enzyme is a catalyst. Catalysts lower the energy needed for a reaction to commence, referred to as the energy of activation. The catalyst is not changed during the reaction and can be recycled over and over again to initiate many more reactions. Thus, catalysts are needed in only small amounts. Enzymes are a conduit. They provide a path through which reactions occur. Enzymes are proteins. Cellular chemistry can proceed at substantially lower temperatures and at substantially greater rates due to the actions of enzyme catalysts. Enzymes are reaction specific. Their names generally, though not always, end in *-ase* and indicate the type of reaction or the substance being acted upon. For example, the group of enzymes known as the proteases is responsible for breaking down proteins. The protease known as pepsin is manufactured in the stomach and catalyzes reactions that break down protein into peptides. *Pepsis* is the Greek word for digestion.

Enzymatic reactions can be catabolic (breaking down) or anabolic (building up). The substance that is acted upon is called the **substrate** (S). The location on the enzyme molecule (E) where a substrate binds is called the **active site**. The binding of a substrate to an enzyme forms an enzyme-substrate complex (ES). This reaction is reversible. When the substrate binds, the activation energy is lowered so that the reaction can proceed. The product (P) or products are then formed and the enzyme regenerated. The general enzymatic reaction equation is:

$$E + S \leftrightarrow \text{ES complex} \rightarrow E + P$$

Enzyme Structure

Each enzyme has a unique amino acid sequence that produces a distinctive three-dimensional structure. The active site can be thought of as a groove or opening in that tertiary structure. Some enzymes have multiple binding sites. The sites in addition to the active site are called the **allosteric** or **regulatory sites**. Allosteric sites provide a place where a molecule other than the substrate can bind. These molecules can be either activators or inhibitors. As long as the substrate has not bound to the active site, these molecules can change the shape of the enzyme so that enzymatic activity is either increased or decreased. If upon binding at the allosteric site, the shape of the enzyme is changed so that the substrate can no longer bind, the molecule is an inhibitor. If upon binding at the allosteric site, the shape of the enzyme is changed so that substrate binding can now occur, the molecule is an activator. After an allosteric activator binds, the active site becomes properly configured to accept the substrate.

EFFECT OF CELLULAR ENVIRONMENT ON ENZYMATIC ACTIVITY

The following describes the effect of the various elements of cellular environment, such as temperature, concentration, and pH, on enzymatic activity.

- **Temperature:** In general, as the temperature increases, chemical reactions speed up. Temperature increases cause the molecules to move faster (increases kinetic energy). This increases the probability that molecular collisions will occur. This is referred to as increasing the **effective collisions**. Within a narrow range (often 0 to 45°C), the rate of reaction is proportional to the temperature. A rough approximation is that each ten-degree increase in temperature doubles the rate of reaction. Just like organisms, each enzyme has an optimal temperature. For most living organisms, 37°C is optimal. Above the optimum temperature the carbon-hydrogen bonds are disrupted, which means that the tertiary structure of the enzyme is disrupted and the protein is **denatured**. Many proteins are denatured by temperatures above 40 to 50°C, but some are still active at 70 to 80°C, and a few can even withstand boiling. At very cold temperatures, molecular motion slows down. Since the substrate and enzyme molecules cannot find one and other, there are no reactions.
- **Concentration:** In general, as you increase either the concentration of the enzyme or the substrate, the chemical reaction speeds up. In both cases the molecular collisions have increased. More collisions

(continued)

EFFECT OF CELLULAR ENVIRONMENT ON ENZYMATIC ACTIVITY *(continued)*

increase the likelihood of enzyme and substrate interacting (effective collisions). When increasing enzyme concentration, there is eventually an optimum point beyond which there are more enzyme molecules available to bind to the substrate than there are substrate molecules, and the reaction rate can be increased no further. Once this saturation point is reached, the rate of the reaction cannot be increased further unless you increase the amount of substrate. When increasing the amount of substrate, the rate of reaction will increase but eventually level off because all of the active sites are filled. Substrates fit into the active site one at a time.

- **pH:** When pH increases, there are fewer hydrogen ions (H^+) in the solution, which can alter the charge on the functional groups of the amino acids. This change in the ionic interactions in the functional group can cause changes to the shape of the enzyme and the active site on the enzyme. When pH decreases, there are more hydrogen ions (H^+) in the solution, which can similarly change the functional groups, alter the shape of the enzyme and the active site, and hinder the active site from binding substrate molecules. Changes in pH can also cause conformational changes in protein and nucleic acid substrates so that they can no longer bind to the active site. Different enzymes have different optimum pHs. Some can endure very acidic or basic environments, for example, pepsin in the stomach (pH 0–1) and trypsin in the small intestine (pH 7–8).

Inhibitors

Inhibitors are molecules other than the substrate that interact with an enzyme to decrease the reaction rate. There are two categories of inhibitors: reversible and irreversible.

Most **irreversible inhibitors** bind covalently to the enzyme, permanently modifying it. They often have functional groups that are highly reactive with the amino acid side chains of enzymes. They usually act on a specific group of enzymes, but not on all enzymes or all proteins. This is in contrast to the nonspecific denaturing effects of high temperature, extremes of pH, and chemical denaturants that are irreversible but act on all enzymes by destroying both the secondary and tertiary structures. Irreversible inhibitors change the structure of the active site so that it can no longer bind with the substrate. This type of inhibition cannot be overcome by adding more substrate, because the active site has been covalently and irreversibly bound. Examples of irreversible inhibitors include many well-known heavy metal poisons, such as lead, mercury, copper, silver, and potassium cyanide.

Penicillin is an example of an irreversible inhibitor referred to as a suicide substrate. It irreversibly binds to the enzyme glycoprotein peptidase which is required for bacterial cell wall (peptidoglycan) synthesis.

There are four types of reversible inhibition.

1. **Competitive inhibitors** are look-alike molecules that compete with the substrate to bind to the enzyme's active site, thus blocking the active site. The enzymatic reaction equation is:

   $E + I_C \leftrightarrow E\, I_C$ complex

   The reaction is reversible, but no product can be formed. However, increasing the amount of substrate molecules can overcome a competitive inhibitor. If the substrate concentration is sufficiently increased, the reaction will proceed and form product at a reasonable rate because the substrate molecules can outcompete or displace the competitive inhibitor.

2. **Noncompetitive inhibitors** bind to an allosteric site, which changes the shape of the enzyme such that the shape of the active site changes and the substrate can no longer bind to it. Many noncompetitive inhibitors act by reacting with amino acid side chains in or near the active site to change its shape or block it. Some inhibitors act by reducing the disulfide bridges (-S-S-) that stabilize the structure of some enzymes. Since they do not compete with the substrate for the active site, increasing the substrate concentration cannot overcome noncompetitive inhibition.
3. **Pure noncompetitive inhibition** is a reversible reaction and binding of the inhibitor does not affect binding of the substrate. The inhibitor binds to both the enzyme and the enzyme-substrate (ES) complex. In fact, it binds to the ES complex just as well as it does to the allosteric site on the enzyme. The enzymatic reaction equations are therefore:

   $E + I_{NC} \leftrightarrow E\ I_{NC}$ complex

   $ES + I_{NC} \leftrightarrow ESI_{NC}$ complex

   Pure noncompetitive inhibition is extremely rare, however. More common is **mixed noncompetitive inhibition** in which the binding of the inhibitor affects the binding of the substrate. Either the binding site for the inhibitor is near the binding site for the substrate (the active site), or when the inhibitor binds, it causes a conformational change in the enzyme. Although the inhibitor can bind with both the enzyme and the enzyme-substrate complex, the binding affinities differ. The inhibitor may be more capable of binding to the enzyme or to the ES complex.
4. **Uncompetitive inhibition** describes the situation in which the inhibitor binds only to the enzyme-substrate complex at an allosteric site. The inhibitor does not compete with the substrate for the enzyme at all. Instead, it attaches to the ES complex.

Feedback inhibition acts on specific metabolic pathways in which several enzymes work together in a specific order. It is a series of linked reactions. Each unique enzyme in the path uses the product from the previous enzyme-catalyzed reaction as its substrate. The product is passed to the next enzyme. The final end product is the inhibitor for the first enzyme in the pathway. This regulates the amount of end product that the pathway can produce. The amount of the end product is regulated by its own concentration. This is a homeostatic device. The cell wants to go from substrate A to product D. This large a change would be dangerous for the cell to do in one step because the reaction would create far too much heat and the cell would explode. Instead, it performs the reaction in a stepwise fashion, and when there is enough D in the system, D reacts with the first enzyme as either a competitive or a noncompetitive inhibitor so that A and D compete for the first enzyme in the pathway. When product D is used up, the pathway is unplugged and begins anew.

Cofactors and Coenzymes

Cofactors are an additional component of some enzymes, which they require in order to become active. Cofactors are nonprotein components, often present at the active site, that make the enzyme take on the correct shape or configuration and assist with substrate binding. Inorganic cofactors include the metal ions, magnesium (Mg^{+2}), potassium (K^{+}), zinc (Zn^{+2}), and iron (Fe^{+2}). These inorganic minerals can be obtained in adequate amounts from the diet. Since only a tiny amount of each recyclable enzyme is needed, only small amounts of minerals are needed in the diet.

The inactive protein when no cofactor is present is referred to as an **apoenzyme**. When the cofactor is present and the protein has converted to an active enzyme, it is referred to as a **haloenzyme**. The enzyme-substrate complex cannot form unless the haloenzyme is present.

Coenzymes are organic cofactors. Coenzymes are relatively small molecules, many of which are derived from vitamins. They transfer a product from one reaction to another, thereby linking together two unrelated molecules. There are four types of coenzymes.

1. **Hydrogen carriers:** Hydrogen carriers form the link between oxidation-reduction (redox) reactions. They can deliver a proton to many different enzymes. One of the most important of these is **nicotinamide adenine dinucleotide** (**NAD^+**), which participates in glycolysis and the Krebs cycle in cellular respiration. NAD^+ is the oxidized form and NADH is the reduced form. Remember that oxidation is the loss of hydrogen or electrons, while reduction is the gain of hydrogen or electrons. If NAD^+ is the reactant, NADH is the product. In glycolysis, NAD^+ is reduced to form NADH and the energy is used to form a molecule of ATP from ADP and a phosphate group. This is called a coupled reaction. The two reactions occur at the same time and one reaction supplies the other with the energy it needs to proceed. NAD^+ also participates in photosynthesis.
2. **Flavin vitamins:** Flavin adenine dinucleotide (FAD) is reduced to $FADH_2$ in the Krebs cycle in cellular respiration. Like the reduction of NAD^+, the reduction of FAD supplies energy to form a molecule of ATP.
3. **Electron carriers:** The electron carriers are molecules that can accept electrons and then donate them on to another electron carrier molecule. One important example is the **cytochromes** (cytochrome oxidases), a protein (enzyme) containing heme that participates in oxidative phosphorylation in cellular respiration. Heme is a helping or **prosthetic group** that has an iron atom in the center of a ring compound that also contains another different element. Cytochromes transfer electrons to one another and other substances by alternating between an oxidation reaction and a reduction reaction. In the process the iron atom in the heme is transferred back and forth from the ferrous (Fe^{+2}) state to the ferric (Fe^{+3}) state. NADH and $FADH_2$ mentioned earlier are also examples of electron carriers.
4. **Coenzymes that carry small organic acids:** The key example is coenzyme A, which carries a necessary small organic acid in cellular respiration. It participates in the oxidation of pyruvate in the Krebs cycle.

Energy

Energy is the ability to perform work. It is measured in calories, which are a measurement of heat. Specifically, it is the amount of heat that must be added to one gram of water (H_2O) to elevate the temperature 1°C. Cells need a lot of energy, so heat is measured in kilocalories. What nutritionists refer to as a calorie is actually a kilocalorie. Adults need 1,600 kilocalories (calories) per day to maintain homeostasis.

There are two states of energy: kinetic and potential. **Kinetic energy** is energy in motion or work being done. **Potential energy** is stored energy. There are four basic forms of energy associated with cells: mechanical energy, electrical energy, light energy, and chemical energy. **Mechanical energy** is used for motion—for example, cytoplasmic streaming and muscle movements. **Electrical energy** is used when electrons change orbitals. The orbitals further out from the nucleus have more energy associated with them. **Light energy** from sunlight starts photosynthesis by activating electrons. At the end of photosynthesis light energy has been converted to **chemical energy** in the form of glucose. The glucose is used to produce other energy-rich molecules such as starch or sucrose. Glucose cannot be produced without sunlight; the ultimate energy source is the sun. Chemical energy is found in food—macromolecules with carbon-hydrogen bonds, where energy is stored in cells. Carbon-hydrogen bonds are potential energy and matter.

The first law of thermodynamics states that energy cannot be created or destroyed, just as matter can neither be created nor destroyed. Energy can only be rearranged or transferred. That is, it can only be converted between the four forms. The amount of energy created when the earth was formed is the same amount of energy present now and the same amount that will be here one million years from now. In other words, there is a finite amount of energy. Matter can be converted into energy, and energy can be converted into matter.

The second law of thermodynamics states that whenever an energy conversion is performed, not all of the energy is converted. Some is always lost as heat. Heat is thermal energy, but it is unusable energy in that it cannot be used to perform useful work. This means that the amount of usable energy is decreasing, which in turn means that in order for an organism to maintain its organization, a constant input of energy is required. Organization must be continually maintained because the natural tendency of any process is toward entropy. Entropy is the lowest level of energy needed or a measure of the degree of disorder or randomness in a system. Entropy always wins in the end. Organisms always die and eventually return to atoms and subatomic particles, the lowest energy states. Life is able to resist the flow toward maximum entropy (disorder, lowest energy) only because of the constant input of energy from the sun.

Biochemical reactions are described as either exergonic or endergonic. **Exergonic** reactions release energy. **Endergonic** reactions store energy. The two major categories of metabolic reaction are catabolism, which is an exergonic reaction, and anabolism, which is an endergonic reaction. Catabolism is based on the concept of oxidation, which is its driving force. Carbon-hydrogen bonds are broken and a hydrogen ion (H^+) is removed. Since carbon atoms require four bonds, carbons are also removed. When a carbon-hydrogen bond is broken, the molecule is made smaller. This is a degradative process that releases energy; thus it is exergonic. There is less energy in the products than there was in the reactant. Heat is released. The reaction has proceeded from a molecule with lots of potential energy to molecules with less potential energy. The main example is cellular respiration. For example, when you exercise, glucose is catabolized to generate ATP and heat is released.

Anabolism is the opposite reaction, reduction. Carbon-hydrogen bonds are built or synthesized. Larger molecules are built. Energy is stored in these larger molecules in an endergonic reaction. Low-energy molecules, for example CO_2 and H_2O, are converted to high-energy molecules, for example glucose ($C_6H_{12}O_6$). The main example is photosynthesis. Anabolic reactions such as photosynthesis require energy to be put into the system. In this case, light is inputted to initiate the energy conversion.

ATP

Adenosine triphosphate (**ATP**) is the molecule of cellular energy. It is a **nucleotide**, which are the units that comprise nucleic acids. Nucleotides are composed of three different constituents.

1. **Pentose:** A pentose is a five-carbon sugar. The pentose in ATP is **ribose**.
2. **Nucleobase:** A nitrogenous or nitrogen-containing base. The nitrogenous base in ATP is **adenine**. A nucleobase combines with a five-carbon sugar to create a **nucleoside**. For ATP the nucleoside that results when adenine is joined to ribose is **adenosine**.
3. **Phosphate groups** (one to three): A phosphate group (PO_4) is also referred to as inorganic phosphate and is notated with the symbol Pi. Phosphate is a salt or ester of phosphoric acid.

> The nucleoside adenosine can be joined to one phosphate group to form **adenosine monophosphate** (AMP), to two phosphate groups to form **adenosine diphosphate** (ADP), or to three phosphate groups to form **adenosine triphosphate (ATP)**.

ATP holds energy for the cell because it is held together by high-energy phosphate bonds. These are covalent bonds, but they are highly unstable; they are easily broken. The instability is caused by the oxygen molecules, which add negative polarity to the molecules.

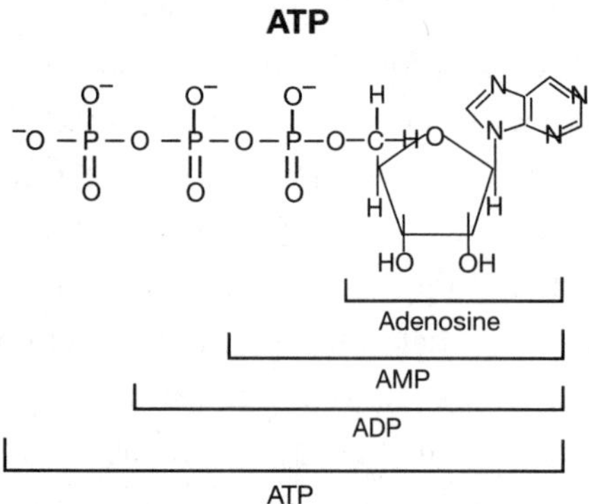

ATP is the energy-holding molecule, because this bond is so easily broken to release energy. At any given moment, there are only a few grams of ATP on hand in the human body. ATP cannot be made or stored by any organ. Each cell must make its own ATP, on demand, as needed to do the work of the cell. When a cell becomes more active, ATP production increases. When a cell becomes inactive, ATP production decreases. ATP cannot be circulated between body tissues or areas. The ability to produce ATP on demand is accomplished by the recycling of the components.

By contrast, energy is stored in carbon-hydrogen bonds, for example in glucose. When this bond is broken, a Pi is transferred onto ADP to make ATP. The C-H bond is broken with enough force to send the phosphate group to a protein—for example, one of the ATP synthase enzymes. This releases an ATP molecule. The ATP then attaches to the protein, causing it to change shape. The phosphate group then detaches because it no longer fits and a molecule of ADP is also released. Work has been done. ATP is potential energy, usable energy with the potential to do work. Kinetic energy is released when a phosphate group is released from ATP to form ADP. Work is being done. A phosphate group is pushed to a protein. ADP is found in muscles after exercise because work has been done.

Phosphorylation is the process by which potential energy is harnessed by an enzyme system to form ATP from ADP + Pi. There are two mechanisms of ATP generation—that is, two ways to add a phosphate group or perform phosphorylation. The first is **substrate-level phosphorylation.** This is the evolutionarily older method for generating ATP. It is less efficient and is performed by all cells in the watery cytosol where there is no membrane present. A phosphate group is directly transferred from a reactive intermediate organic molecule to ADP. This substrate is one of several substances produced as cellular respiration converts glucose to carbon dioxide (CO_2). The bond holding the phosphate group on the substrate is less stable than the new bond holding it to the ATP molecule. Only a very small percentage of ATP is generated by this method.

The second type of phosphorylation reaction is called **chemiosmosis,** and it is part of oxidative phosphorylation. It is the evolutionarily newer, more efficient, and more complex method for generating ATP. It depends on osmotic pressure, so a concentration gradient across a membrane is necessary. There must be a high concentration of solutes on one side of the membrane and a lower concentration on the other side to push on the membrane. Chemiosmosis results in a much higher yield of ATP than substrate-level phosphorylation. In prokaryotes, chemiosmosis occurs in the plasma membrane. In eukaryotes it occurs in the cristae of the mitochondria and in the thylakoid membrane in the chloroplasts of plants. In autotrophs it is driven by the movement of protons through ATP synthase embedded in the thylakoid membrane. The concentration of H^+ is higher in the thylakoid compartment (lumen) than in the stroma. In mitochondria the H^+ concentration is higher in the mitochondrial matrix than in the intermembrane space, so the H^+ moves out through ATP synthase located on the inner membrane to the intermembrane space.

The requirements for chemiosmosis are:

1. A **semipermeable membrane** to serve as the barrier for a hydrogen ion (H^+) concentration gradient.
2. **Two sets of proteins** to be phosphorylated. The first set of proteins spans the membrane. These are the **ATP synthase** complexes. And it is in the membrane that ADP + Pi $\rightarrow$ ATP. The second set of proteins is a series of molecules, one next to the other. These are the electron carriers, including the cytochromes, of the **electron transport system (ETS)**, also referred to as the **electron transport chain (ETC)**.
3. A **hydrogen source** to maintain the concentration gradient. As hydrogen ions leave the cell they must be replaced.

Incoming hydrogen is shredded, and broken down into a proton (H^+) and an electron (é). The electron enters the ETS where the electron carriers are located. When the first electron carrier is forced to accept an electron, it becomes unstable, entering an excited or high-energy state. Molecules are unhappy in an excited state. They strive for stability or the lowest-energy state. Thus, this electron carrier quickly passes the electron on to the next acceptor to return to stability. The second electron carrier in turn enters an excited state and quickly shuttles the electron on to the next acceptor. The initial electron has a lot of energy. When it is pushed to the first molecule, energy is lost. With each step along the chain there is less usable energy. The electron is passed like a hot potato from carrier to carrier. At each step, work is being done. This opens a portal to pump protons (H^+) against their concentration gradient, from the area of low concentration to the area of high concentration. As electrons are passed down the electron transport system, energy is lost; the low H^+ side gets lower and the high H^+ side gets higher, increasing the osmotic pressure. At the final electron acceptor, a molecule is created that is more stable with the extra electron. The electron is no longer a hot potato. The work is now done. The final electron acceptor is a variable. Now the system wants to return to equilibrium. The hydrogen ions want to go to the lower-concentration area. Facilitated transport takes over in the ATP synthase complex. A channel protein allows the H^+ ions to recross the membrane with the gradient. This is where large quantities of ATP are generated from the phosphorylation of ADP molecules.

Photosynthesis

Sunlight (light energy) provides the energy that drives the photosynthesis reaction. The major reactants are carbon dioxide (CO_2), an inorganic carbon source, and water (H_2O), a hydrogen source needed to create an organic carbon compound. The other necessary ingredient is chlorophyll, a photoreceptor. The major products are glucose ($C_6H_{12}O_6$), an organic carbon with chemical energy stored in the carbon-hydrogen bonds, and oxygen (O_2), the waste product of this reaction. Light energy is converted to chemical energy. The creation of glucose derivatives to store energy is the purpose. Plants convert glucose to sucrose or they store chemical energy as starch in amyloplasts or lipids in elaioplasts. There are three accomplishments of photosynthesis that are essential to life.

1. All stored usable energy is from photosynthesis. This underscores the importance of the sun.
2. Oxygen is needed for cellular respiration. Without O_2, ATP cannot be produced in sufficient quantities. Multicellular organisms need massive amounts of ATP, which they could not get

without oxygen. Without O_2, all organisms would have to remain small and unicellular.

3. Photosynthesis is the source of most of our fuels used for heat, transportation, cooking, and so on. Fossil fuels are dead organic matter.

Electromagnetic Spectrum

The electromagnetic spectrum from the least to the most energy (seven waves, from longest to shortest) is as follows:

1. **Radio waves**: These are the longest waves with the least energy.
2. **Microwaves** These are capable of piercing through fog and rain, which makes this portion of the spectrum ideal for transmitting cell phone signals.
3. **Infrared waves**: Infrared waves provide heat and energy and are detected by night-vision goggles to enable night vision.
4. **Visible light**: Photosynthesis must capture visible light. The acronym ROYGBIV is used to remember the order from longest wavelength (λ) to shortest. Visible light runs from approximately 400 nm to 750 nm. Many people with the ability to differentiate colors are unable to distinguish indigo from blue or violet. Indigo (I) may be dropped for this reason.
   400–450 nm = violet
   450–500 nm = blue
   500–570 nm = green
   570–590 nm = yellow
   590–610 nm = orange
   610–750 nm = red
5. **Ultraviolet (UV) light**: UV light can damage DNA and cause mutations, cancer, and death.
6. **X-rays**: X-rays can penetrate soft tissue but not dense tissue like bone. X-ray exposure requires shielding to avoid tissue damage.
7. **Gamma rays**: Gamma rays are used in atomic energy plants and for bombs. These are the shortest waves with the most energy.

Chloroplasts

Chloroplasts are disk-shaped structures ranging from 5 to 10 micrometers in length. Like mitochondria, chloroplasts are surrounded by an inner and an outer membrane. The stroma, a fluid-filled region inside the inner membrane, contains the enzymes for the light-independent reactions of photosynthesis. Infolding of this inner membrane forms the stacks of disks of the thylakoids, often arranged in stacks called grana. The thylakoid membrane encloses the fluid-filled thylakoid interior space, called the **thylakoid compartment** or **lumen**. The chlorophyll and other photosynthetic pigments as well as electron transport chains are on the thylakoid membrane. The light-dependent reactions of photosynthesis occur on the thylakoid membrane.

The outer membrane of the chloroplast encloses the **intermembrane space** between the inner and outer chloroplast membranes. The role of chlorophyll is to absorb light energy. Chloroplasts have photoreceptors, which capture light energy. **Chlorophyll *a*** is very green with a slight blue tint. This means that green wavelengths in the visible light spectrum are not useful for photosynthesis because they are not absorbed; they are reflected back out as the visible color. **Chlorophyll *b*** is also very green, but yellowish. It is an **accessory pigment** that will absorb whatever light chlorophyll *a* cannot to try to maximize light absorbance. It is a helper, but is not necessary. It makes light absorbance more efficient.

Other accessory pigments that help to maximize light absorbance efficiency are the **carotenoids**. The oranges of **carotene** are visible only in the fall when chlorophyll disintegrates. **Xanthophylls** reflect the yellow wavelengths of the visible spectrum. Indigo and violet light are too high-energy, and plants cannot absorb them. The best wavelengths for photosynthesis are red (610–750 nm) and blue (450–500 nm). Chlorophyll molecules plus proteins and other molecules form a complex of all of the pigmented molecules. These complexes absorb the energy from sunlight and are referred to as **photosystems**.

Photosystems work in the opposite direction from electron transport chains or systems. An electron starts with low energy and gains more as it travels through the photosystem. At the final acceptor molecule, the electron has a lot of energy. The absorbed light energy from the sun is converted to chemical energy. There are two photosystems:

1. **PSI (P_{700})**: Photosystem I was the first photosystem discovered. It is evolutionarily the oldest and the simplest. The light-dependent reactions begin in PSII, but P_{700} is named PSI because it was discovered first. The reaction-center chlorophylls are referred to as P_{700} because they have an absorption peak at a wavelength of 700 nm.
2. **PSII (P_{680})**: Photosystem II is the evolutionarily newer and more complex photosystem. Light energy is converted to electrical energy: The reaction-center chlorophylls are referred to as P_{680} because they have an absorption peak at a wavelength of 680 nm.

The role of pigments (photoreceptors) in a photosystem is to absorb **photons** (energy packets) to start the light-dependent reactions. The energy is transferred to a reaction center where an electron is excited. Excitation energy flows randomly from one pigment molecule to the next. With each transfer, energy is lost as heat, until just enough is left that it can be trapped by an acceptor molecule, such as chlorophyll *a*. Acceptor molecules, such as **chlorophyll *a***, do not pass the energy on, but rather give up an electron to start the process of ATP formation.

Light-Dependent Reactions

There are two photophosphorylation pathways, **noncyclic** and **cyclic**. The noncyclic pathway involves both photosystem I and photosystem II. It is the evolutionarily newer pathway and it must operate in order to drive the light-independent (dark) reactions. It occurs in the thylakoid membrane. The overall noncyclic reaction is:

$$\text{Light (Photons)} + H_2O + \text{ADP} + \text{Pi} + \text{NADP} \rightarrow O_2 + \text{ATP} + \text{NADPH}$$

The noncyclic pathway begins in a photosystem II complex when light strikes and the energy is captured. The reaction-center chlorophyll P_{680} absorbs a photon, an energy component that travels in waves λ (**lambda**: the symbol for wavelength) and is measured in nanometers (nm). The reaction center gives up two electrons, which are excited, to the primary electron acceptor protein in the electron transport system. Energy is released by passing through the ETS, and ATP is synthesized via chemiosmosis. At the end of the ETS, an electron must go to a molecule that will be stable when it accepts it. The energy input allows the deficit of electrons to be replenished by triggering the splitting of a molecule of water. **Photolysis** splits it into an oxygen atom (O), which is released into the atmosphere, and a hydrogen molecule (H_2). The hydrogen molecule is split into two protons (H^+) and two electrons.

As electrons travel through the photosystem II ETS, hydrogen ions (H^+) are pumped into the thylakoid compartment, also referred to as the thylakoid lumen. The electrons from photolysis replace those lost by photosystem II that are now passed into a photosystem I complex. Here photon energy provides a boost, allowing the electrons to enter and pass through a second ETS. The reaction-center chlorophyll (P_{700}) is activated, enabling it to accept the electrons from the final electron acceptor in the ETS in the photosystem II complex. The highly excited electrons are transferred to the primary acceptor protein, but this time are passed on to another substance (ferredoxin), and then to the $NADP^+$ reductase enzyme, which uses them to drive the reaction. The excited electrons enter the stroma and release energy by combining with hydrogen ions and attaching to **nicotinamide adenine dinucleotide phosphate ($NADP^+$)** to form NADPH, the reduced form of $NADP^+$. NADP is the final electron acceptor. It accepts two electrons and one proton (H^+) to become NADPH.

Photolysis has caused an accumulation of hydrogen ions (H^+) in the thylakoid compartment (lumen). These protons now flow with or down the concentration gradient via facilitated transport through an H^+ ion channel (channel protein) that has the enzyme ATP synthase complex. The ATP synthase is activated by the ion flow and catalyzes the formation of ATP from ADP + Pi. Since the photosystem II complex replaced its lost electrons from an external source (H_2O), these electrons are not returned to photosystem II as they would in the cyclic pathway. The H^+ ions produced by splitting the H_2O are consumed, leading to a net production of O_2, ATP, and NADPH from the reactants, solar photons and H_2O.

The cyclic photophosphorylation pathway is the evolutionarily older path that supplements the noncyclic pathway. It funnels excess light energy if the light-independent reactions cannot run. The electron flow begins in a photosystem I complex, which absorbs a photon. Excited electrons are passed to the primary acceptor in an ETS and then to ferredoxin. From there they are passed to two cytochromes, and then to another substance (plastocyanin) before returning to the reaction center chlorophyll (P_{700}). This transport chain generates enough energy to produce a concentration gradient and power a proton pump across the membrane, helping ATP synthase to produce ATP during chemiosmosis. Neither oxygen nor NADPH is produced in this pathway. The photons from captured sunlight and ADP + Pi are the reactants, and the product is ATP. Bacteria have only one photosystem, so cyclic phosphorylation must be used.

Light-Independent Reactions

The light-independent reactions occur in the stroma. The reactants are carbon dioxide (CO_2), NADPH, and ATP. The products are glucose, along with $NADP^+$ and ADP to feed back into the light-dependent reactions. The light-independent reactions are sometimes referred to as the dark reactions. This is somewhat misleading because only in crassulacean acid metabolism (CAM) plants does carbon fixation actually take place at night. The stroma receives the products of the light-dependent reactions and uses them to convert CO_2 and other compounds to glucose. There are three parts to the light-independent reactions. The three reactions are called the **Calvin cycle** (C3 cycle). First is carbon fixation in which CO_2 is added to an organic molecule. Second is the actual CO_2-to-glucose conversion, and third is regeneration of the beginning-point molecule so that when CO_2 enters again, the reactions can begin anew. There are three pathways to carbon fixation. C3 is the most common and occurs as the first step of the Calvin cycle in all plants. The other two pathways are C4 and CAM.

The three stages of the Calvin cycle, also referred to as the C3 cycle, are as follows:

1. **CO_2 fixation**: Gaseous carbon is converted to a solid, though unstable, six-carbon compound. CO_2 is taken in from the atmosphere through the plant's stoma and attaches to RuBP (Ribulose-1,5-bisphosphate), a five-carbon molecule. The enzyme RuBisCO (Ribulose-1,5-bisphosphate carboxylase oxygenase) catalyzes a reaction to form a very unstable six-carbon molecule, which spontaneously breaks down into two three-carbon molecules of PGA (3-phosphoglyceric acid).

   $$CO_2 + \text{RuBP} \xrightarrow{\text{RuBisCO enzyme}} 2\ \text{PGA}$$
   (a three-carbon molecule)

2. **CO_2 reduction**: The hydrogen ion source for carbon dioxide reduction is the NADPH from the light-dependent reactions. Since the reaction is proceeding from a high-energy molecule to a low-energy molecule, an input of ATP is necessary. Two-thirds of the ATP from the light-dependent reactions is used. First a high-energy Pi group is transferred from ATP to PGA, and then NADPH donates a proton (H^+). PGA is thus reduced to PGAL (3-phosphoglyceraldehyde), which is user-friendly for the cell, but it is not the ultimate goal; glucose is.

   $$2\ \text{PGA} + \text{ATP} + \text{NADPH} \rightarrow 2\ \text{PGAL} + \text{ADP} + \text{NADP}^+$$

3. **Regenerate RuBP**: The beginning point of the cycle must be regenerated so that when CO_2 enters again it can start over. Most of the newly formed PGAL is converted back to RuBP, which is fed back into the Calvin cycle. One out of every six PGAL molecules is used to make glucose.

   These are referred to as the light-independent reactions because sunlight is not directly necessary, but indirectly it is needed because the NADPH and ATP generated from the light-dependent reactions are used and sunlight is needed in order to produce them.

   The balanced Calvin cycle reactions are as follows:

   $$6\ CO_2 + 6\ \text{RuBP} + 12\ \text{ATP} + 12\ \text{NADPH} \rightarrow 12\ \text{PGA} \rightarrow 12\ \text{PGAL} + 12\ \text{ADP} + 12\ \text{NADP}^+$$
   $$10\ \text{PGAL} + 6\ \text{ATP} \rightarrow 6\ \text{RuBP} + 6\ \text{ADP}$$
   $$2\ \text{PGAL} \rightarrow 1\ \text{glucose phosphate}$$

   Overall, it takes six CO_2 molecules to produce one glucose molecule. It takes six iterations of the cycle to accomplish this.

   $$6CO_2 + 6\ \text{RuBP} + 12\ \text{NADPH} + 18\text{ATP} \rightarrow C_6H_{12}O_2 + 6\ \text{RuBP} + 18\ \text{ADP} + 12\ \text{NADP}^+$$

Photorespiration is the process by which oxygen is added to RuBP rather than to carbon. It is the second reaction catalyzed by RuBisCO. Photosynthesis first evolved at a time when the atmosphere had less O_2 than it does today. RuBisCO is an old enzyme that did not evolve because no mutations could improve upon it. Thus, it violates two of the general rules for enzymes: that they catalyze only one reaction and that they exist in small amounts. RuBisCO is in fact the most abundant protein on Earth, and photorespiration explains why this must be so. The general formula for the reaction is:

$$O_2 + \text{RuBP} \xrightarrow{\text{RuBisCO enzyme}} \text{Unusable carbon molecules}$$

The products are nothing that the plant can use. The amount of CO_2 in the atmosphere is 0.03%. The amount of O_2 in the atmosphere is 21%. If this were the only variable, probability would dictate, therefore, that there would be a far greater chance that photorespiration would occur than the Calvin cycle. However, RuBisCO does have a much higher affinity for CO_2 (about 80 times greater than for O_2). The chance of photorespiration occurring is around 25%. Even so, a plant must have a very large amount of RuBisCO in order to have enough to perform the carbon fixation reaction. This means that the plant's stomata must be open all the time in order to keep pushing in the CO_2 needed for photosynthesis. This is a problem for C3 plants because in the summer months they must shut their stomata to prevent water loss, so they cannot get enough CO_2 to produce glucose. Thus in the heat of summer C3 plants essentially shut down. They must survive on the stored carbon-hydrogen bonds and stop growing. If no photosynthesis is occurring, there can be no growth. Only photorespiration occurs.

C4 plants, also called Hatch-Slack plants, in contrast thrive in the heat even with their closed stomata because they have developed adaptations that minimize the losses to photorespiration. C4 plants include common summer weeds, as well as corn, sugarcane, and sorghum. Rather than the two three-carbon molecules produced in the Calvin cycle, C4 plants form a four-carbon molecule. This is the origin of the terminology. Plants that have only the Calvin cycle are the C3 plants.

The alternative carbon fixation reaction used by C4 plants begins in the mesophyll cells close to the leaf surface. After entering the stomata, CO_2 diffuses here because even though these cells are exposed to high levels of O_2 since they are close to the leaf surface, there is no RuBisCO in these cells so they cannot start either photorespiration or the light-independent reactions of the Calvin cycle. Instead the CO_2 is inserted into a three-carbon compound called phosphoenolpyruvic acid (PEP), forming the four-carbon compound oxaloacetic acid. A different enzyme, PEP carboxylase (PEPCO), is used. The general reaction is:

$$CO_2 + PEP \xrightarrow{\text{PEPCO enzyme}} \text{Oxaloacetate (four-carbon molecule)} \rightarrow \text{Pyruvate (three-carbon molecule)} + CO_2$$

The oxaloacetate is often converted to a different four-carbon molecule, malate (malic acid). Malate is then sent to a nearby bundle-sheath cell that encircles a vascular bundle in a plant leaf and stem. A decarboxylation reaction (removing CO_2) produces the pyruvate, which is returned to the mesophyll cells, and the CO_2, which enters the Calvin cycle. C4 plants thus perform carbon fixation (carboxylation) twice in contrast to C3 plants, which fix CO_2 only once (in the Calvin cycle). This process is less efficient. It takes much longer to make glucose. However, while C4 plants may be slow glucose producers, they finish the job, whereas the C3 plants must stagnate and stop growing in the summer. Then the C4 plants overtake them; for example, the weeds overtake the grass in the heat of August.

Crassulacean acid metabolism (CAM) plants are the succulents, such as cacti and the euphorbias. They are a variant of C4 plants. Since they must live in conditions of not only massive heat, but massive heat changes between day and night, and in conditions with very little H_2O, their stomata must be shut tight in the daylight. At night, the stomata must open wide not only to let the CO_2 in, but to release the built-up heat. The carbon-fixation molecule in CAM plants is a four-carbon malic acid, which lies in wait in the central vacuoles of the plant cells. When the sun comes out, CAM plants enter the light-independent (dark) reactions.

The key difference between C4 and CAM plants is that C4 plants perform carbon fixation and decarboxylation to feed the Calvin cycle in two different types of cells, whreas CAM plants perform carbon fixation at night and decarboxylation in the daytime. CAM plants intake CO_2 when they open their stomata at night. The CO_2 combines with PEP to yield the four-carbon oxaloacetic acid. Oxaloacetic acid is converted to malate, just as it is in most C4 plants. It is stored in the central vacuole of the plant cells. When the stomata close up in the morning, the stockpile of malate exits the central vacuole and decarboxylation takes place. The released CO_2 is taken up into the Calvin (C3) cycle.

Cellular Respiration

There are two types of cellular respiration, aerobic and anaerobic. **Aerobic respiration** requires oxygen and releases lots of energy (ATP). The generalized reaction for aerobic respiration is:

$$C_6H_{12}O_6 + 6O_2 \rightarrow 6CO_2 + 6H_2O$$

The function is to release the energy stored in carbohydrates and lipids during photosynthesis and make it available to living organisms. Glucose is oxidized (loses H^+), and oxygen is reduced (gains H^+). Aerobic respiration can be divided into four steps.

1. Glycolysis
2. A transition reaction that results in the formation of acetyl coenzyme A
3. Krebs cycle (citric acid cycle)
4. An ETS and chemiosmosis

Anaerobic respiration does not require oxygen, but it releases much less energy (ATP) per mole of starting material. Only certain prokaryotic bacteria are capable of anaerobic respiration. The generalized reaction for anaerobic respiration is:

$$\text{Glucose } (C_6H_{12}O_6) \rightarrow 2 \text{ Lactic acid } (C_3H_6O_3) + \text{Energy}$$

Glucose is oxidized, ADP is phosphorylated to produce ATP, and NAD^+ is reduced to produce NADH.

Some prokaryotes are able to carry out anaerobic respiration in which an inorganic molecule other than oxygen (O_2) is the final electron acceptor in an electron transport system. For example, some bacteria called sulfate reducers can transfer electrons to sulfate (SO_4^{2-}), reducing it to H_2S. Other bacteria, called nitrate reducers, can transfer electrons to nitrate (NO_3^-), reducing it to nitrite (NO_2^-). Other nitrate reducers can reduce nitrate even further to nitrous oxide (NO) or nitrogen gas (N_2).

Glycolysis

Glycolysis can be defined as sugar breaking. All cells can perform glycolysis in the cytosol, the soluble portion of the protoplasm in prokaryotic cells and of the cytoplasm in eukaryotic cells. It is a multistep metabolic pathway that involves the partial oxidation of glucose ($C_6H_{12}O_6$). No oxygen is required. The activation steps require the input of two ATP molecules.

$$C_6H_{12}O_6 + 2\ ATP \rightarrow 2\ PGAL$$
(3-phosphoglyceraldehyde)

This is an endergonic reaction. The oxidation steps are about energy capture. Energy is stored in PGAL, also called glyceraldehyde 3-phosphate (G3P). Next are the exergonic steps to release energy. A series of reactions results in two pyruvate molecules, a net gain of two ATP molecules and two NADH molecules. In short, PGAL $\rightarrow$ Pyruvate (pyruvic acid)

The complete reaction is:

$$C_6H_{12}O_6 + 2\ NAD^+ + 2\ ADP + 2\ Pi \rightarrow 2\ NADH + 2\ Pyruvate + 2\ ATP + 2\ H_2O + 2\ H^+$$

The products of glycolysis can be used in either anaerobic respiration or aerobic respiration. In anaerobic respiration, the next pathway is a series of reactions collectively called fermentation. In aerobic respiration, the products of glycolysis are sent to the citric acid or Krebs cycle.

Fermentation

Fermentation refers to the conversion of pyruvate to acetic acid, alcohol, or a number of other organic compounds. Carbon dioxide is often released. Usually, NADH reduces pyruvate and the NAD^+ thus created is recycled back to glycolysis. In simple fermentation, the metabolism of one molecule of glucose has a net yield of two molecules of ATP. Some of the glycolytic reactions are conserved in the Calvin cycle that functions inside the chloroplast. This is consistent with the fact that glycolysis is highly conserved in evolution. It is common to nearly all living organisms, most likely originating with the first prokaryotes 3.5 billion years ago or more.

Fermentation breaks down carbohydrates anaerobically. The final electron acceptor is an organic molecule. There is no electron transport system. Because glucose is only partially broken down, little energy is yielded. A net of two ATP molecules per glucose molecule is yielded by way of substrate-level phosphorylation. Recall that substrate-level phosphorylation refers to the direct transfer in a biochemical pathway of a high-energy phosphate group from an intermediate substrate to ADP. Fermentation involves only glycolysis. It is found in anaerobic and facultative anaerobic organisms. Facultative anaerobic organisms can grow with or without oxygen and can obtain energy from both aerobic respiration and fermentation, if no oxygen is available. Most bacteria are facultative anaerobes.

Glycolysis during fermentation, just as during aerobic respiration, is the partial breakdown of a six-carbon glucose molecule into two three-carbon molecules of pyruvate, two NADH, two H^+, and a net of two ATP as a result of substrate-level phosphorylation. This occurs in the cytoplasm of the cell. The overall reaction is the same.

$$C_6H_{12}O_6 + 2\ NAD^+ + 2\ ADP + 2\ Pi \rightarrow 2\ NADH + 2\ Pyruvate + 2\ ATP + 2\ H_2O + 2\ H^+$$

Many donated protons and electrons from glycolytic intermediary molecules cannot be converted to ATP because there is no electron transport system. Instead, the coenzyme NAD^+ is the final acceptor and is thus reduced to $NADH + H^+$.

The end products of fermentation are the result of reactions that do not produce any further ATP. The two pyruvic acids can yield a number of different organic molecules. For example, lactic acid (lactate) fermentation occurs in certain fungi, prokaryotes, and animal cells. The summary reaction is:

$$C_6H_{12}O_6 \rightarrow \text{Pyruvate} \rightarrow 2 \text{ Lactate} + \text{NAD} + 2 \text{ ATP}$$

The two pyruvic acids are broken down into lactic acid + NAD. Pyruvate is reduced and NADH is oxidized. Lactic acid fermentation also occurs in muscle cells, where an accumulation causes cramps. Some noncellular uses of lactic acid fermentation include the process of rigor mortis, which is the stiffening of the body due to a lack of ATP after death. It is a temporary condition because the body has been accumulating lactic acid through anaerobic respiration. This lowers the pH of the muscles and deteriorates the contraction of the muscles. Eventually, the body loses its rigidity due to the decay of the muscles. Yogurt, cheese, soy sauce, and sauerkraut are all lactic acid fermentation products.

The sewage treatment process includes both aerobic and anaerobic phases. In the aerobic phase, air is bubbled through the sewage to stimulate aerobic bacteria to break down organic material such as human wastes to acids and CO_2. In the anaerobic phase, anaerobic and facultative bacteria decompose the sludge to produce methane gas. Alcoholic fermentation is used to produce beer, wine, distilled spirits, and bread. In alcoholic fermentation, the two pyruvic acids are broken down into ethanol (C_2H_5OH) + CO_2 + NAD.

Important points to remember about fermentation are that it is a primitive anaerobic process possible in all organisms and cells. For some organisms, such as bacteria, it is the only way to produce ATP. For other organisms, it is used to create ATP when the O_2 level is low. In these cases, it is a short-term solution—for example, at the beginning and especially at the end of exercise when oxygen levels are not adequate for muscle contractions. Fermentation is much less efficient than aerobic respiration. Only two 2 ATP are produced. Only 2% of the energy in glucose is captured; the other 98% of the energy is released as heat or used to create organic products. The ATP is created in the first stages of fermentation, in glycolysis, which is always the first step. Aerobic respiration, in contrast, yields between two and 38 ATP molecules per glucose molecule, depending on the precise nature of the electron transport system.

The fermentation reactions continue after ATP production in order to regenerate and run the pathway. The inefficiency of fermentation necessitates a large supply of fuel. To perform the same work, a cell engaged in fermentation must consume up to 20 times more glucose or carbohydrate per second than a cell using aerobic respiration.

Transition Reaction

The transition reaction in aerobic respiration is also referred to as the oxidation of pyruvate. The two molecules of pyruvate from glycolysis enter the matrix of the mitochondria, where they are converted to two molecules of acetyl CoA, a two-carbon molecule. This oxidative decarboxylation reaction will continue as long as there is oxygen supplied to the mitochondria. If not, the pyruvate will be shuttled to the fermentation reactions. The enzyme that catalyzes the reaction is pyruvate dehydrogenase. Two NAD^+ molecules are reduced. Each gains two electrons to yield two NADH and two H^+ molecules. Pyruvate is catabolized in the process, resulting in the release of two molecules of CO_2. The other product of the breakdown, acetyl, instantly bonds with coenzyme A to form acetyl CoA. The acetyl CoA then enters the Krebs cycle. The complete reaction is:

$$2 \text{ Pyruvate} + 2 \text{ NAD}^+ + 2 \text{ Coenzyme A} \rightarrow 2 \text{ Acetyl CoA} + 2 \text{ NADH} + 2 \text{ H}^+ + 2 \text{ CO}_2$$

The Krebs Cycle

The Krebs or citric acid cycle occurs only when oxygen is present. Like the transition reaction, it occurs in the mitochondrial matrix in eukaryotes. In prokaryotes, however, it occurs in the cytoplasm. Acetyl CoA from the transition reaction is oxidized to CO_2 while at the same time reducing NAD^+ to NADH. NADH can then be used by the ETS to create further ATP as part of oxidative phosphorylation. To fully oxidize the equivalent of one glucose molecule, two acetyl CoA molecules must be metabolized by the Krebs cycle. The goal of the Krebs cycle is to completely oxidize the remnants of glucose ($C_6H_{12}O_6$). The final end products are two molecules of ATP, six of NADH, two of $FADH_2$, and four molecules of CO_2. Citrate (citric acid) is both the first and the last product of the cycle. It starts when the acetyl group is transferred to oxaloacetate (four-carbon molecule), creating citrate (six-carbon molecule). It ends when citrate is regenerated by the condensation of oxaloacetate (oxalic acid) and acetyl-CoA.

The sum of all reactions in the Krebs cycle is:

$$\text{Acetyl-CoA} + 3\ NAD^+ + FAD + GDP + Pi + 3\ H_2O \rightarrow \text{CoA-SH} + 3\ NADH + H^+ + FADH_2 + GTP + 2\ CO_2 + 3\ H^+$$

Two carbons are oxidized to CO_2, and the energy from these reactions is stored in GTP, NADH, and $FADH_2$. NADH and $FADH_2$ are coenzymes that store energy and are used in oxidative phosphorylation. GTP is the nucleotide guanosine-5′-triphosphate, which plays roles in the synthesis of RNA and in signal transduction, but here is an energy storage molecule that can be easily converted to ATP.

Electron Transport System

From glycolysis and the Krebs cycle, the high-energy molecules that are produced are four ATP, ten NADH, and two $FADH_2$. Most of the energy harvested from glucose is in the form of the reduced coenzymes (NADH and $FADH_2$). However, only ATP is readily usable to perform cellular work. The job of the electron transport system (ETS), therefore, is to oxidize NADH and $FADH_2$ to produce more ATP. Electrons are removed and shuttled through a series of electron acceptors. Energy is removed from the electrons with each transfer. This energy is used to make ATP. Each NADH yields three ATP. Each $FADH_2$ yields two ATP. Oxygen is the terminal electron acceptor.

$$\tfrac{1}{2}O_2 + 2\ H^+ + 2\ \acute{e} \rightarrow H_2O$$

The electron transport system is located in the inner mitochondrial membrane. A simple explanation for the generation of ATP is that it is the same mechanism as photosynthesis except in the opposite direction. Electrons attract protons (H^+) and pull them through the ETS to the outer compartment of the mitochondria. The hydrogen ions then diffuse back through the ATP synthase channels (channel proteins) producing ATP and H_2O. Thus the overall cellular respiration equation is:

$$C_6H_{12}O_6 + 6\ O_2 \rightarrow 6\ CO_2 + 6\ H_2O + 36 \text{ or } 38\ ATP$$

As electrons are passed through the ETS, high-energy electrons from the H^+ ions are shuttled from acceptor to acceptor in a series of exergonic redox reactions. Energy is released and used to drive the endergonic (energy is stored) synthesis of ATP. The reaction is called oxidative phosphorylation because ATP synthesis is coupled to the redox reactions in the ETS. ATP retains 40% of the energy from glucose; the remaining 60% is lost as heat. This is an exceptionally efficient system with no burnable products.

COMPARISON OF AEROBIC RESPIRATION, ANAEROBIC RESPIRATION, AND FERMENTATION	AEROBIC	ANAEROBIC	FERMENTATION
immediate fate of electrons in NADH	transferred to ETS	transferred to ETS	transferred to organic molecule
terminal electron acceptor in ETS	O_2	inorganic substances such as NO_3^- or SO_4^2	no ETS
reduced product formed	H_2O	relatively reduced inorganic substances	relatively reduced organic compounds (often alcohol or lactate)
mechanism of ATP synthesis	substrate-level phosphorylation and oxidative phosphorylation/ chemiosmosis	substrate-level phosphorylation and oxidative phosphorylation/ chemiosmosis	substrate-level phosphorylation only during glycolysis

Aerobic Respiration and Macromolecules

Aerobic respiration is used in both the catabolism and the anabolism of macromolecules. All reactions are reversible. They are catabolic when ATP is needed—in other words, when cells are doing work. When excess food enters, the reactions reverse to store energy for later use because it is not needed to perform work or no work is being done. Besides the energy production pathways, cells have numerous other metabolic pathways. They must synthesize building-block molecules such as amino acids, purines, pyrimidines, nucleotides, and lipids. There are also metabolic pathways involved in the production of macromolecules, such as DNA, RNA, and proteins. Still other pathways produce cellular structures, such as membranes, cell walls, flagella, pili, mitochondria, and chloroplasts. All of these anabolic pathways are fueled by the energy produced in catabolic ATP-producing pathways. Intermediate molecules in these pathways can either be oxidized to generate ATP or be used to synthesize macromolecule subunits.

Aerobic Respiration, Photosynthesis, Energy, and Matter

The interconnection between energy and matter as it applies to the processes of photosynthesis and aerobic respiration is unambiguous. To begin, the products of one are the reactants of the other. The general reactions:

Photosynthesis: Light energy + $6\ CO_2 + 6\ H_2O \rightarrow C_6H_{12}O_6 + 6\ O_2$

Aerobic respiration: $C_6H_{12}O_6 + 6\ O_2 \rightarrow 6\ CO_2 + 6\ H_2O$ + 36 or 38 ATP

Respiration loses energy in the form of heat. This energy is replaced by the sun in photosynthesis. In photosynthesis, light energy is converted to chemical energy. Carbon-hydrogen bonds are synthesized in glucose. In cellular respiration: chemical energy (C–H bonds) are converted to ATP (P–P bond).

Photosynthesis is the source for glucose production, the genesis of all food. The mass of all multicellular organisms, including humans, comes from food. Autotrophs make their own food. Heterotrophs and decomposers obtain food. Food is used to make ATP. ATP energy is used to make more cells, increasing the mass of organisms. Food will be converted to ATP (burned) only to do work. The excess is stored for later use. If it is never used, mass increases. In order to lose mass, one must exercise and eat less so that the stored food is used to make ATP. Muscle movement requires the ATP produced by cellular respiration. The mass in the respiration reaction is in the $C_6H_{12}O_6$ and CO_2. The H_2O is metabolic water used to replace sweat. ATP is used to power muscle movement. The by-product, heat, is wasted energy. The mass came from glucose, which came from CO_2. Mass is lost when $C_6H_{12}O_6$ is converted back to CO_2. The body has a metabolic pool or reservoir of molecules upon which enzymes can operate. To lose weight there must be more catabolic (breakdown) relationships. Carbohydrates must be catabolized to glucose, glycerol to PGAL, and fatty acids to acetyl groups, and proteins must be deaminated. The amino groups (NH_2) must be removed. All of this must be accomplished aerobically.

Molecular Biology

This section reviews concepts in molecular biology that you should be familiar with for the PCAT exam.

DNA

Deoxyribonucleic acid (DNA) is found in the cell nucleus. It contains the genetic instructions for how all cellular forms of life will develop and grow—specifically, for all of the proteins they will need to produce to form traits and carry on all biological functions. James D. Watson and Francis Crick figured out the structure of DNA based on the work of Rosalind Franklin. It is a long, double-stranded, helical molecule composed of building blocks called deoxyribonucleotides.

Recall that all nucleotides are composed of three parts: a pentose, a nucleobase, and between one and three phosphate groups. The ringed five-carbon sugar (pentose) in DNA is deoxyribose. Deoxyribonucleotides can have one of four nitrogenous bases: **adenine**, **guanine**, **cytosine**, or **thymine**. Adenine and guanine are classified as **purine** bases. Cytosine and thymine are classified as **pyrimidine** bases. One other important pyrimidine base is **uracil**, which replaces thymine in RNA. The purines are composed of two fused aromatic rings. The pyrimidines have only a single aromatic ring. Each nucleotide of DNA has one phosphate group.

The structure of the molecule is visualized following the rules of organic chemistry. Pentose rings are numbered in order going clockwise around the ring from the oxygen atom at the top.

Deoxyribose Ring Numbering

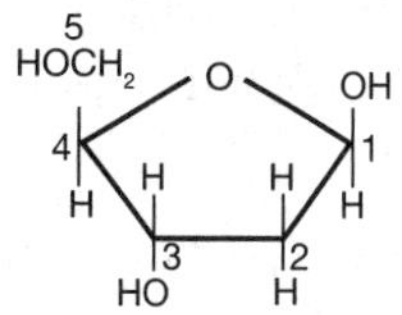

The fifth carbon is a substituent that attaches to the fourth carbon on the ring. They are referred to as the one prime (1′) through five prime (5′) carbons. The nucleobase attaches to the 1′ carbon, and the phosphate group attaches to the 5′ carbon. When DNA is synthesized and a new deoxyribonucleotide is joining the strand, its phosphate group covalently bonds to the 3′ carbon of a nucleotide already on the strand. DNA synthesis is an **addition polymerization** reaction in which monomers are joined together to form polymers (larger macromolecules). The enzyme that catalyzes the polymerization reaction is **DNA polymerase.**

The five prime and three prime carbons of the deoxyribose sugar are also used to describe the molecular structure of the DNA molecule. The 5′ end of the molecule always has a phosphate group attached to the 5′ carbon on its terminal deoxyribonucleotide. The 3′ end of the molecule always has a hydroxyl (OH) on the 3′ carbon of its terminal deoxyribonucleotide. The two strands of a DNA molecule point in opposite directions. One strand runs 5′ to 3′; the opposite DNA strand runs antiparallel, or 3′ to 5′.

DNA replication refers to the synthesis of two chains of deoxyribonucleotides. During DNA replication, the phosphate group at the 5′ end of the new nucleotide is joined to the hydroxyl (OH) group on the 3′ carbon of a nucleotide in the chain. A covalent bond called a **phosphodiester bond** is formed. The DNA molecular structure is often described as being like a ladder. The phosphate of one deoxyribonucleotide binds to the 3′ carbon of the deoxyribose of another to form the sugar-phosphate backbone of the DNA (the sides of the ladder). The rungs of the ladder are formed by complementary base pairs. The complementary base pairs are held together by hydrogen bonds. **Hydrogen bonds** form on molecules that have polar covalent bonds such that one atom carries a partial positive charge and one carries a partial negative charge.

When one charged part of the molecule forms an electrostatic interaction with an oppositely charged part of another molecule, these weak bonds can easily and rapidly form, break, and reform. However, in a molecule such as DNA, even though a hydrogen bond individually is far weaker than a covalent bond or an ionic bond, when there are millions of hydrogen bonds, molecular stability is significantly enhanced. These hydrogen bonds between the complementary base pairs are such a strong force that they keep the two DNA strands securely attached to one another. Additional hydrogen bonds exteriorly with water add further stability. Hydrogen bonds within molecules cause folding, pleating, and other structural changes that create three-dimensional molecular structures. The double-stranded helical shape of DNA is due to the hydrogen bonds between the base pairs. Complementary base pairing refers to the fact that nucleotides with the base adenine hydrogen-bond only with nucleotides with the base thymine (A-T), and nucleotides with the base guanine can form a hydrogen bond only with nucleotides having the base cytosine (G-C).

DNA Replication

The six steps in DNA replication are as follows:

1. The double helix uncoils. These are the two parent strands. The enzyme that catalyzes this reaction is **DNA helicase**. DNA helicase catalyzes the reaction that breaks the hydrogen bonds between the complementary base pairs in the two antiparallel strands. Two Y-shaped **replication forks** form.
2. To ensure that the two strands do not rejoin, **helix destabilizing proteins** bind to the uncoiled strands of the replication fork.
3. Free-floating deoxyribonucleotides hydrogen-bond with the exposed nucleotides on each unwound parent DNA strand. The two new strands are synthesized by complementary base pairing. Replication begins at the **origin of replication**, a specific sequence of bases on the replication fork.
4. **Topoisomerase** enzymes catalyze a reaction that causes gaps in the DNA to alleviate strain on the helical structure while replication is occurring. The same enzyme creates a break and then joins it back as needed.
5. The separated strands continue to unwind in different directions around the DNA molecule.
6. **DNA polymerase** enzymes join the incoming nucleotides to the new strand via phosphodiester bonds. The phosphodiester bonds form between the 5′ phosphate group on the new nucleotide and the 3′ OH group on a nucleotide in the DNA strand. These are actually **deoxynucleoside triphosphates**. The structure consists of the deoxyribose sugar, a nitrogenous base, and three phosphate groups. As the covalent bonds are formed, two of the phosphate groups are removed and their energy is used to fuel the reaction.

In the end, each parent strand serves as a template to synthesize a complementary copy of itself. This results in the formation of two identical DNA molecules.

However, phosphodiester bonds can join the phosphate group only at the 5′ carbon of a new nucleotide to the hydroxyl (OH) group of the 3′ carbon on a nucleotide on the strand. The parent strand, referred to as the **leading strand**, runs in the 3′ to 5′ direction. New nucleotides can directly bond with the leading 3′ end and continue down the strand. The antiparallel strand that runs in the 5′ to 3′ direction is referred to as the **lagging strand**. New nucleotides must join the lagging strand in short sections of around 100 to 1,000 nucleotides each as the DNA unwinds. These sections are referred to as **Okazaki fragments**.

As established, new phosphodiester bonds can only be formed on the hydroxyl group on the 3' carbon of a nucleotide on an established DNA strand. However, DNA polymerase cannot start the synthesis of the new strand unaided. It requires a short ribonucleic acid (RNA) segment referred to as a **primer**. The RNA primer must have complementary bases to the single unwound strands of DNA. The enzyme **primase**, an RNA polymerase, catalyzes the reaction that synthesizes the primer. On one of the unwound single DNA strands, primase adds in complementary RNA nucleotides.

DNA polymerase III then elongates the primer using DNA nucleotides. A primer is needed for both the leading strand and each Okazaki fragment of the lagging strand. Primase is able to join RNA nucleotides without an existing nucleic acid strand, while DNA polymerase is not. **DNA polymerase II** removes the RNA segments and replaces them with the correct DNA nucleotides. **DNA ligase** is the enzyme responsible for ligating the DNA fragments back together.

As complex as this process is, it is accomplished in an incredibly fast time frame. DNA can be synthesized at the rate of 1,000 nucleotides per second, resulting in an exact copy of the molecule in around ten minutes.

Cell Division

In single-celled organisms, the function of cell division is reproduction to create offspring that are identical to the parent cell. In multicellular organisms, by contrast, the function of cell division is growth, the repair and replacement of damaged cells, and the production of gametes via meiosis. All body (somatic) cells contain identical DNA. Single-celled organisms need to pump molecules in and out through the cell wall in order to keep up their metabolism. This exchange gets less efficient as a cell expands, because its volume increases far faster than its surface area. Multicellular organisms can skirt this physical constraint by keeping their individual cells small but gluing them together into big bodies. However, pathways must be kept open to ensure that the individual cells are bathed in the necessary fluids. Single-celled organisms must be generalists that are capable of finding food, defending themselves against parasites and predators, withstanding sudden swings in environment, and creating new copies of themselves. By contrast, multicellular organisms can transform some cells into various types (**differentiation**) to carry out such different tasks as detecting light, digesting proteins, or forming a skeleton. Through evolution, each type of cell, whether it is a nerve cell conducting electrical impulses or a mammary gland cell producing breast milk, can become exquisitely specialized for its job.

Recall that prokaryotic cells do not have a true nucleus. Instead their genetic material is contained in the nucleoid, a single circular molecule of double-stranded, helical, supercoiled DNA. This chromosome is very long in comparison to the length of the organism. Thus, there needs to be a mechanism for allowing this much genetic material to fit within the prokaryotic cell. To make the genetic material more compact, proteins resembling histones are bound to the DNA molecule. This divides the DNA molecule into about 50 chromosomal domains. The molecule is further condensed by supercoiling so that each domain coils around itself. The enzyme **DNA gyrase** catalyzes this reaction. The result is a compacted, supercoiled mass of DNA.

In order for cell division to take place, this supercoiled DNA mass must be unwound, replicated and rewound. The general steps and enzymes outlined for DNA replication in the previous section must all occur. DNA gyrase and DNA topoisomerases play roles in unwinding, duplicating, and rewinding the supercoils. The circle must be cut and rejoined by a topoisomerase.

Unlike eukaryotic cells, prokaryotic cells do not undergo either mitosis or meiosis. These are **haploid** cells. They have only one chromosome. The cytoplasm functions in DNA separation. The process of cell division occurs after replication, recoiling, and DNA separation are complete. Each new DNA circular chromosome is pulled to a pole by the cytoplasm. The cell is pulled and elongates. Finally the cell splits into two complete new cells. This process is called **binary fission**.

Eukaryotic cells have a lot more genetic material. The DNA is enclosed in the nucleus, inside the nuclear membrane, where it is organized into linear chromosomes. These linear chromosomes microscopically resemble rod-shaped, threadlike structures. The chromosomes combine the DNA, with its negative charge from the phosphate groups, with histones, a protein with a positive charge. This forms beadlike structures referred to as **nucleosomes**. The nucleosomes are the repeating unit of the chromatin. They are a packaging unit with the DNA wrapped around the histones. Most of the nitrogenous base pairs are wrapped around the histone core. The rest join to the next nucleosome. This DNA segment of around 60 base pairs is referred to as **linker DNA**.

The linker DNA is also combined with histones, which join adjacent nucleotides to form the **nucleosome thread**. The nucleosome thread becomes a large coiled loop that is fastened together by proteins referred to as **scaffolding proteins**. The coiled loops are compressed during mitosis and can be observed microscopically as condensed chromatin. The **chromatin** refers to all of the DNA and proteins that comprise the DNA. Examination of the chromatin reveals the general structure of the chromosome, but does not reveal the unique properties of individual chromosomes.

The eukaryotic cell nucleus divides by mitosis. In animals, these are **diploid** cells. In plants they can be diploid or haploid depending on the generation. Most protists are haploid. Through mitosis a parent cell produces two identical daughter cells. Either a diploid cell becomes two diploid cells or a haploid cell becomes two haploid cells. Diploid cells have two copies of each chromosome, one from the mother and one from the father. At the end of mitosis there are two genetically identical diploid cells created. Thus a copy must be made of each chromosome.

Chromosome duplication takes place in interphase, the part of the cell cycle before mitosis begins. Interphase is the preparation phase for mitosis. Once there are two identical DNA strands, they are referred to as **sister chromatids**. The sister chromatids are attached in the center at a spot called the **centromere**. The centromeres function in the accurate division of the sister chromatids. The centromere must split so that the sister chromatids can be pulled to opposite poles of the cell. In eukaryotic animal cells, organelles near the nucleus called the **centrioles** form a pair called a **centrosome**, or microtubule organizing center (MTOC). The centrosome synthesizes the microtubules, which become the spindle fibers that attach to areas on the centromere. The centrosome divides, replicates, and each new centrosome moves to opposite sides of the nucleus. Microtubules then grow from the centrosome into the spindle that attaches to the centromere.

Most eukaryotic cells have several areas within the centromere where aggregates of spindle fibers form a structure called a **kinetochore**. The kinetochore is composed of numerous different proteins intertwined with chromatin. The kinetochore captures the spindle fibers to pull the sister chromatids apart at an aggregate that is called the **kinetochore spindle fibers**. Nonattached spindle fibers called **polar spindle fibers** develop across the span of the cell from pole to pole. These polar spindle fibers never attach to the kinetochore; instead, they lengthen, interlock at the equator of the mitotic spindle, slide past one another, and push the poles apart.

At the end of interphase, after chromosome duplication has produced the sister chromatids and centrosome replication has produced two new centrosomes, both the nucleolus and the nuclear membrane disintegrate. At this point the kinetochores develop, the centrosomes begin to move to opposite sides of the cell, and the spindle fibers begin to assemble. The chromosomes line up along the diameter of the now nucleus-free cell. Microtubules attached to the sister chromatids move to opposite ends of the cell, contract, and pull the sister chromatids apart. Once separated, the sister chromatids are referred to as **sister chromosomes**. The cell is now in its elongation phase before cell division. The sister chromosomes continue to be pulled to opposite ends of the cell. New nuclear membranes form around each set of sister chromosomes. **Cytokinesis** is simultaneously proceeding. In eukaryotic plant cells, a new cell wall begins to develop between the two sets of sister chromosomes in their new nuclear envelopes. In eukaryotic animal cells, the cell begins to compress inward in the center where the cell diameter previously existed to separate the two new nuclei. It soon splits in two to create the two identical daughter cells, which each have a perfect copy of the original chromosomes.

Cell Cycle

The cell cycle is the sequence of events that occur in a eukaryotic cell from one cell division to the next. It consists of interphase, mitosis, and usually cell division.

The three phases of the cell cycle are:

1. **G_0 phase**: The G_0 phase is the segment of the cell cycle in which cells exist in a **quiescent** or resting state. G_0 is the no-growth state. Proper nutrition or other growth factors are in short demand, and the cell cycle apparatus is disassembled.
2. **Interphase**: Interphase comprises 90% of the cell cycle timewise. The cell produces enough new organelles for two new cells. Microscopically, the chromosomes cannot yet be seen. The DNA is seen as uncoiled chromatin. Interphase consists of three subphases. In the **G_1 phase**, growth begins. Nutrition and growth factors have been restored. Enzymes referred to as **salvage enzymes** are synthesized. These will become all of the necessary enzymes for cell division. In the **S phase**, DNA is synthesized (replicated). In the **G_2 phase**, the cell prepares for mitosis. This is the second growth phase. The chromosomes have been duplicated and the cell is preparing for the M phase, mitosis.
3. **M phase:** In M phase, nuclear division, or mitosis, and cell division, or cytokinesis, occur.

Mitosis

Mitosis or the M phase (**mitotic phase**) is short and dynamic. Cells are in interphase the vast majority of the time. There are five phases, as outlined, for eukaryotic animal cells:

1. **Prophase**: The chromatin condenses to form the visible, densely packed chromosome. The DNA has already replicated in the S phase of interphase. The sister chromatids, attached in the center at the centromere, are visible. The binding protein in the centromere is **cohesin**. The already duplicated paired centrioles, forming the centrosomes, move to opposite sides of the cell. The mitotic spindle forms. The spindle fibers spread out from each centriole in a starlike pattern that is referred to as an **aster**.
2. **Prometaphase**: Late prophase is sometimes referred to as prometaphase because two distinct events occur. It is now that the nucleolus and nuclear membrane disintegrate. It is also during this phase that the kinetochore (on the centromere) captures some of the spindle fibers so that the chromosomes are attached to the mitotic spindle fiber.
3. **Metaphase:** When metaphase begins, the nuclear membrane is gone, the centrioles are at the poles of the cell, some spindle fibers are connected to the centromeres, and the sister chromatids line

up along the cell equator, also referred to as the **metaphase plate**. The nonattached polar spindle fibers can extend beyond the equator and overlap.

4. **Anaphase**: As anaphase begins, the centromeres holding the sister chromatids together divide. The daughter chromosomes are composed of a centromere and a single chromatid. The spindle fibers lengthen and the kinetochore fibers shorten. These two forces combine to push (spindle fibers) and pull (kinetochore spindle fibers) the daughter chromosomes to the opposite poles of the cell where the centrosomes are located. The kinetochore spindle fibers eventually disintegrate completely. Meanwhile, the polar spindle fibers lengthen and slide past one another. When the daughter chromosomes reach the poles of the cell, telophase begins.
5. **Telophase**: Once the daughter chromosomes reach the centrosomes at the poles of the cell, the nuclear membranes for the two new cells begin to form. The nucleoli reappear. The steps of prophase are undone. The spindles disintegrate and the single chromosomes begin to unwind, elongate, and return to chromatin. Microscopically it is difficult to view the onset of telophase, so its starting point is often marked by the onset of cytokinesis. The cytoskeleton narrows at the metaphase plate and pinches the cell membrane, causing cell furrowing. At the end of telophase, cytokinesis is complete and the two new nuclei look like interphase nuclei. The cell cycle will begin anew in each of the two new cells.

In eukaryotic plant cells, there are some differences. Plant cells do not have centrioles. They have only spindle fibers. Thus, in anaphase, the daughter chromosomes move to the ends of the spindles on the side closest to them rather than toward the centrosomes. Cytokinesis is also different because the new plant cells require a cell wall. First a **cell plate** is deposited over a framework of microtubules and microfilaments called a **phragmoplast**. The cell plate is formed by the new plasma membranes for the two new cells in the center of the old cell. Cellulose is packaged into vesicles and sent from the Golgi apparatus to be inserted between the two adjacent cell membranes. The vesicles merge in the middle of the cell. The two new cells also elongate more than animal cells do. Often an area of active cytokinesis can be observed, particularly in cells located in root tips or the tips of twigs. On one end of the cell there is active cell division, and behind that, active elongation.

The results of mitosis are that a diploid or 2N mother cell generates two sets of chromosomes, which wind up in two diploid daughter cells that are identical both to each other and to the mother cell. If the parent cell is haploid, it generates two identical haploid daughter cells, each containing one set of chromosomes.

Mitotic Errors

One mitotic error is the **failure of mitotic checkpoints**. Mitotic checkpoints are points at which the new cells are examined for damage to the DNA or for malfunctions that have omitted essential procedures. If certain requirements have not been met, the checkpoints will prevent the next cell cycle phase from occurring. For example, if DNA duplication is not complete, a checkpoint will prevent the cell from entering M phase. Or, if the mitotic spindle is not attached to the chromosomes, a checkpoint will prevent the changeover from metaphase to anaphase. If a malfunction is detected, a network of signaling molecules directs the cell to shut down cell division. Signals can be sent to fix the defect or, if it is not repairable, to activate **apoptosis**, or programmed cell death. In this way, defective cells are not reproduced.

Another mitotic error is lack of **contact inhibition**. When cells have filled an area and are encountering other like cells all around them, contact inhibition signals the cells to cease cell division. Cancer cells, however, lack the contact inhibition mechanism. Tumors continue to rapidly perform cell division even when an area is filled and the mass is encountering obstructions such as nearby organs. Cancer cells will even force their way into new cell areas. Lack of contact inhibition also encourages metastasis of cancer cells to other parts of the body.

Cancer cells are thought to arise when mitotic checkpoints fail and do not prevent cell division from proceeding after the first growth phase ($\mathbf{G_1}$). The cells that result have lost their differentiation. They become primitive cells that exhibit excessive replication and growth and excessive chromosomes due to a malfunction in the DNA synthesis phase (S phase).

Meiosis

The life cycle of animals begins with a **zygote** or fertilized egg. This is a diploid (2N) structure. The zygote uses mitosis for growth. Cell differentiation occurs as the animal develops. The sex organs are one of the differentiated cell, or tissue, types. The sex organs produce **gametes**, the haploid (1N) sex cells. They have only one copy of each chromosome. During meiosis, precursor cells have their chromosome number halved by randomly choosing one homologue. Homologues or **homologous chromosomes** are pairs of identical chromosomes. They have the same genes and are the same size, and their centromeres are located in the same place; however, one is maternal and the other is paternal. The genes, although homologous, may code differently from one another. The male gamete is the **sperm** cell produced in the **testes**. The female gamete is the **ova** produced in the **ovary**. **Fertilization** is the union of sperm and egg. This restores the diploid number in the zygote.

Meiosis is the source of the genetic variation that feeds evolutionary change. It is how the gene pool is intermingled and mixed. A different method of cell division is necessary in order to produce the same number of chromosomes in the next generation. The number of chromosomes must be reduced in order to generate a haploid cell. This necessitates two cell division cycles. Interphase is identical in both mitosis and meiosis, but in meiosis, interphase is followed by two cell division cycles, meiosis I and meiosis II. The result is four haploid (1N) daughter cells. The nine steps in meiosis I and II are:

1. **Prophase I**: Similar to mitosis, in prophase I the chromatids condense to form the visible, densely packed chromosomes. The mitotic spindle forms. The already duplicated paired centrioles, forming the centrosomes, move to opposite sides of the cell. In late prophase or prometaphase, the nucleolus and nuclear membrane disintegrate. The difference is that the homologous chromosomes pair up to form what are referred to as either **bivalents** or **tetrads**. *Tetrad* refers to the four sister chromatids. *Bivalent* refers to the pair of homologous chromosomes, each with two homologous nonsister chromatids. Whereas in mitosis the chromosomes line up individually, in meiosis the two chromosomes that constitute a homologous pair line up. **Synapsis** is the process by which homologous chromosomes line up to form a tetrad. Between each pair of homologous chromosomes, a protein structure forms. The function of this structure, called the **synaptonemal complex**, is believed to be to facilitate and manage pairing, synapsis, and recombination. The duplicated chromosomes pair up closely with their homologue and are held tightly together by the synaptonemal complex. When the homologous chromosomes are paired up and tightly bound by the synaptonemal complex, there are points along the bivalents where they touch one another, called **chiasmata**. The chiasmata are points where gene exchange takes place. This exchange of genetic material is called **crossing over**, and it is an additional source of genetic variation.
2. **Metaphase I**: The spindle fiber apparatus is complete. The centrioles are at the poles of the cell. The tetrads line up at the equator.
3. **Anaphase I**: The homologous chromosomes separate and move to the poles.

4. **Telophase I**: The new nuclear membranes form and cytokinesis generates two new haploid cells. Meiosis I is the reduction phase. The DNA is organized in single linear chromosomes. The impetus is to return to two identical DNA, chromatids, attached in the center at the centromere.
5. **Interkinesis**: Interkinesis is the time period between the two cell divisions. During this time, partial elongation of the DNA occurs but the DNA does not replicate.
6. **Prophase II**: The DNA condenses and the nuclear membrane disintegrates. The spindle apparatus forms.
7. **Metaphase II**: The centromeres are attached to the spindle fibers. The centrioles move to the poles and the chromosomes line up at the cell equator.
8. **Anaphase II**: The centromeres divide and the chromatids move to the poles.
9. **Telophase II**: The new nuclei form and cytokinesis occurs. At the end of meiosis II, the same result as in mitosis is accomplished; the chromosomes become chromatids. The result, however, is four haploid daughter cells containing chromatin that makes each cell unique.

Mitosis begins with a diploid mother cell, generates two sets of chromosomes per cell, and ends with two diploid daughter cells that are identical to each other and to the mother cell. Mitosis can also begin with a haploid mother cell and end with two identical haploid daughter cells.

Meiosis begins with a diploid mother cell, generates first two haploid daughter cells with half the number of double-stranded chromosomes at the end of meiosis I, and then four unique haploid gametes with one set of chromosomes each at the end of meiosis II. In sporogenesis (which occurs in many eukaryotic plants, algae, and fungi), four unique haploid spores are formed.

The events in meiosis that contribute to genetic diversity, or mixing the gene pool between generations, are independent assortment, random fertilization, and crossing over. **Independent assortment** refers to the random way in which the homologous chromosomes become oriented on one side of the metaphase plate or the other in metaphase I. The number of possible orientations is 2^n, where n is the haploid number of chromosomes. Since human beings have 46 chromosomes, n equals 23, and 2^{23} equals 8.4 million possible orientations.

Random fertilization refers to the fact that, for example, in humans, any of a male's 8.4 million possible genetic combinations can fertilize any of a female's 8.4 million possible genetic combinations, resulting in a total possible number of combinations of over 70 trillion. Recall that crossing over is when pieces of homologous chromosomes break off and switch places, creating an exchange of genetic material. When crossing over is considered along with independent assortment and random fertilization, the number of possible genetic combinations is nearly infinite.

Spermatogenesis and Oogenesis

Spermatogenesis occurs in the testes beginning in puberty and continuing nonstop 24 hours a day, seven days a week, until 60 to 70 years of age. There are at least 20 million sperm per milliliter (ml) of semen. During meiosis, one diploid primary spermatocyte creates four haploid spermatids. First, a diploid male germ cell increases in size to become a primary spermatocyte. Next, the primary spermatocyte undergoes meiosis and cytoplasmic division to form four haploid spermatids. Finally, each of the haploid spermatids differentiates into a mature haploid sperm. Loose cytoplasm forms around the nucleus to become the head, and an **acrosome** forms around the anterior portion of the nucleus. It contains the enzymes to digest the covering of the egg. A single flagellum is added for a tail, and mitochondria are added for ATP production. The function of sperm is to deliver DNA to the female. The sperm must travel from the vagina through the cervix and uterus and into a fallopian tube (uterine tube) to find an egg.

Oogenesis occurs in the ovaries, which are located in the uterus. At the onset of puberty, each monthly cycle releases one cell, which proceeds to metaphase II. First, a diploid female germ cell increases in size to become a **primary oocyte**, which proceeds to prophase I. The primary oocyte undergoes meiosis and unequal cytoplasmic division to produce one haploid ovum and three polar bodies. The potential egg gets most of the cytoplasm because the fertilized egg must supply nutrients until implantation occurs in about seven days. The three polar bodies disintegrate. Only one functional gamete is produced. Egg fertilization causes the cell to complete meiosis, where more polar bodies are produced along with one fertilized egg.

Karyotypes

A karyotype is an organized profile of a complete set of chromosomes for any living organism. An image is taken of the chromosomes and they are organized from the largest to the smallest. The homologous chromosomes are matched up using size, banding pattern, and centromere position as guides. This array can be used to pinpoint chromosomal variations that may cause a genetic disorder. **Autosomes** are chromosomes that are not sex chromosomes. They are the ordinary paired chromosomes that are the same in both sexes of a species. In humans, there are 22 pairs of autosomes (44 total). The X and Y chromosomes are not autosomal. **Sex chromosomes** are chromosomes whose presence or absence determines the sex of the organism. They are differently shaped (for example, X and Y in humans) chromosomes whose distribution in a zygote determines the sex of the organism. The normal human karyotype has 46 chromosomes—22 pairs of autosomes (containing genes for all functions) and two sex chromosomes (one pair). Female sex chromosomes are denoted XX. Males have the XY chromosomal pair.

Genetic Disorders

The primary techniques for discovering genetic disorders in pregnancy are amniocentesis and chorionic villus sampling. **Amniocentesis** is a process in which a needle is inserted through the mother's abdomen to collect amniotic fluid. It is usually performed around the fourteenth week of gestation. Fetal cells are checked for sex and purified DNA is analyzed biochemically for enzyme or protein abnormalities. Some cells are grown for two weeks in a culture and a karyotype diagram is created. About 40 metabolic disorders can be screened. **Chorionic villus sampling** is a process in which the cells that will develop into the placenta are collected either cervically or transabdominally. These cells are cultured and biochemical tests and karyotyping are performed. This procedure can be done much earlier in pregnancy, but cannot do protein analysis and has a slightly higher miscarriage rate.

The following lists some of the primary causes of genetic disorders:

- **Aneuploidy: 2 N ± 1:** There is a chromosome number that is not a multiple of the haploid number for the species. Either there is only one copy of a particular chromosome or there are three copies of that particular chromosome. Monosomy and trisomy are the two most common aneuploidy conditions.
- **Monosomy: 2N – 1:** There is only one copy of a certain chromosome rather than the usual two.
- **Trisomy: 2N + 1:** There are three copies of a particular chromosome rather than the usual two.
- **Translocation:** DNA from one chromosome attaches to a nonhomologous chromosome. Part of a chromosome breaks off and then reattaches to a different chromosome.
- **Reciprocal translocation:** There is an exchange of DNA between nonhomologous chromosomes. An even swap is made between two chromosomes.
- **Duplication error:** There is one section of a particular chromosome that is duplicated. The

recipient has three copies of this particular DNA segment rather than the usual two. This DNA segment can be on the correct chromosome or it can be on a different chromosome.

- **Nondisjunction:** There are two places where aneuploids can be created: in meiosis I if the homologous chromosomes do not separate or in meiosis II if the sister chromatids do not separate. Mitotic nondisjunction can also occur when the two sister chromatids do not separate. The result is aneuploid cells in which one daughter cell has two chromosomes or two chromatids and the other has none (one daughter cell has both of a pair of parental chromosomes or chromatids and the other has none). When nondisjunction occurs in meiosis I, one cell receives two of the same type of chromosome and the other receives no copy of that chromosome. When the gametes are formed, two will have two copies of the same chromosome and two will have no copies of the chromosome. When fertilization occurs, the fertilized ova will have either three copies of that chromosome or only one copy of the chromosome, depending on which gamete is fertilized or does the fertilizing. The former is trisomy (2N + 1) and the latter is monosomy (2N – 1). When nondisjunction occurs in meiosis II, two normal gametes are produced, but in the other two gametes one cell receives both sister chromatids while the other receives none.
- **Deletions:** A section of a chromosome is deleted; a piece of the chromosome is missing.

Some well-understood genetic disorders or syndromes are as follows:

- **Turner syndrome**: Turner syndrome is an example of monosomy; there is only one X chromosome. In close to 80% of cases, the sperm is lacking a sex chromosome. Therefore the one X chromosome the offspring has is from the egg. Turner syndrome affects one in 2,000 to 2,500 live births. Sufferers are infertile due to a lack of ovarian development. They have wide and short chests and may also have webbed necks and arms that turn out at the elbows.
- **Triple X**: Also called 47 XXX, this syndrome displays three X chromosomes in all somatic cells. Sufferers, who are usually tall, are also referred to as meta-females. They are not sterile and have normal offspring. Some have no symptomology and others display few effects. The serious issues that do display are behavioral abnormalities and developmental delay. Some triple X females display learning disabilities and delayed speech and language skills.
- **Klinefelter's syndrome**: Klinefelter's is a trisomy with one Y chromosome and two X chromosomes (XXY). Boys appear to develop normally but during puberty fail to develop secondary sex characteristics. They may lack axial, facial, and pubic hair and some develop breasts. These males are infertile; they cannot produce offspring. The extra X chromosome has an equal probability of coming from the egg or the sperm.
- **Jacob's syndrome**: Jacob's syndrome is a trisomy with one X and two Y chromosomes (47 XYY). Usually tall, these men often display learning disabilities in childhood and may be developmentally delayed in maturity level. Some data have pointed to an increased probability of incarceration. However, most XYY males are normal. Abnormal sperm formation is the cause. A nondisjunction error occurs during cell division such that the sperm cell contains two Y chromosomes.
- **Down syndrome**: Trisomy 21 involves three copies of chromosome 21. This is also most commonly a nondisjunction error. During meiosis, a paired chromosome does not split up and go to the opposite sides of the cell. Instead, the pair stays together and goes to one side of the cell. The resulting gametes will have 24 and 22

chromosomes. The symptoms are almond-shaped eyes, mental retardation, and heart defect. Sufferers are often more prone to infections, leukemia, and Alzheimer's disease. Down syndrome is correlated to the age of the mother and 90% of the time is due to a nondisjunction error in egg formation.

- **Cri-du-chat syndrome**: French for "cry of the cat," this syndrome results in a distinctive cry in newborns due to abnormal larynx development. Although the cry quickly abates, these newborns are often of low weight and often display respiratory difficulties. This is a rare syndrome seen in only one in 50,000 live births. It is caused by a deletion on the short arm of chromosome 5; 80% of the time, the chromosome with the deletion is in the sperm.
- **Fragile X**: Fragile X syndrome is the second most common cause of mental retardation. It affects both sexes. Sufferers may exhibit only learning disabilities, may exhibit autism, or may be severely mentally retarded. Many males have enlarged ears; some have elongated faces and jutting chins. A variety of connective tissue problems may display, such as problems with the mitral valve of the heart, double-jointedness, flat feet, and ear infections. Skeletal abnormalities are also seen in some patients. Boys may display behavioral abnormalities such as attention deficit disorder or mannerisms such as hand fluttering or hand biting. Girls can display some of the same symptomology; generally their cognitive and behavioral symptoms are less severe, although one-third are severely mentally disabled. The physical symptoms are also usually less severe in females. Fragile X is a duplication error.

Y Chromosome

The Y chromosome is male-determining due to a region on the Y chromosome that is referred to as the SRY gene (sex-determining region). It is the SRY gene that initiates testis development. After the SRY gene is activated and testes development ensues, the testis begins to produce hormones that establish maleness. The testes have specialized cells called the **Leydig cells**, which produce testosterone. Another specialized cell of the testes, the **Sertoli cell**, is a nurse or sustentacular cell of the sperm. In embryonic development, however, it is responsible for producing a substance known as **Müllerian-inhibiting substance (MIS)** or **anti-Müllerian hormone (AMH)**. This hormone prevents the Müllerian ducts from developing into a uterus and female reproductive tract. The best-understood effect is to cause apoptosis of the cells of the Müllerian ducts. This occurs in the first eight weeks of gestation. Another set of ducts, the Wolffian ducts, develops in both sexes into part of the bladder wall. In males, with the Müllerian ducts disposed of and testosterone exposure intact, the Wolffian ducts are free to develop into the male duct system—the testis, prostate, epididymis, vas deferens, and seminal vesicle.

RNA

Ribonucleic acid (RNA) differs from DNA in four ways:

1. Most RNA is single-stranded, not double-stranded like DNA. The exception is double-stranded RNA viruses.
2. RNA has the sugar ribose rather than deoxyribose.
3. RNA has the nitrogenous base uracil in place of thymine. Uracil, like thymine, can form hydrogen bonds with adenine.
4. Unlike DNA polymerases, RNA polymerases can join RNA nucleotides together without requiring a preexisting strand of RNA.

There are three main types of RNA:

1. **Messenger RNA (mRNA):** Messenger RNA copies the genes on a strand of DNA. Complementary base pairing is the mechanism by which the code is copied. Messenger RNA goes to the ribosomes. The ribosomes are the protein factories.

2. **Transfer RNA (tRNA)**: Transfer RNA acquires amino acids and takes them to the ribosomes. Each tRNA carries one amino acid following the code on the mRNA to insert the correct amino acid in the proper sequence to create a polypeptide (protein).
3. **Ribosomal RNA (rRNA)**: Ribosomal proteins plus rRNA combine to form ribosomal subunits.

   There are other RNA transcripts as well: Antisense RNA, microRNA, and riboswitch RNA are some recently discovered iterations of RNA. They have been transcribed from DNA but are not translated to produce proteins. Instead, they perform various functions in gene regulation.

It is the nitrogenous base pairs that form the genetic code stored in DNA. The sequence of the bases along a strand of DNA will ultimately code for the amino acid sequences that comprise a polypeptide chain or protein. The amino acid sequence also determines the three-dimensional shape a protein will assume. This is important for many reasons, including what substrates an enzyme can react with. In order to get from the code stored in the DNA to protein synthesis, the DNA must first be transcribed to an mRNA transcript, and then the transcript, must be translated to synthesize a protein.

Transcription

Messenger RNA (mRNA) is the transcript of the code in a strand of DNA. Complementary base pairing is performed between RNA ribonucleotides and DNA deoxyribonucleotides. RNA polymerase is the enzyme that starts the transcription process. In prokaryotic cells, first, a number of different proteins bind to the enzyme. These proteins are collectively referred to as **sigma factors**. Then, the RNA-protein complex binds to the **promoter region** on a DNA strand. The promoter region is approximately 40 deoxyribonucleotide bases long. This sequence precedes the region that is to be coded. It distinguishes which of the uncoiled strands and the region on the DNA strand that will be transcribed. The DNA template is read from the 3′ to 5′ direction. It is thus synthesized from the 5′ to 3′ direction.

This is the same process that DNA polymerase uses in the process of DNA replication. Nucleic acids are always synthesized in the 5′ to 3′ direction. Recall that the 3′ end has a hydroxyl group (OH), while the 5′ end has a phosphate group (PO_4). The hydroxyl group is unlinked to any further nucleotide. It is attached to the strand to the 3′ carbon of the last deoxyribose sugar. The phosphate group is attached to the 5′ carbon of the sugar on the opposite end. It is also not linked to another nucleotide.

After the RNA polymerase-protein complex locates the promoter region, the sigma factors dissociate from the enzyme. The process of unwinding the DNA strands then begins. The resulting unpaired deoxyribonucleotides function as a template for synthesizing the RNA. The promoter region is not transcribed. A short sequence called a **leader sequence** is transcribed, however. This leader sequence will be transcribed into the ribosome binding site for the mRNA.

After the leader sequence is the coding sequence. It is the coding sequence that will be translated to synthesize the correct protein. Transcribing the DNA code involves ribonucleotide triphosphates forming complementary base pairs through hydrogen bonding with deoxyribonucleotides on the unwound DNA strand. Adenine on the DNA strand is paired with uracil on the RNA strand rather than thymine. Phosphodiester bonds form between the 5′C phosphate group of a nucleotide that is being inserted and the 3′C of the last ribonucleotide on the messenger RNA chain that is being created. As these covalent bonds are formed, two of the phosphate groups are removed and their energy is used to fuel the reaction. RNA polymerase catalyzes the reaction that joins the ribonucleotides and terminates transcription.

In eukaryotic cells, the process is slightly different and more complex. First, transcription is in the cytoplasm in prokaryotes, which have no nucleus. In eukaryotes, transcription is in the nucleus where the DNA is located. Second, in eukaryotes, chromosomes combine the DNA with histones to form the beadlike nucleosomes that are the repeating units of chromatin. This makes the DNA far more difficult for RNA polymerase to interact with.

A number of additional proteins called **transcription factors** are required to coordinate the procedure. **Activator proteins** bind to certain genes. This stimulates them to generate substances that activate other genes that will accelerate the transcription process. These genes are referred to as **enhancers.** Other proteins, called **repressor proteins**, bind to genes called **silencers**. Silencers inhibit activator proteins. Since the enhancer genes are no longer being activated, this retards the transcription process.

Still other proteins, called **coactivators**, synchronize the signals from the activator proteins and the repressor proteins. Coactivators communicate this information to molecules that establish where RNA polymerase should begin transcribing. These molecules, called **basal factors**, position the RNA polymerase at the start of the coding region.

Once transcription begins, the process is the same. Ribonucleotide triphosphates form complementary base pairs through hydrogen bonding with deoxyribonucleotides on the unwound DNA strand. Phosphodiester bonds form between the 5′C phosphate group of a nucleotide that is being inserted and the 3′C of the last ribonucleotide on the messenger RNA chain that is being created. As these covalent bonds are formed, two of the phosphate groups are removed and their energy is used to fuel the reaction. However, in higher eukaryotic cells, there are many regions that are noncoding. These regions, called **introns**, comprise up to 98% of human chromosomes. They are interspersed with the coding regions called **exons**. The introns do not contain code for the protein product. Therefore, an intermediate product is formed called **precursor mRNA**. A modified guanine nucleotide is added to the 5′ end of the precursor mRNA early in the process. This is called a **cap** or **5′ cap**, and it indicates the start sequence. The cap will aid the ribosomes so that they can attach for translation.

Near the end of the process, an addition called a **poly A tail** is added. The poly A tail consists of multiple adenine nucleotides, usually between 100 and 250. The function of the poly A tail, while not entirely clear, appears to be to stabilize the molecule for its trip out to the cytoplasm by aiding in transport and protecting it from degradation. It is also thought that as the length of the tail decreases, the transcript is more likely to be degraded by enzymes. **RNA processing** must occur to transform precursor mRNA into mature mRNA. The introns must be cut out of the precursor mRNA molecule. Then the exons must be spliced together. **Spliceosomes**, complexes of ribonucleoproteins, perform this duty.

Translation

The mature mRNA must now go out to the cytoplasm to the ribosomes. It passes through pores in the nuclear membrane. The molecule will be read as codons. Each codon is three nucleotides long. One codon codes for one amino acid. Since there are four possible nucleotides in RNA, with either adenine, guanine, cytosine, or uracil, there are 4^3 or 64 possible codons. There are 20 amino acids. This means that there are a number of different codons that code for each amino acid. The **start codon** is the sequence AUG. This codon indicates where translation is to begin. The **stop codon** sequences are UAG, UAA, or UGA. These three sequences indicate where translation is to end.

Eukaryotic ribosomes are comprised of a 40S and a 60S subunit. Each subunit is composed of ribosomal RNA and proteins. The small subunit of the ribosome attaches to the mRNA and two RNA binding sites are formed. One site is called the P site or peptidyl site. The other is the A or aminoacyl site.

Transfer RNA is a three-dimensional, inverted cloverleaf-shaped molecule. On the 3′ end, aminoacyl tRNA synthetase enzymes catalyze a reaction to add a specific amino acid. The reaction is **aminoacylation** and is also referred to as charging. Each of the 20 amino acids has a corresponding aminoacyl tRNA synthetase. The tRNA-amino acid complex is called **aminoacyl-tRNA**. The anticodon is on the other end. The **anticodon** is the three bases complementary to the codon on the mRNA. There are no anticodons for the three stop codons. Thus, there are 61 possible anticodons.

Each anticodon on a tRNA can recognize more than one codon on an mRNA. The reading of the third nucleotide is not always exact. However, the correct amino acid is usually still inserted due to the built-in redundancy. Each amino acid except methionine has at least two codons that designate its insertion. The codons that code for the same amino acid have the same two bases in the first two nucleotides. The third nucleotide is the variant. It is at the third nucleotide that translation errors are most likely to occur. The binding affinity is the weakest at the third nucleotide. The built-in redundancy compensates for this problem by ensuring that the correct amino acid will be inserted even for most mistakes in translation that occur at the third nucleotide. In this manner, specific amino acids bind to specific tRNA molecules and are brought to the mRNA attached to the ribosome. The three steps for translation are as follows.

1. **Initiation**: Translation starts when the ribosome attaches to the mRNA. The start codon (AUG) on the mRNA designates the point of attachment. This location is called the **ribosome binding site**. It is the small ribosomal subunit that binds to the mRNA first. The first tRNA comes in at the peptidyl or P site on the ribosome. This initial tRNA must have the anticodon (UAC) for the start codon. The anticodon and the codon bind by complementary base pair hydrogen bonding. The start codon, AUG, codes for the amino acid methionine. Every polypeptide chain will have methionine as its first amino acid. Once the P site is occupied by the initiator tRNA (met-tRNA), the large ribosomal subunit attaches and the **initiation complex** is complete.
2. **Elongation**: Now the appropriate tRNA (the aminoacylated tRNA) with the correct anticodon to bind to the codon at the A site enters and binds. The methionine in the P site and the new amino acid in the A site must be attached by a peptide bond to begin building the polypeptide chain. **Peptidyl transferase** catalyzes this reaction. The two amino acids are now joined together at the A site and the tRNA dissociates from the P site. The ribosome moves down one codon, leaving the other tRNA in the P site and freeing the A site again. In this manner, the polypeptide chain continues to elongate. As new aminoacyl-tRNA enters the A site, peptidyl transferase catalyzes the reaction to join the new amino acid, the tRNA dissociates from the P site, and the ribosome moves down one codon, freeing the A site for another tRNA to attach.
3. **Termination**: When one of the stop codons (UAA, UAG, UGA) is reached at the A site on the ribosome, additional aminoacyl-tRNAs no longer enter. The polypeptide chain is released from the tRNA. The tRNA then dissociates from the ribosome. The large and small ribosomal subunits dissociate from the mRNA.

Genetics

This section reviews various concepts in genetics that you should be familiar with for the PCAT exam.

Mendel's Law of Segregation

An organism's traits are dictated by genes, which are passed on to subsequent generations in a way that can be predicted based on probability. Since each gene can exist in two different forms (alleles), which are segregated during meiosis, each gamete contains only one iteration of the gene. When the gametes unite to form a new organism, the gene is restored to two alleles for each gene, one from the mother and one from the father.

Mendel's Law of Independent Assortment

Gene pair segregation occurs independently from other genes, in an ordered fashion, so as to ensure that each gamete contains one allele for each location on a gene. However, different alleles (at different gene locations) are randomly assorted independently. That is, the inheritance of one trait is independent from the inheritance of another trait. This is due to the homologous chromosomes lining up in metaphase I. However, we now know that there are linked genes that are close to each other on the same chromosome and that the Law of Independent Assortment is completely true only for genes that are located on different chromosomes or those that are far apart from one another on the same chromosome. Linked genes contradict the Law of Independent Assortment because they are transferred together as if they were one gene.

BASIC GENETICS TERMINOLOGY

- **Gene:** A gene is a DNA sequence that creates a hereditary unit on a specific location on a chromosome. Genes determine particular characteristics in an organism.
- **Allele:** Alleles are alternative forms of a gene. There are different gene iterations that can exist at a single locus on a chromosome—for example, a gene for blue eyes and a gene for brown eyes. An allele is one member of a pair of genes for a particular trait.
- **Loci:** The Latin word *locus* translates as place. A locus is the location on a chromosome where a gene occurs. Loci are notated to indicate the chromosome number, whether the gene is on a long arm or a short arm of the chromosome, and the location on the arm. The location on the arm is designated by numbering the bands that are visible when a chromosome is stained starting from the centromere.
- **Genotype:** The genotype refers to the genetic makeup of an organism, as opposed to the physically expressed traits. It is the combination of alleles located on homologous chromosomes that determines all of the characteristics of an organism.
- **Phenotype:** The phenotype refers to the observable physical traits of an organism. Phenotype is determined by genotype plus environmental influences.
- **Homozygous:** Homozygous describes the condition in which there are the same alleles at a particular location on a gene on homologous chromosomes—for example, two alleles for blue eyes.
- **Heterozygous:** Heterozygous describes the condition in which there are different alleles at a particular location on a gene—for example, an allele for blue eyes and an allele for brown eyes.
- **Dominant:** A gene that is expressed phenotypically (visibly) in either heterozygous or homozygous dominant individuals.

(continued)

BASIC GENETICS TERMINOLOGY (*continued*)

- **Autosomal dominant trait:** A trait that is expressed because there is a dominant allele for an autosomal gene. The autosomal genes are all of the trait-determining genes, as opposed to the two sex-determining genes (X and Y). Autosomal dominant genes are always expressed.
- **Recessive:** A type of gene that is not expressed phenotypically as a visible trait unless it is inherited from both parents, creating a homozygous recessive individual.
- **Autosomal recessive trait:** A trait that is only phenotypically visible when there are two alleles of the gene present on an autosomal gene. The organism must be homozygous for the trait.
- **X-linked recessive trait:** A trait caused by a recessive mutant gene on the X chromosome. Since females have two X chromosomes, there must be two alleles for the X-linked recessive trait in order for it to be phenotypically expressed. Since males have one X and one Y chromosome, and the genes on the Y chromosome do not exactly pair up with the genes on the X chromosome, only one allele is necessary in order for the trait to be phenotypically expressed.
- **X-linked dominant trait:** A trait caused by a dominant mutant gene on the X chromosome. X-linked dominant traits are less common than X-linked recessive traits. Both females and males will carry the trait if they inherit an X chromosome with the allele. All females whose father carries the allele will carry the trait because they will inherit the mutated allele on the X chromosome from the father. None of the sons who have only a father with the trait will inherit the trait because they inherit the Y chromosome from their father. The mother of a son with the trait must necessarily be carrying the trait. If the mother is heterozygous for the trait, half of her sons and half of her daughters are likely to carry the trait.
- **Incomplete dominance:** A heterozygous state in which both alleles at a particular location on a gene are partially expressed or blended. This often results in an **intermediate phenotype**, such as pink flowers from crossing red and white flowers.
- **Codominance:** A heterozygous state in which two different alleles for a gene are both expressed phenotypically. The two different alleles are expressed unblended—for example, the AB blood type.
- **Multiple allelism:** The existence of more than two alternative contrasting alleles for a particular gene. For example, blood types are determined by three different alleles, A, B, and O, any two of which can form a pair to determine the phenotype.
- **Mutation:** Mutations are changes in the sequence of nitrogen bases on a DNA strand. They can be caused by errors when the nitrogen base sequence is copied during cell division and by exposure to radiation, chemicals, or viruses. Mutations can result in harmful alterations in the structure and function of an organism or they can be beneficial to the organism.
- **Mutagen:** Mutagens are agents that change the genetic material (DNA) and increase the number of mutations that occur above the normal level that spontaneously occur in nature.
- **Frameshift mutation:** Deletion or insertion of a nucleotide that causes the reading frame for the mRNA to change. When there are more or fewer nucleotides, all of the codons on the mRNA are changed from the point of insertion or deletion onward. If a nucleotide is added or deleted, it can cause an entirely different protein to be made. If the deletion or insertion occurs late in the sequence, it may result in a functioning protein, but it may not. Usually if the mistake is early in the sequence, the protein will be badly damaged or nonfunctional.
- **Point mutation (substitution):** One nucleotide is changed to another. The number of nucleotides stays the same, but it can cause a different amino acid to be synthesized. A single codon on the mRNA is changed.

BASIC GENETICS TERMINOLOGY (*continued*)

Sometimes a codon can be changed and still code for the correct amino acid. This is called a **silent mutation** because no effect is engendered. If the codon causes a different amino acid to be inserted, it can change the structure of the protein such that it malfunctions. This is called a **missense mutation**. A single nucleotide can also cause a stop codon to occur at the wrong location. This is called a **nonsense mutation**. A shortened polypeptide chain is produced that is most often not a complete protein and is nonfunctional.

In general, it can be said that a phenotype is produced by the interaction between the environment and the genotype of an organism. A phenotype may be expressed only in the presence of certain environmental factors, or it can be suppressed in the presence of certain environmental factors. The environment affects gene expression because sometimes the proper environmental conditions are needed in order for a gene to be fully expressed. For example, humans need the proper diet and nutrition in order for the genes for tallness to be fully expressed.

Expressivity is a measure of how fully a gene is expressed. Environmental effects can in essence turn genes on or off. For example, Himalayan and Siamese rabbits have dark fur only on their ears, paws, and noses. This is thought to be caused by a heat-sensitive enzyme that is necessary in order to produce the pigment needed to express the genotype. This enzyme is functional (the gene is turned on/transcribed) only at the lower body temperatures found in the extremities and not in the higher body temperatures of the rest of the body.

Another common example of the environment affecting gene expression is the effect of fertilizer on dwarf wheat varieties. Tall wheat varieties do poorly when fertilized because the additional growth induced by the fertilizer results in increased grain weight, which causes the stalks to bend over. Dwarf wheat varieties, in contrast, have shorter, stronger stalks, so they do well when they are fertilized and produce a larger, heavier grain. Other examples include human fitness training which is more effective in influencing some genotypes over others; the most often cited example is that seeds sprouted in the absence of sunlight will produce yellow leaves because no chlorophyll is produced so that the gene for green pigment can be transcribed.

The laws of probability are used to determine the distribution of hereditary traits. One tool is the Punnett square, which assigns the proper genotypes and phenotypes to the predicted outcomes. The most common allele in a population of organisms is called the **wild type** allele. A single capital letter is used to denote the dominant form of an allele, while a single lowercase letter denotes the recessive form of the allele. A monohybrid cross analyzes a single trait. The initial two parents are referred to as the P generation. The offspring of these two parents are referred to as the F_1 generation. A mating between two members of the F_1 generation results in the F2 generation.

To construct a Punnett square, the genotypes of the parents must be known so that all of the possible gamete combinations can be inserted into the square. The classic example is eye color in which a capital B is used to denote brown eye color, while a lowercase b is used to denote blue eye color. Actually more than one gene is involved in eye color, but this example illustrates how the single allele operates. If one parent is homozygous for the dominant trait, while one parent is homozygous for the recessive trait, what Mendel referred to as **true breeding** varieties, 100% of the first generation displays the dominant trait and the heterozygous genotype:

		Female	
		B	B
Male	b	Bb	Bb
	b	Bb	Bb

However, if two members of the F_1 generation are mated, only 75% of their offspring display the dominant phenotype:

		Female	
		B	b
Male	B	BB	Bb
	b	Bb	bb

The phenotypic ratio is 3:1 brown eyes:blue eyes. The genotypic ratio is 1:2:1, homozygous dominant: heterozygous:homozygous recessive.

A dihybrid cross can also be predicted using a Punnett square. The traits must be unlinked or independent of one another. Once again, all possible gamete combinations must be determined. For example, if tall plants are dominant over dwarf plants, T denotes the dominant tall gene and lowercase t denotes the recessive dwarf gene. If in the same plant white fruit color is dominant over yellow fruit color, W denotes the dominant white allele and w denotes the recessive yellow allele. If two heterozygous plants are crossed and these two traits are independent of one another, the following result will occur:

		Female			
		TW	Tw	tW	tw
Male	TW	TTWW	TTWw	TtWW	TtWw
	Tw	TTWw	TTww	TtWw	Ttww
	tW	TtWW	TtWw	ttWW	ttWw
	tw	TtWw	Ttww	ttWw	ttww

The phenotypic ratio is 9:3:3:1. Tall white fruit:tall yellow fruit:dwarf white fruit:dwarf yellow fruit.

In incomplete dominance, there is a third phenotype created by the blending of an allele. For example, in several flower species the allele for white color is capital W and the allele for red color is capital R since neither is dominant. A monohybrid cross of two true breeding varieties produces the following Punnett square, which shows that 100% of the offspring are pink, a blending of the two dominant alleles:

		Female	
		W	W
Male	R	RW	RW
	R	RW	RW

If two members of the F_1 generation are crossed, 50% will be pink, the blended trait; 25% will be white; and 25% will be red:

		Female	
		R	W
Male	R	RR	RW
	W	RW	WW

In codominance, two different alleles for a gene are both expressed phenotypically. Blood type is an example. Capital I indicates the dominant alleles (A or B), while lowercase i denotes the recessive O allele. If a heterozygous type A female is crossed with a heterozygous type B male, the probability is that 25% of their offspring will be type AB, the codominant blood type in which both the A and B antigens are present on the red blood cells and neither the A nor the B antibodies are present. Another 25% will likely be homozygous recessive type O. Finally, 25% each will be heterozygous type A and heterozygous type B:

		Female	
		I^A	i
Male	I^B	I^AI^B	I^Bi
	i	I^Ai	ii

Examples of autosomal dominant traits include the Rh factor. RH^+ is dominant, while Rh^- is recessive. A homozygous (RH^+–RH^+) individual expresses the RH^+ phenotype. A heterozygous (RH^+–Rh^-) individual expresses the RH^+ phenotype. Only a homozygous (Rh^-–Rh^-) individual expresses the Rh^- phenotype. Huntington's disease is an autosomal dominant trait caused by a mutated gene. There are cytosine-adenine-guanine (CAG) repeats on chromosome 4. These are called **trinucleotide repeats.** People with the disease may have from 40 to over 100 trinucleotide repeats. The good gene that does not contain the repeats is recessive. Individuals who have one of these alleles on chromosome number 4 will display the disease at some point in their lives.

Examples of autosomal recessive traits include Tay-Sachs disease. Infants are primarily affected. It strikes between three and six months of age and is almost always fatal by three to four years of age. The gene involved is called the HEXA gene. It codes for a protein that is used to manufacture the enzyme β-hexosaminidase A. This enzyme is integral to brain and spinal cord function. Lysosomes carry the enzyme to break down a lipid substance called GM2 ganglioside. When the two alleles of the mutated gene are inherited, GM2 ganglioside accumulates and becomes toxic to neurons in the brain and spinal cord. The destruction of these neurons leads to loss of motor skills and eventually seizures, loss of vision, loss of hearing, mental disabilities, and ultimately paralysis. Tay-Sachs is most common in people of Ashkenazi (Eastern and Central European) Jewish descent, some French-Canadian communities, Cajun communities in Louisiana, and some old-order Amish communities in Pennsylvania. When both parents carry one copy of the mutated gene, 25% of their offspring are likely to receive two copies of the mutated gene.

Inheritance Patterns

Pleiotropy is when a single gene affects a number of expressed traits. The word *pleiotropy* is derived from the Greek words for many (*pleio*) and changes (*tropo*). This can cause significant disruptions in certain genetic disorders. If a mutation occurs, at least two and possibly many different phenotypic traits will be affected. For example, in the disease phenylketonuria (PKU), a single gene that codes for the protein phenylalanine hydroxylase has mutated. The gene is called the PAH gene. This enzyme converts the amino acid phenylalanine to the amino acid tyrosine. Since this conversion can no longer take place, the level of phenylalanine in the body builds up and becomes toxic. This mutation has multiple effects, including mental retardation and diminished hair and skin pigmentation. PKU is an autosomal recessive disease. Affected patients carry both copies of the mutated allele.

Sickle-cell anemia is another example of pleiotropy. One amino acid in a β chain that comprises the globin protein in the hemoglobin molecule is mutated, causing the shape of the red blood cell to sickle or become a half-moon shape. This in turn causes problems with multiple organ systems in the body. Sickle-cell anemia is also an example of incomplete dominance. In order to inherit the full-blown disease, patients must have both copies of the mutated allele. These homozygous recessive individuals carry both mutated alleles and have the sickled or flattened red blood cells. Heterozygous individuals who carry one copy of the mutated allele are said to carry the sickle-cell trait. The prevalence of this trait in some populations is thought to be due to its conferring some resistance to malaria. The disease symptoms of sickle-cell trait carriers are generally controllable. Only homozygous dominant individuals are normal. Sickle-cell anemia is a point mutation on the hemoglobin beta gene (HBB) found on chromosome 11. Glutamic acid is produced instead of valine. A single base change results in a host of problematic phenotypic traits.

Another example of pleiotropy is Marfan syndrome. A mutation in a gene named FBN-1, which codes for the protein fibrillin-1, causes multiple problems because fibrillin-1 is an integral part of elastic cartilage tissue. The aorta, eye, skin, and bones are all phenotypically affected. Marfan syndrome is also an example of an autosomal dominant trait. The FBN-1 gene is autosomal dominant, so individuals who inherit one mutated allele exhibit the symptoms of the disease.

Cystic fibrosis is another example of pleiotropy. A mutation in the CFTR gene causes multiple physical symptoms because this gene codes for a channel protein that is needed to create a chloride ion (Cl^-) channel in the plasma membrane of cells. With malfunctioning Cl^- channels, water does not flow properly into tissues. The correct water balance is integral to the production of mucous. This results in cells lining the lungs, pancreas, and other organs manufacturing a mucous that is too thick. Airways and glands become obstructed. Cystic fibrosis is an autosomal recessive trait. Both CFTR genes must have the mutation in order for it to be manifested. If both parents carry one mutated CFTR gene, 25% of their offspring are likely to be homozygous for the recessive gene resulting in the phenotypic expression of the pleiotropy.

Epistasis is when one or more genes inhibit the expression of another gene. The inhibiting gene and the affected gene are on different loci on the genome, although they may be tightly linked. The effect can be either genotypic or phenotypic. One example is albinism. The gene that causes albinism masks the gene that codes for eye color and hair color. Albinism is autosomal recessive.

Another example is the gene that codes for the phenotypic expression of a widow's peak. If the gene for baldness is also present, it masks the gene for the widow's peak. Baldness, the phenotype that is expressed, is **epistatic.** The phenotype for a widow's peak, the phenotype that is masked, is **hypostatic. Hypostasis**, therefore, is when the expression of a gene is masked by an epistatic gene.

Polygenic inheritance is when many genes are involved. Phenotypically expressed traits are caused by the relationships and interactions between a number of genes. Skin color, height, and body shape are all the result of multiple genes interacting. Other phenotypes such as a propensity for high blood pressure are also polygenic. High blood pressure is the result of many genes, including multiple genes that control weight, cholesterol level (metabolism genes), and addiction tendency.

Evolution

Evolution can be described simply as descent with modification. Mutations are the method by which changes or modifications occur. **Microevolution** refers to a change in the gene frequency within a given population of organisms in a particular area. It happens over one or several generations. For example, resistance to pesticides may increase in insect or fungus populations over a single generation. These changes may occur because natural selection supported their inclusion in the genome. **Natural selection** refers to the propensity for better-adapted individuals to survive and thus reproduce. A particular set of genes is passed on because the reproducing individual is adapted to survive and pass on those traits. A new population of pesticide-resistant individuals may have **immigrated** to the group, or one or more mutations may have occurred that changed nonresistant genes to the resistant version. Random **genetic drift** could also explain the increase. Genetic drift refers to random sampling and chance. The alleles that are found in offspring are a result of random sampling. An allele can be eliminated, particularly in a small population, by chance alone.

Adaptations are inheritable traits that increase **fitness** so that the individual will survive and reproduce. An organism with greater fitness passes on more of its genes. Adaptations can be morphological and anatomical—for example, rabbit ear length. Rabbit species have long ears in the desert, but short ears in the Arctic cold. It was a beneficial adaptation to have less surface area exposed to the cold in the Arctic regions. Adaptations can also be biochemical and physiological—for example, poisons in plants and fungi that keep predators at bay. They can also be behavioral. Certain interactions between organisms may prove beneficial to the survival of both individuals and the population as a whole and may be passed down to subsequent generations.

Symbiotic relationships are defined as those in which two organisms live closely together on a long-term basis. **Mutualistic** relationships are symbiotic relationships that benefit both organisms. **Commensalism** is a symbiotic relationship in which one organism benefits and the other is unaffected by the relationship. **Parasitic** relationships are also a type of symbiosis. They are defined by one organism benefiting while the other sustains harm.

Fitness is also contingent upon the ability of an organism to outcompete other individuals and other groups of organisms for food, water, shelter, and other resources. Those better able to compete go on to randomly reproduce, leading to differential reproductive success. The phenotypic variations that have the best reproductive outcomes are perpetuated in the population.

Bacteria demonstrate microevolution because they can exchange DNA within a single generation as well as over several generations. Some bacteria can create a sexual conjugation bridge to exchange DNA. These pili, referred to as F-pili or sex-pili, are used to confer antibiotic resistance and the ability to make F-pili to other bacteria. The recipients can then continue to transfer resistance on to more bacteria. Sometimes bacterial DNA exchange occurs through natural transformations. Bacteria also demonstrate random genetic drift and genetic recombination. These alterations are easy to study in bacteria because they have such a short life span and such a short generation time. Bacteriophages, viruses that infect bacteria, can also cause changes to the genetic code.

Macroevolution occurs over a much longer time frame. The same five mechanisms cause macroevolution.

1. Heritability of traits
2. Migration (gene flow)
3. Natural selection
4. Mutation
5. Genetic drift

However, macroevolution refers to the accumulation of these small population-wide changes over millions of years to produce changes in separated gene pools on an extensive scale. Rather than at the species level, macroevolution focuses on diversity that occurs in families, orders, and classes of organisms and to the organisms with which they interact. Geology, fossil evidence, and living organisms can all be used to reconstruct evolutionary history.

Stasis refers to a lack of change over a long period of time. Some lineages exhibit such extensive stasis that they are referred to as living fossils. **Character change** refers to a change that happens in one direction. The addition of body segments is one example. Several lineages of trilobites added segments over a time period of millions of years. **Lineage splitting**, also called **speciation**, refers to events within a line of descent in which new descendent lineages arise. It is shown as a branching-off point in the phylogenic tree. **Extinction** is when the final organisms in a particular lineage die off. Individual species can become extinct, as can entire lineages of organisms. Extinction can happen infrequently within a lineage, or a mass extinction can occur in which many lineages die out at the same time. **Gene flow** refers to the migration of individuals from one population to another, taking their contribution to the gene pool with them. Emigration away from a population can diminish genetic variation, potentially harming the vitality of the remaining population, just as immigration into a population can enhance genetic variation, potentially increasing the vitality of the gene pool.

The **Hardy-Weinberg principle** posits that the frequency of alleles and genotypes within a population remains constant unless the intervening factors of evolution intercede. In nature, one or more those intervening factors will always be occurring. Other intervening factors include nonrandom mating, restricted population size, and meiotic drive. **Meiotic drive** refers to an event that results in the overrepresentation of certain alleles in the gametes formed from meiosis. Normally, and according to Mendel's law of segregation, the probability is that one-half of the gametes will receive one allele from a pair of alleles from the parent and one-half will receive the other allele. In some cases, one of the alleles is transferred to more than one-half of the gametes.

One example is the segregation distorter gene in the fruit fly *Drosophila melanogaster*. This gene is on a sex chromosome, and it distorts the process such that all sperm without the gene are eliminated and more female progeny are produced. Although the Hardy-Weinberg principle is never fulfilled in nature, it is useful as a tool against which to measure change. The equations are $p + q = 1$ where p is the frequency of the dominant allele and q is the frequency of the recessive allele, and $p^2 + 2pq + q^2 = 1$. Note that $p^2 + 2pq + q^2 = 1$ is the equation used to demonstrate the frequency of homozygous dominant, heterozygous, and homozygous recessive individuals; p^2 represents the homozygous dominant population, $2pq$ represents the heterozygous population, and q^2 represents the homozygous recessive population. The equation is used to work backwards from a known frequency of an allele or a known disease frequency. If any one piece of data is known, the others can be determined.

Two other effects that invalidate the Hardy-Weinberg equation are the founder effect and the bottleneck effect. The **founder effect** is genetic drift that occurs in newly emerging or newly founded populations. When a small number of individuals begin to form a new population, changes in gene frequencies are likely to be found in the succeeding generation simply due to random chance. The small population size means that there will likely be some inbreeding, increasing the frequencies of certain genes. Genetic variation will decrease. The sampling of genes from the original colony from which this small group split is now nonrandom rather than random.

The **bottleneck effect** is another variation of genetic drift. It happens when drastic population reduction occurs. A sudden reduction in the available alleles means that the gene pool is no longer representative of the original population. Genetic drift can cause alleles to be eliminated in small populations by chance alone. This can result in large losses to the genetic variation even if the bottleneck lasts for only a few generations. Whenever genetic variation is diminished, the likelihood of the population being able to withstand new selection pressures is likewise diminished.

There are several mechanisms for natural selection. In general, within any population there are a variety of traits and differential reproduction. No environment can sustain unlimited population growth, because resources are limited. Therefore, not all individuals within a population can reproduce to the extent they are capable. Those individuals who survive to reproduce or who outcompete so that they can reproduce pass on their alleles. The advantageous traits that allowed these individuals to reproduce are carried through to succeeding generations. Trait variety, differential reproduction, and heredity are therefore the components of evolution through natural selection. If there are the usual two phenotypes for a particular trait, it is referred to as **dimorphism**. If, as in the case of incomplete dominance, there are three or more possible phenotypes, it is referred to as **polymorphism**.

Natural selection can favor the extremes of the dominant or recessive phenotype, or it can favor the intermediate phenotype. **Directional selection** is when an allele that is beneficial is passed on in a higher than expected ratio. It is what we think of as natural selection. For example, horses have evolved from small short-limbed creatures that could move easily through woodlands to large long-limbed specimens constructed for maximum speed. Directional selection has selected specific alleles for teeth, toe structure, and leg length that have resulted in the modern horse. **Stabilizing selection** favors the intermediate phenotype over the extreme phenotypes. The extremes are eliminated and the intermediate form persists, diminishing genetic variation in order to promote stability in the population. The most often cited example is human birth weight, which has tended over time to favor intermediate birth weights that facilitate passage through the birth canal and yet promote optimum infant health at birth. **Disruptive selection**, also called **diversifying selection**, is the opposite. It favors the extremes over the intermediates. Genetic variation is enhanced, and two groups begin to emerge that may eventually evolve into separate species.

The supporting evidence for evolution is as follows:

- **Homologies**: Homologies are structures that are atomically alike but can differ functionally due to shared ancestry. The structures may have evolved from a structure in a common ancestor, may have arisen from the same tissue in embryonic development, or may be due to DNA sequences that come from a common ancestor that produce common proteins. Sequence homology may indicate a common function. Conservation of the genetic code occurs to maintain beneficial functionality.
- **Homoplasies**: Homoplasies are structures that are similar but have a different origin. Homoplasies are indicative of convergent evolution in which similar structures independently evolved in different species.
- **Fossils**: Traces of previously existing organisms have demonstrated the changes that have occurred in species. Differences have emerged over time that can be documented. Fossil records reveal physical evidence of both similarities and new differences.
- **Vestigial traits**: Vestigial traits are rudimentary structures that no longer exhibit any functionality or exhibit reduced functionality. They may be homologous to organs or structures in closely related species.
- **Molecular biology**: Molecular biology is used to compare the nucleotide sequences in the DNA and RNA and the amino acid sequences in the proteins of organisms. The more subunit sequences that correspond, the more closely related two species are. DNA nucleotide sequences can also be examined for the number of differences. This can reveal how much time has passed since two species branched from a common ancestor, serving as a **molecular clock.**
- **Biogeography**: The distribution of species throughout history and across geographical areas and the additional consideration of paleobiogeography and plate tectonics have bolstered the supporting evidence for evolution. Fossil history and molecular biology have been used to map the evolution and migration of species as continents split and drifted away from one another.

Ecology

At the cross section between organisms and everything that is external to them (the environment) are the interactions between them. The study of ecology focuses on the living or **biotic** environment surrounding an organism, the nonliving or **abiotic** environment, and the interactions of organisms and populations with one another and the environment. The abiotic environment includes the topographical geology of the area in which the organism lives and the temperature, climate, and access to nutrients, water, and light. The biotic environment encompasses all living organisms that impact the organism's life. This includes those it comes in direct contact with and those whose presence impacts its physical environment in some way. Human beings are almost always the most potent force affecting any organism's environment due to pollution, predation, agriculture, encroachment on habitats and waterways, urban usage, and a myriad of other environmental impacts.

Ecological Organization

The following list provides definitions for basic terminology associated with ecological organization.

- **Organism/species:** An organism is an individual of one particular type. Breeding begins at this level. Organisms are the units of a single population, and they are the fundamental unit of any ecological system.
- **Population:** A population is an individual group of organisms. All organisms are of the same species. They live together in the same location and are affected by the same limitations in the availability of food, water, and shelter. They experience the same geography, climate, temperature, rainfall, and sunlight availability.
- **Community:** A community is all of the populations of different species of organisms living in a particular area. Each group is one population. This includes animal life, plant life, insect life, and bacteria. All kingdoms are likely, but not necessarily, represented: Archaeabacteria, Eubacteria, Protista, Fungi, Plantae, and Animalia. Communities are sometimes referred to as biotic communities to make the clear distinction that communities are living organisms. The ecosystem includes the abiotic environment.
- **Ecosystem:** The ecosystem includes the nonliving environment (the air, water, sun, soil, and topography) as well as the community. The community of organisms impacts the nonliving environment, and the nonliving environment impacts the community of organisms.
- **Biosphere:** The biosphere is the entire planet Earth and all of its communities. The biosphere includes the atmosphere, hydrosphere, and lithosphere. The air, oceans and waterways, and rock and soil composition all both support and impact how the ecosystems operate.

The Environment

The environment in which communities live includes the water, temperature, sunlight, oxygen supply, and soil or rock (substratum of the earth). It also includes how organisms interact and impact one another's existence. The most important constituent of the environment is the availability of water. It dictates what species can inhabit an area. Low water availability necessitates that the species in a community have adaptations that enable them to store and conserve water. Temperature also dictates the species that can inhabit an ecosystem. Extremes of heat and cold also necessitate adaptations to withstand inclemency.

Since all stored usable energy is from photosynthesis, sunlight is necessary to some degree to support life. One exception is the chemoautotrophs, the chemosynthetic bacteria that do not need sunlight to synthesize organic compounds from inorganic raw material. Plant adaptations have evolved to enable some species to thrive in low light environments. Marine life is divided into two zones. The part of the water depth that obtains sunlight is the **photic zone**.

This is the top section in which photosynthesis is possible and where the major productivity of the body of water takes place. When a depth is reached in which less than 1% of light penetrates, the **aphotic zone** begins. This zone is substantial in size in the ocean. Heterotrophic life forms have developed that can live in low to no light. There are a number of species that have developed bioluminescence and can produce their own light.

Oxygen availability is generally not an issue for organisms that live primarily on the land. These terrestrial life forms can obtain their oxygen from the nearly 20% of the air that is comprised of this element. However, aquatic life forms must be able to obtain oxygen in sufficient quantities from the dissolved content in the water. **Dead zones** are becoming disturbingly common in waterways around the world. Sudden oxygen depletion causes mass die-offs of single species or of numerous species of fish and other aquatic life such as crabs, eels, and stingrays. Sometimes it is due to an overpopulation of phytoplankton that thrive on increases in the nitrogen and phosphorous content. When these species of phytoplankton proliferate, an occurrence called **algal bloom** happens. The algae are photosynthetic during the day, but at night, due to their vast numbers, they deplete the oxygen through normal cellular respiration.

When the population dies and bacteria begin to decompose them, oxygen is further depleted. This can be caused by human or **anthropogenic** activities such as fertilizer use and agricultural runoff, sewage runoff, and the environmental degradation that accompanies urban areas, including air and water pollution and hazardous materials. Low tides and high temperatures, changes in wind and water circulation, and stagnant entryways to enclosed bodies of water and the attendant high sedimentation are among the natural causes. Recently, in the British Petroleum oil disaster in the Gulf of Mexico, scientists have been concerned that the oil-eating microbes used to clean the spill could cause a larger than normal dead zone due to their oxygen consumption.

Finally, the substratum of the earth also dictates the species that can inhabit an environment. The soil pH, available minerals, particularly nitrates and phosphates, and the soil texture, composition, and humus content all play a role. Some plants require soil tending toward acidic pH, whereas others require soil tending toward more alkaline pH. Plants that require high water content in the soil cannot thrive in sandy or rocky soils. Soil lacking in minerals can produce weak plants. The species of plants that can grow on beaches are limited by their ability to tolerate that environment. The lower beach lacks plants due to the movement of sand and water. A few plants can grow in pure sand, provided it is stable. Humus, which is generated by decaying plants and animals, has the ability to hold and release soil nutrients due to its high cation exchange capacity. It also helps with water retention and the development of good soil structure.

Populations and the Ecosystem

The populations and communities within an ecosystem interact in various ways that affect the available resources and energy sources. The **habitat** is defined as the natural environment in which a population lives. The **niche** encompasses the habitat plus all functionality of the population, including its nutrient and climate requirements and how it accomplishes the fundamental tasks of life such as nutrient uptake, foraging methods, predation or predator avoidance, mating, and finding or building shelter. It also includes the population's place in the food chain, the parasites and pathogens it deals with and whether those relationships are harmful or beneficial, and how it responds to either an abundance or a scarcity of resources. It encompasses all phases of life and all attributes and qualities of its existence. Two different species cannot occupy the same niche indefinitely. Eventually one will outcompete the other. This is known as the **competitive exclusion principle**.

Even within species there can be two populations that occupy different niches. If two groups in the same species have different migration patterns or different food resources, they occupy two separate niches. Competition within a niche is therefore within the same species. However, two populations can occupy similar niches and competition for resources can overlap. If one population outcompetes the other, the less adept species can be driven to extinction. If one population outcompetes the other only in a certain geographical area and the other species excels in a different environment, they may each be eliminated in the less desirable locale for their species. Finally, under intense competition, there are evolutionary pressures to adapt to conditions and the two species may undergo divergent evolution.

The interactions between organisms vis-à-vis their nutrient uptake methods are discussed toward the beginning of this chapter under the heading "Ecological Classifications." Organisms are classified according to how they obtain their nutrients and what their nutritional requirements are, whether they are producers, primary consumers, or secondary consumers, and how their nutritional requirements intersect with the other populations in the community and with the ecosystem. These designations are: autotrophs, heterotrophs, decomposers, herbivores, carnivores, omnivores, and detritivores.

The populations within a community do not live in isolation. Besides competition for resources, there are interdependencies. These interdependencies are referred to as **interspecific interactions**. The four main categories of interspecific interactions are symbiosis, predation, saprophytism, and scavenging. The three main types of symbiotic relationships were discussed in the "Evolution" section. Predators feed on other living organisms. Carnivores are predators, but herbivores that consume autotrophs are also considered predators. The predator-prey relationship often tends toward an equilibrium in which the predator keeps proliferation of the prey population within the sustenance capacity of the ecosystem. If the prey population grows too large, environmental degradation may result in the total elimination of the prey population. The predator therefore plays a regulatory role. Although this is the most common occurrence, there are instances in which the predator can cause a substantial decrease in the prey population or its geographical distribution, or even cause its extinction.

Saprophytes are the decomposers in the Fungi and Protista kingdoms. They absorb the nutrients from the breakdown of dead matter. Mold, mushrooms, some bacteria, and slime molds are saprophytes. Scavengers eat dead animals. They contribute to the process of decomposition, which the decomposers then complete. Detritivores ingest dead or decaying organisms (mostly plants) and fecal material.

Interactions within the same species can include beneficial and cohesive actions such as cooperation to protect one another from predators, reproduction (although there can be competition for mates), and community building. The main disruptive force is competition for resources. Organisms within the same population must compete with one another for food, water, and shelter. When resources are limited, intraspecies competition can be intense.

Organisms and the Environment

Adaptations to maintain thermoregulation and osmoregulation have enabled organisms to live in challenging environments. For example, saltwater fish must drink lots of water and secrete lots of salt through their gills in order to live in their hypertonic, or hyperosmotic, environment. Freshwater fish, by contrast, must drink very little and absorb salt through their gills in order to live in their hypotonic, or hypo-osmotic, environment. Insects must conserve water, so they excrete solid uric acid crystals rather than liquid urine. The camel is the prototypical example of an organism with adaptations that allow it to live in extremes of heat with limited available water. With food resources scarce in the desert, adipose tissue in the hump can store food for up to two weeks. To conserve water, camels are capable of handling large swings in body temperature. Their body temperature can fluctuate between 94 and 105 degrees Fahrenheit. They do not need to sweat until they reach the upper temperatures in this range.

Recall that cellular respiration is an oxidation reaction in which carbon-hydrogen bonds are broken as a molecule of glucose is catabolized. This degradative process is exergonic. There is less energy in the products, and heat is released. In fact, as energy is transferred into the high-energy phosphate bonds of ATP, approximately 60% of the energy is lost as heat. In cold-blooded or **poikilothermic** animals, this heat is mainly released to the environment. Because the body temperature of poikilotherms is roughly in sync with their environment and metabolism is linked to body temperature, these plants and animals must increase and decrease their activity level in response to changes in temperature. When it gets cold they drastically slow down. Warm-blooded or **homoeothermic** animals have developed adaptations such as hair, fur, feathers, and fat that control heat dissipation. Because they maintain a constant body temperature that is usually higher than the environment and do not need to tailor their activity levels to the outside temperature, homeotherms can live in a wider range of habitats.

Food Chains and Food Webs

Food chains and food webs are methods for charting the energy flow through ecosystems. The energy flow begins with photosynthesis, the source of all stored usable energy, which is stored in the carbon-hydrogen bond. In food chains, energy is depicted as being transferred from the primary producers to the primary consumers, and from the primary consumers to the secondary consumers. If there are tertiary consumers, energy transfer continues to them. The decomposers are the end of the food chain. Each position on the food chain is referred to as a **trophic level**. The trophic level indicates what an organism eats and which organisms eat it.

The primary producers are the autotrophic photosynthetic green plants and algae and the photosynthetic and chemosynthetic bacteria. **Chemosynthetic bacteria** do not use sunlight. The sulfate reducers manufacture carbohydrates from the oxidation of sulfates. The nitrate reducers manufacture carbohydrates from the oxidation of ammonia or nitrates. These chemical compounds seep up from the earth's crust. These ancient life forms live near hydrothermal vents at the bottom of the ocean. The primary consumers include the animals that eat green plants, the herbivores. The secondary consumers are the carnivores, which consume the herbivores. Tertiary consumers are carnivores that eat other carnivores.

The autotrophs, herbivores, and carnivores excrete waste materials during their lifetimes and ultimately perish. The anabolic processes by which their bodies have been built into complex structures must now be reversed.

Entropy continues. At each step in the chain, energy has been lost as it is transferred. Energy has also been used in the procurement of food and for the necessary metabolic processes to continue life against the force of entropy. Each of these activities entails a loss of energy as heat. This is where the decomposers, including the saprophytes, bacteria of decay, and fungi, enter the food chain. Catabolic processes break down waste materials and dead tissues into less complex products, releasing energy yet again. Nitrates and phosphates are returned to the soil to begin the cycle anew.

The food web takes into account the more complex nature of the energy flow through ecosystems. The food chain represents the flow in a linear fashion. In fact, consumption is not linear. Most species are consumed by one or more other species that are not all equals on the ladder. There are in fact branches, and most animals are part of several interconnected food chains. Stability in a community is dependent on the number of branches of the food web. The existence of lots of varied predator-prey branches that link high trophic levels to intermediate and low trophic levels increases food web stability.

Pyramid diagrams are used to represent the flow of a substance through an ecosystem. The pyramid of energy starts at the wide base where the most energy is stored in the photosynthetic green plants. At each level, the amount of energy that is absorbed, the amount of energy that is consumed by the next trophic level, and the amount lost as heat and to the death of organisms are all approximated. A scant 10% to 15% of the absorbed energy is transferred up to the next level. The decomposers are where the least amount of energy is stored. The end products of decomposition will be continually smaller and will continually contain less energy as they are returned to the lowest-energy-level molecules and atoms. However, most pyramids of energy depict the tertiary carnivores at the top supported by all of the higher energy levels.

The pyramid of mass is a representation of the loss of **biomass**. The ecological definition of biomass is the mass of all of the living organisms in an ecosystem at a particular time. From the base upward, each level of the biomass pyramid gets smaller because each level can support a progressively smaller biomass in the level above. The mass of the producers is greater than the combined mass of all of the consumers.

The pyramid of numbers is a representation of the numbers of organisms at each level. The top trophic levels contain consumers that are generally larger and weigh more than the lower-level organisms. However, at the lower levels, the total mass is larger because there are far more total numbers of organisms. The tertiary consumers are at the top with the smallest total mass and the smallest number of organisms. It takes many more of each lower trophic level to support the trophic level above it.

Biomes

Biomes are large communities that have developed adaptations that enable them to survive in a certain climate or under a certain set of environmental requirements. These conditions exist across a wide geographic area. They are named for the chief form of vegetation in the geographical area. This is referred to as the **climax vegetation**. These predominant plant forms will establish themselves after a succession of simpler plants have been briefly established and then replaced by progressively more complex communities of vegetation until the most stable community emerges. The assumption is that no anthropogenic activities have interfered. A **climax animal population** that is suited to this plant community will also emerge. Terrestrial or land biomes include those for deserts, grasslands, tundra, polar regions, tropical rain forests, temperate coniferous and temperate deciduous forest, and taigas.

Desert biomes consist of water-conserving plants and animals that have adapted a superior ability to thermoregulate. There are few mammals or birds, and insects and lizards live underground to survive the harsh temperatures.

Grassland biomes contain relatively higher, but still minimal rainfall adaptive communities. Fire is an important component of this biome as it suppresses woody vegetation. Shelter under trees is not available for animal life. Grassland adaptations include long limbs and hoofs to enable swift ground coverage over flat terrain. The Great Plains of the United States west of the Mississippi and east of the Rocky Mountain range are one example.

Taiga biomes contain communities that can withstand low rainfall and harsh winters. The northern portions of the taiga also have permafrost. Permafrost is soil that has been steadily at or below 0°C (32°F) for two or more years. Ice is usually seen, although it may not be seen if the soil is nonporous. Taiga regions are found in northern Canada and Russia. Evergreen conifers are the dominant tree that can survive these conditions. Several species of fir, spruce, and larch cover the ground with their needles, providing ideal growing conditions for moss and lichens. Animal life consists chiefly of the moose with some black bear and wolf and a few bird species.

Tundra biomes are north of taiga biomes and are frozen plains for much of the year. There is no tree growth due to the frozen conditions in the long winters and the soggy marshy conditions when the ice melts during the short spring and summer. Moisture-loving ground cover such as mosses and lichen predominate. Animal life includes polar bears, musk oxen, and Arctic hens.

The polar region north of the tundra biomes is not a biome. It is frozen year-round such that no vegetation can grow and land animals cannot survive. Aquatic life forms do exist in the polar region.

Tropical rain forest biomes consist of communities that can tolerate massive rainfall and temperatures that remain above freezing throughout the year. Evergreen vegetation provides an impenetrable cover for the forest floor. Closely packed trees are covered in vines and **epiphytes**, air plants that rest atop other plants or the branches of other plants and obtain their water and nutrients from the air, rain, and the surfaces of the plants upon which they grow. The perpetually wet forest floor provides the ideal environment for saprophytic bacteria and fungi. The Amazon river basin and Central America are home to important rain forest biomes. There are also rain forests in Central Africa and Southeast Asia. Rain forests are rife with animal life. Some have not yet been identified or examined. Bird species proliferate. Reptiles and amphibians inhabit the forest floors. Insects abound. Monkeys inhabit the forest canopy and sloths hang by their tails. Iguanas and pythons also live in the canopy. The understory is home to chameleons, a type of lizard, tree frogs, and in the Amazon, jaguars.

Temperate deciduous forest biomes are hospitable to many communities due to their average rainfall amounts. Though the summers are hot and the winters are cold, these are much more favorable climes than the more northerly coniferous forest biome and the taiga and tundra of the far north. The deciduous trees that flourish here include beech, oak, hickory, maple, willow, basswood, linden, walnut, sweet gum, poplar, birch, locust, ash, elm, sycamore, and sassafras. These top-story trees are joined by shorter understory trees such as dogwood and red bud and evergreens such as hemlock and pine. The distribution varies with the particulars of latitude and rainfall. Deciduous temperate forest biomes stretch from southern Ontario in Canada to central and southeastern United States. There are also biomes of this type in Central Europe. Animal life includes squirrels, woodchucks, rabbits, foxes, deer, bobcats, and black bear.

Temperate coniferous forests are further north or in higher-elevation areas. Rainfall is not sufficient for many of the deciduous trees, which are replaced by spruce, fir, pine and cedars. These needle-shaped leaves are a water conservation adaptation. This is a colder biome found in the most northern parts of the United States and in the tallest mountains in North Carolina and in southern Canada. Animal life includes the gray wolf, pine-tar vole, field mouse, jack rabbit, lynx, and weasel.

Aquatic biomes are not classified according to predominant vegetation. Instead they are classified according to saline content. There are two general types of aquatic biomes: freshwater and marine. The importance of aquatic biomes is underscored by the fact that 90% of the oxygen and food for the earth is produced in these areas.

Marine biomes have more stable temperature ranges than terrestrial biomes because water absorbs the heat from the sun without sustaining wide swings in temperature. Nutrient, salt, and mineral contents and oxygen and carbon dioxide levels are also fairly entrenched, conferring a comparatively stable environment. In addition, the dissolved and suspended solutes are largely consistent over wide expanses of water. Despite this consistency, there are still well-defined ocean zones. The **intertidal zone** is the beach area that is revealed when the water level ebbs at low tide. Intertidal zone inhabitants include crabs, starfish, clams, snails, sea urchins, sponges, and algae. The **littoral zone** extends out from the high tide mark at the spray region near the shore and follows the continental shelf outward to the edge of the continental slope. The continental shelf can be from only a few miles wide to over 900 miles wide. The littoral zone reaches depths of 600 feet. Inhabitants include crabs, crustaceans, many fish species and algae.

The **pelagic zone** comprises the ocean that is removed from the shore but not at great depths. It is derived from the Greek word for open seas. The photic and aphotic zones are subdivisions of the pelagic zone. In the topmost **photic zone**, phytoplankton photosynthesize and nekton swim. Nekton are all of the swimming organisms in an aquatic zone. The nekton in the photic zone include sharks, many species of fish, and whales, which eat the plankton. The most common primary producer is an alga called a **diatom**. In the **aphotic zone**, only heterotrophs can live since less than 1% of sunlight penetrates. The inhabitants here have adaptations to withstand cold water, darkness, and high water pressure. Surprisingly, there are substantial competitive forces in play. On the seabed, or **benthic zone**, are the **benthos**, organisms that either are permanently attached (sessile) or can perform crawling movements. They include sea stars, oysters, clams, sea cucumbers, brittle stars, and sea anemones.

Freshwater biomes are found in bodies of water with salt concentrations that are usually less than 1%, such as ponds and lakes, rivers and streams, and wetlands. Rivers brought prehistoric marine life to the land. Some eventually developed land adaptations and emerged from the water. Others developed freshwater adaptations so that they could remain aquatic. Some adaptations were necessary because freshwater is hypotonic to the body cells of the fish. Conversely, the fish cells are hypertonic to the environmental water. There are a lot more solutes inside the cells than there are outside the skin cells in the freshwater environment. Therefore, the osmotic drive is for water to enter the cells. Freshwater fish drink very little, if any, water. The water that enters through the gills and the skin is shuttled to the kidneys and excreted in large amounts of dilute urine. The kidneys have been modified so that they can absorb salts from body fluids before excretion, and changes to the gills enable them to retain salts while still diffusing soluble gases. Freshwater fish also needed to develop strong muscles in order to combat swift currents in rivers and streams.

Freshwater protists such as paramecia and amoebae have large contractile vacuoles to withstand the influx of water. For organisms with cell walls such as paramecia, turgor pressure is the force exerted against the cell wall by fluids inside the cell. Since osmotic pressure is pushing water into the cell, the contractile vacuole is designed to remove it and prevent the cell from undergoing osmotic lysis. Amoebae, which do not have cell walls, also have a contractile vacuole that functions to excrete excess water and waste materials from the cytoplasm. Plants in rushing streams and rivers also have needed to adapt. Those that have survived developed **holdfasts**, rootlike anchoring structures that enabled them to remain sessile, particularly when storms churned up muddy river beds. This is one way in which freshwater biomes contrast with marine biomes with respect to stability.

Freshwater biomes also endure much wider swings in temperature. Smaller bodies of water can freeze in the winter or dry up in the summer. Rivers and streams acquire sediment from upstream at their mouths. Churning sediment prevents light from penetrating, making it more difficult for plant life to flourish. This in turn decreases the oxygen available to fish. Fish such as catfish and carp have adapted to these low oxygen levels and can live here, whereas other fish cannot.

Vertebrate Embryology

The life cycle of animals begins with a fertilized egg or **zygote**. It is a diploid (2N) cell that undergoes mitosis to grow. Cell differentiation occurs as the zygote develops into a multicellular organism. Fertilization occurs in the fallopian (uterine) tubes, also referred to, in particular in nonmammalian vertebrates, as the oviducts. It occurs within 12 to 24 hours after ovulation when a sperm makes its way from the vagina through the cervix and uterus and into a fallopian tube. The enlarged region at the end of a uterine tube is called the **ampulla**. The ampulla ends in an open funnel-shaped structure called the **infundibulum**, which has cilia called **fimbriae** that create a current to draw the egg into the ampulla where fertilization typically occurs.

After fertilization, a process called **cleavage** occurs. This is rapid mitotic cell division with a rapid increase in the number of cells but no cell growth. The result is a ball, called a **morula,** of 16 small cells called **blastomeres.** Since cleavage results in a solid ball of 16 blastomeres equal in size to the original fertilized zygote, a favorable surface area-to-volume ratio enables efficient nutrient and gas exchange. At this point, about three to four days after fertilization, the morula goes to the uterus. Within another day, the morula differentiates, developing an interior space that becomes filled with fluid called the **blastocoel.** After this process, called **blastulation,** has occurred, the now-hollow ball of cells is called a **blastula** or **blastocyst.**

Implantation in the uterine wall can now commence. After implantation, the sphere invaginates such that the single layer of cells that formed the blastula sphere becomes a three-layer ball of cells that is indented to form a cavity in the center. This process called **gastrulation** forms the **gastrula.** The cavity or pouch at the center of the gastrula, where the blastula is invaginated, is called the **archenteron.** It is also called the primitive gut. The opening into the archenteron is the **blastopore.**

The three layers are the **germ cell** layers from which all body tissues descend. The outer layer is the **ectoderm.** The middle layer is the **mesoderm,** and the inner layer is the **endoderm.** Nervous tissue and many tissues of the integumentary system derive from the ectoderm. This includes the epidermis, hair, and nails and the epithelial tissue of the mouth, nose, and anal canal. The lens and retina also arise from the ectoderm. All connective tissue is derived from the **mesoderm.** This includes bone, blood, cartilage, and the extracellular matrix and collagen. Muscles, the excretory system, the gonads and parts of the liver, pancreas, thyroid gland and lining of the bladder also arise from the mesoderm. The endoderm is the germ layer responsible for the epithelial tissue that lines the digestive and respiratory tracts. Parts of the pancreas, liver, lining of the bladder and thyroid gland also arise from the endoderm.

A **notochord** also develops longitudinally under the ectoderm during gastrulation. It signals the ectoderm above it to begin forming the **neural plate,** which folds linearly to form the cylindrical **neural tube.** The neural tube will eventually develop into the brain and spinal cord. The process of **neurulation** is when the edges of the neural folds join to from the neural tube. Cells at the edges of the folds called **neural crest cells** form the roof plate of the neural tube. The neural tube separates from the ectoderm and the neural crest cells go through a process called **epithelial to mesenchymal transition.** Among other effects, this makes the cells mobile. They form four populations of cells, which migrate across the surface areas and differentiate into many different types of cells.

The **cranial neural crest cells** become the cranial ganglia and craniofacial cartilages and bones. They also form parts of the thymus, bones of the middle ear, and the odontoblasts, the stem cells of the dentin that comprises the bulk of the teeth. The **trunk neural crest cells** divide into two groups. One group becomes **melanocytes,** which are found in the deepest layer of the epidermis, the **stratum basale.** Melanocytes manufacture the pigment **melanin,** which gives skin color and protects against ultraviolet (UV) damage. The other group becomes dorsal root ganglia, sympathetic ganglia, the medulla of the adrenal gland, and neurons around the aorta. The **vagal** and **sacral neural crest cells** become parasympathetic ganglia. The **cardiac neural crest cells** become melanocytes, cartilage, connective tissue, neurons of some of the pharyngeal arches, and parts of the heart septum and larger arteries. The neural crest is a defining characteristic of the vertebrate evolutionary path. Neural crest cell differentiation produces many of the structures that are common to the vertebrate monophyletic taxon or clade.

Neurulation is the first step in **organogenesis,** the development of the three germ cell layers into the internal organs. In order for this to happen, cells must differentiate, communicate, transform, migrate, elongate, broaden, invaginate, create linear folds, undergo other shape changes, and multiply. The other stages of internal development are organ growth, which is an ongoing progression through adulthood, and gametogenesis, the production of the gametes in a mature organism.

Amniotes are vertebrates that have a multilayered membrane system to protect the embryo inside the body. The amniotes are mammals, reptiles, birds, and extinct mammal-like reptiles and dinosaurs. All of the tetrapods that are not amphibians are amniotes. Fish, sharks, rays, and amphibians are not amniotes. For these animals, there are also external components to development. They lay their eggs in the water where they are fertilized. Embryos that develop externally in an egg have a yolk. The yolk in **oviparous** (egg-laying) animals is composed of saturated fatty acids, unsaturated fatty acids, and all of the fat soluble vitamins (A, D, E, and K). It also contains phosphorylated proteins that bind to and store iron and calcium to nourish the maturing embryo. Oviparous amniotes (reptiles, birds, and monotremes) are terrestrial.

Monotremes are egg-laying mammals (platypuses and echidnas or spiny anteaters). The egg is fertilized internally prior to laying. **Ovoviviparous** amniotes produce eggs internally. They develop inside the mother's body, where they also hatch. They are nourished on unfertilized eggs in the uterus and born alive. Ovoviviparous amniotes include some fish and some snakes.

All eggs provide shelter. There are four protective egg membranes.

1. **Chorion:** The chorion is the outer membrane that protects the embryo in all reptiles, birds, and mammals. On shelled eggs it is the next layer after the shell. Its function is gas exchange. Fish and amphibians, are not amniotes and do not have a chorion.
2. **Allantois:** The allantois forms a sac. It develops from the posterior of the gastrointestinal (GI) tract of the embryo and is instrumental in gas exchange (O_2 and CO_2), water and salt exchange, and nitrogenous waste removal. Oviparous amniotes (birds, most reptiles, and monotremes) have a large allantois to store waste products. A network of blood vessels performs these tasks, except for marsupials, which have an avascular allantois. In placental mammals, the allantois forms a stalk for the development of the umbilical cord and is part of it. Fish and amphibians do not have an allantois.
3. **Amnion:** The amnion contains the amniotic fluid, which functions as a protective cushion for the embryo. The amnion membrane develops the amniotic sac in reptiles, birds, and mammals. Fish and amphibians do not have an amnion.
4. **Yolk sac:** The final membrane encloses the yolk, which nourishes the egg. A network of blood vessels supplies the embryo with food. Oviparous amniotes have a large external yolk sac that contains nutritional stores. In bony fishes, sharks, reptiles, birds, and lower mammals, the yolk sac is attached to the embryo. In humans, the yolk sac performs all of the roles of the circulatory system before the embryonic circulatory system is functioning. It can be seen at around five weeks of gestation and is the first component of the gestational sac that can be seen on ultrasound. Fish and amphibians have only this membrane surrounding the embryo.

Within the vertebrate clade, some fetuses develop with a placenta and some without. **Viviparous** (live-bearing) amniotes (most mammals and some reptiles) have little or no yolk. They are nourished through the placenta. The placenta has a fetal component and a maternal component. It is comprised of uterine endometrium and some or all of the egg membranes and is the primary site of gas exchange. The maternal component is called the **decidua basalis**. Most placental or **eutherian** mammals have a placenta in which the fetal component is formed by chorion and allantois. In humans, the allantois plays a limited role, furnishing circulation to the chorion (or placenta). Marsupials do not have a placenta. Gas and nutritional exchange between the mother and baby is restricted without a placenta. This leads to premature births. Marsupials therefore incubate their young in a pouch (marsupium).

In human beings, pregnancy is 266 days long, which approximates to the nine-month time period normally cited. It takes the fertilized egg several days to get to the fallopian tube and from six to 12 days for the blastocyst to imbed in the uterus. For developmental purposes, gestation is divided into three trimesters. At three weeks postconception, the embryo is about one week old and the brain, spinal cord, heart, and GI tract have all begun to develop.

When the embryo is between two and three weeks old, the appendages have begun to develop, and at around 22 days the heart begins beating. The eyes and ears begin to develop and there are the beginnings of circulation through the main blood vessels. When the embryo is four weeks old, the lungs, jaw, nose, and palate begin to develop, and the hands and feet are webbed, the rudimentary beginnings of the fingers and toes. Complex brain growth is happening, and the heartbeat may be audible.

When the embryo is five weeks old, all vital organs have started to develop. Hair and nipple follicles, the eyelids, and the tongue have all begun to develop. At gestational week eight, when the embryo is six weeks old, the ears are continuing to develop, the cartilaginous skeleton is turning to bone, and the muscles can already contract. The length of the embryo is around one inch and it is now a fetus. Between seven and 11 weeks, the fetus grows to about three inches long and about one ounce in weight. The gender of the fetus has been established and the genitals are developing. The eyelids close over the eyes and will stay closed until the 28th week of pregnancy.

The second trimester begins in the 14th week postconception when the fetus is 12 weeks old. In the following two weeks the **lanugo**, fine hair, can be seen on the head. Sucking starts and fragments of amniotic fluid are ingested. The fingerprints have formed; the intestinal tract forms meconium, which will be the first bowel movement; and sweat glands have also formed. The pancreas and liver are now making secretions and the approximately four-ounce fetus is about six inches long. When the fetus is between 15 and 18 weeks of age, the eyebrows and eyelashes develop. Fingernails and toenails have started to develop, and the skin is beginning to be covered with **vernix**, a thick white substance that protects the skin from the amniotic fluid. When the fetus is between 19 and 21 weeks old, the adipose tissue under the skin begins to develop and the heretofore transparent skin becomes opaque. The eyes have fully developed and the liver and pancreas are continuing to rapidly develop. The fetus is about ten to 11 inches long and weighs between one and one and a quarter pounds. When the fetus is between 22 and 24 weeks old, the sleep-wake cycles have developed, the startle reflex is evident, and the alveoli in the lungs have begun to develop. There is some nervous system function, and the brain is about to undergo rapid development.

As the third trimester begins, at 28 weeks postconception and a fetal age of 26 weeks, fat storage is rapidly occurring. The fetus now weighs four to four and a half pounds and is about 15 to 17 inches long. Breathing is becoming regular, although the lungs have not completely developed. The bones have ossified to some extent but are still soft. The fetus can now store calcium, iron, and phosphorous and the eyelids reopen. When the fetus is between 31 and 34 weeks of age, it normally turns head downward and rapid weight gain is occurring. When the fetus is between 35 and 38 weeks of age, all organs are developed fully, although the lungs continue to develop until birth. At 38 weeks of age, the fetus is full-term; it is between 19 and 22 inches long and weighs six and a half to over ten pounds. Fetal movement has decreased due to limited room to move around. The mother is sending antibodies to the fetus to safeguard it from disease.

Labor begins with the cervix thinning and dilating. The amniotic sac breaks and amniotic fluid is released. In the second stage of labor, contractions increase in frequency, intensity, and duration. After the baby emerges and the umbilical cord is cut, the third stage of labor soon commences. This is when the placenta and umbilical cord are discharged.

Microbiology

Twenty percent of the questions (about 9 to 19 questions) on the biology section of the PCAT exam will be on microbiology topics.

Microorganisms

There are five basic groups of microorganisms:

1. **Bacteria:** Bacteriology is the study of bacteria.
2. **Viruses:** Virology is the study of viruses.
3. **Fungi:** Mycology is the study of fungi. There are two general groups of fungi based on morphological characteristics: **yeasts** and **molds.**
4. **Algae:** Phycology is the study of algae. Algae have no medical importance.
5. **Protozoa:** Protozoology is the study of protozoa.

Bacteria and viruses are the most important infectious enemies in the United States. Viruses are not classified in a kingdom. They are not alive and thus cannot be killed. They are nonliving and noncellular and thus harder to eliminate. We can only inactivate them or lessen the damage they cause.

Microorganisms have the following general characteristics.

- **Extremely small.** Microscopic organisms are measured in micrometers (1 μm = 10^{-6}m) and nanometers (1 nm = 10^{-9}m).
- **Most are unicellular.** Most are single-celled or acellular, such as viruses.
- **Simplicity.** They are not dependent on any other cell. This self-sufficiency and independence from other cells means that if you leave one survivor, a whole new growth of cells will occur.
- **Tough to attack.** Their simplicity means that they are difficult to destroy. More complex creatures are much easier to kill.

Microorganisms can be classified into three basic categories:

1. **Pathogens:** True pathogens are microorganisms that will always cause some harm. They harm us as they work for their own survival. The amount of harm they inflict is determined by the immune system—how the body is able to respond to their presence.
2. **Opportunistic pathogens:** Normal microorganisms that cause harm when the conditions are right. One such condition would be a suppressed immune system. Another would be that the pathogen has moved to a different location in the body from its usual location, where it can coexist in a symbiotic relationship.
3. **Nonpathogens:** Microorganisms that almost never cause harm. However, even the mildest can cause harm under certain conditions.

Around 99% of microorganisms are nonpathogens. Some are very beneficial. *E. coli* are mainly beneficial; however, they can become opportunistic. For example, *Lactobacillus acidophilus* is a generally beneficial microorganism in the vagina. It maintains the acid environment that prohibits yeast growth. However, under certain suppressed immune system circumstances such as chemotherapy treatment, it can cause serious infections.

Bacteria

Bacteria can be classified by shape, and by oxygen, temperature, pH, and nutritional requirements. This section reviews these classifications, as well as the bacterial growth cycle, the functions of various bacterial structures, such as the bacterial cell wall, cell membrane, flagella, pili, cytoplasm, nuclear material, ribosomes, capsules, and endospores, and concludes with a review of various atypical bacteria.

Bacterial Shapes

There are three main bacterial shapes as outlined. Around 99% of bacteria are these shapes. Rarely, a triangular or other odd shape is seen.

1. **Cocci.** Cocci are spherical. They never have flagella. Their average diameter size is 1 μm.
   - Single cocci: **coccus**
   - Two cells: **diplococcus**
   - Chains: **streptococcus**
   - Irregular bunches: **staphylococcus**
   - Groups of four: **tetrad**
   - Cubes of eight: **sarcina**; average width 2 μm
2. **Bacilli.** Rods that can have flagella. They are only 0.5 μm wide and 1 to 5 μm long.
   - Single cells: **bacillus**
   - Pairs: **diplobacillus**
   - Chains: **streptobacillus**
3. **Spirilla.** These are spirals that can have flagella.
   - **Vibrio:** incomplete spiral; half-moon
   - **Spirillum:** multibending spiral; thick; average width 1 μm; 5 to 50 μm long
   - **Spirochete:** thin and flexible with an average width of 5 μm and a length between 5 and 25 μm long.

Oxygen Requirement Classifications

Different types of bacteria have different oxygen requirements:

- **Obligate aerobe**: Obligate aerobes grow only in the presence of oxygen. They get their energy from aerobic respiration.
- **Microaerophile**: Microaerophiles require only a low concentration of oxygen. They get their energy from aerobic respiration.
- **Obligate anaerobe**: Obligate anaerobes grow only without oxygen. They are inhibited or killed in the presence of oxygen. They get their energy from anaerobic respiration or fermentation.
- **Aerotolerant anaerobe**: Aerotolerant anaerobes cannot use oxygen for growth. They get their energy from fermentation but can tolerate oxygen.
- **Facultative anaerobe**: Facultative anaerobes can grow with or without oxygen but usually thrive better in oxygenated environments. They get their energy from aerobic respiration, anaerobic respiration, or fermentation. Most bacteria are facultative anaerobes.

Temperature Classifications

Different types of bacteria also have different temperature requirements:

- **Psychrophile**: Psychrophiles are cold-loving organisms. Their optimum growth temperatures are between –5°C and 15°C. They are found in Arctic and Antarctic regions and streams fed by glaciers.
- **Mesophile**: Mesophiles thrive in moderate temperatures. Their optimum growth temperatures are between 25°C and 45°C. Most bacteria are mesophilic, including soil bacteria and bacteria that live in and on the body.
- **Thermophile**: Thermophiles are heat-loving organisms. Their optimum growth temperatures are between 45°C and 70°C. They are found in hot springs and compost heaps.

- **Hyperthermophile**: Hyperthermophiles are extreme heat-loving organisms. Their optimum growth temperatures are between 70°C and 110°C. They are usually members of *Archaea* and grow near hydrothermal vents at great depths in the ocean, in hot springs such as those in Yellowstone National Park, and in solfataric fields. Solfataric fields are the soil, boiling mud holes, and surface waters above volcanoes. They contain sulfur, have a low salt content, and are fueled by volcanic fumes.

pH Requirements

The pH of human skin is between 5.00 and 6.00. This is acidic due to the fatty acids on the skin surface. The pH of blood is between 7.35 and 7.45, slightly basic. Bacteria generally prefer a pH between 6.8 and 7.2, so bacteria will not grow effectively in our blood; the logarithmic difference between 7.2 and 7.35 is too extreme a difference. The acidity of the skin surface indicates that skin infections are the exception. Children's skin pH is right around 7. This is why they are more prone to skin infections. Salt, brine, and vinegar are used to preserve food. The food does not decompose because the pickling solutions have a lower pH than bacteria can tolerate.

Nutritional Requirements

Organisms take nutrients (substrates) and break them down into their component parts in order to build them back up into their own cell components. Basic nutrients are the energy source that allows cells to work. This could be from light or chemicals, generally sugars, which are high-energy compounds. Cells that get energy from light are **phototrophs**. Cells that get energy from chemical reactions are **chemotrophs**. Photosynthetic bacteria that get their energy from light and produce their own food using environmental carbon dioxide are **photoautotrophs**.

Photosynthetic bacteria that get their energy from light and produce their own nutrients using carbon from sources other than carbon dioxide are **photoheterotrophs**. Chemotrophs that get their energy from inorganic molecules and use carbon dioxide as their carbon source are **chemoautotrophs**. Chemotrophs that get their energy from inorganic molecules and ingest various organic compounds for their carbon source are **chemoheterotrophs**. Chemotrophs that need whole blood or tissue to get energy are **fastidious chemoheterotrophs**.

Some microorganisms must have living cells and tissue as nutrient source. These are **obligate parasites**. Some use only nonliving material as a nutrient source. These are **obligate saprophytes**. Some can get their nutrients from either living cells or nonliving material. These are referred to as **facultative**. However, facultative organisms always have a preference. **Facultative saprophytes** prefer living cells. **Facultative parasites** prefer nonliving material but will take advantage of a living host when it presents itself.

Bacteria need a source of carbon, nitrogen, hydrogen, sulfur, phosphorus, and oxygen. They also need minerals, including iron (Fe), zinc (Zn), potassium (K), and calcium (Ca). Vitamins including niacin, riboflavin, and vitamin B_6, as well as a water source are mandatory. This is why they prefer to live in hosts: Humans and other hosts provide everything they need. Bacteria also have the ability to compete with hosts for nutrients. Iron **chelators** in the bacterial cell wall bind iron and transport it into the bacterium. The human body produces its own iron chelators, so the concentration in the body of free Fe is very low. Bacterial Fe chelators are able to compete successfully with our iron chelators and with those of normal body flora. This characteristic, the ability to get the iron they need from inside our bodies, may be essential to pathogenic bacteria.

Bacterial Growth Cycle

Bacteria reproduce asexually by binary fission in which they split in two. The time required for bacteria to double is called the **generation time (GT)**. The average GT for bacteria is 20 to 30 minutes. If there is one bacterium to start, in 20 to 30 minutes there will be two and in another 20 to 30 minutes there will be four. If there are one million bacteria, in 20 to 30 minutes there will be two million. This is **geometric** or **logarithmic growth**. Humans reproduce arithmetically. From two, we produce a third. Our GT is hard to define, perhaps 12 to 50 years. One couple could take a lifetime to raise just one child. Bacteria are extremely rapid reproducers. Rapid reproduction ensures survival of the species.

Temperature, oxygen levels, pH, and proper nutrition all contribute to the time line for the bacterial growth cycle. The general outline when these requirements are sufficiently met, however, is the following four stages:

1. **Lag time:** This lasts for 20 to 30 minutes and constitutes the generation time (**GT**). It is when a new colony is establishing and beginning to reproduce.
2. **Logarithmic period of growth:** This lasts for 12 to 24 hours and is when active doubling, or active reproduction, occurs.
3. **Stationary period:** This lasts for 24 to 48 hours. There is an equal rate of growth and death, so overall bacterial numbers stay the same.
4. **Decline or death period:** This lasts for 48 to 96 hours and is when rapid cell death by cell lysis occurs. The colony has reached its maximum capacity given the environmental conditions. Cell lysis is now outpacing binary fission. Spore production commences in spore-forming bacteria.

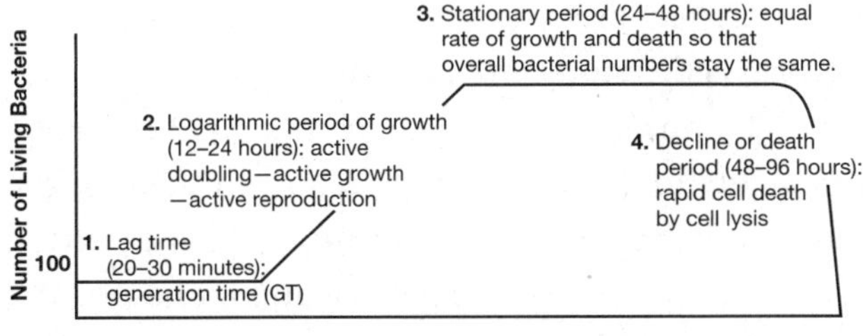
Bacterial Growth Curve
3. Stationary period (24–48 hours): equal rate of growth and death so that overall bacterial numbers stay the same.
2. Logarithmic period of growth (12–24 hours): active doubling—active growth —active reproduction
4. Decline or death period (48–96 hours): rapid cell death by cell lysis
1. Lag time (20–30 minutes): generation time (GT)
Number of Living Bacteria
100
Time

The graph should actually lag and then jump, lag, and then jump. This is what the graph would look like on semilog paper. When the bacteria run out of food and produce waste, the logarithmic period levels off because a lack of nutrients and a buildup of wastes are killing the bacteria. After the stationary period, there is even less food and more waste, leading to the decline period. If the GT were 5 minutes instead of 30, the curve would be even faster or steeper. A shorter GT means a shorter life cycle and a longer GT means a longer life cycle. What antibiotics do is make bacteria die faster, reducing the time it takes to get to the decline period.

Bacterial Cell Wall

The function of the bacterial cell wall is to maintain the size and shape of the bacteria cell and prevent cell lysis. The most important aspect of the chemical composition of the cell wall is the presence of **peptidoglycan** (**PG**). Gram-positive bacteria, which stain dark blue or violet with Gram's staining, has a very thick layer of PG, making the cell wall thicker and more resistant. Gram-negative bacteria, which become decolorized from the Gram's stain, have only a thin layer of PG surrounded by layers of lipoprotein (LP), lipopolysaccharides (LPS), and sugars (polysaccharides). Their cell wall is less durable. The cell wall may or may not play a role in pathogenicity. The cell wall of gram-positive bacteria poses no danger to humans. The gram-negative cell wall, in contrast, can cause harm. The lipopolysaccharide (LPS) layer, which is released when the cell dies, becomes a poison referred to as an **endotoxin**. Endotoxins stimulate inflammation, the body's response to infection, which damages animal cell membranes, causing **necrosis** or cell death. If humans ingest gram-negative bacteria, as they do all the time, the bacteria die in the intestines after two to four days. The endotoxins are released, causing inflammation, which can lead to fluid loss due to diarrhea. Cell necrosis causes bleeding, bloody stool, and scar tissue. About 70% of diarrhea is caused by Gram-negative bacteria. The positive side to this is that it flushes the gastrointestinal tract out. The most common bacterium is Gram-negative *Escherichia coli*. Most strains of *E. coli* are harmless. They are normal flora of the intestines. However, some virulent strains, such as enteroaggregative *E. coli* (EAEC), enterohemorrhagic *E. coli* (EHEC), enteroinvasive *E. coli* (EIEC), enteropathogenic *E. coli* (EPEC), and enterotoxigenic *E. coli* (ETEC), cause serious infections.

The nonpathogenic variety of the gut can also cause infections in other areas of the body. In the gut, a normal manageable endotoxin level has been established. However, if these normal gut flora enter the urinary tract where no level of endotoxins is tolerable, they can colonize the urethra and move upward to the bladder and kidneys or they can infect the prostate in males, causing urethritis, cystitis, nephritis, and prostatitis, respectively. Endotoxins in the bloodstream can cause necrosis of the cells lining the blood vessels, which can lead to hemorrhaging and septic shock (septicemia). The bacterial cell wall is therefore an important target for possible treatments and methods of controlling infections. Penicillins and cephalosporins kill the cell wall by stopping the formation of peptidoglycan (PG). However, they kill only gram-positive bacteria with their thick layer of PG. This is why they are referred to as **narrow spectrum** antibiotics. They are effective only against gram-positive bacteria.

Bacterial Cell Membrane

The main function of the bacterial cell membrane is as the semipermeable barricade for the cell. It regulates the chemicals that enter and leave the cell. It is also the site of cell wall repair. New cell wall pieces, either PG or LPS, are made within seconds to fill in a gap at a damaged site. It is also the site of energy (ATP) production. In bacteria, glycolysis, the Krebs cycle, and the electron transport system all occur on the surface of the cell membrane.

In addition, the cell membrane plays a number of roles in cell division. Bacterial cell division is done by the process of **binary fission**, the simplest form of cell division. The present complement of cytoplasm is split in two. There are two main steps after the DNA is copied. First, the duplicated DNA must separate. The cell membrane chemically attaches to and pulls the copied genetic material apart, separating the DNA copies to opposite sides of the cell. Second, the cell must split in two. The cell membrane forms a new cross wall, called a **septum**, which is an invagination of the membrane from each side of the cell. Next a new cell wall is formed by the membrane. Between the cell wall and the cell membrane is the **periplasmic space**.

The chemical composition of the cell membrane is a phospholipid bilayer, just as it is in all cells. The cell membrane plays no direct role in causing harm. The membrane is not a toxin that is by itself dangerous. Our cell membranes are exactly the same composition as those of bacteria. However, some antibiotics can damage the cell membrane, causing cell leakage. For example, the polymixins, typically found in topical creams used on the skin, are useful against both gram-positive and gram-negative bacteria, because they dissolve the plasma membrane by binding to the phospholipids. Polyene antibiotics such as amphotericin B bind to particular sterols found in the plasma membranes of fungal cells. Other membrane-damaging agents include some disinfectants and some antiseptics.

The difference between antibiotics and **antiseptics** is that antibiotics are generally safe to use on the body. Antiseptics may or may not be safe either on or in the body—for example, bleach and formaldehyde. The more likely use for antiseptics is on surfaces such as table tops. **Disinfectants** such as soaps and detergents work by damaging the cell membranes of bacteria. The method is scrubbing. The soft, scraping abrasive effect of lather action harms the membrane. All soap is therefore antibacterial.

Wounds required the development of synthetic detergents to create chemical action to damage the cell membrane without requiring the lather action that can serve to further open a wound. The first developed were the **quaternary ammonium** compounds, called **quats** for short, which bind to cell membranes and damage them. The active ingredient is ammonium. Second were the **iodophores**, soap plus iodine. These were overused and are potentially detrimental because they destroy not only harmful bacteria but also beneficial bacteria, opening up the possibility for an overgrowth of pathogens. They should be used only for contamination risks such as foods that can harbor pathogenic bacteria, particularly chicken. The third category developed were the **tinctures**, soaps with alcohol. These also damage the cell membrane. Other groups of chemicals that damage the cell membrane are **carbolic acids** (phenols) and **cresols** (methylphenols) found in products such as Lysol, and **hexachlorophene**. When added to soap, these are safe on the skin. Alone they can be used only on surfaces because they are too acidic and are skin irritants.

Bacterial Flagella

Flagella are found on the spirilla and the bacilli, but not on the cocci. Their function is motility. The chemical composition of flagella is a single strand of the protein flagellin. If a bacterium has one flagellum at one end, it is called **polar monotrichous**. Two or more flagella at one end of the cell is **polar lophotrichous**. Two or more flagella at one or both poles is **lophotrichous**. A single flagellum at each pole is **amphitrichous**. If flagella are positioned all around the outside of the cell, it is called **peritrichus** (perimeter). Spirochetes have internally located flagella (**endoflagella**), which wrap around the spirochete toward the middle from both ends. These **axial filaments** are above the peptidoglycan wall but underneath the outer membrane or sheath.

Flagella attach to bacteria by four anchors or rings. From outer to inner, they are classified as the L ring, P ring, S ring, and M ring. The innermost **L ring** attaches to the lipid bilayer. The **P ring** attaches to peptidoglycan in the cell wall. The **S ring** attaches to the periplasmic space, and the **M ring** attaches to the cell membrane. It is mainly Gram-negative bacteria that have flagella. Most cocci are gram-positive. Gram-positive bacteria have flagella with only two rings attached to the plasma membrane, a P ring and an M ring.

Bacterial movement is governed by **taxis**, an innate behavioral response. Bacteria respond to environmental stimuli with directed motility. Positive taxis is movement toward a stimulus, while negative taxis is movement away from a stimulus. **Chemotaxis** describes movement in response to chemicals. **Phototaxis** describes movement in response to light. Bacteria have no sensory structures. They can move away from irritants such as chemicals in the environment or they can move toward certain attractant molecules. The cell membrane is the detector of irritants or attractants. It vibrates. The M ring wobbles, and this is passed throughout the other rings to the flagella, resulting in motility. The bacterium moves either away from the irritant or toward the attractant. Most bacteria move away from light because light gives off heat. In reality they are moving away from the heat. Some cyanobacteria, which are autotrophic, exhibit positive phototaxis, moving toward light. The rings cause a swiveling motion, which causes the flagella to curve around the cell. The flagella must flow one way or the other. The bacterium does not flip; the flagella do. Bacteria prefer dark, damp rooms, which promote growth.

Flagella have no direct role in pathogenicity. However, they can help bacteria to move to places where they can cause harm. Their purpose is to move bacteria through secretions such as those found in the urinary tract. Bacteria with flagella include Gram-negative *Escherichia coli*. Flagella play no role in the treatment or control of bacterial infections. There are no medications to destroy flagella and none being developed, because they would not be useful. Destroying the flagella would not destroy the cell, and furthermore, flagella can regrow. The cell wall can provide the necessary materials to regrow them. Thus, we use antibiotics to kill the cell wall or cell membrane, not the flagella.

Bacterial Pili

Bacterial **pili** or **fimbriae** are structures resembling cilia whose function is attachment. They hold the bacteria securely to a spot. There are three purposes for this action. The first function is to enable bacteria to remain near food sources. For example, in the mouth or intestines many bacteria have pili so that they can hold on to positions where food is readily available; in the mouth, bacterial pili hold on to plaque. The second function is to prevent flushing out. Fluids are the most effective method for removing bacteria, so pili combat this, holding on to the urinary tract, genital tract, respiratory tract, and so on.

The third function is to attach to other bacteria. Using a large pilus, called an **F-pilus**, a DNA bridge is created to transfer genetic material. This process is called **sexual conjugation**. A particular type of bacterium will have **F**$^+$ and **F**$^-$ varieties. F$^+$ have an F-pilus while F$^-$ do not. Contact between the two cells is established using the F-pilus, also called a **sex pilus**. This protein tube is used to pass on antibiotic resistance and the gene, referred to as the **fertility factor** (F-factor), to enable F$^-$ bacteria to make DNA exchanges. How to attack the F-pili or F-factor is one of the top three medical dilemmas.

Pili play no direct role in causing harm. Indirectly they can help bacteria to hold on and to acquire genetic variation.

Gonorrhea is caused by bacteria with pili, *Neisseria gonorrhoeae* (*gono* refers to the genitals, and *rrhea* means discharge). Many diplococcus, such as *N. gonorrhoeae*, are Gram-negative. This is a rare exception to the rule that cocci are mainly Gram-positive. Other Gram-negative diplococci include *Neisseria meningitides*, which causes meningitis, and *Moraxella catarrhalis*, which causes respiratory tract infections. Pili attach bacteria to mucous membranes lining the genital tract, urinary tract, and respiratory tract. *Neisseria gonorrhoeae* attaches to the neutrophils, precluding the neutrophil from phagocytizing the bacterium. More neutrophils are then sent to the area to attack the invader. This vicious cycle creates a massive buildup of neutrophils, which are discharged as pus. In females, 80% of the time gonorrhea is asymptomatic so it goes undetected and spreads. As it continues this cycle of no symptoms, spreading, and no treatment, it eventually reaches the fallopian tubes stuck to the surface of sperm.

Bacterial Nuclear Material

The nuclear material of bacteria is not enclosed in a nuclear membrane. In the cytoplasm, which is 80% water, there are two major structural components, the nuclear material and the ribosomes. The function of the nuclear material is that it determines all cell characteristics and regulates all cell activities. The chemical composition of the nuclear material is deoxyribonucleic acid (DNA), the genetic or nuclear material for all living things. Bacteria have one double-stranded, circular chromosome. If you cut and stretched the circular chromosome out so that it was linear, it would be about 1 mm long. Given that the average bacterium is 1 µm long, this is 1,000 times longer than the bacteria itself. This is an indication of just how tightly packed inside the cell the chromosome is. When the cell dies, the DNA pours out. Bacteria are therefore essentially a package of DNA. DNA, as with all organisms, carries the genetic code for the organisms. The genetic code controls protein production, some of which can become enzymes. Enzymes control all of the chemical reactions in the cell or all cellular metabolism. Through this pathway, DNA determines all cell characteristics.

The role in pathogenicity of DNA is theoretically indirect. However, for example, the DNA in anthrax (*Bacillus anthracis*) directs the production of the poison that when injected into another system causes necrosis. Thus, indirectly, DNA does cause harm. It directs the cell to produce the protein that is detrimental. The role of DNA in possible treatments or control of infections is problematic. Although at present antibiotics are available that can damage bacterial DNA, for example, **quinolones** such as **nalidixic acid**, they are generally not used for the simple reason that humans have DNA, too, so these drugs can harm our DNA as well. They are used only when there are no viable alternatives.

Bacterial Ribosomes

The second major structure in the bacterial cytoplasm is the ribosomes. They are the site of protein synthesis. The chemical composition of ribosomes is protein and RNA. In bacteria the ribosomes are free in the cytoplasm. Microscopically they appear as polyribosomes, long rows joined together. Ribosomes play no direct role in pathogenicity. Indirectly, they make everything the cell uses. Some bacteria produce protein poisons called **exotoxins**, which are released by living bacteria. This is as opposed to endotoxins, which are released from Gram-negative bacteria when the LPS layer of the plasma membrane is released upon cell death. Examples of important exotoxins include **botulism**, **tetanus**, **anthrax**, **cholera**, and **diphtheria**. All of these protein exotoxins are produced in the ribosomes.

The role of ribosomes in the treatment or control of bacterial infections can be both indirect and direct. The major tool we have to treat infections is antibiotics, which can damage ribosomes and therefore interfere with protein synthesis. **Aminoglycosides**, such as streptomycin, kanamycin, and gentamycin; **macrolides**, such as azithromycin, erythromycin, and clarithromycin; and tetracycline and its derivatives, including doxycycline, all damage ribosomes. These are considered **broad spectrum** antibiotics because they will work on both Gram-positive and Gram-negative bacteria. However, these drugs must be used carefully because humans have ribosomes, too. Our eukaryotic ribosomes differ in size and structure from prokaryotic ribosomes, and drugs are designed to exploit these differences. However, kidney damage, auditory nerve damage, and Grey's syndrome, which damages the liver of the fetus during pregnancy, are some of the adverse side effects of ribosome-damaging antibiotics.

Some antiseptics and disinfectants can also damage ribosomes or denature the proteins made by the ribosomes. Alcohols, with their dehydration action, destroy proteins. Tinctures can also damage ribosomes. Heavy metals, which are extremely dangerous to humans, including lead (Pb), argon (Ar), and mercury (Hg), as well as cyanide (CN) have been used. Mercury used in skin antiseptics such as mercurochrome and merthiolate must be diluted so much to make it safe that it is probably of limited usefulness. Silver is used as a 1% solution of $AgNO_3$ (silver nitrate) in the eyes of newborn infants to prevent blindness (ophthalmia neonatorum) caused by passing through gonorrhea discharge at delivery.

Halogens, such as bromine (Br), chlorine (Cl), fluorine (F), and iodine (I) are very effective antibacterials. Bromine is used in hot tubs. Chlorine is used in drinking water and swimming pools. Sodium hypochlorite (NaClO) is bleach and calcium hypochlorite $(CaClO)_2$ is chlorinated lime, used for water treatment. Fluorine is used to disinfect drinking water and in toothpaste to kill tooth decay bacteria. Iodine is used as a skin antiseptic. Aldehydes such as formaldehyde and gluteraldehyde are stronger than bleach. They destroy living tissues and are used to preserve dead tissue. Ethylene oxide gas is used in hospital gas sterilizers to destroy highly infectious waste. It is very toxic and its gas can penetrate where heat cannot to yield total sterilization.

Bacterial Capsules

Bacterial capsules are a mucous complex (slime layers) not produced by all bacteria. For the most part, bacteria that do produce capsules become pathogenic. The main function of capsules is to prevent phagocytosis by neutrophils. If bacteria make a slimy capsule around their outside, the neutrophils cannot attach to them; and if they cannot attach, they cannot ingest them. Other functions of capsules are to aid in the attachment to cells, particularly in the respiratory tract, to help prevent dehydration of the bacteria that thrive in deserts, and to store sugars. Capsules can also prevent viruses from infecting bacteria. The chemical composition of capsules is a mucocomplex made of mostly polysaccharides (complex sugars). Fresh, hydrated capsules are slimy and sticky, but when they become dehydrated, they can help attach to other cells.

The roles of capsules in pathogenicity are thwarting phagocytosis by neutrophils and their ability, when they dry out and become sticky, to fill air spaces, primarily in the bronchi and lungs. This can happen in any space in the body where there are open airwaves. In the lungs, this causes death by drowning in sticky capsules. The role of capsules in possible treatments or control of bacterial infections is nonexistent. We have no anticapsule antibiotics and no anticapsule antiseptics. Destroying the capsule does not kill the bacteria, and the bacteria would likely regrow the capsule too quickly to serve any purpose. Since the capsule does not block antibiotics from entering the bacteria cell, it is more useful to attack the structures that produce capsules.

Bacterial Endospores

Endospores are not produced by all bacteria. They are produced mainly by the genera *Bacillus* and *Clostridium.* **Bacilli** are Gram-positive, aerobic, spore-forming bacteria. The rod-shaped cell produces one spore within the cell. **Clostridia** are Gram-positive, anaerobic spore formers.

The much smaller rod, which is sausage or cigar shaped, produces a tennis racket–shaped cell due to the endospore at one end. The function of endospores is survival, not reproduction like most spores in plants and fungi. Endospores enable bacteria to survive in harsh environments such as extreme heat or cold. Spores do not need nutrients, water, or air. They can survive desiccation and even a variety of chemical and radiation treatments. Depending on whether the bacterium that produces them is an aerobe or an anaerobe, endospores can survive either the lack of O_2 or the presence of O_2. Spores are therefore a survival stage to sustain bacteria, hibernation-like, through a harsh environment.

The composition of endospores begins with DNA duplication and ribosome duplication by **vegetative cells** of bacteria that are actively growing. These copies are surrounded by a membrane and a cell wall, and then this tiny self-replica is surrounded by at least three protective layers. First is the **cortex**, composed of peptidoglycan and calcium. Next is the **spore coat**, composed of protein and **dipicolinic acid** (DPA). Finally, the outer coat is the **exosporium** made mostly of calcium. This process, called **sporulation** (spore production) is performed when conditions are favorable. In a harsh environment, the vegetative cell dies and the spore is released and remains a spore until the environment becomes positive for that species. There are no antibiotics or disinfectants that can kill bacterial spores, but bleach and formaldehyde can eliminate them.

There are five important diseases caused by spore-forming bacteria:

1. ***Clostridium difficile*** **(C. diff.)**: *C. diff* is a major cause of wound infections and gastrointestinal tract infections, especially in compromised persons, including postsurgical patients, the elderly, and post-trauma patients.
2. ***Clostridium botulinin*** **(botulism)**: Spores of *C. botulinin* are found in most large animal intestines, including horses, cows, goats, and pigs. Spores cause no harm to them. *Clostridium* is an anaerobe and there is too much oxygen in a living animal. The spores end up in the feces. Grazing is the method of cyclical transmission. Farming and soil runoff expose the spores. Canning and vacuum packing kill the anaerobic bacteria but not always the spores. The spores germinate bacteria in the anaerobic environment of the can or jar. Bacteria grow and produce the botulism exotoxin and then die. There is no bad odor, no bad taste, and no visible indication. When people ingest this neurotoxin, paralysis and death occur within 24 to 72 hours.

3. ***Clostridium tetani*** **(tetanus)**: Spores of *C. tetani* are also found in large animal intestines. They are anaerobes, so they stay spores and wind up in feces and in the soil. Humans are exposed when they get a puncture wound, which are low-oxygen wounds. Other low-oxygen wounds include burns and hemorrhagic wounds. In the wound, the spores germinate and the bacteria produce the exotoxin (**tetanus toxin**, also called **tetanospasmin**). It enters the blood stream and attacks the nervous system, blocking **cholinesterase** and causing constant muscle contraction and rigidity. The first places affected are the face and neck in symptoms referred to as **lockjaw**. The effects continue to the respiratory muscles and diaphragm, leading to respiratory failure and death. Tetanus vaccines make it appear as if the disease is gone, but these spores are still all around us.
4. ***Clostridium perfringens*** **(gas gangrene)**: *C. perfringens* is one of the decomposer bacteria of dead organisms, including humans. Again, the spores are in large animal intestinal tracts, including humans, and again the spores wind up in the soil. When humans receive an anaerobic wound, the spores germinate. Among the many precursors are car accidents, gunshot wounds, stab wounds, and falls. Once the spores germinate, the bacteria produce a number of **necrotizing toxins** that kill the cells and tissues. The necrotic tissue softens and becomes wet and discolored, turning a greenish brown and black, and emits a foul odor. This odor is due to cells lysing until eventually a gas is produced. The tissue stretches and a bubble forms, and **crepitation** is heard as crackling sounds under the skin. The bacteria spread, eventually reaching vital organs, leading to organ failure and death. This process takes from one to three days. The treatment is antibiotics; however, since antibiotics cannot kill spores, this has no effect pregermination. If the antibiotics are introduced too late in the process, the bacteria have already been producing the exotoxins. Thus, there is a narrow window of opportunity in which antibiotics will work—postgermination and pre-exotoxin production. Wound debridement is also tried to remove the damaged and unviable infected tissue. Sometimes this can help, although other times it leads to a new infection of staph. After crepitation has occurred, amputation is the only sure cure in order to remove all spores and toxins. Tourniquets were a cause of gas gangrene infections in the past, because a tourniquet creates an anaerobic environment. Another possible treatment choice is a hyperbaric oxygen chamber to drastically increase the partial pressure of oxygen in the tissues of the body.
5. ***Bacillus anthracis*** **(anthrax)**: *Bacillus anthracis* is a Gram-positive aerobe. The spores are naturally found in deep anaerobic soil. When humans open up the soil in some manner, most commonly via overfarming and erosion, we bring them to the surface. The spores attach to animal fur, hair, and skin or can be inhaled in dry, dusty, blowing soil particles. The spores germinate and the bacteria produce **necrotizing toxins**. On the skin, this causes blisters and sores from the dead tissue. In the lungs, sores and hemorrhaging result. Pulmonary anthrax has a very high death rate of between 20% and 50%. Genetically engineered anthrax, the weaponized version, has an even higher death rate due to the ease at which it is spread and the strength of the toxin. There has been no proven case of natural anthrax in the United States in over 15 years.

Atypical Bacteria

Bacteria in the genus ***Mycoplasma*** are smaller than most bacteria, generally 0.15 to 0.3 μm long. They do not have a cell wall; thus they lack rigidity and are **pleomorphic**, taking on many different shapes. They are the smallest microorganisms to grow on agar plates, and this growth is very slow, taking up to one week. The name *mycoplasma* comes from the Greek words for fungus (*mykes*) and formed (*plasma*). The name arose in the nineteenth century due to its funguslike characteristics; however, it is not a fungus. Mycoplasmas cause a very common pneumonia, primarily found in hospital patients and infrequently in nonhospital patients. The human immune system can usually fight off these bacteria; however, for compromised patients, mycoplasma infections are grave. These patients acquire infections from healthy caregivers and others.

Mycoplasma infections can also cause **endocarditis**, inflammation of the inside lining of the heart chambers and heart valves. These infections are generally treated with tetracycline or doxycycline, in contrast to most pneumonias, which are treated with penicillin. Penicillin and its derivatives are ineffective against mycoplasmas because they do not have a cell wall.

Rickettsiaceae is another family of bacteria that are smaller than most bacteria, between 0.3 and 0.5 μm long. They have very little peptidoglycan in their cell walls. Rickettsias are **coccobacillary**, a cross between a rod and a sphere that is often oval in appearance. They are **obligate intracellular parasites** that must grow inside the living cells of their host; they cannot be grown in the laboratory on any medium. Rickettsias generally prefer to grow inside cells that line the blood vessels—the endothelial cells. A number of diseases are caused by rickettsias, including **typhus**, **Rocky Mountain spotted fever (RMSF)**, and **Brill-Zinzer disease**, a delayed relapse of typhus.

Ticks and lice are the transmitters (**vectors**) to humans. Both ticks and lice are blood feeders. They have two requisites: a hiding place and a blood supply. The ideal hiding place is the hair on the head (or sometimes pubic hair) close to surface blood vessels. Ticks tend to transmit RMSF, while lice tend to transmit typhus. Rickettsias enter the blood stream at the site of attachment, infect a blood vessel lining, and cause a rash (usually spotted) and a high fever that can induce delirium and eventually cause kidney and brain damage. Despite the name, RMSF is mostly a disease of the eastern United States. The symptoms of typhus are chills, cough, high fever, delirium, joint pain, rash, headache, severe muscle pain, and low blood pressure. The treatment for both typhus and RMSF is tetracycline or doxycycline.

Chlamydiae are also smaller than most bacteria, approximately 0.3 μm in diameter. They also have very little peptidoglycan in their cell walls. They can be coccilike or rodlike. The **elementary body**, found only in the infectious state, is round or, less commonly, pear-shaped. The **reticulate body**, noninfectious and seen in the developmental cycle responsible for intracellular replication, is rectangular and larger, about 1 μm or more in diameter. Chlamydiae are also obligate intracellular parasites, which must grow inside living cells; they cannot be grown in the lab. They cause a number of important infections, including trachoma, psittacosis, lymphogranuloma venereum, and genitourinary infections.

Trachoma is a type of conjunctivitis considered to be the world's leading cause of blindness. It is spread when water that is contaminated with human or animal waste gets into the eye.

Psittacosis is a type of **ornithosis** (abnormal condition of birds). In general, infections do not cross species. Cross-species transfer has not been a problem until now with birds. Psittacosis is also called **parrot fever** because it is a pneumonia of tropical birds such as parrots and parakeets that can be transmitted to humans through aerosol emissions. Humans get a chronic, long-lasting respiratory infection, which can develop into pneumonia. Psittacosis is the reason it is illegal to import tropical birds.

Lymphogranuloma venereum (LGV) is a sexually transmitted disease (STD) that infects the lymph nodes in the groin. Hard, swollen black lumps, or granulomas, develop. It used to be called black syphilis because it resembles syphilis. All three of these infections are treated with tetracycline and doxycycline.

Genitourinary chlamydia infections are caused by *Chlamydia trachomatis*, the same species that causes trachoma. It is the most common STD in the United States. Chlamydiae can cause sterility from cervicitis, pelvic inflammatory disease (PID), and scarring of the fallopian tubes. In males they cause urethritis and prostatitis, which are often asymptomatic.

Fungi

Fungi are eukaryotes, and as such are larger and more complex than bacteria. They are mostly multicellular, although most yeasts are unicellular. They have a nucleus, undergo mitosis, and have more than one chromosome. They do not have peptidoglycan in their cell walls. Instead, they have chitin. There are two main groups of fungi: yeast and molds.

Yeasts

Yeasts were mistakenly called false fungi because they look more like bacteria than molds. They are usually unicellular, generally oval or spherical, and 5–10 μm in diameter, much larger than bacteria. They reproduce asexually by **budding.** First the DNA is replicated in the nucleus. The nucleus then splits into a daughter nucleus, which migrates to the edge of the cell, where the cytoplasm surrounds it. Cell wall material is laid down between the parent cell and the bud. This small bud then continues to grow until it separates from the parent cell when it is fully mature and the same size as the parent cell. Sometimes, as in the case of ***Candida***, the buds remain attached to form fragile branching filaments called **pseudohyphae.** Yeast colonies can appear similar to bacteria colonies on solid media. The cells are much larger under the microscope.

Yeasts are facultative anaerobes. They can get their energy from either fermentation or respiration. The vast majority are nonpathogens. The following are four important yeasts:

1. ***Saccharomyces cerevisiae***: These are oval-budding, beneficial yeasts. They pose no health risk. Examples include **Baker's yeast** and one species of **Brewer's yeast.** They feed on glucose, maltose, trehalose, and other sugars, producing gas or alcohol.
2. ***Cryptococcus neoformus*****:** As the name indicates, ***Cryptococcus neoformus*** was originally thought to be a bacterium. This is the only *Cryptococcus* species. They are oval-budding and produce a capsule that is 5 to 10 μm long. They are pathogenic, causing an infection called **cryptococcosis.** This yeast is found in contaminated soil with certain types of bird droppings, particularly pigeons. Humans can inhale the dust containing *C. neoformus* and develop flulike symptoms, which can progress to pneumonia and eventually lung scarring. Healthy people with strong immune systems may remain asymptomatic. In compromised patients with HIV infections, Hodgkin's disease patients, chemotherapy patients, or people taking high doses of corticosteroids, it can spread through the circulatory system to the meninges and the brain, becoming a **cryptococcal meningoencephalitis.**
3. ***Pneumocystis jirovecii***: *P. jirovecii* affects the lungs, where it causes cysts. For many years it was mistaken as a protozoan and treated with Flagyl, a drug used to treat protozoa. It causes pneumonia primarily in immunosuppressed persons. There are three highly susceptible groups: newborns (rare), cancer patients on chemotherapy, and AIDS patients. It is the leading cause of AIDS death. It is referred to as **pneumocystis pneumonia** or **PCP.**
4. ***Candida***: *Candida* are the most important and most common of all the yeasts, with many species. ***Candida albicans*** is the most common pathogenic yeast, although it exists as a commensal yeast most of the time. Commensal relationships are those in which one organism benefits and the other receives no harm from the relationship. *Candida albicans* causes candidiasis infections. It is a **dimorphic** yeast. It can appear in two forms, as an oval-budding yeast cell or in a moldlike form, producing filaments called **hyphae**, similar to molds. The hyphae help the yeast to invade deeper tissues after it colonizes the epithelium. These long chains of branching cells become multicellular and are

joined together by **pseudohyphae**, budding yeast cells that remain attached to one another. Spores are also formed in clusters along the hyphae, often at branching points. At the ends of hyphae, budding can generate **blastospores**, asexual spores that can break off to become new **chlamydospores**. Thick-walled chlamydospores have the same function as endospores. They ensure the survival of the species in inhospitable conditions. At temperatures of 32°C and up, *C. albicans* is seen in the yeast form. At temperatures below 32°C, *C. albicans* is seen in the moldlike forms.

Candidiasis infections are seen as **thrush** or **oral mucocutaneous candidiasis**, **vaginitis**, **onychomycosis** (an infection of the nails), and **dermatitis**, particularly diaper rash and other infections of moist skin areas. *C. albicans* is the second leading cause of vaginal infection. It causes a creamy white coating and discharge full of yeast cells. It is considered to be an STD with female-to-male transmission. In males it is one of the causes of urethritis.

Thrush is an infection of the mouth and possibly throat that causes a creamy white coating on the tongue and gums. It occurs most frequently in children and immunosuppressed patients.

Candidiasis dermatitis is indicated by an extremely bright, red rash and flaking skin in moist skin areas such as inside the thighs, under the breasts, and in the abdominal folds. **Systemic candidiasis** is seen mainly in immunosuppressed patients. Candida is now the cause of 10% of septicemia cases. Candidiasis of the esophagus, bronchi, or lungs in conjunction with a positive HIV antibody test is one of the indicator diseases for AIDS.

Molds

Molds are usually multicellular and have hyphae. Hyphae of molds, like the mycelial form of *C. albicans* yeast, are long chains of cells with a multicellular surface. They are branching tubular structures from 2 to 10 μm in diameter often divided into cell-like units by cross-walls called **septa**.

Some hyphae grow along the surface and are referred to as **vegetative hyphae**. Some hyphae grow upward, above the surface, and are referred to as **aerial hyphae**. The total mass of hyphae is referred to as the **mycelium**. The portion of the mycelium that anchors the mold and absorbs nutrients is the **vegetative mycelium**. The portion of the mold that grows upward and produces asexual reproductive spores is the **aerial mycelium**. The function of hyphae is to attach the mold to the surface and allow it to obtain nutrients. Most molds are **saprophytes**, which live on dead matter. The aerial hyphae contain the reproductive spores of the mold. For classification purposes, molds can be divided into three groups:

1. **Common nonpathogenic molds**
2. **Dermatophyte molds:** Dermatophyte molds affect the skin, hair, and nails, the locations where keratin proteins are produced.
3. **Systemic molds:** Systemic molds, also called **dimorphic molds**, affect the inside of the body.

There are thousands of common nonpathogenic molds whose growth is regulated by the environment. ***Aspergillus*** species are the most common. Some species may cause problems for people who are allergic to them or if they infect peanuts, which they can contaminate with a **mycotoxin** called **aflatoxin**. Aflatoxin exposure can cause chronic indigestion and has hepatocellular carcinogenic (liver cancer) potential, particularly in animals. It is mostly produced by *Aspergillus flavus* and contaminates food. *Aspergillus* produce white vegetative hyphae and aerial hyphae. The aerial hyphae swell out into specialized structures called **conidiophores**, on which asexually reproductive, nonmotile spores called **conidia** or **conidiospores** are formed. *Aspergillus* conidiospores are usually black and are very resistant to destruction. Even bleach will not completely destroy them.

Penicillium is a mold commonly involved in the spoilage of food. It can grow on fruit. The original strain used to produce penicillin was isolated from a cantaloupe. *Rhizopus* and *Aspergillus* species commonly grow on bread and other starchy substrates. *Penicillium* produces vegetative hyphae (usually white) and aerial hyphae with fingerlike projections called **sterigmata** that look like a series of leaf-shaped protrusions. On top of these are the asexual reproductive conidia or conidiospores, which are found as chains and start out blue, turn green, and then become blue-gray. They are usually nonpathogenic. If a person is allergic to penicillin, he or she is allergic to *Penicillium*.

Rhizopus produces white, vegetative hyphae and aerial hyphae. On top of the aerial hyphae specialized branches called **sporangiophore** emerge. On top of the sporangiophore is a large circular sac called a **sporangium** with brown or black spores inside called **sporangiospores**. *Rhizopus* is a brownish-black mold that is generally nonpathogenic but can cause **mucormycosis** in immunocompromised individuals. Mucormycosis results in sinus infections that may progress to the cranial nerves and sometimes cause thrombosis (blood clots that block blood vessels to the brain). Pulmonary mucormycosis can also occur. This pneumonia can rapidly degenerate in these patients, leading to infections in the chest cavity, heart, and brain. Gastrointestinal (GI) tract, skin, and kidney involvement is also seen. Some uncompromised patients display an allergic reaction to this common inside-the-house mold, and the mold spores are an airborne irritant.

Dermatophytes infect the skin, hair, and nails, locations where keratin is produced. They produce tan or light brown vegetative hyphae, but do not have aerial hyphae. The spores are produced directly on the vegetative hyphae. Dermatophytes have large spores called **conidia** and smaller spores called **microconidia**. There are three main genera of dermatophytes: ***Microsporium***, ***Trichophyton***, and ***Epidermaphyton***. Dermatophyte infections are often referred to as **tinea**. If the dermatophyte mold is on the scalp, it produces a red, circular, raised, itchy rash called **tinea capitus**. The common vernacular for tinea is **ringworm**, though it is not a worm. It is highly contagious. Hyphae and spores in the hairline can be passed along by combs and brushes, hats, and baseball caps. It is more common in children. Ringworm of the chin or face is referred to as **tinea barbae**. It is the same mold, simply now located on the face. Tinea barbae is more common in men because shaving scrapes the spores in. Tinea grow better in melanin, so darker-skinned people are more susceptible. **Tinea inguinale** or **tinea cruris** is groin ringworm, commonly referred to as **jock itch**. **Tinea pedis**, ringworm of the foot, is athlete's foot. Treatment is administered orally using **griseofulvin**, which is derived from the mold *Penicillium griseofulvum*. It binds to keratin precursor cells, conferring resistance to mature keratin cells.

Systemic molds cause mainly respiratory illnesses. Humans breathe in the spores. If ingested, stomach acid will likely destroy them. Systemic molds are **dimorphic**. They have two different growth forms. At higher temperatures, such as inside the body, they look like yeast and are primarily in a single-celled nonmycelial form. This nonmycelial yeastlike form causes lesions called granulomas, which serve to wall off and localize the organism. In immunosuppressed patients they can disseminate to other areas of the body and be life-threatening. Outside the body at lower temperatures, they are more typically seen as molds, producing hyphae and asexual reproductive spores. In the mold form, they are sensitive to the environment. Some like one set of temperatures, moisture levels, and nutrient conditions, whereas others prefer a different set of environmental conditions. Most systemic molds prefer high humidity, but not all. There are three common dimorphic fungal infections in the United States.

1. ***Histoplasma capsulatum***, which causes **histoplasmosis**, produces vegetative hyphae but no aerial hyphae. This is typical of the pathogens. It produces large, rough-edged spores called **tuberculate macroconidia** and small **microconidia**. *Histoplasma* are generally found in the

soil in moist climates, primarily in the Eastern United States, Great Lakes, and the Mississippi and Ohio River valleys. The mold form grows best in soil contaminated with bird droppings or bat droppings, referred to as **guano**. It prefers bird droppings from the crow family, which tend to be scavenger birds that forage in trash. It is also found in chicken droppings. Humans inhale the spores from the contaminated soil, and the spores germinate in the lungs, where the fungus grows as a budding encapsulated yeast. They develop a flulike illness, which can become chronic, causing lung scarring. Histoplasmosis displays tuberculosis-like symptoms, including a persistent cough, malaise, and chest congestion. Human-to-human transmission is rare, though not impossible.

2. ***Coccidioides immitis*** causes **coccidioidomycosis.** The mold form produces vegetative hyphae and no aerial hyphae, as is typical of the pathogens. Fragments of the vegetative hyphae form spores, called **arthrospores**, which are scattered when every other cell swells up and breaks off. It is found primarily in the Southwest United States, including Southern California, Arizona, New Mexico, and Nevada. Humans inhale spores in the dry, dusty air of semiarid desertlike environments. In the body, *Coccidioides immitis* takes on the nonmycelial form and is seen as **endosporulating spherules**. Coccidioidomycosis infections produce a chronic, long-term TB-like illness. It is also referred to as Valley fever, San Joaquin Valley fever, and California disease. Valley fever warnings urge people with respiratory problems or a weak immune system to stay indoors. People who grow up in this region usually have a case as a child and acquire immunity.
3. ***Blastomyces dermatitidis*** causes **blastomycosis.** The mold form produces vegetative hyphae but no aerial hyphae. The small spores, **conidiospores**, develop directly on the vegetative hyphae. In the body, it is in the yeast form with a characteristic thick cell wall. It is found primarily in the Midwest, northern United States, and Canada, proliferating in areas with multiple rivers and lakes, including the Great Lakes region and the Mississippi and Ohio River valleys. Blastomycosis is thought to become a problem when soil is disturbed such that the vegetative hyphae and spores are elevated above the soil surface. Both humans and animals breathe in the spores, which germinate in the lungs to the nonmycelial form. It is seen more often in dogs than in humans but can infect compromised patients and spread to the skin, central nervous system, and bones. Lung infections produce symptoms similar to histoplasmosis and coccidioidomycosis.

Parasitic Protozoans

Protozoa are unicellular, eukaryotic microorganism belonging to the domain Eukarya in the kingdom Protista. The vegetative form of a protozoan is called a **trophozoite**. Trophozoites are motile, feed, and reproduce. A protective or survival form produced by some protozoans that enables them to survive in harsh environments is referred to as a **cyst**. Cysts allow some pathogens to survive when not in a host. When they reenter a host and are once again in an environment that is favorable to them, **excystation** occurs and the protozoan once again becomes a trophozoite.

One of the worldwide scourges, **malaria**, is caused by five species of the protozoan genus ***Plasmodium***. There are 300 million cases per year and between 1.0 and 1.5 million deaths. Malaria is a disease of the tropics and subtropics that can be brought to temperate regions via airplane travelers. The worst form of the disease and the one that is most often fatal is an infection of *Plasmodium falciparum*. The *Plasmodium* genus of protozoa have a life cycle that includes a vertebrate host and an insect vector. The vertebrate hosts are usually humans, but can be higher primates. The insect vector is the female **Anopheline** mosquito, which takes blood meals, whereas the male does not. The recurring fever of malaria is caused by the lysis of infected red blood cells, which causes the release of **merozoites** and their metabolic by-products.

Merozoites are the stage in the life cycle of the plasmodium formed during the asexual division of the **schizont**. The schizont is a cell that reproduces by **multiple fission (schizogony)**. First, the nucleus divides multiple times, and then the cell divides as many times as necessary to house all the nuclei. These merozoites are released and invade other cells.

Entamoeba histolytica is an anaerobic parasitic protozoan that causes **amoebic dysentery**. Approximately 50 million people are affected globally. It is another disease of the tropics, but not due to an endemic vector. Areas of poor sanitation where human feces infected with the cysts contaminate the water or food are the risk factor. The vegetative state is a trophozoite that exists only in the host. It is ingested in its survival form, the cyst. The cysts are found in the soil, in water, and on moist foods. The cysts cannot withstand extremes of temperature and do not survive indefinitely outside the host; they usually survive only for several months. The cysts are ingested, and excystation occurs. The trophozoites then live in the colon and cecum. The trophozoites are mobile because they are equipped with **pseudopodia** (false feet) like all amoebas (amoeboids) These projections of cytoplasm are used to move toward food and to engulf and ingest food, which is packaged into a food vacuole and fused with a lysosome for digestion. *Entamoeba histolytica* reproduces by binary fission. Symptoms of amoebic dysentery are inflamed colon, abdominal pain, and raging, bloody diarrhea leading to weight loss and fatigue. In some cases parasites can reach the bloodstream and migrate to vital organs, including the lungs, liver, spleen, and brain. Liver abscesses are common and can rupture and spread to other organs if left untreated.

Trypanosoma brucei is another member of the kingdom Protista that causes a disease called **African sleeping sickness**. It is a motile flagellate protozoan that has a life cycle that includes a human host and an insect vector. The insect is the **tsetse fly** found only in western and central Africa. When an infected tsetse fly bites a human, the infective **metacyclic trypomastigotes** are injected and develop into **trypomastigotes**, the developmental stage in which the flagellum grows. These leaflike microorganisms have a rounded end and a pointed end where the flagellum develops. They multiply at the injection site and migrate to the blood and lymph, where they further multiply. Later they can infect the heart and central nervous system. The symptoms are fever, lymphadenopathy, and overwhelming lethargy when it reaches the spinal cord and brain, hence the common name.

Giardia intestinalis is another anaerobic, flagellated protozoan that reproduces via binary fission. It causes the illness known as **giardiasis**. It exists as a trophozoite as its vegetative form and as a cyst in its survival form. The cyst is resilient and can live for weeks to months in cold water, is moderately heat tolerant, and will withstand chlorine treatment in water treatment facilities as well as ozonolysis. *Giardia* belongs to a group of flagellates referred to as the **diplomonads**, which have two nuclei in a double cell structure that each have four flagella. The mode of transmission is ingestion of water or food contaminated with the cysts. The cysts can be ingested due to improper hygiene (**fecal-oral transmission**), because there are many asymptomatic carriers of the parasite. *Giardia* trophozoites colonize the small intestine. The symptoms of giardiasis are explosive diarrhea, lethargy, flatulence that can be so severe that it induces vomiting, nausea, bloating, and resultant weight loss. Compromised patients can suffer extended infections. This includes those with immunodeficiency disorders and disorders of the digestive system that result in diminished gastric acid production.

Trichomonas vaginalis is another flagellated, anaerobic parasitic protozoan; however, it exists only in the vegetative trophozoite form. It has no cysts. The trophozoite has five flagella and a sheet of microtubules called an **axostyle**, which is likely used to attach to surfaces and is responsible for tissue damage. *Trichomonas vaginalis* is directly transmitted via sexual intercourse. It divides via binary fission. This occurs more readily when the normally acidic conditions in the vagina (pH between 3.5 and 4.5) are shifted to more basic (pH > 5.9). Direct transmission is related to the fact that it does not form a cyst. Since it does not encyst, there is no fecal-oral transmission. This STD is mainly symptomatic in females. It causes vaginitis, cervicitis, and a greenish yellow discharge. It can make its sufferers more susceptible to cervical cancer and HIV infections and lead to complications of pregnancy, including low-birth-weight babies and premature labor. *Trichomonas vaginalis* can also infect the fallopian tubes and urinary tract and can cause respiratory infections such as pneumonia and bronchitis. Lesions in the mouth are also sometimes observed.

Balantidium coli causes a diarrhea-type infection and is mainly transmitted due to improper hygiene (fecal-oral transmission). It is a ciliated protozoan that exists in both the cyst and trophozoite forms. The cytoplasm of the vegetative cell has a foamy appearance, and it has both a small micronucleus and a large dumbbell-shaped macronucleus. It is the only known cilia-bearing pathogen. *Balantidium coli* is part of the normal flora of the colon and cecum in a number of animal species, most commonly pigs. Cross-species infection is atypical because each animal has different gut flora, creating different home environments. However, it is after a protozoan from one species has adapted to the environment in another species that infestation becomes a problem. Transmission is oral through ingestion of water or food that has been contaminated by the cysts. Humans are infected with the cysts from pig feces. The trophozoites colonize the large intestines. Healthy people rarely become symptomatic. Immunosuppressed patients and people with disorders of the digestive system that result in diminished gastric acid production are most affected. The symptoms for these patients include explosive diarrhea and eventually perforations in the colon.

Viruses

Viruses are the smallest infectious agents. They are about 1,000 times smaller than bacteria. Their nuclear material, either DNA or RNA, is packaged inside a **protein head**, also called a **capsid**.

Viruses require living cells for survival and growth. They cannot reproduce or mutate on their own. It is living cells that reproduce and induce mutations in viruses. They are nonliving, nonactive entities that do not grow on any laboratory medium.

LIVING VERSUS NONLIVING ORGANISMS

LIVING CHARACTERISTICS	NONLIVING CHARACTERISTICS
Can be reproduced at a very rapid rate of one to 50,000 in two to three hours	No cell structures; no cell walls, cell membrane, or ribosomes
Have genetic material	No cytoplasm; carry out no chemical reactions
Can be mutated; undergo genetic change; evolve; adapt to environments	No nutrient or water uptake; no metabolism

Virus Specificity

Viruses are mostly very specific to the organism they infect. Animal viruses infect only animal cells. Plant viruses infect only plant cells. Plant viruses are not harmful to humans except indirectly by, for example, wiping out a particular crop. The first viruses to be studied in detail were bacterial viruses or **bacteriophages**. Fungal viruses are **mycophages**. However, virus mutations and crossovers are now a worry. For example, West Nile disease started in horses, mutated to a form that could infect birds, and now infects humans. Birds seem to be a common crossover vector, though it is not yet known why. Until the present, rabies was the only known virus that could cross species without mutating.

Viruses are also tissue specific. The protein head of a virus has **receptors**, proteins that link to specific proteins on a specific site. For example, respiratory-virus proteins link only to proteins on a lung structure. **Pneumotropic** viruses need lung and respiratory tissue, **dermatotropic** viruses affect only skin, **neurotropic** viruses affect only brain or other nervous tissues, and **lymphotropic** viruses infect only the lymphocytes. This specificity severely limits a virus. Crossovers are occurring due to human involvement. Humans are the vector that is developing new proteins allowing viruses to cross over species and tissue type.

Viruses are difficult to study because they are not living. This is why virus research and development are much slower. The main difficulty is the inability to grow entities that require a living organism in order to thrive. Animal research is problematic due to virus specificity, because how it affects them is not necessarily how it will affect us. The same applies to vaccine development. Most vaccines are **attenuated** or use a weakened virus. Cell cultures, taking infected cells and growing them in solution, is difficult, and they tend to get infected with bacteria. Sometimes viruses can be grown in fertilized chick eggs, but they must be transferred every eight days or so as the chick dies. The bottom line is they are extremely difficult to study.

VIRUS SHAPES AND APPEARANCES

- **Icosahedral:** An icosahedron is a geometric form with 20 triangular faces, 30 edges, and 12 vertices. Most animal viruses are icosahedral. The protein head is hollow. Inside it is either DNA or RNA. Each part of the icosahedral head or **capsid** is a **capsomere**. Sometimes one more protein structure called **spikes** is found at each corner. The function of the spikes is to stick to cell surfaces. Most cold viruses have no spikes, whereas most flu viruses do. This is why the flu is harder to shake.
- **Cylindrical or helical:** Cylindrical viruses are mostly plant viruses. However, lyssaviruses, of the genus *Lyssavirus*, which includes rabies and other animal viruses, are helical. This may help to explain rabies' ability to cross over species without mutating. The rabies virus is bullet-shaped, is enclosed in an envelope, and has a hollow protein head (capsid) that usually contains RNA.
- **Complex shape:** Viruses categorized as having a complex shape are mainly **bacteriophages** and **mycophages**. They are 1 to 3 nm long, 100 times smaller than a bacterium. The protein head is hollow and contains DNA. Attached to the head is a protein coating. Some complex bacteriophages resemble an insect or a plungerlike injection device that is used to push DNA into bacteria. The capsid can be icosahedral or filamentous. It is attached to a hollow tube referred to as the **tail**. The end of the tail has a **base plate** with attached **tail fibers**. The remainder of the tail is covered in a contractile **sheath**. It lands on the bacterial wall with its **tail fibers**, plunges in with **pins** to attach, shoves down, and pushes into the bacterium. The contractile **sheath** acts like the threads of a screw to secure the base plate to the bacterial wall and injects DNA into the bacterium through the hollow tube of the tail.

Phage therapy, which uses bacteriophages to treat bacterial infections in people, is an active area of study. The original study made people sicker because it was attempted on salmonellae, which are Gram-negative bacteria. When the salmonellae phage-killed the bacteria, they released more endotoxins. We already use phages to attack both insects and bacterial infections on plants. For example, bacteriophages have been used to combat two strains of bacteria that cause the disease known as tomato spot.

Virus Life Cycles

Different types of viruses have different types of life cycles.

The **productive life cycle** is the eight-step life cycle of an animal virus, and is as follows:

1. **Attachment**: There are two steps in the attachment process to exposed host cells: First, a non-permanent attachment is formed. This is a reversible attachment, that amounts to instantaneous sticking. In order to form a permanent attachment, the virus must have the correct proteins for that surface. If it does not, it will be shed. If it does, the infection will continue.
2. **Penetration**: On the surface of the cell, the virus is not a problem. It must be inside to cause problems, and the sooner it enters, the safer it is from the immune system. Penetration occurs because the host cell, thinking the virus is a nutrient, takes it into the cell via endocytosis.
3. **Uncoating**: Uncoating releases the viral genome from the remainder of the virus. The host cell digests the protein head of the virus. The purpose of the head is to stick to the host cell and protect the genetic material. When the viral head is destroyed, it releases the viral DNA. The host cell does not destroy the foreign DNA, because it is fooled into thinking it is its own. The first genes are identical to the host's DNA, so the host leaves the viral DNA alone.
4. **Transport of viral DNA to nucleus**: Since the host cell has identified the foreign DNA as its own, it wants to transport it to the nucleus. In the nucleus it is attached to the end of a host cell chromosome at an **operon**, which controls cell division. Now the cell is under the control of the virus. The virus overrides host cell programming; it is partially shut down and taken over by viral DNA. It cannot be totally shut down, however, because the virus needs the living cell to do the work for it. If the cell were totally shut down, the virus would have to leave and find a new host. This is the ideal situation. The host cell can still function, but only for the benefit of the virus.
5. **Replication**: The viral genome now directs the host cell's metabolic machinery (ribosomes, tRNA, nutrients, energy, enzymes, etc.) to synthesize viral enzymes and viral parts. The viral genome is transcribed into viral mRNA that goes to the host cell's ribosomes, where it is translated into viral structural proteins and viral enzymes. The host cell makes copies of viral DNA, 10,000 to 50,000 copies in two to three hours, as well as new viral heads, and if it had them, spikes.
6. **Maturation**: New mature viruses are now assembled by compiling viral DNA and heads together. DNA is inserted into new heads in two to three hours.
7. **Release**: Mature viruses are released from the cell by a process that reverses endocytosis, called **budding out**. The virus nucleoprotein is surrounded by a plasma membrane vesicle, which is released extracellularly.
8. **Reinfection**: The process begins anew with the infection of another cell. Often when a virus leaves a cell, it rips a huge hole in the cell membrane, causing instantaneous host cell death, but enveloping the virus in a sheath of plasma membrane. This covering can help to shield it from the immune system. The only time a virus

can be killed is when it is outside a cell. The end result of the viral life cycle is cell death. Illness is due to all of the cells being destroyed by the viruses.

The **provirus life cycle** is the first four steps of the productive life cycle: attachment, penetration, uncoating, and transport of the viral DNA to the nucleus, where the viral DNA attaches to the host cell chromosome. Then it goes into a latency period. A provirus is an animal virus that has inserted its DNA into the chromosomes of its host cell. It is also referred to as a **virogene**. The virogene is copied any time the host cell replicates. As much as 10% of our genetic code is not human; we are just carrying it. Most of this is viral genes stuck to our chromosomes.

If a virogene detaches or separates from the host DNA, which it could do at any point, it then goes into the productive life cycle. If it jumps from one life cycle to the other, it is classified as a **slow virus disease**. The classic case is a cold sore. When cold sores are active, they have broken out of the latent phase and have resumed the productive life cycle. When the cold sore has healed, some viral cells can get in nerve cells and hide. When a person is immunosuppressed, they again break out. Another example of a life cycle that cycles from productive to provirus to productive is **chicken pox**, which can emerge as **shingles**, usually later in life.

Sometimes when a virogene detaches from the host DNA, it may mutate the host DNA, causing it to undergo rapid cell division and become a tumor cell. Slow viruses can stimulate cancer cell formation. There are at least 30 viruses known to stimulate cancer growth. The key link between infectious **mononucleosis** and **Hodgkin's lymphoma** is the **Epstein-Barr** virus. The latest study showed that people were at increased risk of developing Hodgkin's disease for up to 20 years after having mononucleosis. **Human papilloma virus** (**HPV**) is the precursor to cervical cancer. **Feline leukemia virus** (**FLV**) causes cat leukemia. The mechanism is the same. The provirus detaches from the host cell DNA, mutates the host DNA, and triggers abnormal cell growth.

Viral latency may be caused when the host cell is not producing the proteins the provirus needs to start replicating. Safe within the cell, the provirus cannot be attacked by the immune system; thus it is carried by the host throughout its life. If the host cell is stimulated in some way that causes its DNA to begin production of the lacking proteins, the productive life cycle will kick back in and viral replication will commence.

The **lytic life cycle of a bacteriophage** parallels the eight-step productive life cycle of an animal virus:

1. **Attachment**: The bacteriophage attaches to a specific bacterium. The pins attach specifically to certain walls.
2. **Injection**: The DNA is injected through the hollow tail.
3. **DNA attachment**: The viral DNA attaches to the host cell chromosome.
4. **Shutdown**: The viral DNA partially shuts down and takes over the bacterial cell. It shuts down the host bacterial cell's ability to make DNA, RNA, or proteins.
5. **Replication**: New copies of viral DNA are made. About 100 to 500 new viral heads, tails, sheaths, and so on are made.
6. **Assembly**: New viruses are assembled.
7. **Release**: The bacterium produces an enzyme under the direction of the phage genome, which destroys the cell wall. This causes the bacterium to burst, releasing viruses.
8. **Reinfection**

The end result is cell death. The bacterium is killed and the cycle continues.

The **lysogenic life cycle of a bacteriophage** parallels the four-step provirus life cycle of an animal virus:

1. **Attachment**: The virus attaches to the cell wall of a specific bacterium.

2. **Injection**: The viral DNA is injected into the host bacteria.
3. **DNA attachment**: The viral DNA attaches to the bacterial chromosome.
4. **No shutdown**: No cell takeover occurs. The viral DNA is simply copied every time the bacteria reproduce. A bacteriophage genome has been integrated into the bacterial chromosome, creating a **prophage**. No harm is done to the bacterium unless some stimulus causes a return to the lytic life cycle. If the viral DNA detaches from the bacterial chromosome, cell shutdown will commence because once the prophage detaches, the lytic life cycle resumes, the cellular machinery is taken over, and viral replication begins.

Combatting Viruses

Antibiotics do not work against viruses. They work against living things. We have relatively few antiviral medications. Usually we are simply treating the symptoms. In order to attack a virus, the only thing we can attack is the protein head of the DNA or RNA. The problem is that we also have DNA, so we must be extremely careful. **Protease inhibitors** are used to stop the production of the protein head. Sometimes the virus mutates and produces different proteins. When we get over a virus, it is mainly our immune system that has fought it off.

Antiviral Body Defenses

There are two main antiviral body defenses:

1. **Neutralizing antibodies**: Neutralizing antibodies are proteins made by the immune system, for the most part **B-lymphocytes**, a type of white blood cell that works against a specific virus. Theoretically for each virus we need a different antibody. Antibodies attach to the protein head and, as a result, prevent viral attachment to host cells. Antibodies are not manufactured until we are exposed to a specific virus. Each antibody is specific for a specific infection. B-lymphocytes also produce memory B cells that persist to recognize future infections. This is the principle behind immunizations.
2. **Interferons**: Also referred to as **interleukins**, these antiviral proteins are made by virus-infected cells. They prevent viral replication in other cells. Every cell in the body has the potential to make interferon. Interferons are nonspecific. When they are made by a cell, they enter other cells and protect them from all viruses within a reasonable period of time. However, they are produced only when cells are under active infection, so after a few days there are none left. Interferons are a short-term, general way to fight viruses. For example, beta-interferon is used to shrink tumors in breast cancer and brain cancer. Interferons destroy tumors caused by viruses. They can stop the replication of tumor cells, just as they stop the replication of viruses.

Genetic Recombination in Bacteria

Genetic recombination is the exchange of DNA between two or more bacteria in the same generation. There are three primary methods.

1. **Transformation**: Transformation is the process by which naked DNA, DNA free of associated cells and proteins, passes from one bacterium to another.
2. **Transduction**: Transduction is the process by which DNA is carried by a bacteriophage from one bacterium to another. The vector or carrier is a virus.
3. **Conjugation**: Conjugation is the transfer of DNA from one bacterium to another across an F-pili (DNA bridge between two bacteria).

Transformation

In course of normal bacterial life cycle, a donor bacterium dies after two to four days, the normal life span. It breaks apart and decomposes, including the

DNA, as part of **autolysis**, when pieces of the bacteria explode and burst out. If another bacterium is close by and there is a piece of DNA small enough, it can pass through the cell membrane into the recipient. The recipient can cut out a piece of its own DNA and add in the piece from the donor. The piece that is cut out will be the same number of bases long as the piece that is being added. It is thought that if the piece has a positive effect, it will be added, and if it has a negative effect, it will be destroyed. Both the donor and the recipient are in the same colony in the same genus and species. Thus, most DNA is probably identical and this method is not very likely to cause change. However, transformation can play a powerful role in disease. For example, *Streptococcus pneumonia* is the leading cause of human pneumonia. There are two strains. The **rough** strain cannot make capsules. The **smooth** strain can make capsules, enabling it to resist phagocytosis. Only the smooth strain causes pneumonia.

Transduction

The donor phage (virus) attaches to the cell wall of a bacterium and injects its DNA through its tail. There are two possible choices. The phage can enter the lytic life cycle or the lysogenic life cycle. If it is the latter, the DNA is incorporated into the bacterial chromosome and stays there. If the DNA detaches, it can revert to the lytic life cycle. If during detachment from the bacterial chromosome, the piece of viral DNA breaks away uncleanly, it takes a piece of bacterial DNA with it. When the bacterium bursts and reinfects the surrounding bacteria, it has not only the viral DNA, but a piece of bacterial DNA that now is copied and passed on to the other bacteria.

In transduction, like transformation, the donor bacteria and the recipient bacteria are the same genus and species, because viruses are specific for a particular type of bacteria. This means that transduction has little potential for dramatic change. These are the same bacteria, with nearly identical DNA, so the probability for change is low. However, even bacteria with the same genus and species have slightly different characteristics. For example, *Streptococcus pyogenes* has two important strains. The **toxigenic** strain has the ability to make an **erythrogenic toxin**, which damages and destroys red blood cells. This is the cause of scarlet fever. The **nontoxigenic** strain cannot make the toxin.

Conjugation

The F-pili or sex pili enable DNA to be transferred across a bridge to a donor. The F^+ variety has the gene to make F-pili and the recipient F^- does not. There are actually three types of conjugation:

1. **F^+ conjugation** is the genetic recombination in which there is a transfer of an F^+ plasmid (coding only for an F-pilus), but not chromosomal DNA, from a donor bacterium to a recipient bacterium. **Plasmids** are DNA molecules distinct and independent from the chromosomal DNA that naturally occur in bacteria. They can replicate and are usually circular. The plasmid joins to the F^- bacterium, and one strand of the plasmid is cut and crosses over. The entire plasmid is not donated, just one strand. In each bacterium, complementary base pairing completes the DNA strand. The F^- variety bacterium is converted to F^+. For this individual bacterium, not much benefit is conferred.
2. **High-frequency recombinant (HFR) conjugation** is the process by which pieces of chromosomal DNA from a donor bacterium are transferred to a recipient bacterium. The F^+ bacterium cuts its chromosome, cuts the plasmid, and joins them together. The gene to make F-pili is now attached to chromosomal DNA, creating a **high-frequency recombitant male (HFRM)** donor. When the HFRM attaches to an F^- bacterium, it must now send the whole chromosome. It cuts the main chromosome and starts to send it over the F-pilus. The easiest place to cut is the place the plasmid was just at-

tached. Now the last gene to cross is the F-pilus gene. The F-pilus is actually a fragile structure. It breaks away within a few minutes. Since the F-pilus gene is now last and the F-pili bridge does not stay together long, usually the recipient does not get the last gene. Thus, toxin or antibiotic resistance could cross over, but it is random. Which genes have time to pass over and which ones do not is uncertain, and the recipient is unlikely to get the gene to make F-pili.

3. **Resistance plasmid or R-factor conjugation** is the process by which both F^+ and drug resistance are conferred to a recipient via a **resistance plasmid (R-plasmid)**. One plasmid strand enters the recipient bacterium while one strand remains in the donor. Each strand then makes a complementary copy. The R-plasmid has genes coding for multiple antibiotic resistance and F-pilus formation. The recipient becomes multiple antibiotic resistant and F^+, and is now able to transfer R-plasmids to other bacteria. This is a big problem in treating opportunistic Gram-negative infections such as urinary tract infections, wound infections, pneumonia, and septicemia by such organisms as *E. coli*, *Proteus*, *Klebsiella*, *Enterobacter*, *Serratia*, and *Pseudomonas*, as well as with intestinal infections by organisms such as *Salmonella* and *Shigella*. The fear is that bacteria may selectively pick out genes to transfer. Plasmid transfer is very fast and very specific. R-factor conjugation can happen between two different species. For example, it is nearly certain that *E. coli* has picked up the shigatoxin gene from *Shigella*.

Human Anatomy and Physiology

Twenty percent of the questions (about 9 or 10 questions) in the biology section of the PCAT exam will be on human anatomy and physiology topics.

Body Tissues

Tissue is an ensemble of cells that have the same or similar function. They have the same origin and work in conjunction to accomplish a specific function. There are four basic types.

1. **Epithelial tissue**
2. **Connective tissue**
3. **Muscle tissue**: There are three kinds of muscle tissue. All three muscle tissues contract, but there are differences.
   - **Skeletal**: Skeletal muscle attaches to bone. Movement is the result of these voluntary muscles.
   - **Smooth**: Smooth muscle is found in the organs. These are involuntary muscles. The blood vessels, uterus, stomach, and all digestive tract organs contract by involuntary smooth muscle action.
   - **Cardiac**: Cardiac muscle is heart muscle.
4. **Nervous tissue**: The cell involved in communication is a neuron.

Epithelial Tissue

The functions of epithelial tissue are as follows:

- **Protection**
- **Absorption**
- **Filtration**
- **Secretion**
- **Excretion**
- **Sensory**: This is extremely limited. Debatably, there are a few touch receptors located in epithelial tissues. In general, however, nervous tissue, not epithelial tissue, is sensory.

Epithelial cells have the following characteristics:

- **Extremely cellular appearance**: The proportion that is cell is greater than other tissue types. The ratio of cell to noncell is large. Many cell junctions are seen, particularly tight junctions and desmosomes. In between cells there is a very small amount of intercellular fluid.

- **Many cell junctions**: This is related to the cellularity of the tissues. There are many tight junctions and spot desmosomes.
- **Polarity**: The apical surface and the basal surface display polarity. The upper surface is free and exposed to the exterior lumen of an enclosed body cavity. The lower surface is attached.
- **Avascular**: There are no blood vessels, which means no oxygen, nutrients, or waste removal system. The blood supply for epithelial tissues is deeper. Gases diffuse through the tissue cell layers. The deeper layers are therefore healthier, while the outer layers are naturally dying and sloughing off because they are too far away from the blood supply.
- **Highly regenerative**: If epithelial tissue is damaged, it heals quickly.
- **Associated with basement membrane**: Cells of the epithelial tissue must be supported by something and that structure is the basement membrane. The basement membrane is not cellular. It is proteins and other substances, mostly glycoproteins. It is produced by the surrounding tissues. The basement membrane has two layers. The **basal lamina** is the top layer of the basement membrane. It is produced by the epithelial tissue above it. The **reticular lamina** is the bottom layer of the basement membrane. It is produced by the connective tissue below it.

Epithelial tissue is classified according to the type of cells and the number of layers. The two classifications for the number of layers are either simple or stratified.

1. **Simple epithelia**: Simple epithelial cells exist in a single layer: It is easier for substances to pass through a single layer. This is why simple epithelial cells are found in the alveoli of the lungs and in the capillaries. A single layer facilitates gas exchange.
2. **Stratified epithelia**: There is more than one layer of stratified epithelial cells. Only the lowest layer is attached to the basal membrane.

There are three epithelial cell types. All are six-sided.

1. **Squamous**: Squamous epithelial cells are flat.
2. **Cuboidal**: Cuboidal epithelial cells are cube-shaped.
3. **Columnar**: Columnar epithelial cells are rectangular or column-shaped.

To name single layers of epithelial cells, the classification for the number of layers is stated first, followed by the cell type.

1. **Simple columnar**: one layer of columnar epithelial cells
2. **Simple squamous**: one layer of flat squamous epithelial cells
3. **Simple cuboid**: one layer of cuboid epithelial cells

To name multilayered epithelial tissue, the cell type of the free surface area is examined. The classification for the number of layers is stated first, followed by the cell type of the top layer of cells.

1. **Stratified columnar**: several layers of cells with columnar cells as the top layer
2. **Stratified cuboid**: several layers of cells with cuboid cells as the top layer
3. **Stratified squamous**: several layers of cells with stratified cells as the top layer
4. **Pseudo-stratified**: The nucleus is seen in different planes within the tissue. It looks like stratified tissue but in reality there is only one layer. The nuclei are seen at differing heights, but are only a single layer.

There are three main functions of epithelial tissue, **covering**, **lining**, and **glandular**. Epithelial cells cover all body surfaces. They line blood vessels, the inside of organs, and the digestive tract. There are two main categories of glandular epithelium.

1. **Endocrine**: Glandular endocrine epithelium cells are ductless and produce hormones as part of the endocrine system.
2. **Exocrine**: Glandular exocrine epithelium cells have a duct through which a fluid is excreted. Exocrine epithelial cells can be either unicellular or multicellular. Unicellular epithelial exocrine cells are called **goblet cells**. Goblet cells produce the protein **mucin**. Mucin and water combine to form mucous. Mucous functions in the respiratory tract and digestive tract, cavities that have opening to the outside of the body. **Multicellular** exocrine glands include the lacrimal glands, salivary glands, and mammary glands. These cells are defined by their secretory product and by the type of duct. There are two types of duct structures: **simple duct structure** and **branched duct structure**. There are two main types of secretory structures or units: tubular and alveolar. They vary in complexity and the type of secretory gland.
   - **Tubular**: secretory cells that form tubes
   - **Alveolar**: secretory cells that form small flasklike sacs called **alveoli**. An alveolus forms a small hollow cavity, and is also called an **acinus**. Acinar means berrylike. The secretory unit is an acinus.
   - **Tubuloalveolar**: secretory structures that have both types of secretory unit

The following describes the mechanisms of secretion:

- **Merocrine**: Merocrine glands secrete their product via exocytosis. They have vesicles, which contain the product to be secreted. These glands stay intact and keep working after the product is secreted. Examples include the mammary, salivary, and sweat glands.
- **Holocrine**: In holocrine glands, the cell fills with product until they rupture and release secretions and dead cell fragments. Examples of holocrine glands include the sebaceous glands which produce sebum, a secretion composed of wax and oil.

Connective Tissue

Connective tissue is found everywhere in body. It is the most abundant and widely distributed tissue. All connective tissue is derived from the **mesoderm**. There are three embryonic tissue types:

1. **Endoderm**
2. **Ectoderm**
3. **Mesoderm**

The embryonic cell type of connective tissue is the **mesenchyme**, which are the stem cells of all connective tissue types. Then they differentiate into four different connective tissue types.

1. **Fibroblast**: The suffix *-blast* is the immature form of a cell. When a fibroblast matures it becomes a fibrocyte (*-cyte* means cell).
2. **Chondroblast**: **Chondro-** means **cartilage**. A chondroblast is the immature form of a chondrocyte, a mature cartilage cell.
3. **Osteoblast**: *Osteo-* means bone. An osteoblast is the immature form of an osteocyte, a mature bone cell.
4. **Hematopoietic stem cell**: A hematopoietic stem cell is an immature blood cell. Blood is also connective tissue. Hematopoetic cells become blood cells and macrophages.

Connective tissue has the following characteristics:

- **Common origin**: The common origin of all connective tissue is the **mesoderm** from which the embryonic **mesenchyme** cells arose.
- **Vascular**: The vascular connective tissue supplies the nutrients for epithelial tissue. Vascularity provides a better degree of healing. However, each connective tissue type is vascularized to a different degree. For example, a broken tibia will completely heal so that it is as solid as it was before the break, but a twisted ankle is a stretched ligament and takes much longer to heal. This is because ligament, which connects bone to bone, is much less vascularized.
- **Not highly cellular**: Unlike epithelial tissue, connective tissue has lots of extracellular matrix (ECM).
- **Not layers like epithelium**: Connective tissue is a hodgepodge of substances. There are lots of fibers running through it. There is much matter that is not cellular in appearance. This is extracellular matrix (ECM). An exception is cells of adipose connective tissue which do form a layer.

The composition of the extracellular matrix influences the structure of connective tissue. It is composed of three parts.

1. **Ground substance**
2. **Fibers**
3. **Cells**

The **ground substance** portion of the extracellular matrix determines the structure and physical composition of connective tissue. Some connective tissue is hard—for example, bone. This is determined by the ground substance. Some connective tissue is gellike—for example, adipose tissue and areolar tissue. This is determined by the ground substance. Some connective tissue is fluidlike, such as blood. This, too, is determined by the ground substance.

There are three types of **fiber** in the extracellular matrix.

1. **Collagen fiber**: Collagen fibers are made of a protein called **collagen**. Collagen is extremely flexible and enormously strong, but it does not have the stretch and recoil ability of elastin.
2. **Elastic fiber**: Elastic fiber is composed of the protein **elastin**. Elastin has the ability to stretch and recoil. It can be pulled apart and will come back together in the same shape.
3. **Reticular fiber**: Reticular fiber is made of the protein collagen, but these fibers branch. The advantage to this as opposed to regular collagen is that the strength of the fiber is directional. When collagen is reticulate it has strength in more directions; however, it is not as strong in general as collagen. Reticular fiber is thinner than collagen fiber.

The **cells** in the extracellular matrix are descended from the embryonic cell type fibroblasts, which mature to form fibrocytes. There are two broad categories of connective tissue: **loose** and **dense**. There are three types of loose connective tissue:

1. **Areolar**: Areolar loose connective tissue is the most generalized connective tissue type. All other connective tissue is a variation of areolar.
2. **Adipose**: Adipose loose connective tissue is fat tissue. The majority of the cell is a vacuole for fat storage. All other cellular structures and the cytoplasm are squashed to the side. The large fat vacuole dominates the cell.
3. **Reticular:** Reticular loose connective tissue is composed of a network of reticular fibers. Reticular fibers dominate in this loose connective tissue.

There are two types of dense connective tissue:

1. **Dense regular**: In dense regular connective tissue, the collagen fibers are lined up parallel to one another.
2. **Dense irregular**: In dense irregular connective tissue, the collagen fibers are oriented along multiple planes.

Connective Tissue from Osteoblasts and Hematopoietic Stem Cells

Bone derives from osteoblasts, which develop into osteocytes. **Blood** derives from hematopoietic stem cells, which develop into blood cells or hematocytes. The number of hematopoietic stem cells that become red blood cells is greater than the number that become white blood cells.

There are no fibers in blood, but there is connective tissue. The fibers that define blood as a connective tissue are seen only during blood clotting. Fibrin is suspended in the plasma. When blood vessels are severed, the fibrin becomes fibrous strings.

Cartilage is connective tissue that derives from chondroblasts. There are three types of cartilage.

1. **Hyaline cartilage**: The extracellular matrix of hyaline cartilage has collagen protein fibers and is very uniform, with a glassy, clear appearance. It is found in the ribs where it connects the ribs to the sternum. The cells are found in little compartments called **lacunae**.
2. **Elastic cartilage**: The elastin fibers in the extracellular matrix of elastic cartilage are more clearly visible. Elastin is found in the pinna of the ear and in the epiglottis.
3. **Fibrocartilage**: The fine collagen fibers of fibrocartilage are arranged in layers or bundles, creating a fibrous connective tissue that is arranged in bundles, with cartilage cells between the bundles, surrounded by a concentrically striated area of cartilage matrix.

Epithelial Membranes

Epithelial membranes are composed of epithelial tissue plus connective tissue. This is thus not tissue, but rather a simple organ. Membranes are the first simple organs. There are three types of epithelial membranes.

1. **Cutaneous membrane**: Cutaneous membrane is skin. It is partly epithelial cells and partly connective tissue.
2. **Serous membrane**: Serous membrane is **visceral** (around organs) and **parietal** (lining cavities). It is found in closed body cavities. It is also a combination of epithelial and connective tissue.
3. **Mucous membrane**: Mucous membrane differs from serous membrane in location. It is found in the linings of the open body cavities of the digestive, respiratory, and urogenital tracts.

Tissue Repair

The process of tissue repair consists of five steps.

1. **Macrophages** are sent to the area to phagocytize the cellular debris and pathogens.
2. **Scab formation**: In epithelial layer regeneration, fibroblasts are sent to the connective tissue layer to replace and repair and perform capillary repair.
3. Damaged epithelial tissue is replaced by exactly the same type of cell.
4. Damaged connective tissue is replaced by a **fibrosed** area, which is a different composition from the original tissue. It is **scar tissue** due to the fibrocytes in the fibrosed area. This imparts a relative lack of regenerative ability. Tattoos are permanent because ink is injected into the **dermal** (connective tissue) layer.
5. Blood vessels are regenerative, but sometimes healing cannot seal the end of a damaged vessel. However, new branches can come in to take its place. A capillary is only a single layer of epithelial tissue; therefore, it is regenerative.

Integumentary System

The integumentary system comprises the skin and its appendages.

Skin Structure

The skin is composed of three layers.

1. **Superficial layer**: The superficial layer is the **epidermis**. It is stratified squamous epithelial tissue. It has an apical surface (exposed to air) and a bottom attached surface, the basal surface.
2. **Middle layer**: The middle layer is the **dermis.** The dermis is connective tissue.
3. **Bottom layer**: The bottom layer is the **hypodermis**. It is a layer of fat or adipose tissue. Its function is fat storage, but it also functions as a thermal and protective layer.

Skin Cell Types

There are four cell types in the skin.

1. **Keratinocytes**: Keratinocytes are the most abundant skin cell type. They manufacture the protein **keratin**. The apical squamous epithelial cells are full of dead, flat membranous sacs of keratin, which appear yellow. From the bottom of the epidermis, the keratinocytes sit on the **basal membrane** with connective tissue below. This connective tissue has capillaries. It is vascular, imparting healthy, highly mitotic cells that are rapidly dividing so that new layers of skin are constantly formed on the basal membrane. As you move to the surface, further away from the blood supply, the cells start to die. There is a development process to the dead cells on top. The epidermis has a complete turnover once per month.
2. **Melanocytes**: Melanocytes are found in deepest layer of the epidermis, the **stratum basale.** They manufacture the **melanin** pigments. Pheomelanin is a red-brown pigment. Eumelanin is a brown-to-black pigment that is more photoprotective. It protects from ultraviolet (UV) damage. Suntan is formed when melanocytes go to the surface to try to protect the DNA from sun damage. Dark-skinned people produce more eumelanin; they do not have a greater number of melanocytes. The deepest layers of the epidermis have lots of processes that run between the keratinocytes. The melanin is transported down the projections, released, and taken in by the keratinocytes. Keratinocytes do not produce the melanin, but they contain it. Skin color is therefore defined by three factors. Melanin imparts the brown hues, keratinocytes impart the yellow hues, and the transparency of the epithelial cells allows us to see red blood cells, imparting the pink color of skin in Caucasians.
3. **Langerhans cells**: Langerhans cells are dedicated skin **macrophages.** Their function is endocytosis of cellular debris and pathogens.
4. **Merkel cells**: Merkel cells are **sensory neurons.** Only part of a Merkel cell and its axon is actually in the stratum basale of the epidermis. The dermis has many, many more Merkel cells.

Layers of the Epidermis

From deep to superficial, the following are the five layers of the epidermis.

1. **Stratum basale or germinativum**: The base and the most metabolically active cells are at the bottom.
2. **Stratum spinosum**: Next is the **prickly** layer of the stratum spinosum.
3. **Stratum granulosum**: Next is the **granular** layer of the stratum granulosum.
4. **Stratum lucidum**: Thick skin has a stratum lucidum. Thin skin does not. The only places where this thick skin is found are the palms of the hands and the soles of the feet, the places that sustain the most abrasion.

5. **Stratum corneum**: This layer is **horny**. All of the cells are dead at this layer. It is just sacs of keratin (dead, flattened cells) to protect the body. This is the topmost, most superficial layer, composed of the apical squamous epithelial cells containing dead, flat membranous sacs of keratin.

Dermal Layer

The dermal layer is the connective tissue proper. It is strong and flexible without obvious layers but lots of inclusions. There are three kinds of cells: fibroblasts, macrophages, and **mast cells**, another immune response cell. All three fiber types are also present. Collagen imparts strength. Elastin imparts flexibility and allows stretch. Reticular fibers impart multidirectional strength and support the dermis, which in turn supports the epidermis.

Other structures found in the dermis are the **hair follicles** and **sweat glands**. Hair sits in a follicle that is mainly in the basal layer of the epidermis. The bottom of the follicle is in the dermis. Follicles are epithelial tissue in the connective tissue of the dermis, which is why hair grows. It grows because of the living follicle (epithelial tissue). The hair is nonliving. The part of the hair in the dermis is the **root**. The part that comes out of scalp is the **shaft**. The control mechanism for hair growth, which determines the length of hair, is a cycle with an on phase and an off phase. In the off phase, there is no growth and hair falls out. The relative length of the phases determines hair length.

Hair loss is, to an extent, normal. Hair falls out and new hair is produced. For the eyebrows, the on phase is shorter. This is under the control of hormones, but is also affected by stress and sickness. Chemotherapy causes hair loss because cancer cells are highly mitotic, dividing out of control. The drugs target highly mitotic cells. This is why the highly mitotic epithelial cells of the follicle are killed, too. Hair pigment is the result of melanocytes at the base of the hair follicle. Gray hair occurs when the melanocytes are producing less melanin, resulting in the absence of color. Alopecia, or hair loss, results in baldness. There are two types. **Male pattern baldness** has a strong genetic component through the mother and causes a receding hair line that continues to recede. **Alopecia complete** is when all hair on the body falls out. It is thought to be an autoimmune disease, but this is not known for sure. All autoimmune diseases are more common in women.

Sweat glands are **sudoriferous glands**. They open on epithelial tissue but are located in the connective tissue of the dermis. There are 2.5 million sweat glands, but none on the lip margins, nipple, and portions of the external genitalia. Otherwise, they are everywhere else on the skin.

There are two kinds of sweat glands. **Eccrine sweat glands** are most numerous on the hands, feet, and forehead. They release their product via the merocrine mechanism, exocytosis. They open via a duct to the cell surface. The composition of the sweat is 99% water plus sodium chloride (NaCl). The pH is between 4 and 6, slightly acidic. This acts as protection against bacteria. Sweat also functions in thermal regulation by a process called **evaporative cooling**. Eccrine sweat is under the control of the autonomic nervous system. This is why sweat also occurs when one is scared or nervous.

Apocrine sweat glands are located in the armpits and axillary region and they are not present at birth. They develop at puberty. They do not function in thermoregulation. They release their product into an associated hair follicle. The composition is 98% water plus NaCl, with additional fats and proteins, which are a good nutrient source for bacteria. This is why the armpits attain their distinctive smell—it is from the waste from bacterial metabolism.

In animals, whose primary sense is smell, they play a much more significant role. Apocrine sweat glands release **pheromones**, which are used in communication. The odor is a signal for sexual availability and other messages. Apocrine sweat glands also use the merocrine mechanism, exocytosis. Mammary glands are modified apocrine sweat glands. The **ceruminous gland**, which produces cerumen (ear wax), is also a modified apocrine sweat gland.

Other appendages of the skin are as follows:

- **Nails:** Nails are a scalelike modification of the epidermis. They provide a clear protective covering for the dorsal surface of the fingers and toes. Nails are composed of hard keratin. The half-moon is the **lunula** and the cuticle the **eponychium.**
- **Sebaceous glands**: The sebaceous glands are epithelial tissue that produce oil or sebum, which is important for moisture, pliancy, and its antibacterial properties. The sebaceous glands are directly associated with the hair root and discharge sebum from the same pore as the hair. Sebum is discharged using the holocrine mechanism in which the cell ruptures. They are found everywhere except on the soles and palms.
- **Arrector pili muscles**: These muscles can change the loft of the hair. They are responsible for goose bumps and for standing animal hair up on end in the winter to thicken it and create a thermal barrier. The arrector pili muscles are also responsible for hair standing on end during the fright response.

There are two layers of the dermis.

1. **Papillary**: The papillary layer is composed of papillae or ridges. The pattern of the papillae determines the fingerprints. The epidermal layer is shaped from the papillary layer of the dermis.
2. **Reticular:** The reticular layer is 80% of the dermis. This loose connective tissue is composed of a network of branching reticular fibers that provide multidirectional strength.

The functions of the skin are:

- **Protection**: The skin provides a **physical barrier** against the entry of pathogens. It also provides a chemical barrier as acidic sweat has bactericidal components. The Langerhans cells provide an additional **biological barrier** to pathogens.
- **Thermoregulation**: The inability to sweat impairs the body's cooling ability. Thermoregulation is also achieved through blood supply regulation. More blood is sent to the skin to warm the body.
- **Sensation**: There are cutaneous sensation receptors. The Merkel cells are partly in the stratum basale of the epidermis and mainly in the dermis.
- **Vitamin D synthesis**: The skin requires a little bit of sunlight in order to synthesize vitamin D. A cholesterol precursor (7-dehydrocholesterol) is converted to vitamin D_3 in the presence of UV light.
- **Blood reservoir**: About 5% of blood is in the skin. When blood loss occurs, the skin turns white as the body goes into shock because the blood reservoir is tapped to send to more important areas.

Burns

Burns are categorized based on severity.

1. **First degree**: First degree burns are superficial burns involving the epidermis only. They heal in one to three days.
2. **Second degree**: Second degree burns extend into part of the dermis, forming blisters, which should be kept intact as long as possible to minimize infection. Keeping the epidermis intact provides protection. First and second degree burns are partial-thickness burns. Fluid separates the epidermis from the dermis. They heal in three to seven days.

3. **Third degree**: Third degree burns are full-thickness burns. The entire epidermis and dermis are affected. If they occur over a large part of the body, there are potentially life-threatening risks from excessive water loss, infection due to the loss of the protective barriers, the inability to regulate fluids and thermoregulate, the inability to manufacture vitamin D, the lack of antibacterial properties of acidic sweat, and the lack of Langerhans cells macrophages. The sensory receptors have been burned off so there is no pain. Skin grafts must be performed.

Skeletal System

The skeletal system includes the joints and bones.

Joints

Joints are the sites where two bones articulate. There are two main functions of joints: to give mobility to the skeleton and to hold the skeleton together. However, not all joints are movable. One example of immovable joints is the sutures of the brain. There are two classification methods: structural and functional.

1. **Structural**: The structural classification system is based on how the joint is built.
   - **Fibrous joints**: Fibrous joints are joined by fibrous tissue full of collagen fibers. There is no joint cavity. Most fibrous joints are immovable.
   - **Cartilaginous joints**: Cartilaginous joints are articulating bones united by cartilage. There is no joint cavity.
   - **Synovial joints**: Synovial joints are articulating bones separated by a fluid-containing joint cavity yielding freely moving joints. All joints of the limbs and most joints of the body are synovial.
2. **Functional**: The functional classification system is based on how joints work.
   - **Synarthroses**: immovable
   - **Amphiarthroses**: slightly movable
   - **Diarthroses**: freely movable
   - **Synostoses**: An additional term is used to describe fused bony joints such as when the sutures in the skull become bony and completely fused when the epiphyseal plate is gone after growth is complete.

Structural Joint Types

Fibrous Joints

- **Sutures**: Sutures are fibrous joints found only in the skull. The bones interdigitate or have a double-zigzag holding them together. These are synarthroses, or immovable joints.
- **Syndesmoses**: Syndesmoses are fibrous joints that are held together by ligaments. These joints mostly have only some give. They are synarthroses and sometimes referred to as amphiarthroses, or slightly movable.
- **Gomphoses**: Gomphoses are specialized fibrous joint between the teeth and the mandible and maxilla. These are peg-in-socket joints secured with the periodontal ligament. They are immobile, synarthroses joints.

Cartilaginous Joints

- **Synchondroses**: These are cartilaginous joints in which a bar or plate of hyaline cartilage unites the bones. Almost all are immovable synarthroses. Examples include the epiphyseal plate to the diaphysis and the costal cartilage of the first rib to the manubrium of the sternum. Epiphyseal plates are temporary joints.
- **Symphyses**: These are cartilaginous joints in which the articular surfaces of the bones are

covered with articular (hyaline) cartilage, which is fused to a pad or plate of fibrocartilage to form a shock absorber. These joints have limited movement, or are amphiarthroses. Examples include the intervertebral joints and pubic symphysis, which is made flexible during pregnancy by oxytocin.

Synovial Joints

All synovial joints are freely moving diarthroses joints. They include ball-and-socket, hinge, and pivot joints. They all have a joint cavity. They are continuous with hyaline cartilage and have a synovial membrane. The synovial membrane plus the cartilage define the cavity. The cavity contains synovial fluid produced by the synovial membrane. The hyaline cartilage, synovial membrane, and incompressible synovial fluid act as a shock absorber. Surrounding the synovial membrane is a fibrous capsule. The synovial membrane plus the fibrous capsule forms the articular capsule. The ligament is a part of the joint itself. Synovial joints are much more complex than fibrous or cartilaginous joints. Movement of synovial joints is done by muscles, so the muscle attachment must cross the joint.

MOVEMENTS OF SYNOVIAL JOINTS

- **Flexion/extension:** Flexion decreases the angle of the joint. It is a bending movement that brings the articulating bones closer together. Extension increases the angle of the joint, for example, straightening a flexed neck, body trunk, elbow, or knee. At the shoulder and hip, extension carries the limb to a point posterior to the joint. **Hyperextension** is bending backward, for example, bending the head backward beyond its straight, upright position.
- **Abduction/adduction:** Abduction is away from the body. Adduction is back toward the body. Abduction and adduction typically refer to the appendages and their position in reference to the midline of the body. In reference to the phalanges, abduction is when they are spread apart (away from the midline of the longest digit, while adduction is when the phalanges are brought back together toward the midline, or longest digit.
- **Rotation/circumduction:** Rotation is when a bone is turned around its long axis. The analogy to a pen on a piece of paper is that a dot is created. The radius rotates around the ulna. The first two cervical vertebrae rotate around one another. Another example is the hip which can be directed toward the midline or away from it. Medial rotation is toward the midline. Lateral rotation is away from the median plane of the body. Circumduction describes a cone. The distal end moves in a circle, but the point of the cone at the joint stays more or less stationary—for example, a pitcher winding up to pitch. The analogy to a pen on paper is that a circle is created.
- **Pronation/supination:** Palms up is supination, while palms down is pronation. Pronation also refers to the combined motion of the foot in a normal gait when the outer edge of the heel hits the ground and the foot rolls inward and flattens out. Supination occurs when the heel lifts off the ground and the front of the foot and toes are used to push the body forward.

(continued)

MOVEMENTS OF SYNOVIAL JOINTS (*continued*)

- **Inversion/eversion:** At the ankles, inversion is when the sole of the foot turns medially (inward). Eversion is when the sole of the foot turns laterally (outward).
- **Plantar flexion/dorsiflexion:** The up and down movement of the foot. In plantar flexion, the toes point, like a ballet dancer, downward or away from the body. In plantar dorsiflexion, the toes point up toward the knee.

Synovial Joints Range of Motion

There are six range-of-motion types for synovial joints.

1. **Planar** or **gliding**: The carpals and metacarpals exhibit a gliding or sliding motion.
2. **Hinge**: Uniaxial (single-axis) joints can only be flexed or extended, such as the humerus and ulna at the elbow. The jaw and knee also move like door hinges.
3. **Pivot**: One bone rotates around the other; for example, the radius and ulna rotate around one another at both their proximal and distal ends.
4. **Condyloid**: One bone is concave, the other is convex, and they fit together in an odd shape such as an ellipse—for example, the radiocarpal joint of the wrist.
5. **Saddle**: Saddle joints are so named because they resemble a saddle—for example, the thumb joint or trapeziometacarpal joint.
6. **Ball and socket**: Ball-and-socket joints have the greatest range of motion—for example, the humerus and scapula and the femur and os coxae.

Bones

Bones are a kind of connective tissue. There are two types of bone tissue that comprise bones.

1. **Compact**: Compact bone is superficial or outside dense bone. This is why the outside of bone looks smooth. Compact bone is found covering the epiphyses, both the proximal and distal ends. While the epiphyses themselves are composed largely of spongy bone, thin layers of compact bone cover their surfaces.
2. **Spongy**: Spongy bone is deeper and full of holes. Spongy bone is found on the shaft or diaphysis in the middle of a bone. The outer wall of the diaphysis, however, is compact bone.

There are four bone shapes:

1. **Long bones:** Long bones are longer than they are wide—for example, the femur and the phalanges.
2. **Short bones**: Short bones are cube-shaped, for example, the carpus and tarsus. A special category of short bone is a **sesamoid** (like a sesame seed) bone like the patella (kneecap).
3. **Flat bones**: Flat bones are primarily bones of the skull. They are folded like a sandwich—for example, the sternum, ribs, and most skull bones.
4. **Irregular bones**: Irregular bones are complicated shapes that do not fit into other categories—for example, the vertebra, coccyx, sphenoid, and ethmoid bones.

Bones have the following functions:

- **Support framework**: Bones support the body and cradle the soft organs.
- **Movement**: Bones are the attachment site for muscles. Muscles attach to bones with tendons. Tendons use bones as levers to move body parts.
- **Protection**: The fused bones of the skull protect the brain. The vertebrae surround and protect

the spinal cord. The rib cage protects vital organs in the thorax.

- **Storage**: The long bones store fat in the medullary cavity. The minerals calcium and phosphate are stored in bone. There is a constant flow of deposits and withdrawals of minerals. If dietary calcium is insufficient, the body will remove it from the mineralized matrix of the bone. Important growth factors such as insulin-like growth factor, transforming growth factor, and bone morphogenic protein are also stored in the bones.
- **Site of blood cell formation**: Hematopoiesis occurs in the medullary cavities, also referred to as the marrow cavities, of certain bones.

Compact bone in cross section is highly organized, resembling concentric rings. These are actually cylindrical structures called osteons. **Osteons** are the structural unit of compact bone. The entire network is also called the **Haversian system.** Each osteon is cylindrical, parallel to the long axis of the bone. It is the conduit for nerves, blood vessels, and lymphatic vessels. The other structures within the osteon are as follows:

- **Lamellae**: Each **osteon** has a series of lamellae (layers). This is why compact bone is often referred to as **lamellar bone.**
- **Haversian canal** or **central**: Each osteon has a canal through the core, which runs along the bone axis.
- **Volkmann's canals**: The Volkmann's canals run at right angles, perforating out from the Haversian canals. They connect the blood and nerve supply of the periosteum to the central Haversian canals and to the medullary cavity.
- **Periosteum**: Meaning around bone, the periosteum is the outer fibrous layer of dense, irregular connective tissue on the outside of the bone.
- **Endosteum**: Haversian canals, like all internal bone cavities, are lined with endosteum, a connective tissue lining.
- **Sharpey's fibers**: Sharpey's fibers are fibrous, dense, irregular connective tissue connecting the periosteum to the bone.
- **Osteocytes**: Osteocytes are mature bone cells.
- **Lacunae**: Osteocytes live inside little hollow cavities called lacunae. *Lac* means hollow and *una* means little.
- **Canaliculi**: Hairlike canals connect lacunae to each other and to the central Haversian canal.
- **Medullary cavities**: The medullary cavities are in the middle of the shaft of the bone and house the bone marrow. There are two types of **bone marrow. Yellow** marrow contains adipose (fat) tissue. Long bones in adults typically have yellow marrow, which can be converted to red. **Red** bone marrow, found mainly in flat bones, is involved in blood cell formation (hematopoiesis). Anemia is the reduced ability to carry oxygen. It can be due to low red blood cell count, low hemoglobin, sickle-cell anemia, or many other causes. To get red blood cells in adults, the body taps the reserve in the os coxae.

Spongy bone looks like poorly organized, haphazard tissue resembling a honeycomb. It is composed of small needlelike or flat pieces called **trabeculae,** which line up precisely along the stress lines to help resist stress as much as possible. The trabeculae have irregularly arranged lamellae and osteocytes interconnected by canaliculi. There are no osteons. Nutrients come through the canaliculi from the capillaries in the endosteum.

The composition of bone consists of both organic and inorganic components. **Organic bone** includes the following:

- **Osteogenic cells**: Osteogenic cells are actively mitotic cells found in the periosteum and endosteum. All originate from mesenchyme. Some osteogenic cells produce cells that differentiate into **osteoblasts**, which are the bone builders. Some stay bone stem cells to provide osteoblasts for the future. Others become **osteocytes**, mature bone cells, which secrete a matrix.

- **Osteoclasts**: The third cell type is not connective tissue and did not originate from the mesenchyme. These cells arise from hematopoietic stem cells that produce macrophages. They are giant multinucleate cells that break down bone. They use lysosomal enzymes and hydrochloric acid (HCl) to convert calcium salts to a soluble form. They are phagocytes that phagocytize demineralized matrix and dead osteocytes.
- **Osteoid**: The organic part of the matrix secreted by the osteocytes. It is made of collagen and glycoproteins and provides both strength and flexibility to bones. Collagen provides strength by alternating the direction in which it runs.

The **inorganic** part of the bone matrix is 65% **hydroxyapatites**, which are a mineral salt. Mostly **calcium phosphate**, it is comprised of tightly packed crystals in and around the collagen fibers in the extracellular matrix of the bone. It imparts hardness to the bone so that it can resist compression.

The strength of bones is created by its structure, as follows:

- The structure of the osteon provides strength by alternating the direction that the collagen runs.
- The lamella layers each change the direction of the collagen.
- The collagen fibers in each individual lamella run in the same direction, but in adjacent lamella the collagen fibers run in opposite directions.
- The alternating pattern of the collagen fibers in each adjacent lamella is designed to withstand torsional stress.
- Adjacent lamella reinforce one another to resist twisting.
- The design of the osteon is referred to as the **twister resistor**.
- The crystals of the mineral salts also align with the collagen fibers. They also alternate directions in adjacent lamellae.

Long bone development differs from flat bone development. In the early stages of development all are composed of hyaline cartilage, but long bone starts as hyaline cartilage, whereas flat bone forms from the intramembranous ossification of connective tissue. The hyaline cartilage undergoes **endochondral ossification** from a cartilage template in four steps.

1. The hyaline cartilage structure is supported on the sides by a **bone collar**. Then a **primary ossification** center forms in the middle of the diaphysis (shaft).
2. **Secondary ossification centers** form at the ends, the two **epiphyses**, distal and proximal.
3. The **medullary cavity** forms at the **primary ossification center**. The bone hollows out as ossification of the shaft continues.
4. There is a region between the two ossification centers that is still hyaline cartilage, forming a cartilaginous wedge between the diaphysis and the epiphysis. These are the epiphyseal plates. Ossification of the epiphyses continues. When it is complete, hyaline is only left in the epiphyseal plates.

Bone is a dynamic, constantly changing structure. Osteoclasts, the cells that reabsorb bone, play a vital role in this. There is a dynamic relationship between the osteoblasts and the osteoclasts. Whichever is working harder yields a net buildup or net breakdown of bone. The normal aging process yields a change in the proportion, with much less deposition occurring. The key is the balance of the two cell populations, which determines the relative bone deposition and resorption. The process is under the control of **growth hormone**. There are five zones of the epiphyseal plate.

1. **Quiescent zone**: Abutting the epiphysis, the resting cell zone is full of irregularly scattered cartilage cells. This is the germinal layer that supplies the developing cartilage cells.
2. **Growth zone**: Next is a layer area of rapid mitosis of cartilage cells. New cartilage cells push the epiphysis away from the diaphysis.
3. **Hypertonic zone**: Next is a layer of minimal to no mitosis. As the chondrocytes begin to terminally differentiate they become enlarged, swollen, and vacuolated.
4. **Calcification zone**: Next is an area where lengthwise channels of cartilage matrix become calcified. The chondrocytes have died and prepared the matrix for calcification, which then serves as a template for osteoblastic bone formation.
5. **Ossification zone**: Abutting the diaphysis is the area where new bone formation takes place. When the rate of cartilage formation in the growth zone is greater than the rate of ossification in the ossification zone, bone growth (elongation) occurs. New cells push the epiphysis away from the diaphysis. When the rate of cartilage formation in the growth zone is less than the rate of ossification in the ossification zone, the epiphyseal plate begins to ossify. It eventually disappears and the remaining structure in adulthood is the **epiphyseal line**.

As bone grows, width must be added in addition to elongation at the epiphyseal plate. Changing the shape of bone is called **bone remodeling**. This occurs all throughout the life cycle from growing through aging. Bone deposition and resorption occur both at the surface of the periosteum and at the surface of the endosteum, both on the outside of the bone and on the inside linings. At the articular cartilage, cartilage growth occurs on the outside of the bone. On the inside of the articular cartilage, bone deposition occurs as cartilage is replaced by bone. At the opposite end, abutting the diaphysis, cartilage growth occurs on the inside. On the outside, facing the diaphysis (inside the bone), bone deposition also occurs. Cartilage is replaced by bone. At the same time, bone is resorbed and added on the outside of the epiphysis and diaphysis to reshape the outer contours of the bone. Bone remodeling is controlled by a five-part negative feedback loop hormonal mechanism that regulates and maintains calcium (Ca^{2+}) homeostasis.

1. When the concentration of calcium (Ca^{2+}) decreases, parathyroid hormone (PTH) is released.
2. PTH release indirectly causes osteoclasts to resorb bone. This in turn releases Ca^{2+} into the blood.
3. As the concentration of calcium (Ca^{2+}) in the blood increases, the PTH decreases.
4. As the PTH decreases, the blood concentration of calcium (Ca^{2+}) goes back down to normal.
5. Pressure on the bones also stimulates osteoblasts, which facilitates bone buildup. While the hormonal loop calcium concentration (Ca^{2+}) homeostasis determines whether and when remodeling occurs, it is mechanical stress and weight bearing that determine where bone remodeling occurs. Bone that is the least stressed is considered by the body to be expendable. This is the bone that is resorbed. Mechanical stress is pull from the muscles and from gravity. This is why weight-bearing activity is good for healthy bones.

The following describes the four-step process of bone repair.

1. **Hematoma formation**
2. **Fibrocartilaginous callus formation**: An internal callus of fibrous tissue and cartilage is formed.
3. **Bony callus formation**
4. **Bone remodeling**: Osteoclasts now come in to resorb the bulge at the healed fracture site.

COMMON TYPES OF FRACTURES

There are six common types of bone fractures:

1. **Comminuted:** The bone is broken in three or more pieces. This usually only occurs in aged, brittle bones.
2. **Compression:** In a compression fracture the bone is crushed. This usually occurs only in porous or osteoporotic bones,
3. **Spiral:** Excessive twisting causes a ragged break, often seen in sports injuries.
4. **Epiphyseal:** In an epiphyseal fracture, the epiphysis and diaphysis separate along the epiphyseal plate.
5. **Depressed:** In a depressed fracture, the bone is pushed in. This is the typical skull fracture type.
6. **Greenstick:** A greenstick fracture is an incomplete break in which one side breaks and the other side bends.

Flat bones are formed from fibrous connective tissue. Flat bone development is a four-step sandwichlike process.

1. Central mesenchyme cells cluster and become osteoblasts. They form a **single ossification center** in the middle.
2. Osteoblasts produce osteoid (organic bone matter). The osteoid is mineralized, creating **spongy bone** called **diploë**.
3. Compact bone is laid down on either side of diploë. The periosteum, the outer fibrous layer, forms.
4. Internally, diploë vascular tissue becomes red bone marrow.

Muscular System

This section reviews various elements of the muscle system, including muscle tissue functions, skeletal muscle cells and fibers, muscle attachments, the sliding filament theory of muscle contraction, proteins of the thin and thick filaments, steps in the actin head to myosin binding, the structure of the sarcoplasmic reticulum, excitation contraction coupling, muscle contraction at the muscle level, smooth muscle, and cardiac muscle.

Muscle Tissue Functions

Muscle tissue performs the following functions:

- **Movement**
- **Posture**: maintain posture
- **Joint stability**: hold joints together
- **Produce body heat**

There are three subsets of muscle tissue.

1. **Skeletal**
2. **Smooth**
3. **Cardiac**

There are three organizational levels of study.

1. **Cellular**
2. **Proteins that make up muscle tissue**
3. **Organs**

Skeletal Muscle Cells (Cellular Level)

At the cellular level:

- Each muscle fiber is **multinucleate**.
- Muscle fibers contain proteins, mostly **myosin** and **actin**.
- The plasma membrane of a muscle fiber is called the **sarcolemma**.
- The endoplasmic reticulum is the **sarcoplasmic reticulum** (SER).

Characteristics of Skeletal Muscle Fibers

Skeletal muscle fibers have the following three characteristics:

1. They can contract.
2. They can stretch and recoil.
3. They are excitable. They can receive and respond to electrical stimuli. They can generate action chemicals, signals that allow communication. There are only two categories of excitable cells: muscle cells and neurons.

Structure of Skeletal Muscle Fibers

The following describes the five-level structure of skeletal muscle fibers.

1. Each muscle fiber is wrapped by a connective tissue layer called the **endomysium**.
2. A bunch of endomysium-wrapped muscle fibers are bundled together to form a **fascicle**.
3. Each fascicle (bundle of muscle fibers) is covered by **perimysium**.
4. A bundle of fascicles makes a muscle.
5. The muscle is covered by a top coat connective tissue layer called the **epimysium**.

Muscle Attachments

Muscles can attach in any one of three different ways:

1. **Direct**: Direct attachments are fleshy attachments formed by the muscle **epimysium** (top layer) fused to the **periosteum**, the outer fibrous layer of dense, irregular connective tissue on the outside of the bone.
2. **Indirect**: Indirect attachments are formed when the **epimysium** (connective tissue wrapping) extends beyond the muscle as a ropelike **tendon**.
3. **Aponeurosis**: An aponeurosis is a sheetlike attachment that anchors muscle to the connective tissue covering of bone or to cartilage or to the fascia of other muscles. The **linea alba**, white line, is a tendonous **raphe** or **seam** from the sternum to the pubic symphysis. The **external obliques**, **internal obliques**, and **transverse abdominus**, the abdominal muscles, are joined in the middle at the linea alba. However, they are also joined by a flat tendon sheet, an **aponeurosis**. All of these abdominal muscles have their insertion via aponeurosis into the linea alba.

Elements of the Skeletal Muscle Cell

The following describes the two basic elements of a skeletal muscle cell:

1. **Myofibril**: A myofibril is the next subunit under the cell. It is the next cylinder bundle structure within the muscle fiber cell. Myofibrils are made of **myofilaments** with two different kinds of proteins.
   - **Thin**: mostly actin
   - **Thick**: myosin
2. **Sarcomere**: A sarcomere is a subunit of a myofilament. They are the **basic unit of muscle contraction**.

Myofibrils are an organized pattern of thick myosin and thin mostly actin filaments. They run parallel to the length of the muscle fiber. They are composed of distinct bands and zones, as follows:

- **I-band**: An I-band is a light-colored section of myofibril in which **only thin** filaments are present.
- **A-band**: An A-band is a dark band of myofibril that has **both thick and thin** filaments overlapping.
- **Z-disc**: A Z-disc is the **midline** of an **I-band**. It anchors the thin filaments.
- **H-zone**: An H-zone is the midsection of an A-band. It is named for the word *helle*, which means **bright**. It is composed of **thick filaments only**. The rest of the A band has thin filaments coming in from either side.

- **M-line**: The M-line is a dark line that vertically bisects the H-zone. Myofilaments are connected to the sarcolemma at the Z-discs and M-lines.
- **Sarcomere**: A sarcomere is the **distance from one Z-disc to another**. It is an **A-band** with **half** of an **I-band** on either side.

Sliding Filament Theory of Muscle Contraction

Thin and thick filaments do not change length. They do not shorten, but rather stay the same size. The muscles shorten, but the filaments do not. When the muscle is relaxed, the H-zone, at the midsection of the A-band where the thin filaments do not extend, is present. When a contraction starts, the sarcomere shortens because the filaments change position relative to one another. The following is the four-step process when a contraction starts.

1. The length of the A-band stays the same.
2. The H-zone seems to disappear.
3. The I-band shortens.
4. The sarcomere shortens.

Proteins of the Thin and Thick Filaments

Myosin, the thick filament, has two heads and a tail. The heads are clustered at the ends of the sarcomere. The tails are in the middle. It has two functions.

1. Myosin binds to actin. The myosin heads bind to actin. This is called **cross-bridge formation**.
2. Myosin binds to **ATP**.

Thin filaments actually have three proteins:

1. **Actin**: The actin is called **f-actin** or fibrous actin. There are two strands. It looks like beads on a strung necklace and has a binding site for the myosin head of the thick filament.
2. **Tropomyosin**: Tropomyosin is rod-shaped. It gives the thin filament stability and blocks the binding site on f-actin. It functions with troponin to regulate actin head-to-myosin binding.
3. **Troponin**: Troponin is composed of three polypeptides.
   - **TnI** binds to **actin**.
   - **TnT** binds to **tropomyosin**.
   - **TnC** binds to calcium (**Ca^{2+}**).

Steps in Actin Head to Myosin Binding

The following describes the six steps in actin head-to-myosin binding:

1. At the beginning, before a contraction begins:
   - Actin is bound to troponin I (TnI).
   - TnI is bound to troponin C (TnC).
   - TnC is bound to Ca^{2+} (from the SER).
   - TnC is bound to troponin T (TnT).
   - TnT is bound to tropomyosin.
   - Tropomyosin is blocking the binding site on actin and preventing the myosin head from binding.
2. More Ca^{2+} enters and binds to TnC (troponin C).
3. Calcium-activated troponin undergoes a conformational change.
4. This moves the tropomyosin away from the actin binding site.
5. The myosin head can now bind and cycle.
6. This causes a contraction. The sliding of the thin filaments by the myosin cross bridge begins.

The **cross bridge cycle** begins when the myosin head attaches to the actin myofilament and the cross bridge forms. There are three steps.

1. ADP is lost from the myosin head. This is the **power stroke**. Inorganic phosphate (Pi) generated when the cross bridge was formed is released, initiating the power stroke. The myosin head pivots and bends to a low-energy shape as it pulls on the actin filament sliding it toward the M line.

2. ATP binds to the myosin head, causing the myosin to dissociate from the actin.
3. **ATP hydrolysis** occurs. ATP is split into ADP and P. This energizes the myosin head and cocks it into its high-energy conformation, back to upright.

Structure of the Sarco/endoplasmic Reticulum (SER)

The structure of the sarco/endoplasmic reticulum (SER) consists of 12 parts.

1. The tubules of the SER wrap around each myofibril.
2. The SER stores **Ca^{2+}** in its series of tubules.
3. The broad part of the SER is the **terminal cisternae.** The SER is tubules plus the broad terminal cisternae.
4. The terminal cisternae are at the junction of the A-bands (both thick and thin) and the I-bands (light only thin).
5. The sarcolemma (plasma membrane of the muscle fiber) extends into the center of the cell.
6. The sarcolemma extensions into the center of the cell are called the T-tubules (transverse tubules).
7. The function of the t-tubules is to bring the sarcolemma closer to the center of the cell. When it is closer to all cell parts there is increased communication because it facilitates the movement of ions.
8. The T-tubules run between two terminal cisternae at each A-band to I-band junction.
9. The T-tubules also encircle each sarcomere.
10. The two terminal cisternae with a t-tubule in the middle forms a **triad.**
11. The integral proteins of the T-tubule protrude to form **voltage sensors.**
12. The integral proteins of the SER are called **foot proteins.** They form channels through which Ca^{2+} can be released from the terminal cisternae of the SER.

Excitation Contraction Coupling

Excitation contraction coupling is how the Ca^{2+} is released from the SER. An action potential begins the event. When excitable cells, which include muscle cells, neurons, and endocrine cells, are not active, their plasma membranes maintain what is called a **resting membrane potential (RMP).** This is the voltage or electrical potential energy contained in the membrane. All cells are polarized. The inside of the cell carries a net negative charge compared to the outside. The RMP is determined mostly by the potassium (K^+) concentration. K^+ and protein anions predominate in the cell. Sodium (Na^+) ions predominate in the extracellular fluid, largely balanced by chloride ions (Cl^-). Cells can control, via protein channels, the incoming and outgoing ions. Permeability is changed by opening and closing the channels. In a resting neuron or a resting muscle cell, the charge inside the cell is not equal to the charge outside the cell. Some channels in the plasma membrane are always open.

K^+ is outgoing and Na^+ is ingoing. If left alone in equilibrium, it is not a desirable situation. In excitable cells such as neurons and muscle cells this would mean there was no signaling occurring. There must be a mechanism to maintain the gradient. This mechanism is the Na^+/K^+ pump. It moves K^+ into the cell and Na^+ out of the cell against the gradient. Just right along the plasma membrane there is a –70 mV charge differential between the inside relative to the outside of the membrane. This –70 mV charge therefore represents the electrochemical gradient across the membrane. An **action potential** is a short-lived event in which the membrane potential quickly increases and then decreases. In order for an action potential to occur, the resting membrane potential must be disturbed, causing depolarization to a threshold value of –55 mV. Once the threshold has been met, voltage-gated Na^+ channels open.

The release of the neurotransmitter acetylcholine, which binds to a receptor protein on the sarcolemma, causes a chemically gated Na^+ channel to open. As more Na^+ enters the cell, the voltage inside the cell becomes more positive. At –55 mV, the threshold, the voltage-gated channels open. The cell permeability to Na^+ increases dramatically and membrane depolarization accelerates. At approximately +30 mV, the voltage-gated Na^+ channels close and repolarization begins. Shortly thereafter, the voltage-gated K^+ channels open. Since permeability to Na^+ is up and permeability to K^+ is down and since K^+ is greater inside the cell than outside the cell, K^+ rapidly departs the cell. The K^+ gates begin to very slowly close and hyperpolarization of the membrane to below the RMP occurs. The cell then returns to RMP because all Na^+ and K^+ voltage-gated channels are closed, but the always open channels return the cell to the resting cross-membrane ion concentrations.

With skeletal muscle there must be a relationship with the nervous system. A motor neuron must generate an action potential that through a series of six steps will cause the SER to release calcium.

1. **Signal (action potential)**: The action potential (AP) travels down a motor neuron toward the sarcolemma.
2. **Release of acetylcholine**: When the AP travels down the motor neuron to the sarcolemma, it causes the release of acetylcholine.
3. **Acetylcholine binding**: The acetylcholine binds to a receptor (protein) on the sarcolemma.
4. **Sodium channel opening**: The binding of acetylcholine to the sarcolemma causes a channel to open to allow Na^+ into the cell.
5. **Second action potential**: This causes another AP to travel down the t-tubule.
6. **Calcium release**: This causes the Ca^{2+} release from the SER.

Muscle Contraction at the Muscle Level

At the cellular level, a contraction is all or none. A single muscle fiber with the sarcomeres lined up either does contract or does not; there is no in-between. However, with **muscle organs** there are **intermediates**. How the cellular level is translated to the muscular level hinges on the relationship between the motor neuron and the muscle itself. A **motor unit** is a single motor neuron and all of the muscle fibers it innervates or controls. A single motor unit can activate multiple muscle fibers. There is a wide range of muscle fibers a certain motor neuron can innervate, depending on how many motor neurons are activated.

Concentric contraction involves the force created when the muscle fibers shorten because the force of the contraction exceeds the external force. **Eccentric contraction** involves the force created when the muscle fibers lengthen because the resistance is greater than the force of the contraction. For example, when you land on two feet from a jump and bend your knees, the quadriceps are lengthening, but also creating a force to control the landing. As you spring back from the landing, extending your knees and jumping back up in the air, the quadriceps are shortening as they create force to push you off.

Smooth Muscle

Smooth muscle is found surrounding blood and lymphatic vessels in the bladder, digestive tract, and reproductive tract, as well as in the erector pili of the skin and other parts of the body. In contrast to skeletal muscle, the cells have only a single nucleus. The basic unit of muscle contraction in skeletal muscle, the sarcomere, is not present. Smooth muscle contractions are innervated by the autonomic nervous system. Both sympathetic and parasympathetic prompts cause involuntary contractions.

Smooth muscle is categorized as either single-unit or multiunit. **Single-unit** tissue is innervated at a single cell. This cell lies within a sheet. The action potential, rather than traveling down a motor neuron, is passed via gap junctions to adjacent cells. This causes the entire sheet to contract as a unit. **Multiunit** smooth muscle tissue is found in places where fine motor control is necessary. Individual cells are controlled in a manner similar to skeletal muscle. Smooth muscle contains both actin and myosin in varying ratios depending on the tissue. It can also be **myogenic**, or able to contract without nervous system intervention. The lack of sarcomeres accounts for smooth muscle being referred to as smooth or nonstriated.

Cardiac Muscle

Cardiac muscle is striated and has intercalated discs connecting the ends of adjacent cells. It is organized into sarcomeres. It is found in the heart and the cells are multinucleate. Myocardial contractions are controlled by the autonomic nervous system. Cardiac muscle also contains the proteins actin and myosin. In contrast to skeletal muscles, the myofilaments can be branched rather than only linear. Cardiac muscle requires more calcium than skeletal muscle contraction. This is supplied by extracellular stores of Ca^{+2}. Sodium ions cross the sarcolemma and initiate a second action potential just as in skeletal muscle. However, the additional calcium influx provides cardiac muscle with the ability to sustain depolarization for a longer time period.

Cardiovascular System

There are three components to the cardiovascular system: the blood, the heart, and the blood vessels. All three work together as the cardiovascular system.

The Heart

The function of the heart is to act as a pump to propel blood through the blood vessels so that it can perform all of its functions. It is located inside the **mediastinum**, the medial (central) cavity of the thorax. It is partially covered by the lungs. It is not completely centered in the middle of the body, but rather is slightly left of center. It is pointed toward the left due to a left tilt of the apex. The **point of maximal intensity (PMI)** is at the apex of the heart between the fifth and sixth ribs. This is the point where you can easily feel your heart beating. The heart is enclosed in a double-layered (walled) sac called the **pericardium**. The outermost superficial covering is the **fibrous pericardium**. The functions of the fibrous pericardium are:

- **Protection**: It protects the heart.
- **Anchoring**: It anchors it to surrounding structures.
- **Preventing overfilling**: It prevents the heart from overfilling (filling with too much blood).

The inner layer is the **serous pericardium**, which has two layers of its own.

1. **Parietal layer**: The more superficial layer of the serous pericardium. It contacts the inner surface of the fibrous pericardium.
2. **Visceral layer**: The deep layer of the serous pericardium. It is also called the **epicardium**. It is part of the heart wall.

The **pericardial cavity** is the space between parietal layer of serous pericardium and visceral layer of serous pericardium. It decreases friction because it is filled with fluid. It can become infected and inflamed. If there is too much fluid, it constricts the beating of the heart, causing a condition known as **cardiac tamponade**. The treatment is to insert a needle and remove the excess fluid.

The layers that make up the heart are as follows:

- **Epicardium:** The epicardium is the innermost outer covering of the heart. It is also called the **visceral layer** of **serous pericardium** and is part of the heart wall.
- **Myocardium:** The myocardium is the bulk of heart. It is contractile muscle tissue. The left ventricle is much thicker than right because it must sustain higher pressure. It must pump blood to the body. However, there are always equal amounts of blood on each side even though the sizes and thicknesses differ. One cause of heart attacks or **myocardial infarctions** is when the coronary arteries are blocked and cannot deliver

oxygenated blood. The heart muscle dies and cannot be replaced, but rather is replaced by scar tissue. If the left coronary artery is blocked, the left ventricle will die and death of the individual will ensue. Blockages of coronary arteries are the primary cause of heart attacks.

- **Endocardium:** The endocardium is the innermost part of the heart. It lines the chambers of heart, covers the valves, and is continuous with the blood vessels. It is composed of epithelial and connective tissue.

The following describes the three structures of the heart:

1. The heart chambers consist of two **atria** (left and right) and two **ventricles** (left and right).
2. The **septum** divides the chambers.
   - The **interventricular septum** divides the ventricles.
   - The **interatrial septum** divides the atria. It has a shallow depression called the **fossa ovalis** that is left over from the **fetal** structure that served as the opening for fetal circulation, the **foramen ovale**.
3. The **interventricular sulci** are grooves on the outside of the heart that mark the location of the interventricular septum, which separates the right and left ventricles.

Structures of Atria: The Receiving Chambers

There are two structures of the atria.

1. The **auricles**: These are flaps or appendages on the atria. They increase the amount of blood (blood volume) the atria can hold.
2. The **pectinate muscles**: There is a wall between the right and left atria. On the anterior portion of the right atrium, the wall is ridged by bundles of muscles that look like the teeth of a comb.

There are three vessels of the right atrium.

1. **Superior vena cava:** The superior vena cava delivers blood from everything in the systemic circuit superior to the diaphragm to the right atria.
2. **Inferior vena cava:** The inferior vena cava delivers blood from everything inferior to the diaphragm to the right atria.
3. **Coronary sinus:** The coronary sinus collects blood from the heart muscle, the myocardium. The heart has its own special circulation called the **coronary circuit**.

There are four vessels of the left atrium; all are **pulmonary veins**—two left pulmonary veins and two right pulmonary veins.

Structures of the Ventricles: The Discharging Chambers

The ventricles, which are much bigger than the atria, pump to either the **pulmonary circuit** or the **systemic circuit**. The right ventricle pumps blood into the pulmonary trunk to the pulmonary arteries, which go to the lungs. The left ventricle pumps blood to the aorta. The **trabeculae carne** are ridges in the ventricle walls. The **papillary muscles** work in valve function.

Parts of the Aorta

The aorta has three basic parts:

1. **Ascending aorta:** The ascending aorta receives blood from the left ventricle.
2. **Arch of the aorta:** The aorta arches over and to the left and begins descending right in front of the spinal column.
3. **Descending aorta:** The descending aorta travels through the chest to the abdomen, acquiring other names along the way.

There are three branches off the aortic arch. They are, in order:

1. **Brachiocephalic:** The brachiocephalic artery supplies blood to the head, brain, and right arm.

2. **Left common carotid:** The left common carotid artery supplies blood to the chest and neck.
3. **Left subclavian artery:** The left subclavian artery supplies blood to the left arm. It runs below the clavicle. Branches that arise from it serve the vertebral column, spinal cord, ear, and brain.

As the aorta continues through the abdomen, there are other branches.

The flow of blood through the heart is a closed circuit. The flow proceeds in the following order starting from the body, but you can start anywhere in flow chart.

1. Starting from the body, blood is returned through veins. From the **superior vena cava** and the **inferior vena cava** it flows to the **right atrium** of the heart.
2. From the right atrium blood flows through the **tricuspid** valve, also called the **right atrioventricular (AT) valve**, to the **right ventricle**.
3. From the **right ventricle** blood is pumped through the **pulmonary semilunar valve** to the **pulmonary trunk**.
4. From the pulmonary trunk, blood flows to the **pulmonary arteries**.
5. From the pulmonary arteries, blood flows to the **lungs**.
6. From the lungs, blood flows to the **pulmonary veins**.
7. From the pulmonary veins, blood flows to the **left atrium**.
8. From the left atrium, blood flows through the **bicuspid** or **left atrioventricular (AV) valve**, also called the **mitral valve**, to the **left ventricle**.
9. From the left ventricle, blood flows through the **aortic semilunar valve** to the **aorta**.

Blood Flow through the Heart

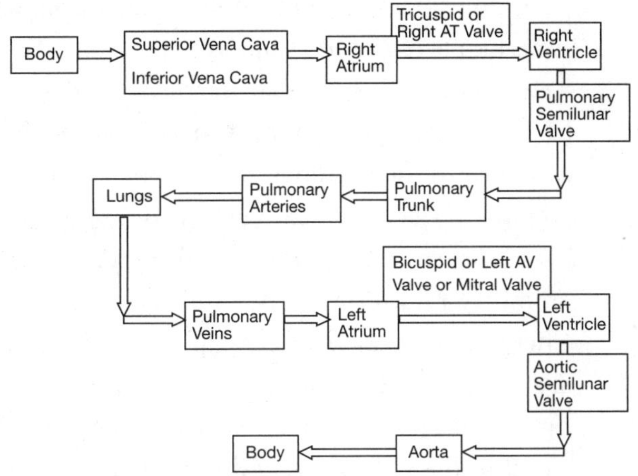

Cardiovascular Circuits

There are three pathways.

1. **Pulmonary circuit**: The pulmonary circuit flows from the heart to the lungs and back to the heart.
2. **Systemic circuit**: The systemic circuit flows from the heart to the body and back to the heart.
3. **Coronary circuit**: The coronary circuit delivers blood to the myocardium, heart tissue. Because it is under so much pressure, the blood the heart is pumping cannot be used for its own purposes.

Vessels

There are four major types of vessels:

1. **Coronary arteries**: The right and left coronary arteries branch off the aorta. They deliver oxygenated blood to heart muscle. They are constricted when the heart contracts such that when the ventricles contract the blood flow is nearly stopped. They deliver blood only when the ventricles are relaxed.

2. **Coronary sinus**: On the venous side, on the posterior surface, blood pools in the coronary sinus and is returned to the right atrium.
3. **Artery**: Blood vessel that carries blood away from the heart, usually oxygenated blood. One exception is the pulmonary trunk, or main pulmonary artery, which carries deoxygenated blood. There are two branches, the left and right pulmonary arteries. The pulmonary trunk emerges at the base of the right ventricle and branches into the two pulmonary arteries. The right pulmonary artery takes deoxygenated blood to the right lung, and the left pulmonary artery takes deoxygenated blood to the left lung. Another exception is the umbilical arteries of a fetus, which carry deoxygenated blood to the placenta through the umbilical cord.
4. **Vein**: Blood vessel that carries deoxygenated blood to the heart. The exceptions are the pulmonary veins, which carry oxygenated blood from the lungs to the left atrium, and the umbilical veins, which carry oxygenated blood from the placenta to the fetus.

The Four Valves

The purpose of the four valves is to keep blood flowing in one direction. There are two types of valves.

1. **Atrioventricular (AV) valves**: The right AV is the **tricuspid** valve. The left AV is the **bicuspid** or **mitral valve**. The function of the AV valves is to prevent backflow into the atria when the ventricles are contracting. A **chordae tendineae** is attached to each AV valve. These are referred to as the heart strings. **Anchor cusps**, flaps of endocardium reinforced by connective tissue, are joined to **papillary muscles** protruding from the ventricle walls. This prevents backflow into the atria; it does not close the valves.
2. **Semilunar valves**: The semilunar valves are between the ventricles and the branches. The right ventricle sends blood to the pulmonary trunk through the pulmonary semilunar valve. The left ventricle sends blood to the aorta through the aortic semilunar valve.

The three steps to open the atrioventricular valves are as follows:

1. Blood returns to heart, filling the atria. This causes pressure on the AV valves, which forces the AV valves open.
2. As the ventricles fill, the AV valve flaps hang limply into the ventricles.
3. As the atria contract, they force additional blood into the ventricles.

The atrioventricular valves open when the blood pressure exerted on their atrial side is greater than the blood pressure on the ventricle side.

The three steps to close the AV valves are as follows:

1. The ventricles contract, forcing blood against the AV valve cusps.
2. The AV valves close.
3. The papillary muscles contract and the chordae tendoneae tighten, preventing the flaps from everting into the atria.

The valves are forced closed when the ventricles contract and the intraventricular pressure rises, moving the blood upward. The papillary muscles and chordae tendoneae keep the valve flaps closed.

The semilunar valves work in two steps as follows:

1. As the ventricles contract, interventricular pressure rises. Blood is pushed up against the semilunar valves, forcing them open.
2. When the ventricles relax, interventricular pressure falls. Blood flows back from the arteries, fills the cusps of the semilunar valves, and forces them closed.

Characteristics of Cardiac Muscle

Cardiac muscles have the following seven characteristics:

1. Cardiac muscle contains short, fat cells and lots of **branching**.
2. The cells are all **interconnected**, which is important so that the heart can contract as a single unit.
3. Cardiac muscle is **striated** like skeletal muscle.
4. The junctions between adjacent cells are **intercalated discs**, where the plasma membranes of the two cells meet.
5. There are **desmosomes** between cells to hold them together during contractions and prevent ripping or tearing of the muscle.
6. There are **gap junctions** that also connect the cells to allow ions and other substances to pass between cells.
7. There are lots of **mitochondria** because the heart must not fatigue.

Cardiac Cell Types

There are two basic types of cardiac cells:

1. **Autorhythmic cells**: These cells do not contract. They depolarize automatically. They are responsible for causing the cells that do contract to depolarize. They depolarize spontaneously and pace the heart. They are part of the **intrinsic conduction system**, which is self-contained and requires no nervous innervation. No hormones are needed. Because it has its own depolarization, the heart can control itself. However, nerve impulses and hormones do influence this. There is no resting membrane potential, so there is no baseline to return to. They are always slightly depolarizing (going through depolarization), which gives them pacemaker potential. It is these depolarizations that initiate the action potential that spreads to the heart.
2. **Contractile cells**: These are the cells that work together as a pump. Contractions are either all or none. Either all cells contract or none contract.

Action Potential of Contractile Cells

The resting membrane potential (RMP) of the contractile cells is –90 mV. The 11 steps to rhythmic contraction are as follows:

1. **Rising phase**: Depolarization opens voltage-gated fast sodium (Na^+) channels. This results in a rise in the action potential (AP) of +30 mV (threshold). This spike, a period of increased Na^+ permeability, is very brief. It is quickly inactivated and the Na^+ influx stops.
2. The depolarization wave travels down the T-tubules and the SER releases Ca^{2+}.
3. **Excitation-contraction coupling:** The influx of calcium (Ca^{2+}) signals for **cross bridge** activation. This couples the depolarization wave to the sliding of the myofilaments. About 10% to 20% of the Ca^{2+} needed for the calcium pulse that triggers contraction enters from extracellular space. This stimulates the SER to release the other 80% of the Ca^{2+}. Ca^{2+} is barred from entering nonstimulated cardiac fibers by the Na^+ influx and membrane depolarization. This provides the necessary stimulation for slow Ca^{2+} voltage-gated channels to open. The slow channels are slightly delayed. Now the Ca^{2+} influx opens nearby Ca^{2+} channels in the SER tubules so that the Ca^{2+} spikes trigger a dramatic rise in the calcium concentration (Ca^{2+}). Sodium (Na^+) permeability is down to resting levels, but the calcium (Ca^{2+}) surge prolongs depolarization. This is the **plateau phase**.
4. During the plateau phase, potassium (K^+) permeability decreases. This also prolongs the plateau, preventing rapid repolarization.
5. As long as Ca^{2+} is entering, the cells continue to contract. Muscle tension develops during the plateau and peaks after the plateau ends.

6. The duration of the AP and the contractile phase is much longer than in skeletal muscle. After 200 ms, the slope of the action potential drops rapidly.
7. The calcium (Ca^{2+}) channels close.
8. The voltage-gated K^+ channels open.
9. There is a rapid loss of K^+ from the cell.
10. The resting membrane potential is restored.
11. During repolarization, Ca^{2+} is pumped back into the SER and extracellular space.

Action Potential of Autorhythmic Cells

For autorhythmic cells there is no resting membrane potential, and the cells are always slightly depolarizing. Depolarization is due to the inward diffusion of calcium (not sodium as in nerve cell membranes). Depolarization begins when the slow Na^+ channels open. This concludes quickly when the fast calcium channels open. Repolarization is due to the outward diffusion of potassium.

1. **Rising phase of the action potential**:
   - Hyperpolarization at the end of the action potential causes the potassium (K^+) channels to close, and the slow Na^+ channels then open.
   - The cell slowly depolarizes. At approximately –40 mV (threshold), the Ca^{2+} channels open, yielding an explosive surge of Ca^{2+} from the extracellular space. At approximately 0 mV, the Ca^{2+} channels close and the K^+ channels open. This starts the falling phase.
2. **Falling phase of the AP**:
   - Repolarization causes Ca^{2+} permeability to decrease and K^+ permeability to increase.
   - When repolarization is complete, the K^+ channels close. Slow Na^+ channels open again and K^+ permeability declines. This yields slow depolarization (pacemaker potential) to the threshold (–40 mV), and the process begins again.

Components of the Intrinsic Conduction System

There are five components of the intrinsic conduction system.

1. **Sinoatrial (SA) node**: The SA node is the pacemaker of heart. It depolarizes faster than any other autorhythmic cells, ~75 times per minute. This is the **sinus rhythm**. It is controlled by the nervous system. If all external neural and hormonal influences were severed, it would depolarize 100 times per minute. The SA node is located in the right atrial wall.
2. **Atrioventricular (AV) node**: A depolarization wave spreads to the AV node via gap junctions and throughout the atria. Above the tricuspid valve, the depolarization wave is slowed. This allows the atria to contract before the ventricles do. The delay is due to smaller-diameter fibers and fewer gap junctions. This ensures that the AV node conducts impulses more slowly, creating a merging area. If the SA node is not working, the AV node takes over as pacemaker, but at a depolarization rate of only 50 times per minute. This is called the **junctional rhythm**.
3. **Atrioventricular bundle**: The AV bundle is also called the **bundle of His**. The impulse surges after the merge to the AV bundle. It is located superior to the interventricular septum. It is the only electrical connection between the atria and the ventricles. If it is severed, there is no longer a way for the impulse to travel to the ventricle.
4. **Right and left bundle branches**: The AV bundle persists only briefly before splitting into these two pathways. The depolarization wave is now traveling through the interventricular septum toward the apex of the heart. Then it starts to curve and travel up along the sides of the ventricles. The depolarization rate is now 30 per minute. This is not enough to sustain life.

5. **Purkinje fibers:** The Purkinje fibers are barrel-shaped cells with few myofibrils. They complete the pathway through the interventricular septum to the apex of the heart. The depolarization wave then proceeds up into the ventricular walls, more on the left side than the right because the left is much thicker. The bulk of ventricular depolarization depends on the Purkinje fibers. The Purkinje fibers directly supply the papillary muscles, which are excited to contract before the rest of the ventricular muscles. The papillary muscles tighten the chordae tendineae before the force of the ventricular contraction pushes the blood against the AV valve flaps. They depolarize at rate of 30 per minute. Ventricular contraction almost immediately follows the ventricular depolarization wave.

Defects of the Conduction System

The following describes defects of the conduction system.

- **Arrhythmia**: Irregular heartbeat is caused when some factor causes cells to depolarize at an irregular rate.
- **Fibrillation**: This is irregular muscle contraction that makes the heart useless as a pump. Defibrillation is a shock to the heart to wipe the slate clean. It gets rid of all of the action potential happening in the hope that the sinoatrial node will take over. There must be some electrical activity in order to shock the heart back to the SA rhythm.
- **Ectopic focus**: Ectopic focus is when there is an abnormal pacemaker. A couple of cells start to depolarize faster than the SA node, causing a bunch of cells to take over the heart. It quickly dissipates and is usually temporary. It can be caused by nicotine or caffeine. The saying "My heart skipped a beat" is referring to these premature contractions.

Electrocardiograph (EKG)

An **electrocardiograph** (EKG; also called an ECG) is an electrical tracing of heart activity, showing the peaks and valleys as waves. It includes the following:

- **P wave**: The first wave constitutes atrial depolarization, which yields atrial contraction. The SA node generates an impulse and atrial excitation begins. An action potential is generated. The impulse is delayed at the AV node, then passed to the heart apex via the right and left bundle branches. Ventricular excitation begins.
- **QRS complex**: Ventricular depolarization yields ventricular contraction. Ventricular excitation completes as the Purkinje fibers spread the action potential depolarization wave up into the ventricular walls and the bulk of ventricular depolarization occurs.
- **T wave**: Ventricular repolarization causes ventricular relaxation in the ST segment. This is when the action potential is in the plateau phase. The entire ventricular myocardium is depolarized. Now, from the apex of the T wave to the beginning of the next P wave, ventricular repolarization completes.
- **Atrial repolarization** is hidden by the QRS complex. It is not seen on the EKG tracing because it happens at the same time.
- **PEA**: Pulseless electrical activity is when there is no pulse but electrical activity of the heart continues. There is electrical activity, but the heart is not pumping. Just because there is electrical activity on an EKG, does not mean there is mechanical function.

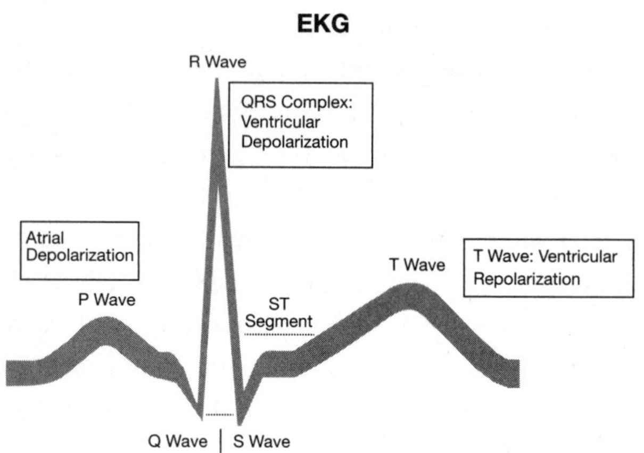

Heart Sounds

The *lub-dub* heart sounds are caused when the valves close. The *lub* sound is when the AV valves close. The *dub* sound is when the semilunar valves close. Abnormal sounds are called murmurs. The sound heard at the top right of the heart is the aortic semilunar valve closing. The sound heard at the top left of the heart is the pulmonary semilunar valve closing. The sound at the bottom left of the heart is the bicuspid or mitral valve (left AV) closing. The sound at the bottom right of the heart is the tricuspid valve (right AV) closing.

Cardiac Cycle

The cardiac cycle is the cycle of contraction and blood flow of one heartbeat. Systole is the contractions; diastole is the relaxations. The mechanical events of the heart slightly follow the electrical events. There are two blood principles. First, blood will always flow down a pressure gradient. The flow is always from higher pressure to lower pressure. Second, blood will always flow through any available opening. The start of the heart cycle is from mid to late diastole (relaxation) in the ventricles.

- **Phase I**: The **first phase** is **ventricle diastole.** The ventricles are relaxing and filling with blood. The AV valves are wide open and blood is flowing in. The semilunar valves are closed. Ventricle blood volume (BV) is increasing. The pressure in the ventricles is fairly low. It is also fairly low in the atria. The P-wave and the contraction of the atria occur (atrial systole). Atrial contraction squeezes the rest of the blood into the ventricle. About 80% of ventricle filling is due to gravity. The other 20% is due to the atria squeezing the rest of the blood into the ventricles.
- **Phase II**: The **second phase** begins with the **isovolumetric contraction** phase. The QRS complex and ventricular contraction occur. As the ventricles start to contract, pressure increases, forcing the blood up against the AV valves and closing them. For a brief split second, the ventricles are completely closed chambers. Now the ventricles have the maximum capacity of blood they can hold. This is called the **end diastolic volume (EDV)**. Ventricular volume does not change, because all of the valves are closed during this phase. Contraction, therefore, is said to be **isovolumic** or **isovolumetric**. The ventricles start to contract. Ventricular pressure goes way up. Pressure in the aorta slightly decreases, although it is for the most part even. When the pressure in the ventricles is greater than the pressure in the aorta, blood is ejected into the aorta through the aortic semilunar valve and to the pulmonary trunk through the pulmonary semilunar valve. The AV valves are still closed. The semilunar valves are still open.
- **Phase II, part II**: The second part of the second phase is **ventricular ejection**. The ventricles contract and squeeze out all of the blood. This is **ventricular systole**. The blood volume in the ventricles decreases rapidly. Blood is returned to the atria, which are relaxed and start to fill with blood (atrial diastole). Then the T wave and ventricular repolarization occur, causing the ventricles to stop contracting and stop forcing blood out. When the pressure in the ventricles is less than the pressure in the aorta, blood flows back into the ventricles. The semilunar valves close. There is another split second in which the

ventricles are completely closed chambers. This is the **dicrotic notch**, an indication of when the semilunar valves snap shut.

- **Phase III, isovolumetric relaxation**: Blood flows backward toward the ventricles. Ventricular pressure decreases. Blood volume goes way down. Now at **end systolic volume (ESV)**, the ventricles are relaxing. They must now begin to fill back up again. The atria have been accumulating more and more blood. Ventricular pressure is less than atrial pressure, causing the AV valves to open. This yields ventricular filling and phase 1 begins again.

The right side of the heart has the exact same cycle as the left side of the heart, but at lower pressure. The pulmonary trunk and pulmonary arteries are the equivalent of the aorta on the right side of the heart. On the right side of the heart, the pressure reaches only 24 mmHg for systole and 8 mmHg for diastole, while the left side of the heart reaches 120 mmHg for systole and 80 mmHg for diastole, the normal blood pressure.

Stroke Volume and Cardiac Output

The following describes the calculation of stroke volume and cardiac output.

- **Stroke volume**: **EDV – ESV = Stroke volume** (SV), the volume of blood pumped from one ventricle of the heart with each beat.
- **Cardiac output**: Cardiac output is the amount of blood pumped out of each ventricle in 1 minute (60 seconds). It is calculated by (**Heart rate**) × (**Stroke volume**).
- As SV decreases, cardiac output decreases. On average, the heart beats 75 times per minute and the average stroke volume is 70 mL/beat or 5,250 mL/minute or 5.25 L/minute.

There are three major factors that affect the amount of blood pumped from the heart or how the stroke volume is regulated.

1. **Preload (Starling's law of the heart)**: The critical factor that controls stroke volume is how much the muscles in the ventricles are stretched. The more blood, the more stretch, and the more blood is pumped out, the greater the contraction, causing the end systolic volume (ESV) to decrease. Anything that speeds the return of the blood to the atria will increase the stretch—for example, exercise.
2. **Contractility**: The greater the contractile force of the ventricles, the more blood is pumped out. This is due specifically to the influx of Ca^{2+}. The greater the influx of Ca^{2+} is, the greater the contraction of the heart. Norepinephrine can also increase stroke volume by increasing contractility.
3. **Afterload**: Afterload is the pressure the ventricles must overcome to eject blood. If the pressure in the aorta is much higher, the ventricles cannot as easily overcome it. High blood pressure lowers the stroke volume because the heart has to work that much harder to overcome the pressure in the aorta.

Other Factors That Control Heart Rate

Other factors that control heart rate are as follows:

- **Nervous system involvement**: The sympathetic division of the nervous system increases heart rate—for example, during the fight-or-flight response. The parasympathetic division decreases heart rate (resting/digesting). The dominant impulse is under resting conditions.
- **Hormones**: Hormones also regulate heart rate. Epinephrine increases heart rate.
- **Ions**: Low blood concentration of Ca^{+2} slows heart rate. High concentration of K^{+} stops the heart.

Tachycardia is a high heart rate, greater than 100 in an adult. **Bradycardia** is a low heart rate, less than 60 in an adult.

The Blood

The blood is connective tissue. It is the only fluid tissue in the body. The functions of the blood fall into three categories.

1. **Distribution**: The blood distributes O_2 to the body cells, CO_2 to the lungs, nutrients to the body cells, and wastes to the kidneys.
2. **Regulation**: The blood aids in body temperature regulation. When it is cold, the blood flow is constricted in the extremities. This is particularly noticeable in fingers and toes and is done to keep the vital organs warm. The blood also functions in the regulation of normal pH in the tissues. It can act as a buffer. The blood also maintains enough fluid in the circulatory system. This is due to salts. Water always follows salts. It moves from an area of low solute (e.g., salt) concentration to an area of high solute concentration. When the solute concentration is the same inside a cell as it is outside (isotonic), water moves into and out of the cell at an equal rate. This keeps H_2O in the bloodstream and excess water out of the tissues. Electrolytes help regulate the osmotic balance of cells.
3. **Protection**: The components for clot formation found in the blood help prevent blood loss. As part of the immune system, the blood carries antibodies and white blood cells that aid the immune system.

Normal Blood Values

The following lists normal blood values.

- **Average blood volume:** approximately 5L
- **Blood pH:** slightly alkaline, between 7.35 and 7.45
- **Density:** denser (thicker) than H_2O (average density of whole blood: about 1,060 kg/M^3)

Components of Blood

Blood has the following components:

- **Red blood cells (RBCs): Erythrocytes** are not true cells because they have no nucleus. They comprise approximately 45% of whole blood. When centrifuged, the bottom layer is the erythrocytes because they are the densest. This constitutes the **hematocrit** or **packed cell volume** in a complete blood count. This is usually a little lower in females, approximately 42%, and a little higher in males, approximately 47%.
- **White blood cells (WBCs)**: Leukocytes are the only true cells in the blood that contain nuclei.
- **Platelets**: Platelets are involved in blood clot formation. They are fragments or pieces of cells.
- **Plasma**: Plasma is the fluid component of blood. It constitutes about 55% of whole blood. It is the least dense and therefore the top layer upon centrifugation.

The next layer in the centrifuge after the erythrocytes is called the **buffy coat.** It consists of **WBCs + platelets** and constitutes approximately 1% of whole blood. The **RBCs + WBCs + platelets** are referred to as the **formed elements.** The top layer is the plasma.

Red Blood Cells

Wright's stain is used to stain blood cells for the microscope. The RBCs are the most numerous and stain pink. The functions of the RBCs are to transport O_2 and CO_2. The **RBC structure** is biconcave. RBCs have a concave surface on each side (like a flattened donut). They have no nucleus and no organelles and are basically little bags of hemoglobin (Hb). The average number of RBCs is 4.3 to 5.8 million/mm^3 of blood. If lower, the blood is too fluid. If higher, the blood is too thick. This is why the body wants to keep the number in this normal range. **Hemoglobin** is the protein that binds O_2 and CO_2. There are two components of hemoglobin.

1. **Globin**: Globin is a protein composed of four polypeptide chains, two alpha chains (α) and two beta chains (β). Each chain binds a heme group.
2. **Heme**: Heme is the red pigment to which the globin is bound. At the center of each heme group is an iron (Fe) atom. Iron is what binds oxygen. Each molecule of hemoglobin can bind four oxygen atoms.

One RBC has 250 million hemoglobin molecules. Each can bind four oxygen atoms. Thus, one RBC can carry 1 billion oxygen atoms. CO_2 does not bind to heme; it binds to the globin protein. It binds better in the absence of O_2, but the binding of oxygen and carbon dioxide are not mutually exclusive since they bind to different portions of the molecule. The normal value of hemoglobin is 12 to 18 g Hb/100 mL blood. About 65% of the body's iron is in the hemoglobin. The rest is stored in the liver and spleen. Free Fe is toxic to the body, so it is stored in iron protein complexes—for example, **transferrin.**

Erythropoiesis occurs in the red bone marrow. In adults this is in the os coxae, the axial/pelvic girdles, both pelvic and pectoral. Generally the hips are the biggest supply to tap into. There is a series of three precursor cells as mature erythrocytes are generated.

1. **Hemocytoblast**: These are the RBC stem cells. They also give rise to the WBC and platelets depending on pathway.
2. **Proerythroblast**: Once a hemocytoblast becomes a proerythroblast, it is a **committed cell.** It cannot go back. It must become an RBC.
3. The developmental pathway then proceeds through three phases.
   - **Phase 1**: The early **erythroblast makes ribosomes.**
   - **Phase 2**: The late erythroblast **accumulates hemoglobin.**
   - **Phase 3**: Now a **normoblast**, the immature erythrocyte ejects the nucleus and becomes a **reticulocyte**.

The reticulocyte is what is released by red bone marrow. The count tells how well the bone marrow is producing new RBC. The reticulocytes persist for two days in the bloodstream and become erythrocytes. The process takes approximately 15 days. RBCs persist for 100 to 120 days. The process must be continuous. The body pumps out two million RBCs per second. Control of the process of erythropoiesis is under the influence of the kidney hormone **erythropoietin (EPO)**. This means that the kidneys must monitor the oxygen level in the blood. When it is low, the kidney makes and releases EPO. EPO targets the bone marrow to make more RBCs.

The reasons for low oxygen levels in the bloodstream, any of which will target the bone marrow to increase the production of RBC, are:

- **Increased RBC destruction** such that destruction is occurring more quickly than construction can replace them.
- **Low Hb**, which can be caused by Fe deficiency.
- **Low oxygen availability**, for example, in high altitudes or due to infections such as pneumonia that decrease lung function (CO_2 exchange).

There are two pathways to red blood cell destruction.

1. They are engulfed by macrophages in the spleen. The **spleen** is referred to as the **RBC graveyard.**
2. Hemoglobin is broken down into heme and globin.
   - Heme is degraded to **bilirubin** (a yellow pigment).
   - Bilirubin goes to the **liver**. It is the liver's job to take care of bilirubin. Bilirubin is a liver function test. If bilirubin is elevated in the blood, it indicates that the liver is not working properly.
   - The liver secretes the bilirubin in the **bile** to the **small intestine.**
   - The globin is broken down into **amino acids** and returned to the blood.

RBC disorders include the following:

- **Anemias**: Anemia is a condition of low oxygen levels in the blood. It is a reduced ability of the RBC to carry oxygen. There are three categories:
  1. **Low number of RBCs**: This can be due to blood loss from an injury, due to ulcers, or because the RBCs are being destroyed too fast and the bone marrow is not producing them quickly enough.
  2. **Low Hb (iron deficiency)**: This can be due to insufficient dietary Fe or not enough B_{12}.
  3. **Abnormal Hb**: There are two reasons for abnormal hemoglobin:
     - **Thalassemia**: Thalassemia is when there is one missing globin chain: Either an α or a β chain is not present.
     - **Sickle-cell anemia**: In sickle-cell anemia, one amino acid in a β chain is mutated, causing the shape of the RBC to become sickled, a half-moon shape. This becomes a problem when the person has a sickle-cell crisis, which can be brought on by stress or exercise. The symptoms include extreme pain in the bones and joints, chest pain, gasping for breath, diminished blood flow, and infection, which can lead to stroke if a pathway to the brain is blocked.
- **Polycythemia**: The overpopulation of RBCs happens when the bone marrow overproduces. This can be due to cancer, but can also happen normally at high elevations. Polycythemia can also be observed in blood doping among athletes. Blood is removed from the body, which begins the process to replace it. EPO comes in and stimulates production. Then the athlete reinfuses the blood. The idea is to trick the body into making more RBCs.

White Blood Cells

Leukocytes are much bigger than RBCs. Some turn purple on staining. They are another of the formed elements. The WBCs comprise less than 1% of blood, fewer by far than RBCs and less than plasma. The normal WBC count is between 4,800 and 10,800/mm^3 blood. WBCs are able to perform **diapedesis**. They can come out of the bloodstream, move like amoebas, and crawl along in connective tissue and other organs. There are two classifications of white blood cells based on visible granules in the cytoplasm.

1. **Granulocytes**: The granulocytes have visible cytoplasmic granules. The neutrophils, eosinophils, and basophils are granulocytes.
2. **Agranulocytes**: The agranulocytes have no visible cytoplasmic granules. The monocytes and lymphocytes are agranulocytes.

There are five types of WBC. From the most to the least abundant, they are:

1. **Neutrophils**: Neutrophils, the most abundant type, comprising 50% to 70% of the WBC population, are granulocytes. They stain purple/lilac, have a multilobed nucleus, and phagocytize bacteria. They live only about six hours to three days, short-lived, because they are constantly encountering bacteria to phagocytize and this process causes death.
2. **Lymphocytes**: Lymphocytes comprise 20% to 45% of the WBC. Two types are agranulocytes, which are easy to identify because they are large and round with a purple nucleus that dominates the cell. The cytoplasm is a lighter purple, thin area surrounding the nucleus. There is also one type of granular lymphocytic cell called a **natural killer (NK)** cell, which destroys cells that do not carry self-markers. Most are not in the bloodstream, but rather reside in the lym-

phatic tissue. The two types of agranulocytic lymphocytes are:

- **T-lymphocytes** or **T-cells**: These phagocytic cells respond to virus infected cells and tumor cells.
- **B-lymphocytes** or **B-cells**: Also part of immune response, these cells make antibodies. They are not phagocytic.

3. **Monocytes**: These agranulocytes comprise 3% to 8% of the WBC population. They are very large cells and are easy to identify due to their purple color and U-shaped nucleus. When they leave the bloodstream, they become macrophages, which attack virus-infected cells and some bacteria. They are important in chronic illnesses such as TB. If the monocyte count is elevated, it could indicate some type of chronic, long-term infection.
4. **Eosinophils**: The granules of these granulocytes stain red, and they have a **bilobed nucleus**. They are not phagocytic. They attack **parasitic worms**, but they cannot engulf them; instead, they release a substance in the granules that contains **digestive enzymes** to dissolve the parasitic worms. They also respond to **allergic reactions** by destroying some of the inflammatory chemicals released during an allergy attack and help to eliminate antigen/antibody complexes formed during an allergy attack. They comprise 2% to 4% of the WBC population.
5. **Basophils**: These granulocytes have dark-staining purplish-black granules and an S- or U-shaped nucleus. They are the least abundant WBC, comprising 0.5% to 1% of the WBC population. They release **histamine**, a chemical used in the inflammatory response that stimulates **vasodilation**, an increase in blood vessel diameter. They also attract more WBCs to infected areas to help remove infection.

The **leukopoiesis** pathway is stimulated by factors called **interleukins** and by **colony-stimulating factors (CSFs)**. Both are made in the bone marrow and in mature WBCs. Mature WBCs can secrete interleukins and CSFs to bring about more WBCs. All WBCs start from hemocytoblasts, just like RBCs. The four steps from hemocytoblast to mature WBCs are as follows:

1. **Hemocytoblasts** differentiate into either **myeloid stem cells** or **lymphoid stem cells**.
   - Myeloid stem cells become **myeloblasts** (the committed cells), which are the precursors of all three granulocytes (eosinophils, basophils, and neutrophils), as well as monocytes.
   - Lymphoid stem cells become lymphoblasts (the committed cells), which are the precursors of lymphocytes.
2. The granulocytes go through a process of development in which the gathering of granules leads to a **myelocyte** distinctive for that type of mature cell: **eosinophilic myelocyte**, **basophilic myelocyte**, and **neutrophilic myelocyte**.
3. Next, the nuclei become arclike and the myelocytes become **band cells**: eosinophilic band cells, basophilic band cells, and neutrophilic band cells. This is the **band cell stage**.
4. Finally, the **nuclei** constrict just before the granulocytes leave the bone marrow and become the mature granulocytes: eosinophils, basophils, and neutrophils.

Platelets

Platelets are cell fragments that stain purple. Their function is clotting. Platelet formation is under the control of **thrombopoietin**. They start from the same stem cells as RBCs and all WBCs, **hemocytoblasts**. Through a series of mitotic divisions, but no cell divisions, a **megakaryocyte** is formed. There are multiple nuclei. When mature, they stick cytoplasmic extensions into the blood flow. These extensions break off, the megakaryocyte seals itself up, and this produces platelets. Other mechanisms are still being studied, but it is known that megakaryocytes are the source of platelets.

Clotting

Hemostasis, the stoppage of bleeding, is a fast, localized, extremely carefully controlled response. There are three steps.

1. **Vascular spasm**: This happens almost immediately. The blood vessels in the area are constricted, slowing the blood flow.
2. **Platelet plug formation**: Normally platelets do not stick. However, when tissues are damaged, they release chemicals that allow them to stick due to the exposure of collagen fibers. Injury causes this to happen. Platelets adhere to collagen fibers and become sticky. This attracts more platelets, and the plug begins to build. Chemicals released by platelets include serotonin, which enhances the vascular spasm, and ADP, a potent aggregating agent. This attracts still more platelets to the area. **Thromboxane A_2**, a short-lived prostaglandin derivative, stimulates both vascular spasm and aggregation.
3. **Coagulation**: This is the actual blood clotting step. There are three steps to blood clotting.
    1. **Formation of prothrombin activator**: Prothrombin activator is formed from **platelet factor 3 (PF3)**, released from platelets in the area, and from **tissue factor (TF)**, released from damaged tissue, calcium, and other clotting factors.
    2. **Prothrombin activator converts prothrombin to thrombin**: Prothrombin is converted to thrombin.
    3. **Thrombin converts fibrinogen to fibrin**: Fibrinogen is converted to fibrin. Insoluble strands of fibrin replace the platelet plug and seal the damaged area. Fibrin strands capture RBCs and WBCs and finish off the seal.

After clotting is complete, the hole or cut is sealed with fibrous tissue.

Plasma

Plasma is the liquid component of blood. It is 90% H_2O with many dissolved solutes. There are over 100 different substances, including proteins. The most important protein is **albumin**, which comprises about 60% of the protein volume. Albumin functions as a carrier. It shuttles substances from place to place and also functions to maintain plasma osmotic pressure by keeping H_2O in the bloodstream. Plasma also contains ions and gases.

Blood Groups

The blood groups are A, B, and O. They are named for the antigens on the surface of RBCs. There are four blood types: A, B, AB, and O.

BLOOD TYPES

BLOOD TYPE	ANTIGEN ON RBC SURFACE	PLASMA ANTIBODY TYPE
A	A antigen	B antibody
B	B antigen	A antibody
AB	both A and B antigens	None; neither A nor B antibodies; this is the **universal recipient**. Type AB people can receive blood from anybody because there are no antibodies to cause clumping.
O	neither A nor B antigens; has other antigens, but not A or B	Both A and B antibodies; this is the **universal donor**. Type O people can give to any other blood type because there are no antigens.

The blood types have opposite antibodies and antigens because antigens and antibodies bind and form clumps, so they must match in this way, as opposites. These preformed antibodies are agglutinins that begin to appear in the plasma about two months after birth. They are the antibodies for the antigens opposite to those the person has on the surface of his or her RBCs. The fact that if the A antibody finds the A antigen it will bind and clump is the basis for blood typing. Type O is the universal donor because there are no antigens. Type AB is the universal recipient because type AB individuals can receive blood from anyone since there are no antibodies to cause clumping.

The **Rh factor** or **D antigen** is either positive or negative. If you are Rh positive, you have the D antigen. If you are Rh negative, you do not have the D antigen. It is usually recorded right after blood type, either (+) or (–). Rh (–) people do not have preformed D antibodies but can form them if they are exposed. The risk in pregnancy involves an Rh (–) mother and an Rh (+) baby. With the first child, there is no problem, but at birth Rh (+) blood cells can pass into the mother from the baby. This is especially true if the placenta detaches from the uterine wall. Then the mother is sensitized due to exposure—the Rh (–) mother forms antibodies against the D antigen. If the second child is Rh (+) again, the mother's anti-Rh antibodies cross the placenta and attack the fetus's RBCs. This can cause fetal death. All Rh (–) mothers get a shot of **Rhogam**, which binds to Rh (+) blood. It seeks out leakers and prevents the mother from forming anti-Rh (anti-D antigen) antibodies. Thus if the mother has another pregnancy, she will not have any antibodies against the D antigen. About 85% of Americans are Rh (+).

BLOOD TYPING

ADD ANTIBODY TO BLOOD SAMPLE		CLUMP?		BLOOD TYPE
antibody (A)	antibody (B)	Yes = Has A antigen	No = Does not have B antigen	A
antibody (A)	antibody (B)	No = Does not have A antigen	Yes = Has B antigen	B
antibody (A)	antibody (B)	Yes = Has A antigen	Yes = Has B antigen	AB
antibody (A)	antibody (B)	No = Does not have A antigen	No = Does not have B antigen	O

This process must be performed before a blood transfusion can be administered. There are two kinds of blood transfusions. **Whole blood transfusions** are rarely used anymore, except in emergency situations. **Packed red cell** transfusions include only RBCs. If the wrong type of blood is given, a reaction will occur—the recipient's blood will be attacked by the transfused blood of the wrong type; clumping can result in clogged arteries and veins. However, the actual lethal component is kidney failure. All the lysed RBCs from the clumps release hemoglobin, and the kidney cannot process the hemoglobin quickly enough. The recipient will need dialysis to prevent kidney failure.

Blood Vessels

There are three classes of blood vessels.

1. **Arteries**: These blood vessels take blood away from the heart. They branch into progressively smaller branches until they become capillaries.
2. **Capillaries**: These are the vessels that are in direct contact with tissue. Thus, they can perform gas exchange and serve the needs of the tissues.

Capillaries become bigger and bigger until they form veins.

3. **Veins**: Veins come together and take blood back toward the heart.

Structure of Arteries and Veins: Common Characteristics

In both arteries and veins three layers surround a central **lumen.** A lumen in general is a space. In this case specifically, it is a space for the blood in the center of a tube. The layers from outer to inner are as follows:

1. **Tunica externa**: The tunica externa is made mostly of collagen fibers. Its function is to protect, reinforce, and anchor the vessel in place by adjoining it to the surrounding tissues.
2. **Tunica media**: The tunica media is composed of smooth muscle and elastin. Muscle activity is very important for **vasoconstriction**, which makes the lumen smaller, and vasodilation, which makes the lumen larger. This layer is largest in the arteries. It is not as thick in the veins, because the arteries are responsible for vasoconstriction and vasodilation.
3. **Tunica intima**: The tunica intima is the innermost layer. It is in intimate contact with the blood. This is **endothelium**, a specific kind of simple squamous epithelium that forms the linings of blood vessels. Endothelial cells line all blood vessels. The cells of the endothelium form a very slick surface so as to minimize friction. Capillaries have only the tunica intima layer. Veins and arteries have all three layers.

Differences between Arteries and Veins

The following describes the three differences between arteries and veins:

1. Arteries have thick, muscular tunica media. Arteries have thick walls, whereas veins have thin walls.
2. Arteries have a small lumen. Veins have a much larger lumen.
3. Veins have valves. They open in only one direction, to help blood get back to the heart. This ensures that there is no backflow in the venous system. Arteries do not have valves.

There are three types of arteries.

1. **Conducting (elastic)**: Conducting or elastic arteries are those closest to the heart. This includes the aorta and the branches off it right near the heart. They must be very elastic in order to withstand the force of the ventricles contracting. They are inactive in vasoconstriction and vasodilation. Conducting arteries do not change the shape of their lumen; they are just conducting tubes.
2. **Muscular** or **distributing arteries**: These arteries deliver blood to specific organs. They are the most numerous. They have thick tunica media, which is why they are named muscular arteries. They are active in vasoconstriction and vasodilation.
3. **Arterioles**: Arterioles are the smallest arteries. They control blood flow to the capillaries. They are composed mainly of smooth muscle. They are active in vasoconstriction and vasodilation.

Capillaries are usually only one endothelial cell thick. They are the smallest vessels. They have external cells called the **pericytes** to provide them support. Pericytes are spider-shaped, with smooth musclelike cells that stabilize the capillary wall. The capillary lumen is extremely small, forcing the RBCs to go through in single file. Some tissues, including the tendons, ligaments, cartilage, cornea, and lens, have no capillaries. There are three types of capillaries.

1. **Continuous**: Continuous capillaries are named after how closely the endothelial cells are packed. Most capillaries are this type. The endothelial cells are so tightly packed that intercellular clefts form to allow the passage of fluids

and solutes but they are not big enough to allow WBCs or RBCs to get out.

2. **Fenestrated**: Fenestrated capillaries have pores, like Swiss cheese. They are more permeable to solutes and fluids and are found only in a few special places. They are necessary in the small intestine for nutrient absorption. They are also found in the endocrine glands to allow the rapid entry of hormones into the blood. The kidney is another location where fenestrated capillaries are found. In the kidney their function is to allow the rapid filtering of blood plasma.
3. **Sinusoids**: Sinusoid capillaries are leaky. They have huge intercellular clefts (huge fenestrations), big enough that RBCs and WBCs can pass out into the tissues. They are found in the liver, bone marrow, and lymph tissue, all places where WBCs come out of the bloodstream and patrol the body.

Capillaries usually form groups in the body that merge into large structures called capillary beds. Capillary beds form an interweaving network in which microcirculation takes place. There are two types of vessels.

1. **Vascular shunt**: A vascular shunt is a short vessel that connects an arteriole to a venule at the opposite ends of a capillary bed.
2. **True capillaries**: True capillaries are the actual exchange vessels. A **precapillary sphincter** (a cuff of smooth muscles) surrounds the root of each true capillary. It acts as valve to regulate blood flow into the capillary. When it is open, it allows blood to go to the true capillaries where gas exchange actually takes place. When it is closed, there is a direct connection between an arteriole and a venule and there is no gas exchange. Whether the precapillary sphincter is open or closed depends on the condition in the surrounding cells. For example, if a person is doing exercise on a particular muscle, the precapillary sphincters must open to allow the true capillaries to be flushed with blood to ensure that the working muscles can receive nutrients and dispose of their metabolic wastes.

Veins

Venules, the smallest vessels in the venous system, come together to form veins. Just like arteries, veins have three layers: the tunica externa, tunica media, and tunica intima. The tunica externa is the largest layer. It holds the largest blood volume (BV). At any one time most of the blood (65%) is in the venous system. This is why it is called upon when blood reservoirs are low. Veins are low-pressure vessels compared to arteries, which are high-pressure vessels. This is because the venous system must fight gravity to get the blood back to the heart. Since it clearly cannot have enough pressure to overcome gravity, it must have other methods:

- **Valves**: The valves in veins are one-way to prevent backflow.
- **Skeletal muscle**: Skeletal muscle contractions squeeze on veins and push blood through the valves, where, once through, it cannot backflow.
- **Breathing**: The process of breathing provides some help. Changes in pressure in the thoracic cavity when people breathe allow blood to flow back into the right atrium.

Blood Vessel Physiology

The following are three important concepts related to blood vessel physiology.

1. **Blood flow**: The volume of blood flowing through any structure, depending on what you are measuring—a vessel, an organ, or an entire system—in a given period to time (usually mL/minute) is the blood flow. The blood flow is equal to cardiac output if you are talking about the entire circulatory system.
2. **Blood pressure**: Blood pressure is the force per unit area on a vessel wall by the blood (mmHg);

99% of time this is equal to **arterial pressure**. Blood moves from high to low pressure.

3. **Resistance**: Opposition to flow is equal to the amount of **friction** blood encounters as it is moving through the blood vessels. It is determined by three factors:
   1. **Viscosity**: Viscosity is thickness. The thicker the blood is, the greater the resistance.
   2. **Vessel length**: The longer the vessel, the greater the resistance.
   3. **Blood vessel diameter**: Blood vessel diameter is the main factor. During vasoconstriction, resistance increases as lumen size is decreased. During vasodilation, resistance decreases as lumen size is increased. There is an equation to relate these three factors: **Blood flow = Change in pressure/Resistance.**

Arterial blood pressure (BP) is usually recorded as systolic/diastolic, which is pressure in heart contraction/pressure in heart relaxation. Normal BP is 120/80.

Pulse pressure is systolic minus diastolic. It is what you can feel at a pulse or pressure point. Using normal BP, normal pulse pressure is 120 minus 80 = 40.

Mean arterial pressure (MAP) is the pressure that propels blood to the tissues. It is calculated as: Diastolic + Pulse pressure/3. Using normal BP and pulse pressure: 80 + 40/3 = 93.33.

Maintaining blood pressure (BP): If you rearrange the blood flow formula and replace blood flow with cardiac output (because they are approximately equivalent if you are talking about total circulation), you get the formula for maintaining blood pressure: Change in pressure = Cardiac output × Resistance.

Mechanisms to Maintain Blood Pressure

Mechanisms to maintain blood pressure include neural controls, baroreceptors, chemoreceptors, and hormonal controls.

- **Neural controls**: Neural controls are used for short-term quick fixes to changes in blood pressure. They work by altering either CO (cardiac output) or resistance. The body can constrict blood vessels when blood volume decreases. The control center for this is the **vasomotor center** in the medulla oblongata in the lower half of the brainstem. Most of the time this keeps the arteries constricted. When it receives inhibitory impulses, it signals for vasodilation to occur.
- **Baroreceptors**: The baroreceptors are pressure (neural) receptors in the aorta and carotid arteries. They cause the vasomotor center to allow dilation.
- **Chemoreceptors**: Chemoreceptors sense O_2 and CO_2 levels in blood. When oxygen decreases or carbon dioxide increases, cardiac output increases and vasoconstriction increases, raising BP. This causes the blood to return to the lungs more quickly, which corrects the low O_2/high CO_2 condition.
- **Hormonal controls**: Hormonal controls are also short-term fixes to changes in BP. **Norepinephrine** and **epinephrine** from the adrenal medulla stimulate vasoconstriction and increase cardiac output. **Atrial natriuretic peptide (ANP)** from the heart antagonizes aldosterone, causing decreased BV, which in turn decreases BP. When blood volume/BP is high, the body does not want more aldosterone. ANP from the heart inhibits its release. In times of major trauma, massive vasoconstriction is undertaken in hopes of getting BP to rise. This is under the control of **antidiuretic hormone (ADH)**. **Angiotensin II**, released from the kidney, also stimulates vasoconstriction so that BP will increase. This long-term mechanism works by altering BV. There is a direct effect in the kidney. High BV causes the kidneys to filter faster, releasing more urine. This brings the BV back to normal. There is also an **indirect mechanism** through **angiotensin II**. BV decreases, causing angiotensin II to be re-

leased. This promotes aldosterone release. Aldosterone causes the kidneys to save more water, causing an increase in BV. **Renin**, a protein released from the kidney, causes an enzyme cascade to form **angiotensin II**. Since angiotensin II is a potent stimulator of aldosterone, renin is released from the kidney when the BP is low.

Hypotension is low BP. Less than 110 systole is possibly problematic but can be considered normal if it is asymptomatic. **Hypertension** is high BP, which is more dangerous. BP that is greater than 140 systole can be problematic. High BP can be caused by diet, age, obesity, heredity, smoking, stress, and sometimes pregnancy.

Blood Flow through the Capillaries

Fluid goes in and out of the capillaries through the **interstitial fluid**. When blood goes through the capillaries, fluid is forced out at the arterial end. It returns back in at the venous end. This is extremely important in determining the relative fluid volumes in the bloodstream and in the interstitial space. In which direction does more fluid flow? Is more entering or leaving? Two pressures determine the direction and amount of **bulk flow** across the capillary walls. **Hydrostatic pressure** is the force exerted by a fluid against the vessel or tissue wall. There are two different hydrostatic pressures.

1. **HP_C Hydrostatic pressure of the capillary** forces fluid out of the capillary.
2. **HP_{IF} Hydrostatic pressure of the interstitial fluid** pushes fluid back into the capillary.

Net HP is the difference between hydrostatic pressure of the capillary and hydrostatic pressure of the interstitial fluid (**$HP_C - HP_{IF}$**).

HP_{IF} is usually 0 because no fluid is in the interstitial fluid. The lymphatic vessels remove it.

Proteins or solutes in a solution cause H_2O to be drawn toward them. Water is free to pass through the capillaries, so osmosis due to solute concentrations occurs and causes **osmotic pressure**.

- **OP_C: Osmotic pressure of the capillaries** is fairly constant at approximately 26 mmHg.
- **OP_{IF}** is approximately 1 mmHg.
- **Net OP = $OP_C - OP_{IF}$**, which equals $26 - 1 = 25$ mmHg.
- **Net filtration pressure** (NFP) = **Net HP – Net OP**.

To figure out how much fluid flows out versus in, calculate at the arterial end and calculate at the venous end. If net HP > net OP, fluids leave the capillary. If net HP < net OP, fluids enter the capillary. Extra fluid is picked up by the lymphatic system. The result is that a constant flow of fluid washes over the tissue cells at the arterial end of the capillary, carrying nutrients and oxygen with it. Most of this fluid is returned at the venous end, thereby depositing wastes into the venous system. Under normal conditions, slightly more fluid leaves than enters the capillaries. The lymphatic vessels absorb this excess fluid and return it to the circulatory system.

Lymphatic System

The functions of the lymphatic system are to transport leaked fluids and proteins back to the blood and as part of the immune system. Lymph vessels collect **interstitial fluids** and **proteins** in a fluid called the lymph. Lymph flows toward the heart. Lymphatic capillaries are the smallest lymphatic vessels. They are found everywhere in the body except in the bone, teeth, and central nervous system (CNS). Lymphatic capillaries are very permeable. They have two structures that allow them to perform their job of picking up interstitial fluid.

1. **Minivalves**: The endothelial cells are not tightly joined. They form flaps called minivalves.
2. **Collagen fibers** anchor the capillary to surrounding tissue. When interstitial fluid pushes

on a lymphatic capillary, it does not collapse. Collagen fibers are the reason why. Once inside the capillary, the fluid is now **lymph.**

Lacteals are special lymphatic capillaries in the intestine that absorb fat. The three main lymphatic vessels are as follows:

1. **Lymphatic vessels.** Capillaries join together to form vessels. Lymphatic vessels have the same three tunics as veins and arteries.
2. **Lymphatic trunks:** Vessels join together to form trunks. Trunks are named for their location, in particular for the body part they drain. The lymphatic trunks are the **lumbar**, **subclavian**, **jugular**, **intestinal**, and **bronchomediastinal.**
3. **Lymphatic ducts:** Lymphatic trunks form ducts. They are the largest lymphatic vessels. There are only two. The **right lymphatic duct** drains the right arm, right side of the head, and right side of the thorax. The **thoracic duct** is bigger and drains more of the body. It drains the left arm, left head and neck, and all of the lower body. Both ducts drain lymph into subclavian veins. The **right lymphatic duct** drains into the **right subclavian vein** and the **thoracic duct** drains into the **left subclavian vein.**

Lymph transport is low pressure like the venous system. It relies on the same mechanisms to overcome gravity, plus two more.

- **Valves:** Valves are one-way-flow mechanisms that prohibit the backflow of venous lymph.
- **Skeletal muscle contractions:** Muscle contractions squeeze on the veins and push lymph through the valves. In the extremities, the activity of the skeletal muscles is an important factor in lymph transport. During contraction of an arm or a leg muscle, the venous and lymphatic systems propel the fluids they contain toward the heart.
- **Breathing:** Changes in thoracic cavity pressure during breathing allow the lymph to flow back into the right atrium by the movements of the diaphragm and by negative pressures within the chest during the breathing cycle.
- **Pulsations from nearby arteries:** Lymph flows only one way, toward the heart. Hence, lymphatic vessels do not form a circuit as the cardiovascular system does. Weak muscle action in the lymph vessels, aided by the pulsation of nearby arteries and the movement of limbs, helps to propel lymph fluid through the system. Any lymphatic vessel blockage causes fluid to accumulate in the affected region, creating a swelling called an **edema.** Lymphatics are usually bundled together in connective tissue sheaths along with blood vessels. Pulsations of nearby arteries promote lymph flow.
- **Smooth muscles** in the walls of ducts and trunks contract rhythmically, helping to pump the lymph along.

Lymph Cell Types

There are four basic types of lymph cells:

1. **Lymphocytes:** Lymphocytes are the main warriors of the immune system. They arise from red bone marrow (like all formed elements). They mature into either **T-lymphocytes** (T-cells) or **B-lymphocytes** (B cells). They **protect** the body against **antigens**, any foreign substance. **T-cells** are **phagocytes** for **viruses** and **tumor** cells. B-cells are the producers of plasma cells that secrete antibodies. The lymphocyte population is constantly changing to respond to the body's needs.
2. **Macrophages:** Macrophages play a crucial role in body protection and the immune response. They phagocytize foreign substances. They also help activate T-cells. They prefer to stay on the reticular stroma.

3. **Dendritic cells**: Dendritic cells are spiny-looking cells that also help to activate T-cells. They immobilize antigens by capturing them and bringing them back to the lymph nodes.
4. **Reticular cells**: Reticular cells are fibroblast-like cells that produce the **reticular stroma**, a network of fibers upon which other cells, such as macrophages, like to stay and live. This network supports other cell types in the lymphoid organs.

Lymphoid tissues house and provide a proliferation site for the phagocytic lymphocyte cells. They furnish an ideal surveillance vantage point for lymphocytes and macrophages. **Diffuse lymphatic tissue** is found in every organ as scattered reticular tissue. Larger collections are found in the **lamina propia** of **mucous membranes** and in lymphoid organs. **Lymphoid follicles** are tightly packed reticular tissue, forming a solid mass. They are found in lymphoid organs such as **lymph nodes** and in **Peyer's patches** and the **appendix**.

Lymphatic System Organs

Lymph nodes are the principal organs of the lymph system. They cluster around lymphatic vessels. There are many of these scattered all over the body. Lymph is filtered through a lymph node before it returns to the blood. There are large clusters in certain areas. The **axillary** lymph nodes are in the armpit. The **inguinal** lymph nodes are in the groin. The **cervical** lymph nodes are in the neck. There are two functions of lymph nodes: **filtering** and helping to **activate the immune response.** Lymph nodes filter so that macrophages can remove any pathogens before lymph is returned to the blood. **Sinuses** are open spaces within a lymph node through which lymph flows. The **capsule** is a structure that surrounds each lymph node. Dense, fibrous connective tissue called **trabeculae** extends inward from the capsule and divides the node into compartments.

There are two main regions of a lymph node.

1. **Cortex**: The cortex is the outer portion of a lymph node. It has densely packed follicles and houses B-lymphocytes (B-cells) and dendritic cells.
2. **Medulla**: The medulla is the inner portion that contains B-cells, T-cells, and plasma.

The following describes the four-step flow of lymph through the lymph node.

1. Lymph enters the node through a series of **afferent** vessels. There are many afferent vessels leading in.
2. Next, it enters the **subcapsular sinuses**.
3. Next, it proceeds through **smaller sinuses** and exits.
4. Finally, it exits the lymph node through **efferent** vessels at the **hilum**. There are only two efferent vessels exiting. This slows the flow of lymph through the node so that macrophages and lymphocytes can survey the lymph for pathogens and foreign bodies.

Lymph capsules can pick up proteins, cells, and bacteria, resulting in swollen glands because this cellular debris gets stuck. They can also pick up cancer cells, which travel and establish themselves there. This is one of the ways cancers metastasize. Swollen nodes that do not hurt can be a sign of cancer of the spleen.

Another organ of the lymphatic system is the **spleen**. Located on the left side of abdomen, it is the largest lymphoid organ. The functions of the spleen are as follows:

- Lymphocyte proliferation
- Immune surveillance
- Processes old RBCs (saves Fe from hemoglobin)
- Site of RBC production in the fetus
- Stores blood platelets

There are two main structural differences in the spleen.

1. **White pulp**: The white pulp is where lymphocytes are found on reticular fibers.
2. **Red pulp**: The red pulp has macrophages, lymphocytes, dendritic cells, and reticular cells. It is where RBCs are processed.

There is also a very thin fibrous **capsule** that surrounds the spleen. It is prone to damage. The treatment has been to remove the spleen because the liver and bone marrow will take over its functions. However, new studies have demonstrated that damaged spleens will in fact heal themselves.

Another organ of the lymphatic system is the **thymus**, which secretes the hormones **thymopoeitin** and **thymosin** that target T-cell maturation. The thymus becomes progressively smaller with age. It atrophies to become mostly fibrous and fatty tissue. The cells of the thymus are mostly T-cells.

The final organs of the lymphatic system are the **tonsils**, which are tissue found in certain areas of the throat. They are named by their location. The **palatine** tonsils are located at the posterior end of the oral cavity on both sides. The **lingual** tonsils are located at the base of the tongue. The **pharyngeal** tonsils, also called the **adenoids** when they are enlarged, are located on the posterior wall of the **nasopharynx**.

Tonsillar crypts are structures that all tonsils have. Tonsils are not fully encapsulated. Epithelium overlying the tonsils invaginates deep into the interior, forming these blind-ended enclosures. Bacteria and other particulate matter get stuck in the crypts and make their way into the tissue of the tonsils, where macrophages will then destroy them. These are also memory cells that are said to invite infection in. This is one of the body's calculated risks. The process produces a wide variety of immune cells that have a memory for the trapped pathogens and can be reproduced if needed to fight infection later. The risk is mainly undertaken during childhood for the benefit of heightened immunity and better health later.

Two other lymphoid configurations are **Peyer's patches** and **mucosa-associated lymphatic tissue (MALT)**. Peyer's patches are located in the wall of the **small intestine** and **appendix** (a small offshoot of the large intestine). They have lymph follicles that are useful for destroying large numbers of bacteria. They also generate memory to the lymphocytes for long-term immunity. Peyer's patches, the appendix, tonsils, some walls of the bronchi, and the genitourinary organs comprise MALT.

Nervous System

The nervous system consists of the brain, spinal cord, nerves, and sensory receptors. The function of the nervous system is to take sensory input and process it, or integrate the signals sent to it, to generate decisions that result in motor output. The brain and the spinal cord are the integrative and control centers that comprise the **central nervous system (CNS)**. Signals are sent to and from the brain and spinal cord to the **peripheral nervous system (PNS)**. The peripheral nervous system consists of the cranial nerves and spinal nerves, which are the communication lines between the CNS and the body. There are two divisions of the peripheral nervous system.

1. **Sensory or afferent**: The afferent division consists of the somatic and visceral sensory nerve fibers. It conducts impulses from receptors to the CNS.
2. **Motor or efferent**: The efferent division consists of the motor nerve fibers. It conducts impulses from the CNS to the **effectors**, the muscles and glands. There are two divisions of the motor division.
    1. **Somatic**: The somatic division provides the motor innervations for skeletal muscles. It is also called the **voluntary** nervous system.
    2. **Autonomic**: The autonomic nervous system is the autopilot. It conducts impulses from the CNS to the cardiac muscles, smooth

muscles, and glands. There are two divisions of the autonomic nervous system.

1. **Sympathetic**: The sympathetic nervous system is often referred to as the fight-or-flight division.
2. **Parasympathetic**: The parasympathetic nervous system is often referred to as the resting, digesting division.

Neurons

Nervous tissue is highly cellular—it is about 80% cells. The singular cell of the CNS is the **neuron.** Its function is communication. There is also a population of cells for support. These are the **glial** cells. They work for the neuron to provide nutrition and the proper pH, among other duties. There are three main parts of a neuron.

1. **Cell body**: The cell body is the hub for incoming and outgoing nerve impulses. Most cell bodies are inside the CNS. Clusters of neuron cell bodies called **ganglia** are found in the autonomic nervous system, a division of the efferent division of the peripheral nervous system.
2. **Axon**: The axon is a long, slender, and often highly branched extension from the cell body that is sometimes referred to as the nerve fiber. The axons carry messages. The **axon terminals** are the ends of the axon, where the secretory components are located. There **axon hillocks** are the sites where action potential is originally generated to travel down the axon.
3. **Dendrites**: The dendrites are the main receptive input regions. They are highly branched. They are usually twice or three times the diameter of the axon.

There are three categories of neurons, classified according to the number of axons and dendrites.

1. **Unipolar**: Unipolar neurons have one process that extends from the cell body to form central and peripheral processes, which together amount to one axon. Unipolar neurons are afferent (sensory) neurons. They send signals to the CNS.
2. **Bipolar**: Bipolar neurons are neurons of the special senses. They are very rare in humans and are found only in the retina of the eye, in olfactory tissue, and in the vestibulocochlear nerve of the ear. They have one axon on one end and one dendrite on the other end.
3. **Multipolar**: All motor neurons are multipolar. Multipolar neurons have many processes. They have one axon and many dendrites.

Neurons can be either **myelinated** or **unmyelinated.** Myelinated neurons have a covering or sheath of myelin. Myelin is composed of lipids and lipoproteins. The speed of action potential propagation is controlled by the diameter of the axon and the myelination. The greater the diameter of the axon, the greater is the speed of propagation. There are spaces between the myelin called the **nodes of Ranvier**. In a myelinated axon, the signal jumps from node to node, which increases the speed of signal propagation. Thus, myelinated axons are intrinsically faster than unmyelinated axons.

Neurons are also classified according to function.

- **Sensory or afferent**: Afferent neurons are unipolar neurons that conduct nerve impulses to the CNS. The cell body is outside the CNS. Sensory neurons are not found in the brain or spinal cord. Cell bodies of unipolar neurons are clumped together in structures called a **dorsal root ganglion.** A ganglion is a cluster of cell bodies outside the CNS. If the central axons enter the spinal cord it is a **spinal ganglion.**
- **Motor**: Motor (**efferent**) neurons are multipolar and they conduct nerve impulses away from the CNS. Their cell bodies are inside the CNS. They conduct impulses from the CNS to the effectors (muscles and glands). Motor neurons are myelinated.

- **Interneurons**: Interneurons, also called association neurons, are multipolar neurons that function in signal integration. Their role is in the evaluation process. They lie between the afferent (sensory) and the efferent (motor) neurons and are completely inside the CNS. About 99% of all neurons are association neurons. They are unmyelinated.

Neurons are poorly regenerative. This is why the outcomes from spinal cord injuries are so poor.

Glial Cells

However, this is not true of the glial cells. The support cells can regenerate. A **glioblastoma** is the most common form of brain cancer because these are the brain cells that have the capability to rapidly regenerate. There are four types of CNS glial cells.

1. **Astrocyte**: Astrocytes lie between capillaries and neurons. They have lots of projections as they wrap around the capillary and attach to the dendrites. Their functions are to help buffer ions such as potassium (K^+) and sodium (Na^+) and to recycle neurotransmitters.
2. **Microglial cell**: Microglial cells are a branch of the immune system in the CNS. They are the CNS macrophages. They were unknown until about 15 years ago because they do not look like typical round lumpy macrophages. In the typical process of cell death, when they are in their active form, however, they do round out to engulf dead cells.
3. **Ependymal cell**: These cells line the brain and spinal cord. Both the brain and the spinal cord have fluid-filled cavities. In the brain there are four such spaces called the ventricles. They are filled with cerebrospinal fluid (CSF) CSF is a blood-derived product. The components are selectively chosen. Ependymal cells are responsible for this process.
4. **Oligodendrocyte**: These glial cells form the myelin sheath for axon in the CNS. The myelin sheath wraps axons to increase the velocity of signal transmission.

There are also two types of glial cells in the peripheral nervous system.

1. **Schwann cells**: Schwann cells myelinate the axons of motor neurons in the PNS. In muscular sclerosis, an autoimmune disease, the immune system attacks the Schwann cells that myelinate the axons of motor neurons, causing muscle paralysis due to slowing down the muscle signals. Other Schwann cells can rewrap the axons, though, and this is why MS can be cyclical.
2. **Satellite cells**: Satellite cells help control the chemical environment for neurons.

In the CNS, in general **gray matter** refers to cell bodies and unmyelinated axons, while **white matter** refers to myelinated axons and glial cells. Developmentally, the CNS is a simple neural tube in utero. The fully developed spinal cord has a central canal with cerebrospinal fluid (CSF).

Brain Stem

The brain stem has three regions.

1. **Medulla oblongata**: The first section up from the spinal cord, the medulla oblongata is continuous with the spinal cord. The function of the most inferior portion is to maintain primitive basic life functions. It controls heart rate, blood vessel diameter (and thus how much blood goes to a particular organ), respiration, and protective mechanisms such as swallowing, vomiting, sneezing, and coughing. These activities help to eliminate noxious substances and foreign objects. The medulla oblongata does not control these activities exclusively, but rather

plays a role. Cranial nerves VIII through XII leave the brain through the medulla oblongata.

2. **Pons**. The middle section is the pons. It is a bridge that connects the higher brain centers of the cerebral hemispheres to the lower brain centers in the medulla oblongata. The pons attaches to the cerebellum. The pons is also involved to some extent with controlling respiratory rate and with sleep cycles. Cranial nerves V through VII exit the brain at the pons.
3. **Midbrain**: The last section of the brain stem is the smallest. Cranial nerves III and IV exit the brain at the midbrain. In the midbrain there are four collections of cell bodies that lie within the CNS. Collections of cell bodies within the CNS are called **nuclei**. These four nuclei are called the **corpora quadrigemina**. They are four dome-like protrusions on the dorsal surface of the midbrain. The top two are the **superior colliculi**, which are visual reflex centers. The bottom two are the **inferior colliculi**, which are part of the auditory relay from hearing receptors of the ear to the sensory cortex. Also embedded in each side of the midbrain white matter are two pigmented nuclei called the **substantia nigra**. They are black due to a high content of melanin. Melanin is a precursor of dopamine, the neurotransmitter released by the substantia nigra. In Parkinson's disease, there is a problem with dopamine production. Normally the substantia nigra prevent extraneous unwanted movements. They play an inhibitory function that is interrupted with Parkinson's disease, resulting in tremors that cannot be controlled. These are **resting tremors**. The drug L-dopa is given to stimulate dopamine production at the synapse, but over time the body adapts to the increased level and it no longer works. The midbrain connects to the **diencephalon**, which is referred to as the between brain or **interbrain**. It is the back section of the forebrain. There are three parts of the diencephalon:

- **Thalamus**: The thalamus acts as an afferent (sensory) relay station. Afferent impulses come into the thalamus from all parts of the body. Neurons are synapsing with numerous other neurons, and signals are sent to different parts of the brain. For example, light impulses are sent to the cerebral cortex and other parts of the brain that control the sleep-wake cycle.
- **Epithalamus**: The important structure in the epithalamus is the pineal gland. Deep inside the brain, this endocrine gland produces melatonin, a hormone that functions in sleep-wake cycles. At night the levels of melatonin increase to make you sleepy. Melatonin is also thought to be involved in inhibiting puberty onset and to play a role when it does occur.
- **Hypothalamus**: The hypothalamus is part of the autonomic nervous system. It is an autonomic control center for blood pressure, heart rate regulation, digestive tract functions, and respiration rate. It has many overlapping functions with the medulla oblongata and the two often work together. The hypothalamus is also part of the **limbic system**, which is involved in emotional responses. Many parts of the brain are involved with the limbic system, which deals with pain, sexual drive, and feelings of pleasure. The hypothalamus is also involved in controlling body temperature, in maintaining H_2O balance, and in sleep-wake cycles in conjunction with the pineal gland. As part of the endocrine system, the hypothalamus is also involved in hormone production and release.

The Brain

The parts of the brain are the cerebellum and the cerebrum.

- **Cerebellum**: The cerebellum is referred to as the little brain. It is located at the back, at the bottom of the brain. It is involved in balance and coordinates voluntary movement. It produces smooth motor coordination. It also has a comparator function. It compares data from two places and sends data out to coordinate the two. Every time muscles move, there are special receptors called **proprioceptors** in use. The proprioceptors send sensory data to the cerebellum. The cerebellum comparator function discerns what the motor cortex of the cerebrum meant the body to do—for example, when you suddenly step downward when you have not seen a step or a curb. It compares the sensory input from the unexpected movement and sends data back to the motor cortex to adjust the motion. When disorders occur with the cerebellum it can result in tremors, problems with muscle tone, loss of balance, and overshooting when reaching for objects. The tremors that occur with cerebellum disorder are **intention tremors**, unlike the resting tremors caused by Parkinson's disease. When the cerebellum malfunctions, the tremors are associated with the intention to make a movement that can now not be coordinated properly.

- **Cerebrum:** The cerebrum is where all activity of the conscious being is located. It is the two cerebral hemispheres that differentiate humans from other animals. It is at the top front of the brain. Different parts of the brain have different sensitivities to reduced oxygen levels. The cerebral hemispheres are extremely sensitive to decreased oxygen. This is in contrast to the medulla oblongata, which can endure diminished oxygen for longer periods of time. This is why sometimes after a stroke or other traumatic event, the heart is still beating and breathing continues but there is no consciousness left. Only the primitive basic functions continue, but oxygen deprivation has destroyed the cerebrum.

  On the medulla oblongata there is a region of axons of motor neurons that creates raised lumps called the **pyramids**. The cell bodies are in the cerebral hemispheres. Just above the medulla oblongata–spinal cord junction, most of these fibers cross over to the opposite side before continuing into the spinal cord. This crossover point is called the **decussation of the pyramids**. The result of this crossover is that each cerebral hemisphere chiefly controls the voluntary movements of muscles on the opposite side of the body.

The brain is protected by several layers. The skin of the scalp covers the outer periosteum of the flat bones of the skull. After the inner periosteum of the skull bones are the **meninges**, protective structures between the skull and the brain. The first meningeal layer is the **dura mater** (tough mother). The second meningeal layer is the **arachnoid mater**, which is followed by a space, the **subarachnoid space**, which provides a path for cerebrospinal fluid flow. After the subarachnoid space is the **pia mater**. It follows all of the folds of the brain and is tightly adhered to it. The meninges also surround the spinal cord. Cerebrospinal fluid (CSF) is produced in the **choroid plexus**, which has leaky capillaries and ependymal (glial) cells. The leaky capillaries make it possible for blood plasma, ions, nutrients, and small proteins to be incorporated into the CSF.

There are four choroid plexus in each of the four **ventricles** of the brain. The four ventricles describe the organization of the open spaces that are filled with CSF in the brain. There are two lateral (side) ventricles on each side of the brain. They connect to the third ventricle, which is in the middle of the brain via the **interventricular foramina**. The fourth ventricle is in the back of the brain. The third ventricle connects to the fourth ventricle via the **cerebral aqueduct** or **aqueduct of Silvius**, a small channel. The fourth ventricle is continuous with the central canal of the spinal cord.

The brain is the most sensitive organ in the body to changes in set point. It is the most homeostatically controlled organ. The pH level and glucose level must be strictly controlled. The brain requires glucose. It cannot break down glycogen. In the choroid plexus, there is no control over the leakiness of the capillaries, but the ependymal cells control the process of manufacturing CSF. They put the nutrients and ions into CSF and send the waste back into the blood. A choroid plexus in each of the four ventricles is always making new CSF. It must also get rid of some of it to avoid overpressure from fluid on the brain. H_2O is not compressible, but the brain is. If H_2O is allowed to build up, it will push against the brain in a condition called hydrocephalus. Hydrocephalus occurs with increased probability in premature infants. But in infants, fluid can fill up and spill out through the fontanel.

Pressure inside the brain also pushes up on the skull bones, which can expand in infants. In adults the sutures are fused so that the bones cannot expand. This causes the brain to be squished, compressing blood vessels and crushing soft nervous tissue. The treatment is to insert a shunt to drain off the excess CSF into the peritoneal cavity, where it is absorbed.

The body's mechanism for handling excess CSF is a series of channels. Two **lateral apertures** (openings), one on the left and one on the right, and a **median aperture** from the middle of the fourth ventricle drain the CSF into the subarachnoid space. Small bulges in the subarachnoid space called **arachnoid villi** jut into the **superior sagittal sinus**, a large venous space that runs from the front of the brain to the back. The CSF is transported through this vein to create a constant flow system. The flow of CSF through the brain is from the lateral ventricles through the interventricular foramina to the third ventricle through the cerebral aqueduct to the fourth ventricle. From the fourth ventricle it flows through the lateral aperture, and then through the median aperture to the central canal of the spinal cord.

The final protective mechanism is the **blood-brain barrier**. Typically, most brain capillaries have lots of tight junctions so that nothing can leak out. This is a way to ensure that what does exit is highly controlled in order to control the blood components that end up going to the brain. The exceptions to the blood-brain barrier rule are the choroid plexus, which requires leaky capillaries in order to produce CSF, and the hypothalamus, which must be able to release hormones, almost all of which function through negative feedback loops or set point mechanisms, so there must be methods of monitoring hormonal blood levels.

The cerebrum is divided into the hemispheres by the **longitudinal fissure**. Each hemisphere is divided into four lobes. The cerebrum is highly convoluted due to **gyri** and **sulci**. Gyri are grooves and sulci are furrows. A fissure is a deeper groove. The **transverse fissure** divides the cerebrum from the cerebellum. The cerebrum is divided into front and back, the frontal lobes and the parietal lobes, by the **central sulcus**. The bones of the skull correspond to the lobes of the brain. The frontal bone covers the **frontal lobes** and the parietal bone covers the **parietal lobes.** The other two lobes are the **occipital lobes** and the **temporal lobes**. The frontal lobe is divided on the bottom (inferiorly) from the temporal lobe by the **lateral fissure**, also called the **fissure of Sylvius.** The temporal lobes are underneath the frontal and parietal lobes anterior to the occipital lobes. The occipital lobes are the smallest lobes at the back of the brain (the most posterior lobes).

The cerebral hemispheres have components of gray matter (unmyelinated axons) that are superficial, on the outside of the cortex. The **cortex** is the outermost neural tissue. White matter (myelinated axons) is found deeper and in the medulla oblongata. The cortex is the center of all conscious thought and all awareness. The **prefrontal cortex** is the most anterior (frontmost) part of the brain. It is considered to be the part that makes us human, including such aspects as the intellect, personality type, mood, and motivation. There is communication from the cortex between different areas of the brain along **fiber tracts.** A **tract** is a bundle of axons inside the CNS, as opposed to a bundle outside the CNS, which is a ganglion. There are three types of fiber tracts that provide communication within the brain.

1. **Association fibers**: Association fibers connect areas of the cortex within the same hemisphere.

2. **Commissural fibers**: Commissural fibers connect one hemisphere to the other.
3. **Projection fibers**: Projection fibers are nerve fibers that connect the cerebral cortex with subcortical centers, the brain stem, and the spinal cord. Projection fibers enter the hemispheres from lower brain or spinal cord centers and leave the cortex to travel to lower areas, tying the cortex to the rest of the nervous system and to the body's receptors and effectors. Projection fibers run vertically, while association fibers and commissural fibers run horizontally.

The **corpus callosum** is the most important commissural fiber. It is myelinated white matter that runs under the cortex at the longitudinal fissure that divides the hemispheres. It facilitates communication between the hemispheres. In severe epilepsy it is severed as a last-ditch effort to stop the seizures, with remarkably few side effects.

The **peduncles** are three paired fiber tracts that connect the cerebellum to the brain stem. The bottom pair are the **inferior peduncles**, which connect to the medulla oblongata and send data about the position of body parts. The middle pair are the **middle peduncles**, which connect to the pons and send data about the desired position of these body parts. The top pair are the **superior peduncles**. The data from the inferior and middle peduncles are integrated, and the cerebellum sends this information to the midbrain through the superior peduncles. Efferent impulses are then sent through the pons and medulla oblongata to the spinal cord. From the spinal cord they are sent to the appropriate effectors to either innervate or inhibit skeletal muscle movement.

There are three functional areas of the cortex: motor areas, sensory areas, and association areas. All neurons in the cortex are interneurons. The motor areas control voluntary movement and lie in the posterior of the **frontal lobe**. The motor cortex is located at the **precentral gyrus**, which is directly anterior to the central sulcus. All motor output is initiated here. There are four motor (efferent) areas.

1. **Primary motor cortex**: The primary motor cortex (**somatic motor cortex**) is only an output center. It does not control how to do an action but only that the action occurs. It is strictly concerned with output control.
2. **Premotor cortex**: The premotor cortex is responsible for organizing movement. It is also the site where data is stored about learned motor skills—for example, complex organizations of movement such as typing or playing a musical instrument.
3. **Broca's area**: Broca's area is the center for motor speech, the organization of speech, and language comprehension. It directs the muscles involved in speech production.
4. **Frontal eye field**: The frontal eye field is superior to Broca's area and anterior to the premotor cortex. It controls the voluntary movement of the eyes.

There are six sensory (afferent) areas. They are located at the **postcentral gyrus**, which is directly posterior to the central sulcus.

1. **Somatosensory areas**: The **primary somatosensory cortex** receives data from touch receptors from the skin and muscles (mainly the skin). Data interpretation does not occur here, only data reception. It is in the parietal lobes. Also in the parietal lobes, the **somatosensory association cortex** is responsible for evaluating input. It takes in data you feel. There are lots of integration interneurons that can analyze objects you feel and identify their size, shape, and texture. The input from the touch receptors goes first to the primary somatosensory cortex, but in the somatosensory association cortex that data is evaluated to determine what an object is.

2. **Visual areas**: These areas of the cortex are in the **occipital** lobes. There is a **primary visual cortex** and a **visual association area.** Visual input goes from the eyes first to the thalamus and then to the primary visual cortex and pineal gland to deliver sleep-wake cycle data. We are not aware of this, because it is not in the cerebral cortex. The third stop is the visual association area, which is involved in recognition. To put it simply, seeing a cat occurs in the primary visual cortex and recognizing that it is a cat occurs in the visual association center.
3. **Auditory areas**: There is a **primary auditory cortex** and an **auditory association area**. Input goes to the primary auditory cortex in the **temporal** lobe first. This is where the actual hearing takes place. Sound waves are interpreted as vibrations by the tympanic membrane in the middle ear. The vibrations are transferred to the inner ear and are converted to electrical signals by the cochlea. Those signals eventually make their way to the primary auditory cortex. The auditory association area is where the interpretation of what is heard takes place.
4. **Olfactory areas**: Also in the **temporal** lobes, the **olfactory cortex** is responsible for receiving smell input and interpreting it. Smell is routed through the thalamus first, as are all of the other special senses.
5. **Taste areas**: The **gustatory cortex** is in the **parietal** lobe.
6. **Wernicke's area**: In the left temporal lobe there is a second area involved in speech comprehension. Stroke patients with a Broca's disruption will be able to understand the spoken word but are motor impaired and have difficulty speaking. Wernicke's aphasia, by contrast, causes patients to lose the ability to understand speech inputs, and sentence formation may be impaired such that sentences cannot be understood by others.

An additional part of the brain, the emotional component, adds information to an event. This explains why eyewitness accounts of the same incident can differ widely. The emotional components add individuality to the responses. The complexity of the recognition process varies greatly based on personal experiences.

Spinal Cord

The spinal cord is encased in vertebrae. At L2, the second lumbar vertebra, a cone-shaped structure called the **conus medullaris** is where the spinal cord terminates. The spinal cord must be anchored in place so that it is not jostled by body movements. A fibrous connective tissue called the **filum terminale** is continuous above with the pia mater and enclosed within the dura mater as it projects upward to close to S2, the second sacral vertebra. Going downward, it clings to the dura mater and attaches to the first section of the coccyx. The spinal cord is not uniform in diameter. There are two enlargements: the **cervical enlargement** and the **lumbar enlargement** where the nerves for the upper and lower limbs arise because innervations are needed for the appendages.

In cross section, the spinal cord is white matter (myelinated) superficially, with two gray matter (unmyelinated) butterfly-shaped sections in the middle. This is the opposite of the brain, which is gray matter superficially and white matter deeper. The two lateral gray masses in cross section are connected by the **gray commissure**, which encloses the central canal. Tracts (axons within the CNS) run the length of the spinal cord. Ascending are the afferent (sensory) tracts to the brain. Descending are the motor (efferent) tracts away from the brain.

The inferior end of the vertebral canal looks like a horse's tail and is called the **cauda equina**. Information is sent to the CNS from the **dorsal root**. This is the afferent root that at the distal end has a prominent enlargement to house the cell bodies outside the CNS, the dorsal root ganglion. These cell bodies are just outside the spinal cord. The ventral root carries signals away from the CNS. This is the efferent motor root. However, information is so important that there cannot be only a single route.

Alternate routes go through a **plexus**, an area of branching spinal nerves. There are four regions of complicated branch patterns: the **cervical plexus**, the **brachial plexus**, the **lumbar plexus**, and the **sacral plexus**. The cervical plexus has a main route from the phrenic nerve to the diaphragm, among a number of other branches. The brachial plexus has three main trunks: the **axillary nerve**, the **ulnar nerve**, and the **radial nerve**, which innervate the shoulder, forearm, and hand respectively. The lumbar plexus includes the femoral nerve, which innervates the quadriceps femoris muscles for thigh flexion and knee extension. The sacral plexus includes the sciatic nerve, which innervates the hamstring muscles (semitendinosus, semimembranosus, and biceps femoris long head and short head).

Reflexes

Reflexes are controlled by a five-part neural pathway called the **reflex arc** that does not go to the cortex of the brain.

1. Receptor
2. Sensory (afferent) neuron (in the spinal cord gray matter)
3. Association neuron (interneuron)
4. Motor (efferent) neuron
5. Effector

An example is withdrawing a hand from a hot fire or stove. This is a muscular response mediated exclusively at the level of the spinal cord. This is why the reaction is fast and reflexive. It does not have to go all the way to the cortex. Sometimes there are no interneurons involved in integration at all. Reflexes are either monosynaptic or polysynaptic. When there is only one synapse between an afferent and an efferent neuron with no association neuron, the reflex is **monosynaptic**. When an association neuron is involved, it is **polysynaptic**. Reflexes can also be either ipsilateral or contralateral. **Ipsilateral** responses such as the knee-jerk reflex are responses on the same side of the body. **Contralateral** responses are responses on the opposite side of the body.

Immune System

There are two branches of the immune system: the **innate** or **nonspecific immune system** and the **adaptive immune system**.

Innate or Nonspecific Immune System

The innate immune system consists of surface barriers and internal defenses.

Surface Barriers

The first lines of defense are surface barriers. First among these is the **skin**, the first contact for many bacteria and pathogens. The skin presents both a physical and a chemical barrier. Slightly acidic secretions inhibit bacterial growth. The **mucosa** are also on the first line of defense. Any mucous membranes, and all cavities that open to the outside lined with them, including the respiratory, digestive, and genitourinary tracts, play specialized roles in defense. The respiratory system mucosa have **cilia** to trap dust and other particles and move them toward the throat so they can be swallowed. The mucosa of the stomach have glands that secrete **hydrochloric acid** (HCl) to kill bacteria. The salivary and lacrimal glands have mucosa that contain **lysozyme**, an antibacterial agent. **Body fluids** such as tears, saliva, urine, and vaginal secretions all play roles in diluting, washing away, and flushing out irritants and preventing colonization by microbes.

Internal Defenses

Internal defenses include the following:

- **Phagocytes**: The next lines of defense, if the skin and mucosa are breached, are the phagocytes. **Macrophages** are the chief phagocytes. They derive from monocytes, which through the process of diapedesis leave the bloodstream. There are two types of phagocytes. **Free phagocytes** are wanderers. **Fixed phagocytes** are in specific organs. For example, **Kupfer cells** are macrophages that stay in the liver. Neutrophils also phagocytize bacteria, though not as well as macrophages because neutrophils are killed in the process whereas macrophages can keep on working. **Eosinophils** are not phagocytes, but they release their granules to destroy parasites.
- **Natural killer (NK) cells**: **Natural killer** cells are responsible for targeting cancer cells and body cells infected with viruses. They work in the nonspecific immune system, targeting some of the same cells that the adaptive immune system will, but will do so with specificity. NK cells are a type of nonphagocytic lymphocyte. They look for lack of self-antigens or **major histocompatibility complex (MHC proteins)**. All body cells are marked with MHC proteins specific to that individual. Thus, NK cells know that if a cell does not have MHC, something is amiss. NK cells use direct contact with **perforin.** Perforin perforates the plasma membrane of the target cell, causing an influx of H_2O that causes cell lysis. NK cells also secrete chemicals that enhance inflammation.
- **Antimicrobial proteins**: **Bacteriocins** in the large intestine inhibit the growth of *Salmonella* and *Shigella*. Antimicrobial proteins also include **interferons**, which are released from virus-infected body cells. They move to noninfected areas because the body is trying to stop the spread of the virus. In the noninfected cells, they interfere with viral replication in order to stop the virus from taking over the genetic machinery of the cells for their own replication. They also activate macrophages and NK cells. The **complement system** is a group of between 20 and 30 plasma proteins that circulate in the blood in an inactive state. Their job is to amplify all aspects of inflammation through two different cascade pathways.
- **Normal microbiota**: Normal body bacteria are antagonists to pathogens, competing with them and disallowing them from growing. For example, normal microbiota in the vagina inhibit the growth of *Candida albicans.*
- **Fever**: Fever is a systemic response to infection caused by **pyrogens**. Pyrogens are released by white blood cells (WBCs), causing body temperature to increase. High fevers are dangerous because they denature proteins. If proteins are denatured, the body cannot function properly. However, mild fevers are beneficial. They cause the liver and spleen to hold on to Zn and Fe, which bacteria need in order to reproduce. If the liver and spleen store zinc and iron, bacteria have decreased access to them. This is the body's way of slowing down bacterial replication. It also encourages inflammation.
- **Inflammation**: There are three functions of inflammation: to prevent the spread of damaging agents or localize the infection, to dispose of cell debris (both dead body cells and dead microbes), and to promote healing. The signs of inflammation include redness, heat, swelling, pain, and sometimes, if the infection is in or around a joint, immobilization of the joint.

Process of Inflammation

The process of inflammation is directed by chemicals. Macrophages release **cytokines**. Mast cells and basophils, which become mast cells, release **histamine**. Other phagocytes and lymphocytes release **kinins**, **prostaglandins**, **leukotrienes**, and **complement** to start the inflammatory response. These chemicals cause vasodilation, which leads to **hyperemia**, increased blood flow to the area, which causes heat and redness. This in turn leads to increased temperature and metabolic rate, which causes increased O_2 and nutrients to be sent to the area. This promotes healing.

Chemicals also cause increased capillary permeability. This results in fluid from the blood, with clotting factors and other proteins, leaking into body tissues. This creates swelling (**edema**), and the increased pressure causes pain and possibly joint immobilization. When increased capillary permeability sends clotting proteins to tissues, it also results in a temporary fibrin patch (clot formation) to prevent the spread of bacteria.

In the inflammatory response, phagocytic mobilization occurs in four steps.

1. **Leukocytosis**: When tissue injury occurs, WBCs are released from the bone marrow in response to the release of **leukocytosis-inducing factor** released by the injured cells. The neutrophils are first, followed by the monocytes, which become macrophages. They enter the bloodstream and migrate to the injured area.
2. **Margination**: Neutrophils roll along blood vessel walls looking for **selectins**. Selectins, which are **cell adhesion molecules (CAMs)**, indicate the injury site to the neutrophils. When they encounter selectins, neutrophils cling to the capillary wall in the process known as margination.
3. **Diapedesis**: The neutrophils squeeze through the capillary walls.
4. **Chemotaxis**: Out in the tissues, inflammatory chemicals act as chemotactic agents, directing the neutrophils where to go. The neutrophils are seeking out inflammatory chemicals. Once there, they can phagocytize the pathogens. The **monocytes/macrophages** come in second and stay around longer. In severely infected areas, the battle takes a toll on both sides, yielding a buildup of pus, which is composed of dead and dying neutrophils, broken-down tissue cells, and both living and dead pathogens. If the inflammatory mechanism fails to clear the area of debris, a sac of pus can be walled off by collagen fibers, creating an **abscess**.

Mechanism of Phagocytosis

The following describes the four-step mechanism of phagocytosis.

1. The phagocyte must bind to the bacterium or other microbe.
2. The phagocyte forms **cytoplasmic extensions** to surround the microbe. Once engulfed, the bacterium inside the phagocyte is called a **phagosome**.
3. The phagosome fuses with a lysosome and is now a **phagolysosome**.
4. The microbe is digested by **hydrolytic enzymes** in the phagolysosome followed by exocytosis of any unused particles.

Phagocytes are able to recognize bacteria because bacteria have different markers on their cell membranes. These are usually carbohydrate molecules that project from the cell membrane. However, there are some bacteria that a phagosome cannot recognize by itself. Antibodies and complement can bind to these microbes so the phagocytes can recognize that they need to be destroyed. This process is called **opsonization**, which means to make tasty. The antibodies and complement also create handles for the phagocytes to grab onto so that they can engulf and destroy the bacteria.

Adaptive Immune System

There are three characteristics of the adaptive immune system.

1. **Specific**: It is directed against specific pathogens.
2. **Systemic**: It is not limited to the infection site, as are some of the innate immune system responses.

3. **Memory**: After an initial exposure, the next time the same pathogen enters it can mount a stronger attack.

The adaptive immune system has two branches: **humoral** and **cellular**. Humoral responses are by B-cells. They are **antibody mediated**. Cellular responses are by T-cells, which directly contact pathogens. These responses are **cell mediated**. The adaptive immune response takes about one week. It is much slower than the innate response.

Antigens

Any substance that mobilizes the immune system and provokes an immune response is an antigen. They are usually large, complex molecules that are not normally present in the body and thus are considered nonself or foreign. They enter from outside the body. Proteins are the strongest antigens and the most common, but antigens are not always proteins. Antigens trigger the production of antibodies. There are two main types of antigens.

1. **Complete antigens**: Complete antigens have two characteristics:
   - **Immunogenicity**: They will stimulate production of specific lymphocytes and antibodies. They, in effect, turn on the immune system.
   - **Reactivity**: They can react with activated lymphocytes and antibodies.
2. **Incomplete antigens**: **Haptens** are usually smaller molecules such as short peptides, nucleotides, or hormones. They do not have immunogenicity by themselves. They can cause a reaction, but they cannot stimulate the immune system. However, they can combine with self-proteins (MHC proteins) or antigens, and the immune system can then recognize the combination as foreign. They borrow some of the body's proteins so they can turn on the immune system; for example, poison ivy hypersensitivity is when the immune system overreacts to a hapten that is formed by the oxidation of urushiol. This is an example of an allergic response.

Antigenic determinants are certain parts of the entire antigen that are immunogenic. There can be more than one, which is beneficial, because one antigen can be recognized by hundreds of different lymphocytes, depending on how many antigenic determinants it has. Some antigens mobilize more than one lymphocyte population. This is one reason plastics are used for implants. Plastic is a polymer of repeating units, which means that there may be only one, and certainly are not many antigenic determinants, so they will only mobilize at most one lymphocyte population.

Self-antigens are **major histocompatibility complex** (**MHC**) proteins. All nucleated body cells are coated with them. They are foreign to another person. Everyone's MHC proteins are individual. They are identical only in identical twins. There are two types.

1. **Class I MHC proteins** are on every body cell except red blood cells (RBCs).
2. **Class II MHC proteins** are on only cells of the immune response.

Cells of the Adaptive Immune System

The lymphocytes (the B-cells and T-cells) must be educated before they can do their jobs in the adaptive immune response. The thymus educates T-cells. The bone marrow educates B-cells. Not much is known about how the mechanism in the bone marrow works. The education of T-cells in the thymus depends on immunocompetence and self-tolerance. **Immunocompetence** is the ability to recognize a specific antigen. T-cells must be able to recognize antigens. **Self-tolerance** is the ability to be unresponsive to self. T-cells must be unresponsive to self so they do not attack their own body cells. They must be able to recognize MHC proteins. If they cannot, they are eliminated. Additionally, if they bind too strongly to MHC and cause a reaction, they must be eliminated. The only T-cells that make it through the education process are those that bind to MHC but do not cause a reaction. This is only about 2% of all T-cells. When they are released into bloodstream, they are **naive T-cells**, those that have not yet been exposed to an antigen. Antigen challenges usually occur in a lymph node or in the spleen. Antigen binding to immunocompetent lymphocytes happens after they are released into the bloodstream. This is called **antigen activation**. The body is preprogrammed by DNA to a set of likely exposures. Thus, the body knows what lymphocytes to make before it is exposed to a particular antigen. Only some lymphocytes will ever be activated. The rest sit idle in the body forever. It is our DNA, not the antigen, that determines what lymphocytes are made.

Antigen-presenting cells (APCs) engulf antigens and present them to the T-cells. There are three types of APC.

1. **Dendritic cells**: Dendritic cells are the best APCs. They engulf antigens and migrate to the lymphatic system to make sure T-cells see the antigen.
2. **Macrophages**
3. **B-cells**

Humoral Immunity (B-Cell Antibody-Mediated Immunity)

Naive B-cells are released from the bone marrow. **Challenges** by antigens occur in the spleen or lymph node. This provokes the humoral immune response, which is to produce antibodies against the antigen challenger.

- **Initial encounter with antigen**: The antigen binds to a receptor on specific B-cells. Immunocompetent but naive B-cells are activated, which stimulates them to complete differentiation. B-lymphocytes with noncomplementary receptors remain inactive.
- **Clonal selection**: The activated B-cells grow and rapidly divide, making multiple copies, or clones, of themselves. The majority become plasma cells, which make lots of antibodies for four to five days and then die. The clonal selection process has essentially created antibody-producing machines. This is the **primary response** to a first-time infection. There is a five-day lag period until the plasma cells begin producing antibodies. During this time the B-cells begin clonal selection. It takes three to six days for them to start producing antibodies. The antibody level peaks at approximately the tenth day. The key point is that for a first-time infection it takes some time before the adaptive immune system response kicks in.
- **Memory B-cells**: Some B-cells that do not differentiate into plasma cells will become memory cells, which are long-lived. These are the cells that will mount the attack for subsequent exposures. The **secondary response** with memory B-cells is much faster. The antibody level rises much more rapidly and attains a higher peak. There is no lag time. The antibody level also remains high for a much longer period of time. The secondary response is prolonged, more effective, and quicker. Antibodies can be made within hours versus the five-day lag period in the primary response.

There are two types of humoral immunity. **Active** humoral immunity is the process just described in which B-cells encounter antigens and make antibodies. **Passive** humoral immunity is when B-cells are not challenged and no memory is made. The two types can be either naturally acquired or artificially acquired. **Naturally acquired active** immunity is when you get an infection. **Artificially acquired active** immunity is when you receive a vaccine. Vaccines can be either dead or weakened pathogens that activate B-cells so that they can make memory cells of the exposure, but you do not have to go through the illness. **Naturally acquired passive** immunity is acquired from the mother's antibodies through the placenta or breast milk. The baby borrows antibodies from the mother for the first few months of life. **Artificially acquired passive** immunity is acquired when antibodies are given to a patient. This fixes the immediate problem but no memory cells are created.

Antibody Structure

The following describes the basic six-part structure of an antibody monomer.

1. The basic structural unit of an antibody is composed of four chains, two light and two heavy. These four chains comprise one antibody monomer.
2. Within each chain there is one **constant region** and one **variable region.**
3. Heavy chains also have a **hinge region** that allows bending so that antibodies can assume a Y shape.
4. Disulfide bonds between the antibody chains hold the monomer together.
5. The **variable region** is the place that changes to allow a specific antibody to bind to a specific antigen. It is an antigen binding site.
6. There are therefore two binding sites on each monomer.

Antibodies are also called **immunoglobulins** (Ig). There are five classes of antibodies that determine the other proteins with which the antibodies can interact. For example, to activate complements or macrophages, on the constant region of heavy chains there is a complement binding site and a macrophage binding site.

1. **Immunoglobulin A (IgA)**: IgA is a monomer or dimer. It is secretory and found in mucous, sweat, saliva, urine, spinal fluid, and genital secretions. It prevents pathogen entry into the body.
2. **Immunoglobulin D (IgD)**: IgD is seen only as a monomer. It is always attached to a B-cell surface. It is an antigen receptor and as such is important in B-cell activation.
3. **Immunoglobulin E (IgE)**: IgE is also a monomer. It is the troublemaker antibody, involved in allergies and parasites. It works with basophils and mast cells to release histamine.
4. **Immunoglobulin G (IgG)**: IgG is the most abundant antibody. It is also a monomer. It crosses the placenta, giving passive natural immunity to the fetus. It activates the complement system. IgG are the main antibodies of the late primary and secondary response. IgM come first and then IgG take over.
5. **Immunoglobulin M (IgM)**: IgM can exist as a monomer or can link up with others to create a pentamer. When B-cells are activated and turn into plasma cells, IgM are the first antibodies released. They are particularly good at forming clumps of antigens, acting as a potent **agglutinating agent**. IgM also readily fix and activate complements.

Antibody Function

Antigens and antibodies form a complex called the **immune complex.** There are four different avenues to the immune complex.

1. **Neutralization**: Antibodies bind all around the antigen and mask the dangerous parts. Once the antibodies cover the antigens, they can be phagocytized. Neutralization also enhances phagocytosis.
2. **Agglutination**: Antibodies bind to a cell-bound antigen and clump.
3. **Precipitation**: Antibodies bind to a soluble antigen and cause it to precipitate out of solution. This also enhances phagocytosis.
4. **Activate complement**: The most common method, this is when antibodies bind to an antigen and change shape slightly to expose a **complement binding site.** This allows the complement system to target antigens for lysis. This

membrane attack complex (**MAC**) creates an insertion pore or pathway such that a massive influx of H_2O causes lysis of the antigen.

Cellular Immune Response or Cell-Mediated Immunity (CMI) (T-Cells)

T-cells are responsible for two main types of immune response based on **glycoprotein surface receptors**: **CD4 helper T-cells** ($\mathbf{T_H}$) and **CD8 cytotoxic T-cells** ($\mathbf{T_C}$). T-cells respond to antigens that have been processed by MHC proteins. They cannot recognize antigens in their natural state. This is in contrast to B-cells, which just respond to the antigen. The T-cell must accomplish **double recognition.** It must recognize nonself and self (MHC proteins). This is why T-cells cannot recognize free-floating antigens.

Class I MHC proteins can bind to and display **endogenous antigens**, foreign proteins that are synthesized inside a body cell—for example, virus or cancer proteins. Class I MHC proteins that carry these **antigenic peptides** are recognized by CD8 cytotoxic T-cells (T_C). T_C can hide within a body cell and look for this self/nonself combination, the Class I MHC protein/antigenic peptide complex. The four-step process with **body cells** is as follows:

1. An endogenous antigen is degraded by protease.
2. Endogenous antigen peptides enter the ER via a **transport protein associated with antigen processing (TAP)**.
3. The endogenous antigen peptide binds to a Class I MHC protein.
4. The Class I MHC complex migrates to the plasma membrane of a cell and displays the antigenic peptide self/nonself combination to the T_C.

T_C directly attack and kill cells to which they have bound. This includes cells that are virus-infected, bacteria-infected, or cancer-infected, and foreign cells such as grafts and implants. They work through two mechanisms to kill target cells. The first mechanism involves binding to the target cell through self/nonself (antigen) recognition. Two substances are then released, **granzymes**, which degrade cellular machinery, causing apoptosis, and **perforin**, which causes cell lysis. The second mechanism involves binding to a membrane receptor called a **Fas receptor** on the target cell. This stimulates apoptosis. T_C also release **cytokines**, which contribute to their killing ability.

Class II MHC proteins, which are found on antigen-presenting cells (B-cells, macrophages, and dendritic cells), are recognized by CD4 helper T-cells ($\mathbf{T_H}$). Class II MHC proteins can display **exogenous antigens**, foreign antigens that they have engulfed and broken down in a phagolysosome vesicle. Class II MHC proteins have a protein called an **invariant chain**, a coupling that prevents the MHC protein from binding to an antigenic peptide. It prevents self from being seen so that it does not bind to an antigen unless the invariant chain has been removed. The four-step process with cells of the immune system is as follows:

1. An extracellular antigen is phagocytized.
2. A lysosome merges with the phagosome to become phagolysosome and the antigen is degraded.
3. A class II MHC protein (synthesized in the ER) migrates in a vesicle and fuses with the phagolysosome. The invariant chain is removed and the antigen is loaded.
4. The class II MHC complex migrates to the plasma membrane of an APC (B-cells, macrophages, dendritic cells) and displays to T_H.

CD4 helper T-cells (T_H) bind to a class II MHC receptor. They are the most important cell of the adaptive immune response. They also help to activate cytotoxic T-cells (T_C). They cause dendritic cells to release different molecules that will then activate T_C. In a process called **co-stimulation**, T-cells bind to other receptors on the cell, which causes T-cells to proliferate. Helper T-cells also help activate B-cells, causing them to produce more and more antibodies. Almost all antigens require T-cell help to activate B-cells. These are called **T-cell dependent antigens**.

Once activated, the antigen binds to the B-cell and the B-cell produces antibodies. **T-cell independent antigens**, which do not need helper T-cells to stimulate B-cells, usually stay in the system longer because they withstand degradation. This means that they will continue to stimulate an immune response; however, the response is weak and short-lived. The B-cell binds directly to the antigen. Some activated T-cells also become memory cells, which persist.

Regulatory T-cells (T_{REG}), formerly called suppressor T-cells, dampen or slow the immune response. They release **cytokines** to do this. **Immune surveillance** is performed by T_C and NK cells of the innate immune system. These two types of cells wander the body and examine cells for markers. NK look for lack of MHC proteins. T_C look for the class I MHC protein/foreign antigen complex.

Respiratory System

The most important function of the respiratory system is gas exchange. It must bring in O_2 and remove CO_2. It also functions in the processes of speech and smell. There are four processes that comprise respiration.

1. **Pulmonary ventilation** is the process of breathing, or bringing air into and out of the lungs.
2. **External respiration** is moving O_2 from the lungs to the blood and CO_2 from the blood to the lungs.
3. **Transport of respiratory gases:** O_2 must be transported from the lungs to tissue, and CO_2 must be transported from the tissue back to the lungs. This is a function of the cardiovascular system because blood is used as the transport medium.
4. **Internal respiration:** O_2 must be transported from the blood to tissue and CO_2 from tissue cells to the blood.

Anatomy of the Respiratory System

There are two zones. The **conducting zone** is comprised of the passageways that get air into and out of lungs: the nose, mouth, pharynx, larynx, trachea, and terminal bronchi. The **respiratory zone** is where the gas exchange actually takes place. It starts where the terminal bronchioles end and includes the respiratory bronchioles, alveolar ducts, and alveolar sac.

Nose

The **nose** is the only passageway that can be seen from the outside. Its functions are to moisten and warm air as it enters, filter the air of dust and particles, act as the resonator in the process of speech, and act as an organ involved in the sense of smell. It houses **olfactory epithelium.**

The nose is divided into two parts: the **external nose** and the **internal nose.** The root of external nose is bounded by the **frontal bone** of the skull superiorly. Also superiorly, the **nasal bones** comprise the bridge. It is bounded laterally by the **maxillary** bones and inferiorly by a bunch of **hyaline** cartilage. The internal nose, or **nasal cavity**, is divided by the **nasal septum.** The roof of the nasal cavity is made up of the **ethmoid** and **sphenoid** bones of the skull. The **floor** of the nasal cavity is the **palate**, which separates the nasal and oral cavities. The **hard palate** is anterior to the palate where the palate is supported by the maxillary processes and the palatine bone. The **nasal septum** is composed of the **ethmoid bone**, the **vomer bone**, and **cartilage.**

The **nasal vestibule** is at the opening of the **nares.** It is lined with hairs to filter out large particles such as dust and pollen. The rest of the nasal cavity is lined with one of two sets of mucosa. **Olfactory mucosa** are smell receptors. **Respiratory mucosa** are ciliated in order to move dust, pollen, and debris toward the pharynx so it can be swallowed and digested. When it is very cold outside and you get a runny nose, it means that the cilia are not working. It is also a function of increased mucous production and condensation. The nasal cavity is also lined with nerves that initiate the **sneeze reflex** to expel whatever has been inhaled. There are three projections called **nasal conchae** or **turbinates**, which increase the surface area of respiratory mucosa. The conchae and the mucosa are involved in filtering, heating, and making air moist. The **posterior nasal apertures** or **choanea**, which means **funnels**, are the passageways from the back of each side of the nasal cavity to the pharynx.

Pharynx

The pharynx connects the nasal cavity and mouth to the **esophagus** and **larynx**. There are three divisions of the pharynx tube. The **nasopharynx** is directly behind the nasal cavity. Normally this is only an air passageway because the **uvula** on the **soft palate** blocks liquid and food from entering the nasal cavity. What happens when you laugh and **liquid** comes out your nose is that the uvula flips open.

The **oropharynx** is behind the oral cavity. It is a common passageway for both air and food. There are no longer any cilia at this point in the conducting zone. The tissue becomes stratified squamous epithelial tissue in order to deal with the increased friction. The **laryngopharynx** is directly posterior to the epiglottis. It is also a common passageway for both air and food, and is also stratified squamous epithelial tissue to deal with the increased friction.

Larynx

The larynx is the next place air enters. This is the **voice box**. It functions in maintaining an open airway by directing food and air down the correct paths through the use of the epiglottis. When you swallow, the epiglottis flips and covers the larynx to block food. When you are not eating, the epiglottis stays open. The functions of the larynx are as a **patent airway**, as a switching mechanism to route air and food, and in **voice production**, because it houses the vocal cords. There are nine cartilages of the larynx.

- **Thyroid cartilage**: The largest of the nine, it has a structure called the **laryngeal prominence** **(Adam's apple)** composed of hyaline cartilage.
- **Cricoid cartilage**: Inferior to the thyroid cartilage, the cricoid cartilage is also hyaline cartilage.
- **Series of three pairs of cartilages**: The three pairs are two **arytenoids**, which anchor the vocal cords and are composed of hyaline cartilage; two **cuneiforms**, also composed of hyaline cartilage; and two **corniculates**, also composed of hyaline cartilage.
- **Epiglottis**: The ninth cartilage, composed of elastic cartilage, is the epiglottis.

The **vocal cords** are housed in the larynx. There are two types. **True vocal cords** are involved in sound production and are also called the **vocal folds**. The true vocal cords plus the opening between the two infoldings of the vocal folds is the **glottis**. They vibrate as air is rushing up from the lungs to produce sound. The length of the vocal cords changes based on the **laryngeal muscles**. This changes how wide open the glottis is. Deep tones are produced when the glottis is wide open. High-pitched sounds are produced when the glottis is narrow. Loudness depends on the air stream or amount of air rushing through. The vocal cords actually produce buzzing sounds. All of the chambers above (the mouth, lips, tongue, etc.) amplify sound to produce speech. The **false vocal cords** are vestibular folds that do not produce sound. They close the glottis when you swallow. Below the vocal cords, tissue is lined with ciliated epithelium in order to move dust and particles up toward the pharynx so the debris can be swallowed.

Trachea

The larynx leads into the trachea or windpipe. The trachea leads from the larynx to the bronchi. The trachea has three layers.

1. **Mucosa**: The mucosa layer is ciliated. Cilia move up toward the pharynx.
2. **Submucosa**: The submucosa layer has **glands** that produce **mucous**.

3. **Adventitia**: The outside layer is a layer of connective tissue reinforced with C-shaped rings of hyaline cartilage that help keep the airway open. These are not complete rings, to accommodate for the esophagus. The esophagus must be able to expand when food is swallowed.

Bronchi

The trachea leads to the bronchial tube, which splits into the left and right **primary** or **main bronchi**. The left and right primary bronchi enter the lungs at a structure called the **hilum**. The right primary bronchus is larger. There are more documented cases of foreign objects stuck here. Air is warm, clean, and moist when it reaches here. The next series of branching from the primary bronchi are the **lobar** bronchi, which in turn branch into the **segmental** bronchi. The branching continues 23 times, getting progressively smaller and smaller and forming a bronchial tree. **Bronchioles** are passages smaller than 1 mm. They end at **terminal bronchioles**, which are the smallest at approximately $\frac{1}{2}$ mm diameter. From the nose to the terminal bronchioles is the conducting zone. No gas exchange has occurred yet.

There are structural changes as the branching occurs. The cartilage rings are replaced, first by scatterings of cartilage, and then when they reach the smallest bronchioles, there is no cartilage left. The cartilage diminishes as the branches get smaller and smaller, but elastic cartilage is found all the way through. Cilia and mucous-producing epithelium disappear as branching continues. Debris is removed by macrophages. At the lowest level, there is no longer any cilia or mucous. Smooth muscle increases with branching. The bronchioles are more smooth muscle than the bronchi.

When the terminal bronchioles end and the respiratory bronchioles begin, the respiratory zone also begins. This is where the gas exchange actually takes place. The respiratory bronchioles have alveoli scattered on them. The respiratory bronchioles lead to the alveolar ducts, which lead into alveolar sacs. There are two alveoli cell types. **Type I alveoli cells** are squamous epithelium surrounded by a thin basement membrane covered with pulmonary capillaries. Alveolar and capillary walls and their fused basement membranes form an approximately 5 μm thick air-blood barrier with gas on one side and blood on the other. This is the **respiratory membrane**. It is composed of alveolar epithelium, the fused basement membranes of the alveolar epithelium and the capillary endothelium. On the alveolar side is gas. On the other side of the respiratory membrane is the capillary and blood. O_2 enters the blood. CO_2 returns from the blood.

Type II alveoli cells are **surfactant-secreting** cells. They are scattered in alveoli and secrete a substance that decreases surface tension so that lungs do not stick together and make it impossible to inflate them. Surfactant can be a problem in premature infants. They often do not have enough and therefore cannot breathe. Surfactant allows the inner surface of the lungs to expand properly. It lowers the surface tension within alveoli, the tiny air sacs within the lungs. By doing so, it prevents the alveoli from collapsing during exhalation, and eases the work of breathing.

Alveoli are surrounded by fine elastic fibers, the same type that surround the entire bronchial tree. They have open pores called alveolar pores that connect adjacent alveoli. This is important in equalizing lung pressure and in bypassing damaged alveoli if the bronchi collapse due to disease. Alveoli also have macrophages to dispose of any debris that make it this far. Since the respiratory zone is a dead end, macrophages must be prevented from accumulating. Most are swept up by the **ciliary current** of superior regions. They are carried passively to the pharynx and swallowed, at a rate of about two million alveolar macrophages per hour.

Lungs

The lungs have two main lobes, the right lung and the left lung. The right lung has three lobes—a superior lobe, a middle lobe, and an inferior lobe. The left lung has two lobes—a superior lobe and an inferior lobe. The **cardiac notch** on the left lobe makes room for the heart. The lungs consist mostly of air spaces and elastic connective tissue. They are very spongy and have two blood supplies.

The pulmonary arteries carry deoxygenated blood to pulmonary capillaries. O_2 exchange occurs from the pulmonary arteries to the pulmonary capillaries. The pulmonary capillaries then replenish the pulmonary veins with freshly oxygenated blood to return to the heart. Lung tissues are served by bronchial arteries, which supply all lung tissues with blood except the alveoli.

The alveoli get their blood supply from the pulmonary capillary networks that surround them. Pulmonary capillary networks are formed as pulmonary arteries branch profusely along with the bronchi. Bronchial veins return deoxygenated blood to the venous system, where they meet up with pulmonary veins and deposit deoxygenated blood into them.

The coverings of the lung, **pleurae**, are double-layered serosa. The **parietal pleurae** line the thoracic cavity and diaphragm. The **visceral pleurae** cover the lungs. The **pleural cavity** is the space between the two serosa. It is filled with **pleural fluid**, which allows the lungs to glide over the thorax wall during breathing. **Adhesion** between the parietal and visceral pleurae, due to the fluid in the pleural cavity, causes the lungs to expand or contract based on changes in the size of the chest. Although pleurae slide easily across each other, their separation is strongly resisted by the surface tension of pleural fluid. Thus, lungs cling tightly to the thorax wall and are forced to expand and passively recoil as the volume of the thoracic cavity increases and decreases during breathing. The visceral pleurae are stuck to the lungs. The parietal pleurae are stuck to the thoracic cavity. They are separated by the pleural cavity, which is filled with fluid. With the layers fixed and with fluid between them, they are forced to expand and recoil with breathing.

Physiology of the Respiratory System

Pressures in the thoracic cavity are measured relative to atmospheric pressure (1 atm = 760 mmHg). **Intrapulmonary pressure (P_{pul})** inside the alveoli in the lungs is always 760 mmHg. It goes up and down with breathing but always equalizes at 760 mmHg. It is written as 0 mmHg relative to atmospheric pressure. **Intrapleural pressure (P_{ip})**, the pressure inside the pleural cavity (between the visceral and parietal pleurae), is always 4 less than atm pressure (756 mmHg). It is written as **–4 mmHg.**

The lung's natural tendency is to collapse. Lungs are very elastic and always want to recoil and collapse. The surface tension of alveolar fluid also causes lungs to want to collapse. The opposing force is the elasticity of the chest wall, which is working to expand the lungs. In healthy individuals, neither wins. This is the normal intrapleural pressure.

Transpulmonary pressure is intrapulmonary pressure minus intrapleural pressure **(P_{pul}) – (P_{ip})**. This is the pressure that keeps air spaces in the lungs open, which keeps the lungs from collapsing. Trauma that equalizes (P_{pul}) and (P_{ip}) causes the lungs to collapse. **Pneumothorax** is the term for collapsed lung. It is caused by an accumulation of air or gas in the pleural cavity. The treatment is to insert tubes to allow the pleural cavity to fill back up with fluid.

Ventilation is a mechanical process based on changes in volume in the thoracic cavity. **Boyle's law** is **$P_1V_1 = P_2V_2$**. Pressure varies inversely with volume. In breathing, as volume changes in thoracic cavity, the pressure changes. Gases move down their pressure gradients to equalize pressure. **Inspiration** is controlled by two muscles that increase the size of the thoracic cavity. The **diaphragm** moves inferiorly while the external intercostals lift the rib cage. Both movements together increase the volume of the thoracic cavity. The five-step process of inspiration is as follows:

1. The diaphragm and external intercostals contract. The diaphragm pushes down and the rib cage pushes up.

2. Thoracic cavity volume increases.
3. The lungs are stretched such that intrapulmonary volume (V_{pul}) rises.
4. This causes intrapulmonary pressure (P_{pul}) to decrease to –1 mmHg.
5. This causes air to enter the lungs (down the pressure gradient) until (P_{pul}) = 0 mmHg.

The five-step process of expiration is as follows:

1. The inspiratory muscles relax. The diaphragm moves upward and the rib cage downward due to the recoil of the costal cartilages.
2. Thoracic cavity volume decreases.
3. The elastic lungs recoil passively and intrapulmonary volume (V_{pul}) decreases.
4. Intrapulmonary pressure increases (P_{pul}) to +1 mmHg.
5. This causes air to be pushed out of the lungs until (P_{pul}) = 0 mmHg.

All of this is based on changes in volume, normally approximately 500 mL of air. There are a number of factors that affect ventilation. **Airway resistance** is the resistance to gas flow or friction of respiratory passages. As resistance rises, gas flow decreases. The equation is F (gas flow) = $\Delta P/R$. Gas flow equals change in pressure divided by resistance. Gas flow changes inversely to resistance.

Resistance, just as in the cardiovascular system, is determined by the diameters of the conducting tubes. **Airway resistance** is insignificant because the airway diameter in the first part of the conducting zone is huge relative to the low viscosity (resistance to flow) of air. As the airways become smaller, there are more branches. Even though individual bronchioles are tiny, there are an enormous number of them so the total surface area is still great. The greatest resistance to flow, therefore, is at the medium-sized bronchi. At the terminal bronchioles, the gas flow stops. Diffusion takes over as the driving force of gas movement. Resistance is no longer an issue. The diameter of the bronchi can change under neural controls. The parasympathetic nervous system can cause constriction and the sympathetic nervous system can cause dilation.

Alveolar surface tension also affects ventilation. When faced with a gas, a liquid is always drawn to another liquid. The lining of the alveoli has alveolar fluid, which is mainly H_2O. The alveolar fluid is always acting to constrict the alveoli so less surface area is exposed to gas. Surfactant from type II cells also reduces surface tension. Without surfactant, the alveoli would completely collapse with each breath. Surfactant acts like a soapy detergent to break up the cohesiveness of the H_2O molecules. This reduces the surface tension of the alveolar fluid so that less energy is needed to overcome these forces to expand the lungs and discourage alveolar collapse.

Healthy lungs are very elastic and stretchy. This is referred to as **lung compliance**. The higher the lung compliance, the more stretchy the lungs and the easier it is to expand the lungs. Lung compliance is determined by two factors: the **elasticity of the tissue** and alveolar surface tension. If the elasticity of the tissues is diminished—for example, in TB patients—when elastic tissue is replaced by scar tissue, lung compliance decreases.

Respiratory volumes are measured with a **spirometer. Tidal volume** equals 500 mL. This is the amount that is breathed in and out in a normal resting state (based on normal, healthy 18-year-old man in peak physical condition). The **inspiratory reserve volume** equals 3,100 mL. This is the volume you can forcefully inhale after a normal tidal volume inhalation. **Expiratory reserve volume** equals 1,200 mL. This is the volume you can forcefully exhale after a normal tidal volume exhalation. **Residual volume** equals 1,200 mL. This is the volume remaining in the lungs after forced exhalation. It is the volume in the lungs that prevents collapse. It cannot be expired unless the lungs are punctured or some other trauma or abnormality occurs.

Respiratory capacities with which you should be familiar are as follows:

- **Total lung capacity** is approximately 6 L (6,000 mL). It is all of the volumes added up (vital capacity (4,800) + residual volume (1,200).
- **Vital capacity** is 4.8 L (4,800 mL). It is the maximum amount of air that can be expired after a maximum inspiratory effort. It is 80% of total lung capacity and it equals tidal volume + inspiratory reserve volume + expiratory reserve volume (500 + 3,100 + 1,200 = 4,800 mL).
- **Inspiratory capacity** is 3,600 mL. It is the maximum amount that can be inspired after a normal expiration.
- **Functional residual capacity** is 2,400 mL. It is the volume of air remaining in the lungs after a normal tidal volume expiration. It is the expiratory reserve volume plus the residual volume (1,200 + 1,200 = 2,400).

Respiratory volumes and respiratory capacities are diagnostic tools to determine obstructive disease and other abnormalities.

There is also a phenomenon referred to as **dead space**. When you breathe in, not all air reaches the alveoli. Some is still in the conducting zone, approximately 150 mL. Thus, the actual tidal volume is only 350 mL, the amount that actually makes it to the respiratory zone.

Digestive System

The functions of the digestive system are nutrient uptake, nutrient breakdown, nutrient absorption, and ridding the body of waste. There are two groups of organs: the gastrointestinal (GI) tract and the accessory organs. The GI tract is the alimentary canal, a continuous digestive tube that is also continuous with the outside of the body. Food in the GI tract is continuous with the outside of the body. The functions of the GI tract are to digest food and absorb nutrients. The organs of the GI tract are the mouth, pharynx, esophagus, stomach, small intestine, and large intestine. Accessory organs aid the GI tract organs mostly through secretions or in helping to break down food. The accessory organs are the teeth, tongue, salivary glands, gallbladder, liver, and pancreas.

There are six digestive processes.

1. **Ingestion** is nutrient intake.
2. **Propulsion** is moving food via swallowing and peristalsis.
3. **Mechanical digestion** has three stages.
   1. **Chewing** occurs in the mouth.
   2. **Churning** or mixing occurs in the stomach.
   3. **Segmentation** occurs in the small intestine. This is a specialty type of mechanical digestion. The small intestine contracts rhythmically to churn, mix, and break down food.
4. **Chemical digestion** occurs from the mouth to the small intestine. **Enzymes** chemically break down food.
5. **Absorption** occurs mainly in the small intestine. A small amount occurs in the mouth.
6. **Defecation** is ridding the body of waste as feces, and this occurs from the large intestine.

Structural Commonalities of the Digestive System

The digestive system has the following two structural commonalities:

1. **Peritoneum**: The peritoneum is the serous membrane that forms the lining of the abdominal cavity. Its functions are to support the abdominal organs and to supply them with blood, lymph, and nerve impulses from the vessels it contains. The visceral peritoneum covers the organs. The parietal peritoneum lines the abdominopelvic cavity. Not all digestive organs are in the abdominopelvic cavity—for example, the mouth, esophagus, and pharynx—but most are.

2. **Mesentery**: The mesentery is a double layer of the peritoneum, fused back to back, from the body wall to the organs. It anchors organs in place and provides a foundation for blood, lymphatic, and nerves vessels. It is referred to as greasy mesentery because it stores fat.

Circulation through the Digestive Tract

Splanchnic circulation includes the arteries that come off the descending aorta—the **hepatic artery**, **splenic artery**, **gastric artery**, and the **superior** and **inferior mesenteric arteries**, which serve the small intestine and the large intestine. Approximately 25% of cardiac output goes to the GI, and after a meal this percentage increases. **Hepatic portal circulation** collects nutrient-rich blood from all digestive organs and delivers it to the liver. The liver absorbs and stores nutrients through the blood and then releases them back to the bloodstream for general cellular use.

Gastrointestinal (GI) Tract Layers

There are four GI tract layers.

1. **Mucosa**: The innermost layer is responsible for secreting mucous that contains digestive enzymes and hormones. It also plays roles in absorption of the end products of digestion and in fighting off infection. There are three sublayers.
   - **Epithelium**: The innermost sublayer has lots of **goblet cells**, which make mucous.
   - **Lamina propria**: The middle layer is connective tissue with lots of capillaries that work in absorption. It is also the sublayer that has the **MALT system** and immunity functions.
   - **Muscularis mucosa**: The outermost sublayer is a scant layer of smooth muscle cells that produces local movements; for example, via twitching it dislodges food particles that have adhered to the mucosa.
2. **Submucosa**: The submucosa layer is connective tissue that is moderately dense. It allows distention and then regaining of shape after distention—for example, in order to store a large meal.
3. **Muscularis externa**: This layer is responsible for **peristalsis** and **segmentation**, propelling food through the GI tract and churning. There are two layers of the muscularis externa.
   - **Circular**: The inner layer is smooth muscle cells.
   - **Longitudinal**: The outer layer is smooth muscle cells.
4. **Serosa**: The outermost layer is the connective tissue protective layer, also known as the **visceral peritoneum**, which is the layer that covers all digestive organs.

Gastrointestinal (GI) Tract Organs

GI tract organs include the following:

- **Mouth**: The oral or **buccal cavity** is composed of **stratified squamous epithelium** to withstand the friction from food. There are five parts of the mouth.
  - **Lips and cheek**: The borders of the mouth keep food in its place, between the teeth. The buccal cavity also plays a role in speech production.
  - **Palate**: The roof of the mouth is composed of the **hard palate** and the palatine and palatine processes of the maxillary bones anteriorly and the **soft palate** posteriorly. The **uvula** on the soft palate closes the nasopharynx when you swallow to stop food from entering the nasal cavity.
- **Tongue**: The tongue is an accessory organ of the digestive system. It forces food up against the hard palate during chewing. The palate is thus involved in the process of food breakdown. The tongue is skeletal muscle that manipulates and

maneuvers food for chewing, mixing food with saliva to create a **bolus**. It also initiates swallowing by forcing the bolus posteriorly. There are two types of muscles in the tongue.

1. **Intrinsic**: Intrinsic muscles are solely in the tongue itself. There is no bone attachment. This allows the tongue to change shape.
2. **Extrinsic**: Extrinsic muscles are attached to bone. They are used to change the position of the tongue forward, backward, up, and down.

There are two main anatomical characteristics of the tongue.

1. **Lingual frenulum**: This fold of mucosa secures the tongue to the floor of the mouth and limits posterior movement of the tongue. This is important to prevent the tongue from being swallowed.
2. **Papillae of the tongue**: There are four types of papillae.
   - **Filiform**: Filiform papillae are the most numerous. They provide roughness for friction to help move and process food.
   - **Fungiform**: Fungiform papillae are the **taste buds**. They are scattered around the tongue.
   - **Circumvallate**: The circumvallate papillae form a V-shaped taste bud site at the back of the tongue.
   - **Foliate**: Found on the sides at the back of the tongue, these papillae are more important in taste in infancy and early childhood.

- **Salivary glands**: Another accessory organ of the digestive tract, the salivary glands are responsible for cleaning the mouth and helping to dissolve food chemicals. Saliva contributes to moistening the food to help create the bolus. It also contains enzymes for the digestion of starchy foods. **Salivary amylase** is the first enzyme that attacks food, specifically carbohydrates. There are several salivary glands.
  - **Parotid gland**: Located anterior to the ear, this salivary gland expels saliva through the parotid duct, which discharges at the upper jaw by the second molar.
  - **Submandibular gland**: This gland, along the mandible, empties under the tongue by the lingual frenulum.
  - **Sublingual gland**: The sublingual gland empties under the tongue.
- **Teeth**: The teeth are also an accessory organ of the digestive tract. There are four types of teeth.
  1. **Incisors**: The incisors are the cutting or snipping teeth.
  2. **Canines**: The canines are the tearing or piercing teeth.
  3. **Premolars**: The premolars are grinding teeth.
  4. **Molars**: The molars also are grinding teeth.

  Baby teeth are referred to as **deciduous** or milk teeth. There are 20 deciduous teeth. There are 32 permanent or adult teeth. The roots of deciduous teeth are reabsorbed. This is why baby teeth fall out; permanent teeth do not in fact push out the baby teeth. There are two main regions of the tooth. The **crown** is the exposed upper portion. It is covered in **enamel**, the hardest substance in the body, composed mostly of calcium salts. The cells that make enamel die when the tooth erupts through the gum. This is the origin of cavities. Under the enamel is **dentin**, which is found in both the crown and the root. It is the hard, bonelike material that forms the **bulk** of the tooth. The cells that make dentin are **odontoblasts**. Inside the dentin there is an open cavity called the **pulp cavity**. It contains blood vessels and nerves (the pulp) that extend all the way to the root canal. When you get a root canal operation, the pulp cavity is drilled out all the way through the root canal. Beneath the gum line is the root. It is anchored in bone. Some teeth (incisors, canines) have one root. Others (molars/premolars) have more than one root. The root is surrounded by **cementum**, calcified connective tissue that cements the tooth to the **periodontal ligament**. The periodontal ligament anchors the tooth to the jawbone. At the apex of the root, a small hole, called the **apical foramen**, allows for the passage of blood vessels and veins. It is a constricted region between the root and the crown. **Cavities** or dental caries occur when the enamel and dentin are demineralized, broken down by bacteria. Acid produced by bacteria when food is metabolized in the mouth causes this demineralization.

- **Pharynx**: There are three regions of the pharynx.
  1. **Nasopharynx:** The nasopharynx plays no digestive role. There is only air in this portion of the pharynx.
  2. **Oropharynx:** The oropharynx is involved in digestion. It has muscles that propel food.
  3. **Laryngopharynx:** The laryngopharynx also has muscles that propel food.

  The **epiglottis** is the ninth cartilage of the larynx, made of elastic cartilage. The larynx maintains an open airway by directing food and air down the correct paths through the use of the epiglottis. When you swallow, the epiglottis flips and covers the glottis, or middle of the larynx between the vocal folds, to block food. When you are not eating, the epiglottis stays open. The pharynx forces food into the esophagus.
- **Esophagus**: When there is no food, the esophagus is a closed tube. It flattens and folds in on itself. It runs from the pharynx to the stomach. The esophagus enters the stomach at the **cardiac sphincter**, also called the **gastroesophageal sphincter**. Failure of this sphincter causes heartburn or acid reflux, which can lead to **gastroesophage reflux disease (GERD)** in which stomach acid backs up into the esophagus and burns it.

Saliva

The salivary glands secrete one and a half liters of saliva per day. Salivary secretions are controlled by the parasympathetic nervous system. When food enters the mouth or you smell or even think about food, a signal is sent to the pons in the medulla that triggers increased saliva secretion. The composition of saliva is as follows:

- Saliva is composed mainly of H_2O.
- It is slightly acidic.
- It contains **salivary amylase** for starch digestion (carbohydrate or CH_2O).
- It contains **mucin**, the precursor to mucous.
- It contains **lysozymes**, an antibacterial agent.
- It contains **IgA antibodies**, the secretory antibodies.
- It contains **metabolic wastes** such as urea and uric acid.

Digestive Phases

There are four phases in the digestive process.

1. The mouth is responsible for ingestion, mastication (chewing), the mechanical breakdown of food, and the beginning of the chemical breakdown through the salivary amylase. Some drugs can be absorbed in the mouth; for example, nitroglycerin tablets can be absorbed sublingually.
2. The mouth, pharynx, and esophagus are all involved in the first phase of swallowing, called the **buccal phase**. This is voluntary swallowing of the bolus. Humans voluntarily choose the items they put in their mouths and choose to force the bolus with their tongue to the oropharynx.
3. The pharynx and esophagus are involved in the second phase of swallowing, the **pharyngeal/esophageal phase**. This is the involuntary swallowing phase. There is no conscious control once food enters the pharynx. The epiglottis closes, the uvula closes, and there is no other way for the bolus to go but to the esophagus. Peristalsis moves the bolus down the esophagus. Just before the bolus is going to reach the stomach, the cardiac sphincter opens to accept it.

4. The stomach is involved in the chemical breakdown of proteins and lipids. **Lingual lipase** catalyzes lipid breakdown. The source of this enzyme is the mouth, but it works in the stomach. In the stomach, the food, which was a bolus, is now converted to **chyme**, a creamy paste.

Stomach

The stomach can hold up to four liters of food. The empty stomach has folds called **rugae**. There are four regions of the stomach.

1. **Cardiac**: The cardiac region is the area by the cardiac sphincter.
2. **Fundus**: The fundus is the dome-shaped extension above the cardiac region, underneath the diaphragm.
3. **Body**: The body of the stomach is the bulk of the organ. It is the midportion of the stomach.
4. **Pylorus** or **pyloric region**: The pyloric region is by the pyloric sphincter that connects to the first part of the small intestine, the duodenum.

The stomach has three surfaces.

1. **Greater curvature**: The greater curvature is the outer convex curve that runs laterally.
2. **Lesser curvature**: The lesser curvature is the inner medial concave curve.
3. **Omenta**: The omenta are the mesenteries extending from the greater and lesser curvatures that help tether the stomach to other digestive organs.
   - **Lesser omentum**: The lesser omentum runs from the liver to the lesser curvature.
   - **Greater omentum**: The greater omentum runs from the greater curvature to cover the coils of the small intestine.

The GI tract layers have certain modifications within the stomach. The third or innermost layer of the GI tract, the muscularis externa, has a third sublayer. In addition to the usual circular (inner) and longitudinal (outer) sublayers, there is a third and innermost layer called the **oblique layer**. The oblique layer helps churn food. The structures of the stomach are as follows:

- **Gastric pits**: The gastric pits lead into the gastric glands. Cells in the gastric pits are mostly goblet cells to produce mucous.
- **Gastric glands**: The gastric glands produce **gastric juice**. There are four types of gastric gland cells.
  1. **Mucous neck cells**: Located in the upper part of gastric glands, these cells make specific acidic mucous which has a purpose as yet unknown.
  2. **Parietal cells**: Parietal cells secrete HCl and are involved in activating the enzyme pepsin. HCl kills bacteria and helps to break down proteins. Parietal cells also secrete **intrinsic factor**, which is necessary for the absorption of vitamin B_{12} in the small intestine.
  3. **Chief cells**: Chief cells produce **pepsinogen**, the inactive form of pepsin. Pepsinogen is converted to pepsin in the presence of HCl. Pepsinogen is activated by HCl to convert to pepsin. Once pepsin is present, it catalyzes the reaction of pepsinogen to pepsin.
  4. **Enteroendocrine cells**: Part of the gut endocrine system, enteroendocrine cells secrete hormones that act as local messengers, including histamine, serotonin, and gastrin, which regulates stomach secretions and motility.
- **Stomach mucous wall**: This extremely thick wall has a thick coat of bicarbonate-rich mucous to counteract the HCl. The cells have very tight gap junctions to prevent leakage of gastric juices. The surface epithelium is renewed every three to six days to help ensure that gastric juice stays in the stomach.

The three processes in the stomach are as follows:

1. **Digestion**: Pepsin catalyzes protein digestion.
2. **Mechanical digestion**: The stomach produces churning movements.
3. **Absorption**: There is very little absorption in the stomach. Alcohol and aspirin are absorbed in the stomach.

There are three phases in the release of gastric juices.

1. **Cephalic reflex**: The cephalic reflex occurs before food enters the stomach. It is triggered by food in the mouth or before this through the smell, sight, or thought of food. It is a conditioned reflex that lasts for only a couple of minutes.
2. **Gastric phase**: The gastric phase lasts for about four hours. It provides about two-thirds of the gastric juice released. The stimulus for the gastric phase is stomach distention. Peptides enter the stomach and distend it. This activates stretch receptors, which release acetylcholine. The release of acetylcholine triggers the release of more gastric juices. Low acidity and peptides both trigger gastrin release. Gastrin targets the parietal cells to make more HCl. Gastrin also triggers the release of histamine. Histamine also targets the parietal cells to make more gastrin.
3. **Intestinal phase**: The final phase of gastric secretion occurs in the small intestine. There are two components.
   - **Excitatory phase**: In the excitatory phase, food enters the duodenum, which initially starts more gastric secretions.
   - **Inhibitory phase**: Then, the **enterogastric reflex** kicks in as the duodenum starts to get too acidic from all the acidic chyme coming in. High acidity in the duodenum inhibits the pyloric sphincter, which prevents passage into the small intestine. This causes gastric secretions to decrease.

The following three chemicals cause inhibition of gastric secretions.

1. **Secretin**
2. **Cholecystokinin (CCK)**: The origin of this chemical name is Greek. *Chole* means bile; *cysto* means sac, and *kinin* means move—hence, move the bile sac (gallbladder). CCK is a peptide hormone. It triggers fat and protein digestion. It is secreted in the duodenum and triggers the release of digestive enzymes from the pancreas and bile from the gallbladder. It also acts as a hunger suppressant.
3. **Vasoactive intestinal peptide (VIP)**: VIP causes inhibition of gastric acid secretion and absorption from the intestinal lumen.

Stomach actions include the following.

- **Receptive relaxation**: Receptive relaxation is the initial stomach filling. It allows expansion and is coordinated through the brain with swallowing. Upon swallowing, the stomach knows to relax.
- **Plasticity**: The smooth muscle of the stomach stretches. There is no increase in tension or no tension buildup to cause a contraction. The stomach is designed to hold food and relaxes to accommodate it.
- **Stomach contraction**: Peristalsis begins at the gastroesophageal sphincter (cardiac sphincter) and moves in waves. There are gentle rippling movements of the thin stomach wall. The body and fundus of the stomach are large enough so that the food in them does not move as rapidly. Most of the force of the peristaltic wave is put on the pylorus so that it will force the food into the small intestine. The stomach musculature is thicker at the pyloric antrum, which takes a pummeling due to the lively mixing at the pylorus.
- **Stomach emptying**: Three mL of chyme is forced through with each contraction. These are small squirts with each contraction. The rest of

the chyme is forced back into the stomach where it undergoes more mixing and is squirted through with each wave. This happens for four to six hours. The rate of the waves is three times per minute. It takes the stomach a very long time to empty, up to four hours. Fluids move faster than solids because they do not need as much mixing and churning. The duodenum works against emptying. Fatty meals can remain in the stomach for six hours. Digestion in the duodenum slows down with fatty meals. The stomach and duodenum are coupled. If the duodenum slows down, food backs up into the stomach.

Small Intestine

The small intestine extends from the pyloric sphincter to the ileocecal valve. There are three sections.

1. **Duodenum**: Approximately the first ten inches of the small intestine comprises the duodenum. It receives secretions from the **bile duct** from the **liver** and the **gallbladder**, the **pancreatic duct**, the **cystic duct** from the gallbladder, and the **hepatic duct** from the liver. The left and right hepatic ducts merge to form the **common hepatic duct**, which exits the liver and joins with the **cystic duct** to form the **common bile duct**. The common bile duct joins the **pancreatic duct** to form the **hepatopancreatic ampulla**, which enters the duodenum.
2. **Jejunum**: The next approximately eight feet is the jejunum.
3. **Ileum**: The next approximately 12 feet is the ileum, which joins the large intestine at the **ileocecal valve**.

Small Intestine Modifications of the GI Tract Layers for Absorption

- **Plicae circulares**: These deep, permanent, circular folds of the **mucosa** and submucosa layers help slow down chyme as it enters the small intestine. This allows longer time for absorption by increasing the surface area.
- **Villi**: These fingerlike projections of the **mucosa** layer are specialized cells for absorption.
- **Lacteals**: These special lymphatic capillaries in the small intestine absorb fat. At the core of each villus there is a wide lymph capillary bed and a dense capillary bed.
- **Microvilli**: These tiny projections of the plasma membrane of the villi give the mucosal surface a fuzzy appearance called the **brush border**. The brush border is involved in digesting proteins and carbohydrates. These reactions are catalyzed by **brush border enzymes**.
- **Intestinal crypts**: Between the villi are cells that secrete between one and two liters of intestinal juice every day. Intestinal juice is mostly water with some mucous, but no enzymes. It is a carrier fluid only that functions to absorb nutrients from chyme. Stem cells are also found in the intestinal crypts. These rapidly dividing cells renew the villus epithelium every three to six days.
- **Peyer's patches**: In the **submucosa** layer, Peyer's patches increase in abundance toward the end of the small intestine. This region has a huge numbers of bacteria that must be prevented from entering the bloodstream.
- **Brunner's glands**: Also called the **duodenal glands**, these glands produce alkaline mucous to neutralize stomach acid.

The four-step digestion process in the small intestine is as follows:

1. **Chemical digestion**: Chemical digestion is accomplished by the digestive enzymes, bile, and bicarbonate ions.
2. **Absorption**: Absorption is accomplished by the villi and microvilli.
3. **Movement through the small intestine**: Movement is accomplished by **segmentation**, which consists of back-and-forth contractions. It is

faster in the duodenum and slows as it progresses through the small intestine. There is also continued **peristalsis** in the small intestine that occurs only after absorption.

4. **Motilin**: The small intestine also releases motilin, a hormone from the intestinal crypts, which functions in sweeping everything from the small intestine to the large intestine.

Liver

The liver is an accessory organ of the digestive tract that makes bile, a fat emulsifier. The structures of the liver are as follows:

- **Lower lobules**: The lower lobules are the functional units of the liver. They are hexagonally shaped, sesame-seed-sized structures consisting of plates of liver cells or **hepatocytes**.
- **Central vein**: In the center of each lobule, hepatocyte plates radiate outward from central veins.
- **Portal triad**: At each corner of the liver is a portal triad that consists of a branch of the hepatic artery, a branch of the hepatic portal veins, a branch of the bile duct, and lymphatic vessels.
- **Sinusoids**: The spaces between the hepatocytes are the sinusoids. Blood from the portal triads enters the sinusoids, goes to the central vein, continues to the hepatic veins, and proceeds to the inferior vena cava.
- **Kupffer cells**: Star-shaped Kupffer cells form part of the sinusoid walls. They remove debris, including bacteria and worn-out blood cells. Kupffer cells are the macrophages of the liver sinusoids.

The hepatocytes make bile, process nutrients, store glucose as glycogen, and use amino acids to make plasma proteins. They are also involved in fat-soluble vitamin storage and in detoxifying the blood (ammonia removal). Between adjacent hepatocytes, tiny canals called **bile canaliculi** carry secreted bile to bile duct branches in the portal triad. Bile leaves the liver via the common hepatic duct toward the duodenum. This is the opposite direction from the blood flow.

Bile is a yellow-green alkaline solution composed of bile salts, bile pigments, and cholesterol. Bile salts aid the digestive process and are recycled. The chief bile pigment is bilirubin, a waste product of the heme portion of hemoglobin. Bilirubin is formed from the breakdown of worn-out erythrocytes. They are absorbed from the blood by the hepatocytes and excreted into bile.

Bilirubin is metabolized in the small intestine by resident bacteria. It is not recycled. There is one breakdown product, **stercobilin**, which gives feces their brown color. Cholesterol and its derivatives are fat emulsifiers. They are recycled through enterohepatic circulation and reabsorbed in the ileum. Then they are returned to the liver and made into new bile. Bile also contains triglycerides, phospholipids, and a variety of electrolytes. Phospholipids also aid the digestive process.

Gallbladder

The gallbladder is another accessory organ of the digestive system. It is a muscular sac that stores bile. It concentrates bile by removing H_2O. Bile is released from the gallbladder under the control of CCK from the small intestine.

Pancreas

Yet another accessory organ of the digestive tract is the pancreas, which produces 1.2 to 1.5 liters of pancreatic juice per day. Pancreatic juice is released via an exocrine function into a duct. The digestive function of the pancreas is to neutralize chyme. Bicarbonate ions make pancreatic juice alkaline with a pH of around 8. The pancreas also produces proteases in their inactive form. This prevents the pancreas from self-digestion.

The pancreatic proteases are activated in the duodenum, where they will perform their work. For example, **trypsinogen** is produced in the pancreas.

Trypsinogen is the inactive form of **trypsin**. It is activated in the duodenum by **enteropeptidase**, a **brush border protease**. Trypsin, in turn, activates two other pancreatic proteases, **carboxypeptidase** and **chymotrypsin**. Other pancreatic enzymes are released in their active forms. Amylase catalyzes starch breakdown. Lipase catalyzes lipid breakdown, and nucleases catalyze the breakdown of nucleic acids.

The release of pancreatic juices is under the control of the small intestine. Specifically, there are two intestinal hormones that regulate their release. **Secretin** is released in response to HCl in the intestine. It targets duct cells to release bicarbonate-rich pancreatic juice. **CCK** is released in response to the entry of proteins and fats. It stimulates the release of enzyme-rich pancreatic juice. Pancreatic juice drains into the **pancreatic duct** which fuses with the **bile duct** to enter the duodenum of the small intestine at the **hepatopancreatic ampulla**.

Large Intestine

The large intestine runs from the ileocecal valve to the anus. The large intestine performs some water absorption and eliminates food residue. Food remains in the large intestine for 12 to 24 hours. Three longitudinal smooth muscle bands, the **teniae coli**, or **ribbons of the colon**, cause the large intestine to form pockets called **haustra**. These pocketlike sacs are caused by muscle tone of the teniae coli. The regions of the large intestine are as follows:

- **Cecum**: The cecum is a saclike section below the ileocecal valve. It is the first part of the large intestine.
- **Appendix**: The **vermiform** (wormlike) **appendix** hangs off the cecum. It is masses of lymphoid tissue and is part of the MALT system of the immune system.
- **Colon**: There are six regions in the colon.
  1. **Ascending colon**: The ascending colon runs up the right side of the abdominal cavity to the level of the right kidney and makes a right turn.
  2. **Hepatic flexure**: The ascending colon makes its right turn into the hepatic or **right colic flexure**, which is the right-turn portion of the colon anterior to the right kidney.
  3. **Transverse colon**: As it makes its way across the abdominal cavity, this section of the colon is called the transverse colon.
  4. **Splenic flexure:** The splenic or **left colic flexure** is the left-turn portion of the colon anterior to the spleen.
  5. **Descending colon**: The descending colon runs down the left side of the abdominal cavity posterior to the abdominal wall.
  6. **Sigmoid colon**: The end of the large intestine is the sigmoid colon, an S-shaped portion that enters the pelvis and posteriorly leads to the rectum.
- **Rectum**: The rectum has a thick muscularis externa and no haustra. There are three transverse folds, the **rectal valves**, which separate feces from flatus. This stops feces from being passed along with gas.
- **Anal canal**: The last segment of the large intestine is the anal canal located in the perineum. It is entirely external to the abdominopelvic cavity and has two sphincters.
  1. **Internal anal sphincter**: The internal anal sphincter is smooth involuntary muscle.
  2. **External anal sphincter**: The external anal sphincter is voluntary skeletal muscle. The two sphincters act in concert like purse strings to open and close the anus.

The processes of the large intestine include the following:

- **Motility**: The large intestine is inactive much of the time. When it is presented with food residue, it becomes motile. The contractions are sluggish and short-lived.
  1. **Haustral contractions**: Haustral contractions are the movement most often seen in the large intestine. They are slow segmenting

movements that occur every 30 minutes for a duration of about one minute each. Food enters, one haustra contracts, and the food then proceeds to the next haustra.

2. **Mass movement**: Mass movement occurs across the whole colon three to four times per day. This occurs after eating and forces food into the rectum. The presence of food in the stomach activates the **gastroileal reflex** in the small intestine and the **gastrocolic reflex** in the colon. These are propulsive reflexes.

- **Defecation**: The process of defecation is as follows:
  1. The rectum is normally empty until mass movement occurs and feces are forced into it.
  2. When it is full, the defecation reflex occurs. The defecation reflex is a spinal-cord-mediated parasympathetic reflex that causes the sigmoid colon and the rectum to contract.
  3. After the sigmoid colon and the rectum contract, the internal sphincter relaxes.
  4. Next the external sphincter contracts.
- **Bacterial flora**: There are over 700 species of bacterial flora in the large intestine. They produce gas and make vitamins. Mucous has dendritic cells to keep bacteria in the large intestine.

Chemical Digestion and Absorption Physiology

- **Carbohydrate digestion:**
  1. Carbohydrate digestion begins in the mouth with salivary amylase.
  2. It continues in the small intestine with pancreatic amylase from the pancreas.
  3. In the small intestine, **brush border enzymes** continue carbohydrate digestion.
     - **Lactase**: Lactase catalyzes reactions that break down lactose.
     - **Maltase**: Maltase catalyzes reactions that break down maltose.
     - **Sucrase**: Sucrase catalyzes reactions that break down sucrose.
     - **Dextrinase**: Dextrinase catalyzes reactions that break down dextrins.
     - **Glucoamylase**: Glucoamylase continues the breakdown of amylase and amylopectins.
- **Absorption**:
  1. **Monosaccharides**: Glucose and galactose are absorbed via co-transport with Na^+ ions. They enter the capillary blood in the villi and are transported to the liver via the hepatic portal vein.
  2. **Fructose**: Fructose is absorbed via facilitated diffusion.
- **Lipid digestion**:
  1. Lipid digestion begins in the small intestine where bile salts ducted in from the liver perform emulsification.
  2. Also in the small intestine, pancreatic lipase is involved in lipid digestion.
  3. **Absorption**:
     - Fatty acids and monoglycerides enter the intestinal walls via diffusion. They then combine with proteins within the cells to form **chylomicrons** (small milky globules of fat and protein), which are extruded.
     - The chylomicrons enter the lacteals of the villi and are transported to the systemic circulation via lymph in the thoracic duct.
     - Glycerol and short-chain fatty acids are absorbed into the capillary blood in the villi and transported to the liver via the hepatic portal vein.
- **Protein digestion**:
  1. Protein digestion begins in the stomach. The chief cells produce pepsinogen, which is activated by HCl to convert to pepsin.
  2. Protein digestion continues in the small intestine with the pancreatic enzymes **trypsin**, **chymotrypsin**, and **carboxypeptidase**.
  3. Also in the small intestine, the brush border enzymes **aminopeptidase**, **carboxypeptidase**, and **dipeptidase** continue protein breakdown.

4. **Absorption:**
   - Amino acids are absorbed via co-transport with Na^+ ions.
   - They enter the capillary blood in the villi.
   - They are transported to the liver via the hepatic portal vein.

- **Nucleic acid digestion:**
  1. Nucleic acid digestion begins in the small intestine with **pancreatic ribonuclease** and **deoxyribonuclease.**
  2. Also in the small intestine, brush border **nucleosidases** and **phosphatases** continue nucleic acid breakdown.
  3. **Absorption:**
     - The products of nucleic acid breakdown are transported via active transport with membrane carriers.
     - They are absorbed into the capillary blood in the villi.
     - They are transported to the liver via the hepatic portal vein.

Urinary System

The urinary system is the major excretory system of the body. It filters approximately 200 liters of fluid from the plasma in the bloodstream every day. It removes toxins such as waste products, excess ions, and any other unnecessary substances such as salts. The urinary system is responsible for maintaining blood volume and the chemical makeup of blood. It uses H^+ and HCO_3^- ions to control pH. The kidney is located in the retroperitoneal space (behind the peritoneum). The external kidney anatomy is as follows:

- **Hilum:** The hilum is the area where the blood vessels and lymphatic vessels enter the kidney.
- **Coverings:** There are three coverings of the kidney.
  1. **Fibrous capsule:** The deepest layer is also called the **renal capsule.** It is very thin and it functions to prevent infections that can spread to the kidney.
  2. **Perirenal fat capsule:** The perirenal fat capsule is a layer of fat that attaches to the posterior wall of the abdomen and serves to cushion the kidney.
  3. **Renal fascia:** The outermost connective tissue layer anchors the kidney to surrounding structures.

The internal kidney anatomy has two major layers.

1. **Cortex:** The outer layer is the cortex.
2. **Medulla:** The inner layer is the medulla. The medulla is composed of seven to 18 cone-shaped subsections called the **medullary** or **renal pyramids.** The base of the pyramid faces the renal cortex.
   - **Apex** or **papilla:** The apex or papilla is the point of a pyramid. It points inward.
   - **Collecting ducts:** The collecting ducts give the medullary pyramids their striations. There are two cell types.
     1. **Intercalated cells:** The intercalated cells maintain the acid-base balance in the blood.
     2. **Principal cells:** The principal cells maintain the H_2O-Na^+ balance in the blood.
   - **Renal columns:** The renal columns are extensions of the cortical tissue that come down between each renal pyramid, separating them from one another.
   - **Renal pelvis:** This large structure is continuous with the ureter and is where urine collects before it exits. The renal pelvis is composed of the **major calyces** and the **minor calyces.**

Urine flows through the collecting ducts to the papilla (apex) of the pyramid through the minor calyces to the major calyces and on to the renal pelvis, and from there to the **ureter.** From the ureter, urine flows to the **bladder**, where it is stored for excretion through the **urethra** to the exterior of the body.

The **nephron** is the major functional unit of the kidney. There are one million nephrons per kidney, two million in total. The nephron is composed of two structures.

1. **Renal corpuscle**: The first filtering device at the start of the nephron is the renal corpuscle. It filters out large solutes and sends water and small solutes to the renal tubule. It is composed of the following.
   - **Glomerulus**: The glomerulus is a capillary bed with the following distinguishing characteristics:
     - **Endothelium**: The endothelium lining the capillaries is fenestrated. It has numerous pores.
     - **Filtrate**: The filtrate in the glomerulus is solute-rich but virtually protein free. It flows from the blood into the Bowman's capsule. The filtrate is the raw material that the renal tubules will use to form urine.
     - **Afferent arteriole**: Blood enters the glomerulus of the nephron through an afferent arteriole.
     - **Efferent arteriole**: Blood exits the glomerulus through an efferent arteriole.
   - **Bowman's capsule**: This cuplike sac is also called the **capsula glomeruli (glomerular capsule)**. It has two layers.
     1. **External parietal layer**: This layer has no function except for simply providing structure.
     2. **Visceral layer**: The visceral layer clings to the glomerulus capillaries. It has specialized cells called **podocytes** that send out cytoplasmic extensions called **foot processes.** The spaces between the foot processes are **filtration slits** through which filtrate moves to get to the capsular space.
2. **Renal tubule**: The renal tubule of the nephron is the tube through which the filtrate passes to the collecting ducts. It consists of the following:
   - **Proximal convoluted tubule** (PCT): The PCT is the portion of the renal tubule that leaves the Bowman's capsule and runs to the loop of Henle. It is distinguished by its cuboid epithelium cells with microvilli. The microvilli increase the surface area for absorption.
   - **Loop of Henle** (LOH): The **descending loop of Henle** is composed of simple squamous epithelial cells and is extremely permeable to water and relatively impermeable to solutes such as Na^+ and Cl^-. The **ascending loop of Henle** is composed of cuboidal or columnar epithelium and is impermeable to H_2O but relatively (through active transport) permeable to NaCl.
   - **Distal convoluted tubule**: The DCT is composed of cuboidal epithelium with no microvilli.

Between the blood and the interior of the Bowman's capsule, the **filtration membrane** is composed of three structures: the endothelium of the glomerulus, the podocytes (in the visceral layer of the Bowman's capsule), and a basement membrane consisting of the fused basement laminae (membrane) of the endothelium of the glomerulus and the podocytes. Fluid passes from the plasma through fenestrations on the ends of the glomerulus and through the podocytes. There are two types of nephrons.

1. **Corticoid nephron**: About 85% of nephrons are corticoid nephrons. They are found mostly in the cortex of the kidney with some in the loop of Henle, where it dips into the medulla.
2. **Juxtamedullary nephron:** Juxtamedullary nephrons are found closer to the junction between the cortex and the medulla of the kidney.

Nephron Capillary Beds

There are three types of nephron capillary beds.

1. **Glomerular capillary bed**: The capillary bed in the glomerulus is where filtrate is formed from everything pushed out of the blood. It is fed by an afferent arteriole and drained by an efferent arteriole. It is the highest-pressure capillary bed in the body. The diameter of the afferent arteriole is larger than that of the efferent arteriole. Thus, more fluid can enter than can drain out, yielding high pressure.
2. **Peritubular capillary bed**: The peritubular capillary beds pick solutes back up and reabsorb them. They arise from an efferent arteriole and run all along the renal tubules. They are low-pressure capillary beds that absorb solutes and H_2O from the renal tubules. There is one exception: Juxtamedullary nephrons do not have peritubular capillary beds.
3. **Juxtamedullary nephron capillary beds**: Rather than peritubular capillary beds, juxtamedullary capillary beds have a **vasa recta**. Vasa recta are more ordered and more perpendicular to the loop of Henle. They function in helping to concentrate the urine.

The **juxtaglomerular apparatus (JGA)** is located where the ascending loop of Henle (LOH) touches the afferent arteriole. Specialized granular cells in the afferent arteriole release the hormone renin, which causes an enzyme cascade to form angiotensin II, a potent stimulator of aldosterone. Renin is released from the kidney when the blood pressure is low and needs to be raised. In the ascending LOH, **macula densa**, a group of chemoreceptor cells, respond to changes in NaCl in the filtrate.

Kidney Physiology

The blood plasma is filtered 60 times per day in the kidney. The kidney uses between 20% and 25% of all oxygen in the body when it is at rest. This small organ accounts for massive oxygen use. The filtrate consists of everything from the blood plasma except the proteins. Urine is filtrate that has lost most of its H_2O and nutrients (glucose, ions, etc.) back to the body. Filtrate is not urine until it reaches the end of the collecting ducts. We produce one and a half liters of urine per day. Filtration occurs in three segments: glomerular filtration, tubular resorption, and tubular secretion.

The sites of resorption are the proximal convoluted tubule, the loop of Henle, and the distal convoluted tubule. Most resorption occurs in the PCT. All glucose, all amino acids, 65% of H_2O, 65% of Na^+, 60% of Cl^-, 55% of K^+, urea, and bicarbonate ions are resorbed in the proximal convoluted tubule. In the loop of Henle, water is reabsorbed in the descending loop, but not solutes. H_2O reabsorption is not linked to any other reabsorption. The ascending loop, however, is permeable to solutes, but not H_2O. In the distal convoluted tubule, almost everything that has needed to be resorbed already has been. In the ascending loop, adjustments are made by hormones. Aldosterone regulates Na^+ uptake. Parathyroid hormone alters Ca^{+2} uptake. Antidiuretic hormone (ADH) can regulate water uptake.

Urine Composition and Urination

Urine gets its pigment from urochrome. The yellowing is from the destruction of hemoglobin. The pH is acidic, approximately 6. The specific gravity (mass of substance/mass of an equal volume of distilled water) is always higher than water, which has a specific gravity of 1. Due to the solutes, urine is between 1.001 and 1.035. The more concentrated urine is, the higher the specific gravity. Urine is 95% H_2O and 5% solutes. Those solutes consist of nitrogenous wastes such as urea, creatinine, and uric acid.

The **ureters** connect the kidney to the bladder and contract to propel urine. This is why kidney stones can be so painful to pass. The urinary bladder is an 800 to 1,000 mL storage sac. The **urethra** is the tube that runs from the bladder to the outside. In females it is shorter than in males. Males also use the urethra for sperm passage.

Urine passage is controlled by two sphincters. The **internal sphincter** is **involuntary**. It keeps the urethra closed when urine is not being passed. The relaxed state is when the urethra is closed. When it contracts, the urethra opens. The **external sphincter** is **voluntary**. You can choose to keep it closed and postpone bladder emptying until eventually the urge to void becomes irresistible. Urination is also referred to as **micturition**. Voiding is based on the distention of the bladder. It activates stretch receptors, and signals are sent to the pons to keep the internal sphincter closed (relaxed) temporarily and stimulate contraction of the external sphincter.

Endocrine System

The endocrine system is a series of ductless glands that produce and secrete hormones. These hormones control the activity of body cells. Hormones are chemical messengers that travel through the blood long distances. They are usually longer-acting than neurotransmitters, but they take longer to initiate a response, unlike neurotransmitters, which initiate a response almost immediately. Hormones bind to an organ or to the cells they affect. Thus, there are target organs or cells, and the target organ must have receptors for the hormone.

There are three major endocrine organs in the head: the **pineal gland**, the **hypothalamus**, and the **pituitary gland**. There are two in the neck: the **thyroid gland**, and on the dorsal aspect of the thyroid gland there are around four bumps referred to as the **parathyroid glands**. The **thymus** is a lymphoid organ in the upper anterior portion of the chest cavity just behind the sternum. The **adrenal glands** are on top of each kidney. The **pancreas**, **ovary**, and **testis** are also endocrine hormone-producing glands. All three are also exocrine glands that release other products through a duct. The pancreas releases digestive juices through a duct. The ovary releases an ovum through a duct, and the testis releases sperm through a duct.

There are two distinct groups of hormones: **amino acid–based hormones** and **steroid-based hormones**, which are formed from cholesterol, a lipid. Steroid-based hormones are produced in the gonads and the adrenal cortex. Each of these groups has distinct mechanisms by which they control the release of hormones.

- **Amino acid–based mechanism**: This mechanism relies on secondary messengers that yield an amplification effect. Not much hormone is needed in order to create an enormous amount of product. Amino acid–based hormones cannot enter the cell. A receptor must be on the plasma membrane of the target cells. The exception is the thyroid hormones, which use the lipid-based hormone mechanism, even though they are amino acid–based (from the amino acid tyrosine). The secondary messenger is generated by an effector enzyme that is activated by a **G-protein** that can be either off or on. It is off when it is bound to guanosine diphosphate (GDP) and on when it is bound to guanosine triphosphate (GTP). There are two kinds of G-protein. $\mathbf{G_S}$ stimulates **adenylate cyclase.** $\mathbf{G_I}$ inhibits adenylate cyclase. The protein **kinase** brings about the final response. The six steps are as follows:
  1. A hormone, the first messenger, binds to a receptor site.
  2. Binding causes the receptor to change shape. Now it can bind to a nearby active G-protein (a G-protein bound to GTP).
  3. The activated G-protein moves along the plasma membrane and binds to the effector enzyme, adenylate cyclase. Eventually the GTP on the G-protein is hydrolyzed to GDP and the G-protein is back in the inactive state.
  4. If activated, adenylate cyclase generates a second messenger, cyclic AMP (cAMP) from ATP.

5. cAMP is free to diffuse through the cell, and it triggers a cascade of chemical reactions, the first of which is the activation of a protein kinase.
6. Kinase is an enzyme that phosphorylates various proteins (many are other enzymes). This activates some proteins and inhibits others such that a variety of reactions may occur in the same target cell at the same time. Kinase mediates the cellular responses to the hormone.

- **Lipid-based mechanism**: The steroid hormones and the thyroid hormones (the exceptions) use a direct gene activation mechanism. They can cross the plasma membrane because the receptors are inside the cell. Since they are lipid-based, they can pass through the phospholipid plasma membrane. There are no secondary messengers. The seven steps are as follows:
  1. A lipid-soluble hormone (or thyroid hormone) diffuses through the plasma membrane.
  2. It binds to a receptor, a **chaperonin complex**, in the nucleus.
  3. The chaperonin dissociates from the receptor.
  4. The hormone receptor complex binds to a specific DNA sequence.
  5. This initiates transcription of a certain gene.
  6. mRNA is formed during transcription and migrates to the cytoplasm to direct the synthesis of a specific protein.
  7. A third signaling mechanism, a **PIP-calcium signal mechanism**, is initiated.

A number of factors influence how the target cells are activated. The more receptors, the stronger the response will be. The higher the hormone level in the blood, the stronger the response will be. The greater the affinity of the hormone for its receptor, the stronger the effects will be. **Up regulation** is an increase in the hormone receptor number in response to a higher hormone level in the blood, which causes a sustained reaction. **Down regulation** is a decrease in the hormone receptor number in order to lessen the effects when there has been a sustained overexposure. This is usually long-term and is the body's first attempt to fix the problem. There are three categories of hormone activity.

1. **Permissiveness**: Permissiveness is when one hormone is needed in order to bring about the full effect of another hormone. One hormone cannot exert its full effect without another hormone. For example, thyroid hormone is needed to bring about the full effect of sex hormones or full maturation would not occur at puberty.
2. **Synergism**: Synergism is when two hormones work together to produce the same effect or a combined effect that is greater than if only one hormone were acting alone. For example, glucagon and epinephrine both cause release of glucose from the liver to raise the blood glucose level.
3. **Antagonism**: Antagonism is when hormones produce opposite effects. For example, insulin lowers blood glucose levels by forcing the storage of glucose in the liver and muscle cells in the form of glycogen, and glucagon raises blood glucose levels.

Stimuli that cause the release of hormones can be of three different types. They are not exclusive. Hormone release can be controlled by all three or by just one or just two. The nervous system can come in and override any of these three responses if it does not deem it correct.

1. **Humoral:** A humoral stimulus triggers a response to the concentration in the blood of ions or other substances.
2. **Neural:** A neural stimulus triggers nerve fibers to stimulate hormone release.
3. **Hormonal:** A hormonal stimulus triggers the release of other hormones. These are called **tropic hormones** and they target endocrine glands.

ENDOCRINE ORGANS, GLANDS, AND HORMONES

PRODUCING ENDOCRINE ORGAN/GLAND	RELEASING ENDOCRINE ORGAN/GLAND	HORMONE	STIMULUS	TARGET	EFFECT
Hypothalamus	Posterior pituitary gland	Oxytocin	Neural stimuli: uterine stretching from labor and suckling infant	Uterus and breast	Uterine contractions and milk ejection; the let-down reflex
Hypothalamus	Posterior pituitary gland	Antidiuretic hormone (ADH)	Neural stimulus: increased osmolality of blood (more Na^+, Ca^{2+}, etc. ions in the blood); low blood volume and the need to conserve H_2O	Kidney	Decrease urine production
Hypothalamus	Hypothalamus	Growth hormone-releasing hormone (GHRH) and growth hormone-inhibiting hormone (GHIH)	Neural stimuli: need for growth or need to curtail growth	Anterior pituitary gland	Release growth hormone (GH) or inhibit its release
Hypothalamus	Hypothalamus	Prolactin-releasing hormone (PRH) and prolactin inhibiting-hormone (PIH); PIH is more important as it is on all the time; when the effect of PRH is needed, PIH levels decrease and PRH levels increase.	Neural stimuli: need for milk production or to curtail milk production	Anterior pituitary gland	Release prolactin or inhibit prolactin release
Hypothalamus	Hypothalamus	Thyrotropin-releasing hormone (TRH)	Neural stimuli: need for increased metabolic activity	Anterior pituitary gland	Release of thyroid hormones
Hypothalamus	Anterior pituitary gland	Corticotrophin-releasing hormone (CRH)	Neural stimuli: fever, stress, hypoglycemia (low blood sugar)	Anterior pituitary gland	Release of adrenocorticotropic hormone (ACTH)
Anterior pituitary gland	Anterior pituitary gland	Growth hormone (GH), anabolic (tissue-building) hormone	Hormonal stimulus: growth hormone-releasing hormone (GHRH)	Most body cells, primarily the liver, bone and muscles	Increase in size; mitosis and cell division to make more; promotes protein synthesis; uses stored fats to make proteins; also breaks down glycogen to glucose and releases glucose 99 to the bloodstream

(continued)

ENDOCRINE ORGANS, GLANDS, AND HORMONES *(continued)*

PRODUCING ENDOCRINE ORGAN/GLAND	RELEASING ENDOCRINE ORGAN/GLAND	HORMONE	STIMULUS	TARGET	EFFECT
Anterior pituitary gland	Anterior pituitary gland	Prolactin	Hormonal stimulus: prolactin-releasing hormone (PRH); inhibited by prolactin-inhibiting hormone (PIH) and dopamine; dopamine is the major prolactin-inhibiting factor. It is secreted into portal blood by hypothalamic neurons and inhibits both the synthesis and secretion of prolactin. When dopamine secretion or receptor binding is inhibited, prolactin secretion is enhanced.	Breast	Milk production; unknown in males
Anterior pituitary gland	Anterior pituitary gland	Luteinizing hormone (LH); tropic hormone	Adrenocorticotropic hormone (ACTH); tropic hormone	Testes or ovaries	Stimulates testes or ovaries to produce gonadal hormones; testosterone in M and estrogen and progesterone in F; synergist with FSH and estrogen to help bring about maturation of follicles; in females, LH triggers ovulation
Anterior pituitary gland	Anterior pituitary gland	Thyroid-stimulating hormone (TSH) also called thytrophin; tropic hormone	Hormonal stimulus: gonadotropin-releasing hormone (GnRH); inhibited by: gonadal hormones, estrogen, and progesterone in F and testosterone in M	Thyroid gland	Stimulates activity of thyroid gland
Anterior pituitary gland	Anterior pituitary gland	Follicle-stimulating hormone (FSH); tropic hormone; FSH and LH together are sometimes called the gonadotropins.	Hormonal stimulus: thyrotropin-releasing hormone (TRH); inhibited by growth hormone-inhibiting hormone (GHIH)	Testes or ovaries	Stimulates gamete production; also synergist with LH to help bring about maturation of

ENDOCRINE ORGANS, GLANDS, AND HORMONES *(continued)*

PRODUCING ENDOCRINE ORGAN/GLAND	RELEASING ENDOCRINE ORGAN/GLAND	HORMONE	STIMULUS	TARGET	EFFECT
					follicles, immature eggs in F; in M aids in sperm production
Anterior pituitary gland	Anterior pituitary gland	Thyroxine (T_4) and Triiodothyronine (T_3); T_4 has four bound iodine atoms and is the predominant form secreted by the thyroid; the target organs convert it to T_3, the much more active form with three bound iodine atoms; after T_4 and T_3 are formed, they are packaged into lysosomes and transported.	Hormonal stimulus: gonadotropin-releasing hormone (GnRH); inhibited by: gonadal hormones, estrogen and progesterone in F and testosterone in M	Adrenal cortex of adrenal glands	Release of adrenal cortex hormones (aldosterone, cortisol, and testosterone)
Anterior pituitary gland	Thyroid gland	Calcitonin	Hormonal stimulus: corticotrophin-releasing hormone (CRH)	Three targets: Skeleton: takes Ca^{2+} out of bony matrix; stimulates osteoclasts to digest or reabsorb bony matrix; Kidneys: increase Ca^{2+} absorption; less to urine; Small intestine: reabsorb Ca^{2+} during digestion	Increased metabolic activity; produces body heat; also involved in maintaining BP and in the normal growth and development of the reproductive, skeletal, and nervous systems
Thyroid gland	Thyroid gland	Parathyroid hormone (PTH)	Hormonal stimulus: thyroid stimulating hormone (TSH); both require iodine to work correctly	Kidney; renal tubules	Lowers Ca^{2+} in bloodstream
Thyroid gland	Parathyroid glands	Mineral corticoids; the main one is aldosterone.	Humoral stimulus: when Ca^{2+} in the bloodstream is high (approximately 20% above normal)	Body cells	Raises Ca^{2+} in bloodstream

(continued)

ENDOCRINE ORGANS, GLANDS, AND HORMONES ***(continued)***

PRODUCING ENDOCRINE ORGAN/GLAND	RELEASING ENDOCRINE ORGAN/GLAND	HORMONE	STIMULUS	TARGET	EFFECT
Parathyroid glands	Adrenal glands; adrenal cortex	Glucocorticoids; the main one is cortisol.	Humoral: stimulus: when Ca^{2+} in the bloodstream is low; inhibited by high concentration of Ca^{2+} in bloodstream	Reproductive organs; ovaries and testes	Stimulates kidney renal tubules to reabsorb Na^+ and excrete K^+; by reabsorbing Na^+ this causes the resorption of H_2O (H_2O follows Na^+).
Adrenal glands; adrenal cortex	Adrenal glands; adrenal medulla	Gonadocorticoids; sex hormones; mainly androgens; which are converted to estrogen and testosterone after release; only small amounts are released.	Four mechanisms of stimulus: 1. Humoral stimulus: high K^+ in bloodstream or low Na^+. 2. Hormonal stimulus: Adrenocorticotropic hormone (ACTH) from anterior pituitary; only stimulates aldosterone under stress. 3. Renin: Protein released from the kidney causes an enzyme cascade to form angiotensin II, a potent stimulator of aldosterone; renin is released from the kidney when the BP is low. 4. Atrial natriuretic peptide (ANP), a hormone released from the heart when blood volume and BP are high inhibits aldosterone release.	Variety of organs; same ones as sympathetic nervous system: heart: lungs, liver, and circulatory system	Creation of glucose from nonglucose sources; breaks down fats and proteins; cortisol also inhibits inflammation and the immune system response
Adrenal glands; adrenal cortex	Adrenal glands; adrenal medulla	Two hormones; epinephrine (adrenaline) and norepinephrine (noradrenaline); slightly different but grouped together; part of the sympathetic nervous system; fight or flight response	Hormonal stimulus: ACTH (from the anterior pituitary)	Almost every cell; exceptions are the brain, spleen, testes, uterus, and itself (thyroid)	Thought to be responsible for the onset of puberty; jump-start the ovaries and testes; also thought responsible for female sex drive (libido) and estrogen production postmenopause

ENDOCRINE ORGANS, GLANDS, AND HORMONES *(continued)*

PRODUCING ENDOCRINE ORGAN/GLAND	RELEASING ENDOCRINE ORGAN/GLAND	HORMONE	STIMULUS	TARGET	EFFECT
Adrenal glands; adrenal cortex	Adrenal glands; adrenal medulla	Insulin	Hormonal stimulus: ACTH (from the anterior pituitary)	Three targets: skeleton: puts Ca^{2+} into bony matrix; stimulates osteoblasts to build bony matrix; kidneys: puts Ca^{2+} into urine; if the body cannot use it, it is shuttled to a waste product; small intestine: lowers Ca^{2+} absorption so that when digesting food, calcitonin inhibits Ca^{2+} absorption if it is not needed.	All are a reaction to stress; effects mimic sympathetic nervous system activation; raise heart rate and BP; dilate bronchioles; increase respiration rate, raise blood glucose level, redirect blood flow to the heart and muscles and away from the digestive system.
Adrenal glands; adrenal medulla; inner nervous tissue	Pancreas; beta cells; islets of Langerhans are circular bodies inside the pancreas tissue that produce two populations of cells; beta cells produce insulin; alpha cells produce glucagon.	Glucagon	Neural stimuli: preganglionic fibers of sympathetic nervous system; synergist with glucagon	Variety of organs; same ones as sympathetic nervous system: heart, lungs, liver, and circulatory system	Lower blood glucose levels
Pancreas; beta cells	Pancreas; alpha cells	Two hormones: thymosin and thymopoietins; immune response	Humoral stimulus: blood glucose level rises; antagonist to glucagon	Two targets: 1. All body cells: uptake glucose. 2. Liver: inhibits glycogen breakdown; do not want more glucose released so insulin comes in and keeps the glycogen as glycogen.	Raise blood glucose levels
Pancreas; alpha cells	Thymus; the size of the thymus decreases	Melatonin	Humoral stimulus: blood glucose level drops;	Liver; glycogen converted to glucose	Stimulates maturation of T-cells

(continued)

ENDOCRINE ORGANS, GLANDS, AND HORMONES ***(continued)***

PRODUCING ENDOCRINE ORGAN/GLAND	RELEASING ENDOCRINE ORGAN/GLAND	HORMONE	STIMULUS	TARGET	EFFECT
	with age as it turns into adipose and fibrous tissue; hormone release is correspondingly diminished.		antagonist to insulin; synergist with epinephrine		
Thymus	Thymus		Immune system	T-cells (T-lymphocytes)	Cyclic levels; low in A.M., high in P.M.; sleep/wake cycles; stimulated by the amount of light; this is why highest at night; regulation of biological clock; possibly onset of puberty
Pineal gland	Pineal gland		Humoral stimulus: indirectly from visual pathways (retina to suprachiasmatic nucleus of hypothalamus to superior cervical ganglion to pineal gland) about intensity and duration of daylight		Inhibits mineral corticoid (aldosterone) production; decreases blood volume, which in turn decreases BP
Heart	Heart	Atrial natriuretic peptide (ANP)	Humoral stimulus: when blood volume and BP are high, do not want more aldosterone; ANP inhibits its release; aldosterone antagonist	Adrenal cortex	RBC production
Kidneys	Kidneys	Erythropoietin (EPO)	Feedback mechanism that measures blood oxygenation	Stem cells in red bone marrow	
Gastrointestinal (GI) tract	Gastrointestinal (GI) tract	Hormones that aid digestion; work locally; released and work in the GI			Stimulates the retention of the corpus luteum; corpus luteum then secretes progesterone to promote the enrichment and

ENDOCRINE ORGANS, GLANDS, AND HORMONES *(continued)*

PRODUCING ENDOCRINE ORGAN/GLAND	RELEASING ENDOCRINE ORGAN/GLAND	HORMONE	STIMULUS	TARGET	EFFECT
					retention of the endometrial lining to maintain a pregnancy; after the third month of pregnancy, the placenta takes over in maintaining pregnancy.
Placenta	Placenta	Human chorionic gonadotropin (HCG); the pregnancy test hormone; also produces estrogen and progesterone	Pregnancy	Corpus luteum of the ovary	
Female gonads	Ovaries	Estrogen and progesterone	Hormonal stimulus: gonadotropins: follicle-stimulating hormone (FSH) and luteinizing hormone (LH)	Uterus, ovaries, and breast	Controls menstrual cycle (uterine/ovarian cycle); responsible for maturation of eggs and follicles and for development of secondary sex characteristics and pubic hair; progesterone is responsible for maintaining pregnancy.
Male gonads	Testes	Testosterone	Hormonal stimulus: gonadotropins: follicle-stimulating hormone (FSH) and luteinizing hormone (LH), which stimulate gamete production and the production of gonadal hormones; these in turn were stimulated by gonadotropin-releasing hormone (GnRH).	Male reproductive organs	Testes maturation; sperm production; male secondary sex characteristics; axillary, pubic, and facial hair

Reproductive System

The function of the reproductive system is to produce offspring. The primary sex organs are the gonads. The function of the gonads is to produce gametes. In the male, the testes produce sperm. In the female, the ovaries produce eggs. The gonads also produce sex hormones. Everything else is performed by the accessory sex organs.

Male Anatomy

The main structures of the male anatomy are as follows:

- **Testes**: The testes are the gonads of the male. They have two coverings or tunics.
  1. **Tunica vaginalis**: The outside covering of the testes is a continuation of the peritoneum.
  2. **Tunica albuginea**: The inside covering is fibrous connective tissue. The testes are divided into structures called **lobules** by the **septula testes**. The fibrous septa run between the **mediastinum testis**, a network of fibrous connective tissue, and the tunica albuginea. Each lobule contains a series of tubules, called the **seminiferous tubules**, where sperm is produced. There are two cell types.
     1. **Myoid cells**: The cells that surround the seminiferous tubules are little **muscular** cells that help move sperm out of the testes.
     2. **Interstitial cells**: The cells that make testosterone are found sporadically around the seminiferous tubules.
- **Spermatic cord**: The spermatic cord is a collection of nerves, blood vessels, and lymphatic vessels, plus the ductus deferens that travels from the epididymis through the inguinal canal to each testicle.
- **Scrotum**: The scrotum encloses the testes. It is a sac of skin outside the abdominopelvic cavity. Its function is to hold the testes at a temperature lower than body temperature so that sperm can be more accurately produced.
- **Ducts**: The ducts deliver sperm to the epididymis. In the order of the sperm flow the four ducts are as follows.
  1. **Epididymis**: The epididymis is composed of three sections: the head, the body, and the tail. Most of the epididymis is highly coiled. **Microvilli** absorb excess testicular fluid. Sperm in epididymis are nonmotile when they enter. Sperm mature here. It takes approximately 20 days for them to gain the ability to swim. Sperm can be stored for several months in the epididymis before it is ejaculated from the epididymis. After several months, sperm is broken down and reabsorbed if it is not ejaculated.
  2. **Ductus deferens**: The ductus deferens is also called the vas deferens. It is the next stop as sperm travels. It is part of the spermatic cord. It enters the pelvic cavity and loops up over the ureter. At the end of the ductus deferens is an enlarged area called the **ampulla**. It joins with a short duct to form the ejaculatory duct. A vasectomy is when the ductus deferens is cut inside the scrotum so that sperm can no longer get into the pelvic cavity.
  3. **Ejaculatory duct**: The ductus deferens plus a duct from the seminal vesicle form the ejaculatory duct. Peristalsis moves sperm during ejaculation.
  4. **Urethra**: The urethra receives sperm from the ejaculatory duct. In males, the urethra is part of both the urinary and reproductive systems. The urethra carries both urine and sperm. There are three parts of the urethra.
     1. **Prostatic urethra**: The prostatic urethra is surrounded by the prostate gland.
     2. **Membranous urethra**: The short membranous urethra is in the **urogenital diaphragm**, the layer of the pelvis that

separates the deep perineal sac (the partially enclosed space in the perineum above the perineal membrane) from the upper pelvis.

3. **Spongy** or **penile urethra**: The spongy urethra is in the penis. It leads to the external urethral orifice.

- **Glands**: The glands help with semen formation by contributing secretions.
  - **Seminal vesicles**: There are two seminal vesicles on the posterior bladder surface. They produce a yellowish alkaline fluid that contains fructose, ascorbic acid, prostaglandins, and other substances that enhance sperm motility. The secretions from the seminal vesicles comprise 60% of semen volume.
  - **Prostate**: The single prostate gland is immediately inferior to the bladder. The secretions from the prostate gland enter the prostatic urethra. The secretions from the prostate gland comprise about one-third of semen volume. The prostate gland produces a milky, acidic fluid that contains citrate, enzymes, and **prostate-specific antigen (PSA)**, which is used as a clinical marker for prostate cancer diagnosis.
  - **Bulbourethral glands**: These small glands inferior to the prostate gland produce a thick, clear, alkaline mucous that is thought to neutralize the acidic urethra (urine). It lubricates the glans penis.

Sperm

Sperm are made at the end of the testes lobules in the seminiferous tubules. They then travel to the epididymis through the **tubulus rectus**, the **rete testes**, and the **efferent ductules**. Sperm composition is in general alkaline to protect it from two acidic places: the male urethra and the female vagina. **Seminal plasmin** destroys bacteria. Two to five mL of semen is expelled during each ejaculation. One mL has 20 to 150 million sperm. Sperm are produced in a process called **spermatogenesis**. It takes between 64 and 72 days to produce sperm in the seminiferous tubules. The process starts at puberty (approximately 14 years of age). After puberty has been reached, 400 million sperm are formed each day. The process begins with stem cells called **spermatogonia** at the basal laminae of the seminiferous tubules. They undergo mitosis to produce two types of cells.

1. **Type A**: Type A cells stay at the basal lamina and remain part of the stem cell populace to continue the process of producing type A and type B cells. They maintain the germ cell line.
2. **Type B**: Type B cells are pushed toward the lumen (open space in seminiferous tubule), where they become **primary spermatocytes.** Primary spermatocytes undergo meiosis I to become **secondary spermatocytes**. Secondary spermatocytes undergo meiosis II to become **spermatids.** One stem cell yields four spermatids.

Spermiogenesis is the process of differentiation that spermatids undergo to become sperm. There are three regions on the sperm.

1. **Head**: The head of a sperm cell contains the nucleus with the genetic information (DNA). The **acrosome** is a specialized piece on the head that has enzymes to digest the covering of the egg so that it can enter.
2. **Midpiece**: The midpiece provides the fuel. It is the metabolic portion containing many mitochondria.
3. **Tail**: The tail provides movement.

Sustentacular or **nurse cells** in the seminiferous tubules surround the developing sperm and help them to mature. The seminiferous tubule has two compartments. The sustentacular cells divide the tubule. Sustentacular cells are bound to each other laterally by tight junctions. It is these tight junctions that form the division between the two compartments.

1. **Basal compartment**: Closest to the basement membrane, this compartment is where the spermatogonia (stem cells) are located.
2. **Adluminal compartment**: Everything from primary spermatocyte (from type B cells), secondary spermatocyte (after meiosis I), spermatid (after meiosis II), and sperm (after spermiogenesis) is pushed here to undergo the differentiation process.

The tight junctions between the sustentacular cells form the **blood-testis barrier**. This prevents the membrane antigens of differentiating sperm from escaping through the basal lamina into the bloodstream, where they could activate the immune system. This is necessary because sperm are not present until puberty. They were therefore not present when the immune system was developing in the first month after birth when the self-inventory occurred. Anything present in the body in the first month of life is identified as self. Anything entering afterward is identified as an antigen. **Spermatogonia**, which were present at birth, are outside the blood-testis barrier in the basal compartment. They can therefore be influenced by blood-borne chemical messengers that prompt spermatogenesis. After they undergo mitosis, the tight junctions open, allowing the primary spermatocytes to enter the adluminal compartment across the blood-testis barrier. Now the spermatocytes are nearly enclosed in sustentacular cells so they are safe from attack by the immune system, which will perceive them as antigens. Sustentacular cells provide nutrients and essential signals to the dividing cells to move them to the lumen. Sustentacular cells also secrete testicular fluid, the transport medium to move immature sperm to the epididymis. There they mature and gain increased motility and fertilizing power.

Hormone Regulation

The **brain-testicular axis** refers to the interactions among the hypothalamus, anterior pituitary gland, and the testes that regulate spermatogenesis and androgen production. The hypothalamus releases GnRH, which controls the release of FSH and LH, to the anterior pituitary via the hypophyseal portal system. The anterior pituitary then secretes FSH and LH (the gonadotropins). The testes release testosterone. FSH causes the nurse cells (sustentacular cells) to release **androgen-binding protein (ABP)**. ABP causes spermatogenic cells to concentrate testosterone and be more receptive to testosterone. LH stimulates interstitial cells to make more testosterone. Concentrated testosterone stimulates spermatogenesis. Testosterone also inhibits further release of GnRH from the hypothalamus. When the sperm count is high, the nurse cells release **inhibin**, which inhibits the anterior pituitary from releasing FSH and LH.

Testosterone, a steroid hormone, promotes spermatogenesis. It also promotes the development of all male sex organs, including the ducts, glands, testis, and penis, as well as the development of facial hair, pubic hair, and axillary hair. Other effects include the voice deepening, bone and muscle growth, and the basis for the sex drive.

External Male Genitalia

The following structures comprise the external male genitalia.

- **Penis**: The function of the penis is to deliver sperm to the female. There are three regions of the penis.
  1. **Root**: The root is attached to the body.
  2. **Shaft or Body**: The shaft is the free-hanging portion of the penis.
  3. **Glans penis**: The glans penis is the expanded end of the penis. The **foreskin** covers the glans penis if circumcision has not been performed.

The penile (spongy) urethra is the section of the urethra contained in the penis. There are three bodies of cylindrical tissue that run the length of the penis. This is connective tissue with spaces that fill with blood during an erection.

- **Corpus spongiosum**: This body of connective tissue surrounds the urethra. Its function is to keep the urethra open during an erection.
- **Corpus cavernosa**: These two bodies of connective tissue form the bulk of the penis. They are the two lateral sides of the penis.

Female Reproductive System

The gonads of the female reproductive system are the ovaries. A series of ducts carry the egg. The uterine or fallopian tubes lead to the uterus, which leads to the vagina. The ovaries are suspended on each side of the uterus. There are two regions of the ovary.

1. **Cortex**: The outer region of the ovary is involved in forming gametes. The structures of the cortex are as follows.
   - **Follicles**: Follicles are immature eggs (oocytes). They are surrounded by one or more layers of cells. If only one layer of cells surrounds the oocyte, they are **follicle cells.** If two or more layers of cells surround the oocyte, they are **granulosa cells**. There are four follicle types.
     1. **Primordial follicle**: Primordial follicles have one layer of cells around the oocyte (follicle cells) and they mature into primary follicles.
     2. **Primary follicles**: Primary follicles have two or more layers (granulosa) and they mature into secondary follicles.
     3. **Secondary follicles**: When a fluid-filled space called an **antrum** appears, the follicle is now a secondary follicle and will become a vesicular follicle.
     4. **Vesicular follicle**: When the antrum is so large that the oocyte is pushed to one side of the follicle, it is a vesicular or **Graafian follicle.** The secondary oocyte will be ejected in the process of **ovulation**. The remaining cells left after the secondary oocyte is released form the **corpus luteum**, responsible for the production of progesterone and estrogen.
2. **Medulla**: The medulla is the inner part of the ovary that contains the blood vessels and the nerve supply. It runs through the middle of the ovary.

After ovulation, the egg enters one of the **uterine tubes**. The uterine tube is the site of fertilization. The enlarged region at the end of the uterine tube is called the **ampulla**. The ampulla ends in an open funnel-shaped structure called the **infundibulum**. The infundibulum has fingerlike projections with cilia on them called **fimbriae** that drape over the ovary, but do not actually come in direct contact with it. The fimbriae create a current that draws the egg into the uterine tube. Not all eggs make it to the uterine tube. This is why ectopic pregnancies occur in the uterine tube or abdomen. They usually result in miscarriage. If not, the pregnancy must be terminated or the uterine tube will burst and the mother will die.

The fimbriae anatomy is necessary because the female duct system is not continuous like that of the male. The male duct system is a closed circuit, but the female duct system is not. The fact that uterine tubes are not continuous with the ovaries creates both the risk of ectopic pregnancy and the risk of **pelvic inflammatory disease (PID)**. Infections that spread into the peritoneal cavity from other parts of the reproductive tract can cause PID, which can lead to scarring of the uterine tubes and ovaries and sterility.

The next stop for the egg is the **uterus** or **womb**, a thick-walled muscular organ. Its functions are to receive, retain, and nourish the embryo. There are three regions of the uterus.

1. **Body**: The body is the main part of the organ.
2. **Fundus**: The rounded part above the entrance of the uterine tubes is the fundus.
3. **Cervix**: The region that extends into the vagina and that dilates during childbirth is the cervix. In the mucosa of the cervical canal, **cervical glands** produce mucous. A **mucous plug** plugs the hole between the vagina and uterus, preventing bacteria from entering. It can also prevent sperm from entering, so it disappears when ovulation has occurred in the hope that the sperm can enter and fertilize the egg.

The four layers of the uterine wall from the outermost to the innermost are as follows.

1. **Perimetrium**: The outermost layer is part of the peritoneum.
2. **Myometrium**: This muscle layer makes up the bulk of the uterus. It is the muscle that is used to expel the baby during childbirth.
3. **Endometrium**: The innermost layer is a mucosal lining with two sublayers or strata.
   1. **Stratum basalis**: The deepest sublayer forms a new functional layer after menstruation.
   2. **Stratum functionalis**: The surface layer is shed during menstruation (only the stratum functionalis is shed during menstruation, not the entire endometrium).

The next part of the duct system is a thin-walled tube called the **vagina**. It connects the uterus to the outside of the body and is also called the birth canal. It has an acidic pH, making it a hostile environment to sperm. The **hymen** is a layer of mucosa that covers the opening of the vagina. It is ruptured at some point during the lifetime, whether through sports, feminine product insertion, or sex. The cervical glands provide some of the lubrication for the vagina.

External Female Genitalia

The following four structures comprise the female external genitalia.

1. **Mons pubis**: The mons pubis is a fatty lump over the pubic bone.
2. **Labia**: Two flaps of skin and adipose tissue extend and cover the external genitalia. There are two layers.
   1. **Labia majora**: This layer is homologous to the male scrotum. It derives from the same tissue developmentally and is hair covered.
   2. **Labia minora**: This layer is two soft skin folds that are not hair covered and that surround the opening to the vagina.
3. **Vestibule**: The vestibule contains the openings to both the urethra and the vagina. Females have a completely separate urinary system and reproductive system. This is the opposite of the male, in which the urethra carries both sperm and urine. The **greater vestibular glands** secrete a thick mucous. They are homologous to the bulbourethral glands in the male.
4. **Clitoris**: The clitoris is the erectile tissue. It is homologous to the penis.

The **mammary glands** are present in both sexes, but are functional only in the female and only in the third trimester of pregnancy and postbirth. They are modified sweat glands and as such are part of the integumentary system. The size is dependent on the amount of fat deposited. The mammary glands are divided into **lobules**, which contain **alveoli** that produce milk. Milk goes from the alveoli through the lactiferous duct to the lactiferous sac, where it accumulates. It is expelled out the nipple.

Oogenesis

The egg supply is set at birth when the total supply for a lifetime is present. This is very different from the male, who produces 400 million per day postpuberty. Eggs form during the fetal period and develop into primary oocytes, which are found in primary follicles. Development is then stopped in prophase I in meiosis I, and the oocytes wait for 10 to 14 years for puberty. After puberty, each month several oocytes are selected, one of which completes meiosis I to produce two cells: a **polar body** (nonfunctional cell) and a secondary oocyte. The secondary oocyte is arrested in metaphase II. The secondary oocyte is ovulated from the secondary follicle and will complete its development only if sperm penetration occurs. If a sperm penetrates, it completes meiosis II to yield two cells: a polar body (may or may not form two more polar bodies) and an **ovum** (egg). The result is one to three nonfunctional polar bodies and one functional ovum. There are approximately 250,000 oocytes, but during a lifetime only about 500 are released.

Ovarian Cycle

The ovarian cycle is approximately 28 days long. There are two phases.

1. **Follicular phase**: The first phase (days 1 through 14) follows the development of the follicle until ovulation. Ovulation signals the end of the follicular phase. The steps are as follows:
    1. GnRH from the hypothalamus stimulates FSH and LH from the anterior pituitary.
    2. FSH and LH stimulate the primordial follicle to grow into the primary follicle.
    3. Connective tissue condenses around the primary follicle, producing the **theca folliculi**, a box around the follicle. It is targeted by LH.
    4. Primary follicles with two or more layers (granulosa) are targeted by FSH.
    5. The cells start producing estrogen. As the estrogen level rises, it inhibits FSH and LH in order to prevent other follicles from developing.
    6. Estrogen continues to rise as more and more estrogen is produced in the ovary. The primary follicle continues to develop and the granulosa starts to develop the liquid antrum space. Now it is a secondary follicle.
    7. The antrum continues to grow. More fluid fills the follicle and the oocyte becomes isolated to one side of follicle. This causes the oocyte to be surrounded by a set of cells called the **corona radiata**. Now it is a vesicular (Graafian) follicle.
    8. Estrogen levels peak or reach a critical level. Now FSH is no longer inhibited. Instead it initiates a positive feedback loop that results in an LH surge close to day 14.
    9. The primary oocyte finishes meiosis I to become a secondary oocyte. The secondary oocyte in a vesicular follicle is ovulated on day 14.
    10. Ovulation expels the secondary oocyte and its surrounding tissues (the corona radiata).
    11. Postovulation, the estrogen levels decrease because the follicle has been broken apart and is no longer producing estrogen.
2. **Luteal phase**: The second phase is from days 15 to 28.
    - LH transforms the vesicular follicle into the corpus luteum, which starts to produce estrogen and progesterone, but mostly progesterone.
    - If pregnancy does not occur, the corpus luteum degenerates, usually within 10 days, leaving behind the **corpus albicans** (white scar tissue).
    - If pregnancy does occur, the corpus luteum grows, causing more progesterone to be produced because it is needed to maintain the pregnancy until the third month. After this

the placenta takes over progesterone production to maintain the pregnancy.

- During the first three months of pregnancy, the corpus luteum is producing estrogen and mostly progesterone. Both hormones inhibit FSH and LH, but the corpus luteum needs LH in order to continue to grow. As LH drops, it is replaced by HCG (human chorionic gonadotropin), an LH-like hormone that prompts the corpus luteum to continue secreting progesterone and estrogen.
- If pregnancy does not occur, the LH levels drop and the corpus luteum degenerates, causing the levels of estrogen and progesterone to drop. With FSH and LH no longer inhibited, the cycle starts again.

Uterine or Menstrual Cycle

The uterine cycle is also 28 days long and is coordinated with the ovarian cycle to receive an egg, approximately six to seven days postovulation. This is how long it takes for an egg to travel through the uterine tubes. There are three phases.

1. **Menstrual phase**: In days 1 through 5 the uterus sheds the stratum functionalis.
2. **Proliferation phase**: In days 6 through 14, at the same time as the follicular (first) phase in the ovarian cycle (days 1 to 14), the endometrium rebuilds the stratum functionalis stimulated by rising estrogen levels.
3. **Secretory phase**: In days 15 through 28, the endometrium prepares for implantation. If an egg implants, it is during this phase that progesterone from the corpus luteum acts on endometrium to maintain it. If there is no implantation during the secretory phase, the corpus luteum degrades and endometrial cells start to die off. As they start to slough off, it is once again day 1 of the menstrual phase.

At puberty, gonadotropin-releasing hormone (GnRH) controls FSH and LH release. It takes approximately four years to establish the two cycles. In addition to FSH and LH, females need fat, which is particularly important for the neural development of the fetus because myelin is composed largely of lipids. Fat needs the hormone **leptin**. If there is not enough fat in a female to support a pregnancy, there is no reason for the body to turn on the cycles. This is why young female athletes may be amenorrheic.

Effects of Estrogen and Progesterone

Estrogen stimulates the growth and development of the uterine tubes, uterus, and vagina. It also affects the development of the external genitalia, the growth of the breasts, and the deposit of fat, particularly at the hips. The widening of the pelvis and the facilitation of the uptake of Ca^{+2} are also the result of estrogen. Progesterone establishes and regulates both the ovarian and the uterine cycles. It is also the hormone that maintains pregnancy.

Special Senses

Special senses include hearing, smell, taste, and vision.

Hearing

There are three functions performed by the ear. Receptors for each are found in different parts of the inner ear.

1. **Hearing**
2. **Dynamic equilibrium**: Dynamic equilibrium is the sensation of **rotational movement**—for example, when you are spinning.
3. **Static equilibrium**: Static equilibrium is movements that are up and down and side to side.

The seven structures of the ear are as follows:

1. **External (outer) ear**: The shell-shaped projection surrounding the ear is called the **pinna** or **auricula**. This plus the external acoustic meatus (auditory canal), which includes an osseous

portion that runs through the temporal bone, comprise the external ear. The external acoustic meatus is lined with skin, sebaceous glands, and sweat glands (ceruminous glands) that produce cerumen, a yellow-brown waxy substance that forms a sticky trap for foreign bodies and serves as an insect repellent.

2. **Cochlea**: The cochlea is the portion of the ear where hearing occurs. It transforms sound vibrations into nerve impulses.
3. **Semicircular canals**: The three semicircular canals (lateral, anterior, and posterior) maintain dynamic equilibrium. They sense movement in three spatial planes.
4. **Vestibule**: The vestibule maintains static equilibrium.
5. **Tympanic membrane**: The eardrum is connective tissue covered by skin externally and by mucosa internally. It is shaped like a flattened cone. The apex protrudes medially into the middle ear. It passes vibrations to the middle ear.
6. **Tympanic cavity** or **middle ear**: This air-filled, mucosa-lined cavity is in the petrous portion of the temporal bone.
7. The three bones of the middle ear are the **malleus** or **hammer**, which connects to the eardrum; the **incus** or **anvil**, which is the middle bone; and the **stapes** or **stirrup**, which is the third bone.

The following describes how hearing works in nine steps.

1. Sound comes through the air and enters the external acoustic meatus.
2. It moves to the tympanic membrane (eardrum).
3. Vibrations of the eardrum pass sound to the bones.
4. The bones vibrate. The function of the middle ear is to amplify the signal.
5. The stapes sits against a membrane called the **oval** or **vestibular window**. This is the entrance to the inner ear.
6. Sound from the stapes goes to the cochlea.
7. In the cochlea, which is filled with fluid, there are three compartments.
    1. **Scala vestibuli**: The top compartment is filled with **perilymph**, a fluid with a composition similar to blood plasma and cerebrospinal fluid.
    2. **Scala tympani**: The bottom compartment is also filled with **perilymph** because the two compartments are connected in a loop.
    3. **Scala media**: The middle compartment, also called the cochlear duct, is filled with a different fluid with a high potassium content called **endolymph**. The stapes vibrating causes movement of the fluid. This distorts and changes the shape of the membrane that separates the scala tympani from the scala media, the **basilar membrane.** Low notes are distributed to the apex. Waves take a complete route through the cochlea, up the scala vestibuli, around, and back toward the round window (where the scala tympani terminates). These waves are below the threshold of hearing. High notes are distributed to the other end, the base of the cochlea. They create pressure waves and take a shortcut, and are transmitted through the cochlear duct (scala media) into the perilymph of the scala tympani.
8. The actual sound receptor, the **organ of Corti,** sits inside the scala media. It is located on the basilar membrane. There is also a membrane or root on the top of the organ of Corti called the **tectorial membrane** (*tector* means root). It is covered with ciliated cells. These hair cells on the organ of Corti are the **mechanoreceptors.** The vibration of the basilar membrane depresses the membrane of the round window (at the termination of the scala tympani). Since fluid is noncompressible, it must move over, causing the basilar membrane to be pushed up. Now the cilia on the tectorial mem-

brane make contact with the basilar membrane. When the cilia move, the disturbance sends a signal down the **cochlear nerve**. This is how the mechanoreceptors send a signal to the brain that activity has occurred.

9. The signal is sent to the temporal lobe in the brain, where hearing is located.

Damage to the ciliated cells from loudness causes hearing loss because the hair cells do not reproduce. There are notches of cells according to frequency, which if damaged will result in no longer being able to hear the corresponding frequencies. When sound is transmitted to the cochlear nerve, it undergoes transduction. Transduction is a mechanical or visual stimulus converted to an action potential. The cilia in the basilar membrane are like strings on a harp. Near the oval window they are short and stiff and resonate to high frequencies. On the basilar membrane they are longer and floppy and resonate to lower frequencies.

Dynamic Equilibrium

The semicircular canals have three different planes or axes. When you spin, the fluid sloshes and imparts the perception of rotational movement. This disturbs the **crista ampullaris**, the receptor organ for dynamic equilibrium. There is one pair in each ear. Each crista is composed of supporting cells and hair cells. A single taller cilia is called a **kinocilium**. A cluster of many cilia is called a **stereocilium**. The crista ampullaris is a cupula, a gelled mass that looks like a pointed cap. Cilia project into this gelled mass. Dendrites of the vestibular nerve encircle the base of the hair cells. Fluid moves the cilia of the hair cells, and they touch the cupula. Hair cells in the crista ampullaris are the mechanoreceptors. When you stop spinning, fluid is still moving. There is a disconnect from sensory input. The semicircular canal still conveys rotational movement. The eyes, however, convey dizziness.

Static Equilibrium

Static equilibrium is planar movement. The vestibule sits between the semicircular canals and the cochlea. There are two parts: the **utricle** and the **saccule**. Each utricle and each saccule has a sensory receptor called a **macula** inside it. The macula is the receptor organ for planar movement. Again, there are hair cell clusters that are not uniform in length—kinocilium and stereocilium. These scattered receptor cells are embedded in the **otolithic membrane**. On top of that there are salt crystals called **otoliths**. When you tilt your head, the crystals slide on the membrane and move the **kinocilium** in one direction or the other. If you bend your head toward the kinocilium, it causes an increase in the frequency of action potential generation. If you bend your head away from the kinocilium, it causes a decrease in the frequency of action potential generation. The utricle responds to horizontal acceleration, such as forward and back or left and right movement. The saccule responds to vertical, or up and down, accelerations.

Smell

The receptor organ for smell is the **olfactory epithelium**. The receptor cell is the **olfactory receptor cell**. Chemicals must be dissolved in H_2O. This is why moist mucous membranes are required to moisten the tongue and nasal passageways, which if they are dried out, do not work well. The **olfactory apparatus** is on the roof of the nasal cavity. The dorsal surface is associated with the **cribriform plate** of the **ethmoid** bone, where some receptor cells for smell are found. The top is the **olfactory bulb**, which is at the end of **olfactory tract**. It is axons of neurons inside the central nervous system. Next is the **olfactory gland** and then the **olfactory epithelium**, which covers the superior nasal conchae on each side of the nasal septum and contains the olfactory receptor cells.

The olfactory receptor cells are **bipolar neurons**, which are rare. The axons of the olfactory neurons protrude through holes on the cribriform plate to the olfactory bulb. Here olfactory receptor cells synapse on structures called **glomeruli**, which are bundles of cell bodies inside the central nervous system (nuclei). They synapse on cells in the glomeruli called **mitral cells.** The turnover rate, if any, for neurons is very slow. This is why olfactory receptors are unusual among neurons. There is a high turnover rate of approximately once every 60 days. These receptors are inundated with lots of input and wear out; then they must be replaced. The **olfactory tract** action potentials go via the thalamus to the cortex. We know how things smell due to conscious awareness. The information is also sent to the hypothalamus and to the limbic system. This is why we respond emotionally to smells.

Taste

Maps of tongue sensitivity to taste have turned out to be false. The taste buds can detect all of the five tastes more or less equally regardless of where they are on the tongue. The five distinct identifiable tastes cannot be recognized with smell. They include sweet, sour, bitter, salty, and **umami**, which means savory. The latter was discovered by the Japanese and is elicited by the amino acids glutamate and aspartate, which give the beef taste to steak.

Foods must be dissolved and be wet. If they are dry, taste differences cannot be perceived. Taste and smell are completely related. For example, when you are sick, you cannot smell or taste food or it does not taste good because you cannot smell it.

Taste buds are in depressions on the tongue called papillae. The papillae are described in the digestive system section. The **gustatory receptor cells** are the receptors for taste on the epithelial cells on the taste buds. Turnover is fast. The taste buds on the circumvallate papillae are completely replaced every few weeks. Cranial nerves VII, IX, and X are involved in taste. Signals from these cranial nerves go through the medulla oblongata to the thalamus and then to the cortex. From the cortex the signals proceed to the hypothalamus and the limbic system. Different ion channels are involved in transducing taste—for example, Na^+ channel for sour because these are acid ions.

Vision

Sight involves a complex structure and path. The ten parts of the eye area as follows:

1. **Cornea**: The most superficial region on the eye is the cornea.
2. **Iris**: The colored portion of the eye is the iris.
3. **Pupil**: The pupil looks black but is actually an opening. There is no light inside the eye to illuminate this opening. The ophthalmologist shines a light in to see how the hole contracts in response to light.
4. **Lacrimal apparatus**: The lacrimal glands produce tears, and the lacrimal ducts release them onto the eye surface each time you blink your eye. The purpose is mainly to reduce friction on the cornea to prevent it from getting scratched. However, the cornea is also the most highly regenerative eye structure.

   Just as with the continuous production of cerebrospinal fluid, the fluid must drain somewhere. It drains through the lacrimal punctum, the lacrimal canaliculus, and the nasal lacrimal duct, the structural connection between the eye and nose. When you cut an onion or are sad and cry, the tears cannot all drain. Your nose becomes stuffy because you are maximizing the amount of fluid that can pass.
5. **Extrinsic eye muscles**: These six muscles have the smallest motor units yielding the most precise control.
   1. **Lateral rectus**: These muscles move the eye laterally. The controlling nerve is nerve VI, the abducens nerve.
   2. **Medial rectus:** These muscles move the eye medially. The controlling nerve is nerve III, the oculomotor nerve.

3. **Superior rectus**: These muscles move to elevate the eye and turn it medially. The controlling nerve is nerve III, oculomotor.
4. **Inferior rectus**: These muscles depress the eye and turn it medially. The controlling nerve is nerve III, oculomotor.
5. **Inferior oblique**: These muscles move to elevate the eye and turn it laterally. The controlling nerve is nerve III, oculomotor.
6. **Superior oblique**: These muscles depress the eye and turn it laterally. The controlling nerve is nerve IV, trochlear.

6. **Tunics**: The layers of the eye are called tunics. There are three tunics.
   1. **Fibrous tunic**: The first, most superficial tunic is on the outside and it consists of two parts.
      1. **Cornea**: The cornea is clear. Anteriorly, light must pass through it. It is highly regenerative. There are no blood vessels associated with it. Therefore, cells of the immune system cannot identify it. This is why corneal transplants are so successful.
      2. **Sclera**: The sclera is the white of the eye.
   2. **Vascular tunic**: The second tunic is pigmented. It has bits of color associated with it. There are three regions.
      1. **Choroid**: The choroid region has many blood vessels. Some contain a brown pigment to absorb light so that it does not bounce off the inside of the eye.
      2. **Ciliary body**: The ciliary body is another vascular layer filled with many blood vessels. It is very thin and is involved in the control of the iris. It is also responsible for accommodation, which adjusts the focus of the lens by changing its shape through a ligament that attaches to the iris.
      3. **Iris**: The iris gives color to the eye. The most anterior portion can change shape to allow more or less light in.
   3. **Sensory tunic** or **retina**: The third tunic is where the process of vision occurs. It is the innermost layer. Cells in the retina called photoreceptors respond to light. There are two kinds.
      1. **Rods**: The rods sense only black and white. They respond to a single photon of light, unlike cones, which need tens to hundreds of photons in order to be activated. This sensitivity to a single photon of light as well as their mode of operation makes rods the low-light vision receptors. Rod cells unite at a single interneuron. These association neurons collect and amplify the signals, making night vision possible but at the cost of sharpness. Because the data from each rod is combined, vision is less well-defined than it would be if each photon was received and passed to an interneuron individually. Rods also do not react as quickly to light as cones do. Thus, rods are sensitive to small amounts of light, but visual acuity suffers. At dusk, this is why everything begins to look gray. This is rod-induced vision that does not provide sharp focus.
      2. **Cones**: The cones are involved in color vision. There are three populations for different wavelengths. They are activated quickly by high light levels. Vision from activated cones provides very clear focus, which is why objects are clearer in bright light. Blue cones receive wavelengths of 420 nm. Green cones are active at 530 nm and red cones are active at 560 nm. The highest density of cones is on the **macula lutea** and **fovea centralis** of the retina. When you want to see something clearly, you want light to focus on the fovea centralis. However, you are completely unaware that you move your eyeball using the extrinsic eye muscles to always get

sharp focus and exclude the periphery. Toward the outside of the retina, there is a decrease in cones and an increase in rods.

7. **Lens**: The lens is behind the iris. It is involved in the refraction of light. Light enters through the cornea to the pupil and then hits the lens. Light is reflected onto the back of the retina. The lens shape can change for near or far vision. With age, the lens becomes less flexible. Presbyopia is a disease of old age that makes people unable to focus.
8. **Optic nerve**: The place where the optic nerve, also called the cranial nerve, leaves the eye is the region in the retina where the blind spot is located. There are no photoreceptors at this spot, also called the optic disc. The rods and cones are at the back of the retina. The first layer is a layer of ganglion cells. The axons of ganglion cell bodies are what make up the optic nerve. The second layer is bipolar neurons. The third layer is the photoreceptors (rods and cones). Activation is from back to front. The light goes to the receptors, then to bipolar neurons, and finally to the ganglion cells, which generate action potential.
9. **Anterior cavity**: The eyeball does not collapse because it has several important fluid-filled compartments. In front of the lens, the fluid-filled compartment is the aqueous humor. Aqueous humor fluids are constantly produced, The **canal of Schlemm** is the drainpipe for the fluid. Sometimes the canal gets blocked or too much aqueous humor fluid is produced, and pressure builds up in the anterior compartment, causing the condition known as glaucoma.
10. **Posterior cavity**: The fluid-filled compartment behind the lens is the **vitreous humor**, which is thicker or more viscous. The vitreous humor does not turn over. Sometimes bits of choroid layer tissue from the vascular tunic or from the retina float in the vitreous humor, causing dark spots in the vision (floaters). These do not go away because there is no turnover of this gel-like, mostly water, collagen-infused, avascular, and mainly acellular mass.

Vision Problems

The **emmetropic eye** is the normally shaped eye with the proper focus. Convergence occurs on the retina at a single point of light. **Axial myopia**, one type of nearsightedness, occurs when there is an elongated eyeball front to back. **Refractive myopia** is caused by excess refractive power, which can be due to excess curvature of the cornea or lens. In either case, light is refracted by the lens and focuses on a spot that is anterior to the cells of the retina. Light converges, but it converges in front of the retina and then spreads out again at the retina. Vision is corrected with a concave lens. **Hyperopia**, or farsightedness, occurs when light hits the retina before it has converged. The point of focus has yet to occur. It is behind the retina wall outside of the eye. Vision is corrected with a convex lens. The corrections for both hyperopia and myopia yield a focal point where the rays do converge on the back wall of the retina.

Cataracts are a problem of the lens in which the vision becomes foggy. The lens can be surgically replaced with a plastic lens. **Astigmatism** is a condition in which rather than the eyeball being equally arced, the anterior portion is uneven. With age, although the eyeball shape does not change, there is a decreased ability of the lens to change shape.

Image Transmission

The optic nerve crosses the optic chiasma. This crossing is complicated. The lens systems of each eye reverse all images. The **medial half** of each retina receives light from the temporal (lateralmost) part of the vision field (from the far left or far right), not from straight ahead. The **lateral half** of each retina receives an image of the nasal (central) part of the visual field. The result is that the left optic tract carries and sends a complete representation of the right half of the visual field, and the right optic tract carries and sends a complete representation of the left half of the visual field. The paired optic tracts sweep posteriorly around the hypothalamus and send most of their axons to synapse with neurons in the **lateral geniculate body** of the thalamus. The lateral geniculate body of the thalamus maintains the fiber separation established at the chiasma, but balances and combines the retinal input for delivery to the visual cortex.

Practice Questions

1. The type of bacteria that can grow with or without oxygen but usually thrive better in oxygenated environments are
a. microaerophiles.
b. obligate anaerobes.
c. facultative anaerobes.
d. obligate aerobes.

2. The cell walls of Gram-negative bacteria are harmful to humans because
a. Gram-negative cell walls pose no danger to humans.
b. they release exotoxins such as botulism, anthrax, cholera, and diphtheria.
c. they produce a slimy surface that prevents neutrophils from being able to phagocytize them.
d. when the Gram-negative bacterial cell dies, the lipopolysaccharide (LPS) layer is released and becomes an endotoxin that causes inflammation, cell necrosis, bloody stool, and fluid loss.

3. The scientific name *Trichomonas vaginalis* refers to this protozoan's
a. kingdom and phylum.
b. genus and specific epithet.
c. family and order.
d. class and family.

4. Protozoa are
a. unicellular prokaryotes belonging to the domain Archaea in the kingdom Archaeabacteria.
b. multicellular eukaryotes belonging to the domain Eukarya in the kingdom Plantae.
c. unicellular prokaryotes belonging to the domain Eubacteria in the kingdom Eubacteria.
d. unicellular eukaryotes belonging to the domain Eukarya in the kingdom Protista.

5. The molds that are potentially the most harmful to humans are
a. systemic molds.
b. saprophytic molds.
c. dermatophyte molds.
d. *aspergillus.*

6. The two main genera of bacteria that produce endospores are
a. *Rickettsia* and *Chlamydia.*
b. *Bacillus* and *Clostridium.*
c. *Neisseria* and *Moraxella.*
d. *Proteus* and *Pseudomonas.*

7. Which cell type has the highest number of mitochondria?
a. cardiac muscle cells
b. sperm
c. keratinocytes
d. osteogenic cells

8. The division of the peripheral nervous system that conducts impulses from receptors to the central nervous system (CNS) is
a. motor or efferent division.
b. somatic division.
c. sensory or afferent division.
d. sympathetic nervous system.

9. The class of antibodies that are the first antibodies to be produced in response to exposure to an unfamiliar antigen are
a. IgM.
b. IgA.
c. IgG.
d. IgE.

10. Carbohydrate digestion begins with two amylases, salivary amylase in the mouth and pancreatic amylase from the pancreas in the small intestine. The next enzymes that continue carbohydrate digestion are
a. pancreatic proteases in the duodenum, the first section of the small intestine.
b. the brush border enzymes lactase, maltase, sucrase, and dextrinase in the small intestine.
c. pepsin in the stomach.
d. the brush border enzymes aminopeptidase, carboxypeptidase, and dipeptidase in the small intestine.

11. Which of the following does NOT function in body temperature regulation?
a. hypothalamus
b. blood
c. skin
d. secretin

12. Which is the structure responsible for dynamic equilibrium?
a. tympanic membrane
b. vestibule
c. cochlea
d. semicircular canal

13. Which hormone decreases urine production?
a. prolactin
b. antidiuretic hormone (ADH)
c. adrenocorticotropic hormone (ACTH)
d. follicle-stimulating hormone (FSH)

14. During the ovarian cycle, which hormone(s) stimulate the primordial follicle to grow into the primary follicle?
a. estrogen and progesterone
b. GnRH
c. FSH and LH
d. oxytocin

15. Traits that existed in the ancestral species that are still seen in all of the descendant groups are
a. shared derived characters or synapomorphic characters.
b. homoplasies.
c. homologies.
d. shared ancestral characters or plesiomorphic characters.

16. What is the term that refers to a single gene affecting a number of expressed traits?
a. pleiotropy
b. epistasis
c. incomplete dominance
d. polygenic inheritance

17. The human universal recipient is which of the following blood types?
a. type A
b. type O
c. type AB
d. type B

18. Which of the following organelles is responsible for the digestion of macromolecules?
a. Golgi complex
b. peroxisome
c. vacuole
d. lysosome

19. Where do the light-independent (dark) reactions of photosynthesis take place?
a. chlorophyll
b. stroma
c. thylakoid membrane
d. photosystems

20. During which phase of the mitotic cycle do the nuclear membranes for the two new cells begin to form?
a. metaphase
b. prophase
c. telophase
d. anaphase

21. During which phase of the mitotic cycle do the centromeres holding the sister chromatids together divide?
a. metaphase
b. prophase
c. telophase
d. anaphase

22. During which phase of the mitotic cycle does the chromatin condense to form the chromosomes?
a. metaphase
b. prophase
c. telophase
d. anaphase

23. During which phase of the mitotic cycle do the sister chromatids line up along the cell equator?
a. metaphase
b. prophase
c. telophase
d. anaphase

24. Which is the process by which homologous chromosomes in meiosis line up to form a tetrad?
a. apoptosis
b. contact inhibition
c. chiasmata
d. synapsis

25. Which of the following is the general condition in which the chromosome number is not a multiple of the haploid number for that species?
a. translocation
b. aneuploidy
c. trisomy
d. monosomy

Answers and Explanations

1. **c.** Facultative anaerobes can grow with or without oxygen but usually thrive better in oxygenated environments. They get their energy from aerobic respiration, anaerobic respiration, or fermentation. Choice **a** is incorrect: Microaerophiles require only a low concentration of oxygen. They get their energy from aerobic respiration. Choice **b** is incorrect: Obligate anaerobes grow only without oxygen. They are inhibited or killed in the presence of oxygen. They get their energy from anaerobic respiration or fermentation. Choice **d** is incorrect: Obligate aerobes grow only in the presence of oxygen. They get their energy from aerobic respiration.
2. **d.** The lipopolysaccharide (LPS) layer of the Gram-negative bacterial cell wall is released when the bacterial cell dies and becomes a poison referred to as an endotoxin. Endotoxins stimulate inflammation, which damages animal cell membranes, causing cell necrosis. Choice **a** is incorrect: Gram-positive cell walls pose no harm to humans. Choice **b** is incorrect: Exotoxins are released by living bacteria. They are proteins that are produced in the ribosomes. Choice **c** is incorrect: Bacterial capsules produce a slimy surface around the outside of the bacterial cell wall so that neutrophils cannot attach and phagocytize them.
3. **b.** The first name identifies the organism's genus. It is capitalized. The second name indicates the specific epithet or specific name (species). It starts with a lowercase letter. In the system of binomial nomenclature, Latin words ensure that the name is universally recognized across language barriers. Choice **a** is incorrect: Kingdom and phylum are the topmost taxonomic categories under domain and as such are among the broadest or most general taxa. Choices **c** and **d** are incorrect: The levels of taxonomic classification are domain, kingdom, phylum, class, order, family, genus, and species.
4. **d.** Protozoa are unicellular, heterotrophic, eukaryotic microorganisms belonging to the domain Eukarya in the kingdom Protista. Protozoa are typically motile and are known as the animal-like protists. Choice **a** is incorrect: Unicellular prokaryotes in the domain Archaea in the kingdom Archaeabacteria can perform more advanced protein synthesis than the Eubacteria and are often bacteria that can live in extreme conditions such as extreme alkalinity or acidity. Choice **b** is incorrect: Members of the Eukarya domain in the kingdom Plantae are multicellular autotrophs. They are the photosynthetic green plants. They produce a multicellular embryo inside an archegonium. Choice **c** is incorrect: The Eubacteria kingdom contains small, simple, single-celled prokaryotes. They have peptidoglycan (mucoprotein) in their cell walls. Most are decomposers, some are photosynthetic autotrophs, and some are parasitic and pathogenic.

5. a. Systemic molds are mainly respiratory. They are dimorphic, having two different growth forms. At higher temperatures, such as inside the body, they look like yeast and are primarily in a single-celled nonmycelial form. This nonmycelial yeastlike form causes lesions called granulomas, which serve to wall off and localize the organism. In immunosuppressed patients they can disseminate to other areas of the body and be life-threatening. Choice **b** is incorrect: Most molds are saprophytes, that live on dead matter. This includes some of the dermatophytes which cause nail infections. Choice **c** is incorrect: Dermatophytes infect the skin, hair, and nails, locations where keratin is produced. Dermatophyte infections are often referred to as tinea. Treatment is administered orally using griseofulvin, which is derived from the mold *Penicillium griseofulvum*. It binds to keratin precursor cells, conferring resistance to mature keratin cells. Choice **d** is incorrect: *Aspergillus* is the most common of the common nonpathogenic molds. It is a problem only for people who are allergic to it or if it infects peanuts, where it can contaminate them with a mycotoxin, called aflatoxin. Chronic aflatoxin exposure is potentially carcinogenic for the liver.

6. b. Endospores are produced mainly by the genera *Bacillus* and *Clostridium*. *Bacillus* are Gram-positive aerobic spore-forming bacteria. The rod-shaped cell produces one spore within the cell. *Clostridium* are Gram-positive anaerobic spore formers. The much smaller rod, which is sausage- or cigar-shaped, produces a tennis racket–shaped cell due to the endospore at one end. The function of endospores is survival, not reproduction as spores are in plants and fungi. Endospores enable bacteria to survive in harsh environments such as extreme heat or cold. Choice **a** is incorrect: *Rickettsia* and *Chlamydia* are both atypical bacteria. *Rickettsia* are coccobacillary, a cross between a rod and a sphere. Diseases caused by *Rickettsia* including typhus and Rocky Mountain spotted fever. *Chlamydia* can be coccilike or rodlike. They cause a number of important infections, including trachoma, psittacosis, lymphogranuloma venereum, and genitourinary infections. Both are obligate intracellular parasites, which must grow inside living cells. They cannot be grown in the lab. Choice **c** is incorrect: *Neisseria* and *Moraxella* are Gram-negative diplococci bacteria that have pili that enable them to attach to neutrophils, preventing phagocytosis, and to the genital tract, meninges, and respiratory tract. Choice **d** is incorrect: *Proteus* and *Pseudomonas* are genera that cause opportunistic Gram-negative infections such as urinary tract infections, wound infections, pneumonia, and septicemia.

7. a. There are lots of mitochondria in cardiac muscle cells because the heart must not become fatigued. Mitochondria are the powerhouses of the cell, manufacturing ATP to fuel cell activity. All muscle cells have more mitochondria than other cell types. Choice **b** is incorrect: While the midpiece of a sperm contains many mitochondria to provide metabolic fuel for sperm activity such as swimming and digesting the egg covering so that it can enter, the energy needs of a sperm do not approach those of a cardiac muscle cell. Choice **c** is incorrect: Keratinocytes are the most abundant skin cell type. They manufacture the protein keratin. The apical squamous epithelial cells are full of dead flat membranous sacs of keratin, which appear yellow. From the bottom of the epidermis, the keratinocytes sit on the basal membrane with connective tissue below. Choice **d** is incorrect: Osteogenic cells are actively mitotic cells found in the periosteum and endosteum. All originate from mesenchyme. Some osteogenic cells produce cells that differentiate into osteoblasts, which are the bone builders. Some stay bone stem cells to provide osteoblasts for the future. Others become osteocytes, mature bone cells, which secrete a matrix. While there are activities that require ATP, the needs are not as extensive as in muscle cells and particularly cardiac muscle cells.

8. c. The sensory or afferent division consists of the somatic and visceral sensory nerve fibers. It conducts impulses from receptors to the CNS. Choice **a** is incorrect: The motor or efferent division consists of the motor nerve fibers. It conducts impulses from the CNS to the effectors, the muscles and glands. There are two divisions of the motor division. Choice **b** is incorrect: The somatic division is a subdivision of the motor division of the peripheral nervous system. It provides the motor innervations for skeletal muscles. It is also called the voluntary nervous system. As part of the motor division it conducts impulses from the CNS to the skeletal muscles. Choice **d** is incorrect: The sympathetic nervous system is a subdivision of the autonomic nervous system. It is often referred to as the fight-or-flight division. It conducts impulses from the CNS to the cardiac muscles, smooth muscles, and glands.

9. a. Immunoglobulin M (IgM) can exist as a monomer or can link up with others to create a pentamer. When B-cells are activated and turn into plasma cells, IgM are the first antibodies released. They are particularly good at forming clumps of antigen, acting as a potent agglutinating agent. Choice **b** is incorrect: Immunoglobulin A (IgA) antibodies are secretory and found in mucous, sweat, saliva, urine, spinal fluid, and genital secretions. They prevent pathogen entry into the body. Choice **c** is incorrect: Immunoglobulin G (IgG) is the most abundant antibody. It crosses the placenta, giving passive natural immunity to the fetus. IgG are the main antibodies of the late primary and secondary response. IgM come first and then IgG take over. Choice **d** is incorrect: Immunoglobulin E (IgE) is the troublemaker antibody, involved in allergies and parasites. It works with basophils and mast cells to release histamine.

10. b. In the small intestine, brush border enzymes continue carbohydrate digestion. Lactase catalyzes reactions that break down lactose. Maltase catalyzes reactions that break down maltose. Sucrase catalyzes reactions that break down sucrose. Dextrinase catalyzes reactions that break down dextrins, and glucoamylase continues the breakdown of amylase and amylopectins. Choice **a** is incorrect: Proteases break down proteins. The pancreatic proteases include trypsin, carboxypeptidase, and chymotrypsin. Trypsinogen, the inactive form of trypsin, is produced in the pancreas. It is activated in the duodenum by enteropeptidase, a brush border protease. Choice **c** is incorrect: Pepsin catalyzes protein digestion in the stomach. Choice **d** is incorrect: In the small intestine, the brush border enzymes aminopeptidase, carboxypeptidase, and dipeptidase continue protein breakdown.

11. d. Secretin is not involved in body temperature regulation. It is one of two intestinal hormones that regulate the release of pancreatic juices. Choice **a** is incorrect: The hypothalamus is involved in controlling body temperature, maintaining H_2O balance, and in sleep-wake cycles in conjunction with the pineal gland. It is often referred to as the body's thermostat because it receives feedback from temperature receptors throughout the body. Choice **b** is incorrect: The blood aids in body temperature regulation. When it is cold, the blood flow is constricted to the extremities. This is particularly noticeable in fingers and toes and is done to keep the vital organs warm. Choice **c** is incorrect: The skin is involved in thermoregulation. The sweat glands are located under the skin. The inability to sweat impairs the body's cooling ability. The erector pili muscles under the skin surface can either relax to make the hair on the skin lie down so that heat is not trapped or contract to lift the hairs upright so that they insulate and trap heat.

12. d. The semicircular canals maintain dynamic equilibrium. Choice **a** is incorrect: The tympanic membrane or ear drum is connective tissue covered by skin externally and by mucosa internally. It is shaped like a flattened cone. The apex protrudes medially into the middle ear. It passes vibrations to the middle ear. Choice **b** is incorrect: The vestibule maintains static equilibrium. Choice **c** is incorrect: The cochlea is the portion of the ear where vibrations are transformed to nerve impulses

13. b. Antidiuretic hormone (ADH) decreases urine production. Choice **a** is incorrect: Prolactin stimulates milk production in females. Choice **c** is incorrect: Adrenocorticotropic hormone (ACTH) stimulates the release of the adrenal cortex hormones, aldosterone, cortisol, and testosterone. Choice **d** is incorrect: Follicle stimulating hormone (FSH) stimulates gamete production. It is also synergist with luteinizing hormone (LH) to help bring about the maturation of follicles, immature eggs in the female. In males it aids in sperm production.

14. c. Follicle-stimulating hormone (FSH) and luteinizing hormone (LH) stimulate the primordial follicle to grow into the primary follicle. Choice **a** is incorrect: After the primary follicle has developed, estrogen inhibits follicle-stimulating hormone (FSH) and luteinizing hormone (LH) to prevent other follicles from developing. It also contributes to further development of the primary follicle and the development of the granulosa as the secondary follicle is formed. Progesterone is released by the corpus luteum to maintain the pregnancy if fertilization occurs. Choice **b** is incorrect: GnRH (gonadotropin-releasing hormone) from the hypothalamus stimulates follicle-stimulating hormone (FSH) and luteinizing hormone (LH) release from the anterior pituitary. Choice **d** is incorrect: Oxytocin is produced in the hypothalamus, is released by the posterior pituitary gland, targets the uterus and breast, and stimulates uterine contractions and the milk letdown reflex. It is not involved in the ovarian cycle.

15. d. Shared ancestral or plesiomorphic characters are traits that existed in the ancestral species that are still seen in all of the descendant groups. Choice **a** is incorrect: Shared derived characters or synapomorphic characters are characteristics shared by two or more taxa that are found in their most recent common ancestor. Depending on how broad or narrow the taxon being looked at is, the same trait may be classified as plesiomorphic or synapomorphic. In a broad structured group, the trait may be derived, whereas in a narrower taxon it is an ancestral trait. Choice **b** is incorrect: Homoplasies are analogous biological traits or functions that are similar in two groups of organisms, but were not inherited from a common ancestor. Convergent evolution has occurred, and the trait or function is an environmental adaptation that both species converged upon despite having different heredity. Choice **c** is incorrect: Homologies are structurally or anatomically similar structures in two or more species that originated from a common ancestor. They do not necessarily share the same function.

16. a. Pleiotropy is when a single gene affects a number of expressed traits. Choice **b** is incorrect: Epistasis is when one or more genes inhibit the expression of another gene. The inhibiting gene and the affected gene are on different loci on the genome, although they may be tightly linked. Choice **c** is incorrect: Incomplete dominance is a heterozygous state in which both alleles at a particular location on a gene are partially expressed or blended. This often results in an intermediate phenotype, such as pink flowers from crossing red and white flowers. Choice **d** is incorrect: Polygenic inheritance is when many genes are involved. Phenotypically expressed traits are caused by the relationships and interactions between a number of genes. Skin color, height, and body shape are all the result of multiple genes interacting.

17. c. Type AB blood has both the A and B antigens. It has neither A nor B antibodies. This is the universal recipient. Type AB people can receive blood from anybody because there are no antibodies to cause clumping. They cannot donate to type A, because the B antigen will clump with the B antibody. They cannot donate to type B, because the A antigen will clump with the A antibody. They cannot donate to type O, because the A and B antigens will clump with the A and B antibodies in type O blood. The only type they can donate to is their own. Choice **a** is incorrect: Type A blood has the A antigen on the red blood cell surface and the type B antibody in the plasma. Like all blood types, it has the antibodies for the antigen opposite to those on the surface of the RBC. Type A cannot receive type B or type AB blood, because the B antibody will bind to and agglutinate when exposed to the B antigen on the surface of the RBC on type B and type AB blood. Type A can receive blood only from another type A or from the universal donor, type O, which has no antigens. Choice **b** is incorrect: Type O blood has neither the A nor the B antigen. It has both the A and B antibodies. This is the universal donor. Type O people can give to any other blood type because there are no antigens. It is not the universal recipient because the A and B antibodies will bind to and form a clump with the A antigen found on the surface of the RBC in type A blood, the B antigen on the RBC in type B blood, and both the A and B antigens on the RBC in type AB blood. Type O can receive blood only from another type O. Choice **d** is incorrect: Type B blood has the B antigen on the surface of the RBC and the A antibody in the blood plasma. It cannot receive blood from either type A or type AB, because the A antibody will clump with the B antigen. It can receive blood only from another type B or from the universal donor, type O, which has no antigens.

18. d. Lysosomes are a type of membrane-bound vesicle that are referred to as a suicide sac or destruction vacuole. They contain digestive enzymes to break down macromolecules. They are synthesized by the endoplasmic reticulum and the Golgi complex and can break down nucleic acids, proteins, and polysaccharides. They take in and break down older nonfunctioning or sick cells and organelles so that the products can be reused to make new organelles. Choice **a** is incorrect: The Golgi complex is the packaging center for storage, distribution, and excretion. These organelles are responsible for sorting proteins and lipids received from the RER and the SER. They also modify certain proteins and glycoproteins and fold polypeptides to create proteins. These molecules are sorted and packaged into vacuoles and vesicles for storage, transport to other parts of the cell, or for secretion. Choice **b** is incorrect: Peroxisomes are a type of membrane-bound vesicle that contain enzymes that catalyze a variety of metabolic reactions. They use oxygen to detoxify harmful substances such as alcohol and hydrogen peroxide. Choice **c** is incorrect: Vacuoles are a type of vesicle that contains mostly water. Vacuoles are large and there is only one or a few in a cell. Amoebas have a food vacuole that contains any food item that the amoeba has recently consumed. Plant cells have a central vacuole that contains water and substances such as amino acids, sugars, and other compounds that the plant needs. It also provides turgor pressure to support the plant cell, providing it with rigidity and structure.

19. b. The light-independent (dark) reactions of photosynthesis occur in the stroma where photosynthetic enzymes are stored. The stroma, a fluid-filled region inside the inner membrane, contains the enzymes for the light-independent reactions. Infolding of this inner membrane forms the stacks of disks of the thylakoids. Choice **a** is incorrect: The role of chlorophyll is to absorb light energy. Chloroplasts have photoreceptors, which act like antennae to capture light energy. Choice **c** is incorrect: The light-dependent reactions of photosynthesis take place in the thylakoids where chlorophyll and other photosynthetic pigments are stored. The thylakoid membrane encloses the fluid-filled thylakoid interior space, which contains chlorophyll and other photosynthetic pigments as well as electron transport chains. The light-dependent reactions of photosynthesis occur in the thylakoid membrane. Choice **d** is incorrect: Photosystems are complexes of all of the pigmented molecules formed by chlorophyll molecules. They absorb the energy from sunlight and work in the opposite direction from electron transport chains systems. An electron starts with low energy and gains more as it travels through the photosystem. At the final acceptor molecule, the electron has a lot of energy.

20. c. In telophase, the daughter chromosomes have reached the centrosomes at the poles of the cell. Then the nuclear membranes for the two new cells begin to form. The nucleoli reappear. The steps of prophase are undone. The spindles disintegrate and the single chromosomes begin to unwind, elongate, and return to chromatin. Microscopically it is difficult to view the onset of telophase, so its starting point is often marked by the onset of cytokinesis. Choice **a** is incorrect: When metaphase begins, the nuclear membrane is gone, the centrioles are at the poles of the cell, some spindle fibers are connected to the centromeres, and the sister chromatids line up along the cell equator, also referred to as the metaphase plate. Choice **b** is incorrect: In prophase, the chromatin condenses to form the visible, densely packed chromosome. Choice **d** is incorrect: As anaphase begins, the centromeres holding the sister chromatids together divide. The daughter chromosomes are composed of a centromere and a single chromatid. The spindle fibers lengthen and the kinetochore fibers shorten. These two forces combine to push (spindle fibers) and pull (kinetochore spindle fibers) the daughter chromosomes to the opposite poles of the cell where the centrosomes are located.

21. d. As anaphase begins, the centromeres holding the sister chromatids together divide. The daughter chromosomes are composed of a centromere and a single chromatid. The spindle fibers lengthen and the kinetochore fibers shorten. These two forces combine to push (spindle fibers) and pull (kinetochore spindle fibers) the daughter chromosomes to the opposite poles of the cell where the centrosomes are located. Choice **a** is incorrect: When metaphase begins, the nuclear membrane is gone, the centrioles are at the poles of the cell, some spindle fibers are connected to the centromeres, and the sister chromatids line up along the cell equator, also referred to as the metaphase plate. Choice **b** is incorrect: In prophase, the chromatin condenses to form the visible, densely packed chromosome. Choice **c** is incorrect: In telophase, the daughter chromosomes have reached the centrosomes at the poles of the cell. Then the nuclear membranes for the two new cells begin to form. The nucleoli reappear. The steps of prophase are undone. The spindles disintegrate and the single chromosomes begin to unwind, elongate, and return to chromatin. Microscopically it is difficult to view the onset of telophase, so its starting point is often marked by the onset of cytokinesis.

22. b. In prophase, the chromatin condenses to form the visible, densely packed chromosome. Choice **a** is incorrect: When metaphase begins, the nuclear membrane is gone, the centrioles are at the poles of the cell, some spindle fibers are connected to the centromeres, and the sister chromatids line up along the cell equator, also referred to as the metaphase plate. Choice **c** is incorrect: In telophase, the daughter chromosomes have reached the centrosomes at the poles of the cell. Then the nuclear membranes for the two new cells begin to form. The nucleoli reappear. The steps of prophase are undone. The spindles disintegrate and the single chromosomes begin to unwind, elongate, and return to chromatin. Microscopically it is difficult to view the onset of telophase, so its starting point is often marked by the onset of cytokinesis. Choice **d** is incorrect: As anaphase begins, the centromeres holding the sister chromatids together divide. The daughter chromosomes are composed of a centromere and a single chromatid. The spindle fibers lengthen and the kinetochore fibers shorten. These two forces combine to push (spindle fibers) and pull (kinetochore spindle fibers) the daughter chromosomes to the opposite poles of the cell where the centrosomes are located.

23. a. When metaphase begins, the nuclear membrane is gone, the centrioles are at the poles of the cell, some spindle fibers are connected to the centromeres, and the sister chromatids line up along the cell equator, also referred to as the metaphase plate. Choice **b** is incorrect: In prophase, the chromatin condenses to form the visible, densely packed chromosome. Choice **c** is incorrect: In telophase, the daughter chromosomes have reached the centrosomes at the poles of the cell. Then the nuclear membranes for the two new cells begin to form. The nucleoli reappear. The steps of prophase are undone. The spindles disintegrate and the single chromosomes begin to unwind, elongate, and return to chromatin. Microscopically it is difficult to view the onset of telophase, so its starting point is often marked by the onset of cytokinesis. Choice **d** is incorrect: As anaphase begins, the centromeres holding the sister chromatids together divide. The daughter chromosomes are composed of a centromere and a single chromatid. The spindle fibers lengthen and the kinetochore fibers shorten. These two forces combine to push (spindle fibers) and pull (kinetochore spindle fibers) the daughter chromosomes to the opposite poles of the cell where the centrosomes are located.

24. d. Synapsis is the process by which homologous chromosomes line up to form a tetrad in prophase I of meiosis. Choice **a** is incorrect: Apoptosis is programmed cell death. Choice **b** is incorrect: Contact inhibition is the process that occurs when cells have filled an area and are encountering other like cells all around them so the cells are signaled to cease cell division. A mitotic error occurs with cancer cells, in which the contact inhibition mechanism is not triggered. Choice **c** is incorrect: Chiasmata are points along the bivalents where they touch one another and gene exchange takes place during the time when the homologous chromosomes are paired up and tightly bound by the synaptonemal complex.

25. b. Aneuploidy is $2N \pm 1$. There is a chromosome number that is not a multiple of the haploid number for the species. Either there is only one copy of a particular chromosome or there are three copies of that particular chromosome. Monosomy and trisomy are the two specific aneuploidy conditions. Choice **a** is incorrect: Translocation is when DNA from one chromosome attaches to a nonhomologous chromosome. Part of a chromosome breaks off and then reattaches to a different chromosome. Choice **c** is incorrect: Trisomy is $2N + 1$. There are three copies of a particular chromosome rather than the usual two. It is one of the two specific types of aneuploidy. Choice **d** is incorrect: Monosomy is $2N - 1$. There is only one copy of a certain chromosome rather than the usual two. It is one of the two specific types of aneuploidy.

CHAPTER 7

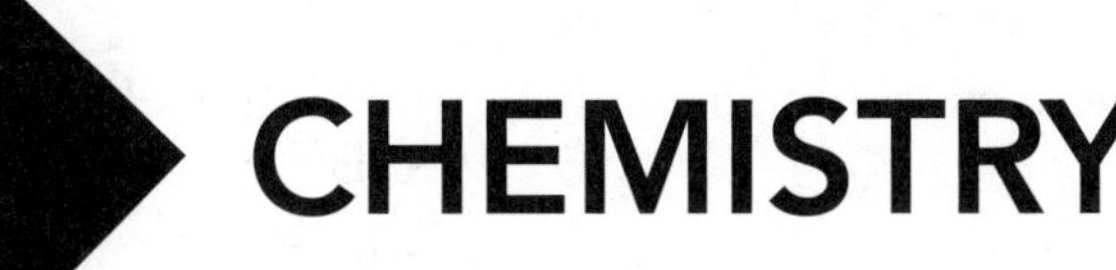

CHEMISTRY

The Chemistry section of the PCAT test consists of 48 questions. About 60% of the questions will be on general chemistry concepts and around 40% on organic chemistry concepts. You will not be allowed to use a calculator, nor will you be provided with a copy of the Periodic Table of the Elements.

The roots of chemistry lie in the ancient world. Early civilizations tried to classify the substances they found around them, often using philosophy or religion to explain observed phenomena. The Greeks divided their material world into the four classical elements of earth, water, air, and fire. (Aristotle posited a fifth element, aether, which was neither hot, cold, wet, nor dry.) Early Arab, Persian, and later European alchemists expanded our empirical knowledge of matter and its interactions. Today, the study of chemistry continues this exploration of matter and its interactions, and provides the bridge between the physicist's study of subatomic particles and the biologist's study of larger, complex organic systems.

Properties of Matter

Matter is commonly defined as anything that has mass and occupies space. Matter is comprised of smaller units called molecules, which themselves are comprised of atoms—the elements found in the Periodic Table. Chemistry's primary focus is to understand the behavior of these atoms and molecules. Chemical substances are described by properties that fall into two categories:

1. **Physical properties**—those properties that can be determined by observation (qualitative properties) or measurement (quantitative properties) without altering the chemical identity of the substance. Color, taste, density, boiling point, freezing point, and solubility are all examples of physical properties. Saying that something is colored red would be a qualitative observation; defining the precise shade of red (via some standardized measuring technique) would be a quantitative observation.
2. **Chemical properties**—those properties of a substance that become evident when the substance undergoes (or fails to undergo) a chemical reaction. Flammability, heat of combustion, and ionization energy are examples of chemical properties. We can describe how wood appears to our eyes, and we can weigh it to determine the mass, but these are both physical properties; the fact that wood is (generally) flammable is a chemical property.

Changes in chemical substances can be physical (e.g., cutting, freezing, melting, hammering into a different shape, and boiling) or chemical (e.g., oxidation, being burnt, etc.). Physical changes do not alter the composition of a substance. A gold nugget that is hammered into gold foil is still gold. Chemical changes (which occur during chemical reactions) do change the composition of a substance; they create another unique substance. When water freezes (physical change), the ice created remains H_2O. However, when iron rusts (oxidizes; chemical change) the resulting iron oxide is a different substance, distinct from the original material.

States of Matter

Chemical substances can exist in any of four states, called phases, depending on a number of factors. These factors include the chemical nature of the substance, the temperature of the substance, and pressure applied to the substance. The phases are:

- **Solid.** Intermolecular forces (electronic interactions between neighboring, but separate atoms or molecules) keep the matter in a fixed volume and shape (e.g., ice).
- **Liquid.** Intermolecular forces keep the matter in a fixed volume, but the substance will flow to take the shape of its container (e.g., water).
- **Gas.** Intermolecular forces have limited effect in a gas and the substance will expand to fill its container (e.g., steam). The minimal intermolecular forces give gases unique properties that will be discussed later.
- **Plasma.** High temperatures can cause gas molecules to ionize. This creates a distinct fourth state of matter that is not common under normal conditions on Earth, and is therefore of little interest to most chemists.

While some properties of the substance change with changes in state, the composition of the substance does not change unless some type of chemical reaction was the cause of the change. Note the terms associated with phase changes depicted in the following diagram. The inverse effects of temperature and pressure on the state of a substance can be visually depicted in the form of a graph called a phase diagram.

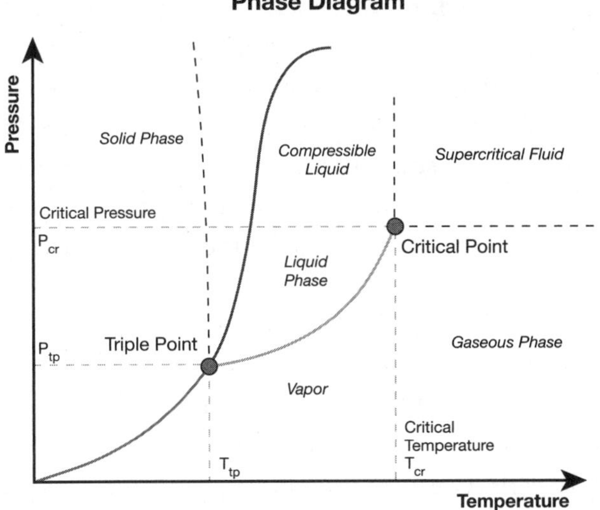

A unique point on the graph exists called the triple point; the placement is different for each substance. The triple point is where the combination of temperature and pressure allows three phases (solid, liquid, and gas) of a substance to simultaneously coexist in thermodynamic equilibrium. It is a phenomenon not commonly seen in everyday life, as it requires exacting temperatures and pressures that are usually not close to standard conditions.

Classification of Matter

Developments in the late 1700s and early 1800s greatly influenced our modern classification of matter. During the late 1700s, Antoine Lavoisier, often considered the father of modern chemistry, performed some of the first quantitative chemical experiments. Quantitative experiments entail keeping careful track of the relative masses that disappear of form during the course of a process. By weighing reactants and products, Lavoisier found that for a given reaction, the total mass of the reactants equaled the total mass of the products. He published this principle, the **law of conservation of mass**, in 1789. Lavoisier went on to define an **element** as a substance that cannot be decomposed by chemical means. He proposed that all **compounds** were formed from the combination of two or more elements. Two other laws were proposed shortly thereafter:

1. **The law of definite proportions.** Joseph Proust determined that a given compound always contains the same elements in the same mass percentages (aka Proust's Law). The corollary, the **law of constant composition**, states that a given chemical compound always has the same elemental composition. In other words, water is always H_2O, no matter the source of the water.
2. **The law of multiple proportions.** John Dalton determined that when elements combine, they combine in a ratio of small whole numbers, and if two elements form more than one compound, the ratios of the mass of the second element relative to the mass of the first element will be small whole numbers. In other words, oxygen and hydrogen may combine in different, but always small, whole number proportions (e.g., water, H_2O; hydrogen peroxide, H_2O_2). This law prohibits the existence of a molecule such as $HO_{\frac{1}{2}}$. Oxygen is an atom, and insofar as chemical reactions are concerned, cannot split into "half of an oxygen."

These laws form the basis of a concept called **stoicheometry** that will be covered later.

Combinations of substances that vary in composition are called **mixtures**. Salt and sand can be mixed in any proportion and, while the mix may be hard to separate, close inspection will still reveal the original substances to be chemically unchanged. The two laws have not been violated, because the mixtures are not single compounds; they are simply physical mixtures. Such mixtures are described as being **heterogeneous**. Solutions created by dissolving solutes in solvents (salt water, for instance) are examples of **homogeneous** mixtures as long as everything is fully dissolved. Slurries of undissolved compound make the solution heterogeneous; if there are no visible undissolved solids, it is considered homogeneous. These mixtures can be separated into their components without a chemical reaction simply by using physical means. Salt water, for example, can be heated until all the water has boiled away, leaving behind the (previously dissolved) salt.

Classification of substances can be summarized as follows:

Pure Substances

- **elements**—substances that cannot be further decomposed into simpler components via chemical means. A list of known elements can be found in the Periodic Table of the Elements.
- **molecules, also sometimes called compounds**—combinations of two or more elements that chemically combine in definite proportions

Mixtures—combinations of two or more distinct substances that physically mix, but do not form chemical bonds or chemically react. They retain their chemical identities.

- **homogeneous mixtures**—mixtures of two or more substances that yield no discernible phase boundaries
  - **solution**—mixture of a solute in a solvent (including gas mixtures)
    - **alloy**—metals that are mixed together while in their liquid form, then allowed to cool
    - **amalgam**—mixture of mercury with another metal
- **heterogeneous mixtures**—mixtures of two or more substances that show distinct phase boundaries
  - **colloids**—visually homogeneous mixtures in which the particles are too small to settle, but simultaneously too large to be considered dissolved
    - **emulsions**—Liquid-in-liquid mixtures (e.g., mayonnaise)
  - **dispersions**—visually heterogeneous mixtures
    - **suspensions**—Solid-in-liquid dispersions where the particles are large enough that they will eventually settle

Atomic Theory

While early Greek philosophers postulated that all matter was comprised of tiny particles (atoms), key tenets of modern atomic theory weren't formalized and put on a solid foundation until the eighteenth century. Building on the understanding of compounds versus mixtures, John Dalton articulated the basis for our modern atomic theory in 1803. His theory is summarized in five points:

1. Elements are composed of particles called atoms that cannot be created, destroyed, or altered by chemical means.
2. All atoms of a given element are identical, possessing identical properties.
3. Atoms of one element are different from the atoms of any other element, and these different atoms can be distinguished by their atomic weights.
4. Atoms of one element can combine with the atoms of other elements to form chemical compounds, and these compounds always have the same, fixed atomic composition.
5. Chemical reactions merely involve the rearranging of atom combinations and do not create or destroy atoms.

Nuclear Theory of the Atom

Observations of chemists and physicists during the 1800s revealed that matter could exhibit electrical and radioactive properties. These observations hinted at the existence of both subatomic particles and subatomic forces. In 1897, the physicist J.J. Thomson observed rays emitted by negative electrodes (cathodes) in a vacuum tube, also called a cathode ray tube. By measuring the deflection of these rays under varying applied electric and magnetic fields, he determined that the rays were composed of negatively charged particles approximately 1,840 times lighter than the mass of hydrogen. These rays behaved the same regardless of the cathode material. These negatively charged particles were called electrons. Subsequent oil-drop experiments by Robert Millikan (published in 1911) led Millikan to determine the elementary charge of a single electron (a value we now denote as *e*): 1.602×10^{-19} coulombs.

If atoms are neutrally charged, then the negative particles (the electrons) must be offset by an equal number of positively charged particles (which are called protons). In 1896, physicist Henri Becquerel discovered naturally occurring radioactive substances. Ernest Rutherford, considered the father of nuclear physics, built on this discovery of radioactivity. Rutherford observed what he termed *alpha rays* being emitted during the natural decay of uranium; the uranium slowly transformed itself into the element thorium. He also witnessed alpha rays being emitted during the decay of radium to radon gas.

He determined that these alpha rays behaved like doubly-charged helium ions (He^{2+}). By targeting these alpha particles at gold foil (the Geiger-Marsden experiment), the expectation was that these large, heavy alpha particles would go right through the gold with little resistance, due to the low mass of the electrons in the target and the very heavy alpha particles. Instead, it was observed that several of the alpha particles were deflected at large angles; some flew back almost 180°, toward the alpha particle source. Rutherford determined that the only possible explanation was that the target atoms contained a small but incredibly dense positively charged nucleus surrounded by a vastly larger, seemingly empty, cloud of negatively charged electrons. This theory, published in 1911, constitutes the Rutherford model, or planetary model, of the atom. Rutherford later theorized that neutrally charged particles must be required in the atomic nuclei to compensate for the repelling force that would exist between positively charged particles. These neutral particles clumped together with the protons at the atom's nucleus were called neutrons, and are also quite heavy compared to electrons.

Subatomic Particles

The subatomic particles that form an atom are summarized in the following paragraphs. Chemical reactions cannot alter these particles; however, nuclear reactions, or radioactive decay, can alter these particles (to be discussed later).

Protons

The positively charged subatomic particles in the atomic nucleus are called protons. Protons have a +1 elementary charge and a mass of approximately one atomic mass unit (see "Atomic Mass Units" sidebar). While the proton has an equal, but opposite, charge from an electron, the proton has 1,836 times more mass. An element's **atomic number (Z)** is defined as the number of protons in each atom of the element. Each element has a unique atomic number, as shown in the Periodic Table of the Elements (discussed later).

The proton is essentially a positive hydrogen ion (one proton, no neutrons, and no electrons: H^+). When this species exists in water, it reacts with the water molecule to become H_3O^+, sometimes written simply as $H^+(aq)$, and is called a hydronium ion. We'll discuss this more when we review acid-base reactions. To gain a sense of proportion, the diameter of the hydrogen atom is 145,000 times larger than the hydrogen ion (proton), as the nucleus (just a proton, in this case) is very small compared to the size of the electron cloud that normally surrounds the nucleus.

Electrons

Electrons have a –1 elementary charge, exactly opposite that of a proton, and a mass of approximately $\frac{1}{1,836}$ atomic mass units. Electrons are believed to be elementary particles because they have no known components. In a neutral atom, the atomic number (Z) will indicate the total number of electrons since the number of protons must equal the number of electrons. While the Rutherford atomic model says nothing about the orbits and energy levels that the electrons occupy, quantum mechanics addresses these issues (to be discussed later). Without going further at this time, know that the electrons in the outermost orbit of an atom are called **valence electrons.** The ease with which an atom attracts or gives up valence electrons greatly determines atomic reactivity. The process of losing or adding electrons is called **ionization**, and the resulting atom is called an **ion.** An atom that loses an electron has a net positive charge and is called a **cation**. Conversely, an atom that gains an electron has a net negative charge and is called an **anion.**

Neutrons

In 1932, James Chadwick confirmed the existence of the neutrally charged subatomic particles that Rutherford had expected. These neutrons have a mass slightly greater than a proton. Neutrons can decay into protons in a process known as beta decay. While the number of protons in an atom of an element does not vary, the number of neutrons in an atom of an element can vary. The quantity of neutrons in an atom, known as the **neutron number**, defines the **isotope** of an element.

Mass Number and Isotopes

Protons and neutrons are collectively known as nucleons. The **mass number (A)**, also called the nucleon number, is the total number of protons and neutrons in an atom. The following formulas summarize this relationship, stating the same thing in two ways:

Mass number = Total protons + Total neutrons

Mass number = Atomic number + Neutron number

Isotopes are identified by their mass number. To specify a particular isotope, the mass number is appended after the element name, or the mass number is written over the atomic number before the element symbol as in ${}^{M}_{Z}X$ for a given element X. (The symbols for all the elements appear in the Periodic Table of the Elements that will be discussed later.) Since the atomic number is always the same for a given element, the atomic number may be omitted. Carbon-12, ${}^{12}_{6}C$, and ${}^{12}C$ all refer to the most common isotope of carbon that has six protons and six neutrons. A common radioisotope of carbon has eight neutrons; this radioactive isotope is called carbon-14 (${}^{14}C$). Carbon-14 goes through beta decay to become nitrogen-14 and can be formed from the action of gamma rays in the atmosphere. The archaeological analysis technique called radiocarbon dating relies on the trace occurrence of carbon-14 in organic materials. The chemical properties of most isotopes of an element differ negligibly (as chemical behavior is largely dependent on electrons); however, the nuclear stability of an element's isotopes can vary significantly.

Atomic Mass—Atomic Weight

Naturally occurring elements are a mix of one or more naturally occurring isotopes, both stable and unstable (radioactive). Radioactive isotopes may persist in natural samples either because they have long decay periods (long half-lives) or because they may get created through absorption of cosmic rays that reach the earth (as in the case of carbon-14 mentioned previously). Because the protons and neutrons in the nucleus of an atom make up 99.9% of the mass of an atom, differences in the neutron number among isotopes of an element greatly affect the naturally observed atomic weight of an element. To address this issue, chemists define two specific terms, atomic mass and relative atomic mass (also called standard atomic weight).

The **atomic mass** (m_a) is defined as the mass of an atom (one isotope of an element) relative to the mass of a carbon-12 atom and is expressed in atomic mass units (amu, or more correctly, just u—see "Atomic Mass Units" sidebar). One **atomic mass unit (amu)** is defined as one-twelfth of the mass of an unbound carbon-12 atom. Since carbon-12 has six protons and six neutrons plus an essentially negligible (in terms of mass) 12 electrons, the atomic mass unit represents a mass somewhere between the mass of a proton and the mass of a neutron. Atomic mass is a physical constant for a given atom; however, samples of naturally occurring elements rarely have such isotopic purity.

The **relative atomic mass** (A_r) is an average of the atomic masses of the isotopes of an element as the element is observed in nature (the average of the naturally occurring isotopes). The relative atomic mass, or average atomic mass, is not a physical constant, but rather an accepted standard. Standard samples of elements are analyzed to determine the **natural abundance** (relative abundance) of the isotopes of elements. The International Union of Pure and Applied Chemistry (IUPAC) publishes the accepted sample averages and determines the generally accepted relative atomic mass for each element. The relative atomic mass for each element is listed in the Periodic Table of the Elements.

For example, hydrogen has three naturally occurring isotopes: protium (^1H), deuterium (^2H), and tritium (^3H). The relative atomic mass calculation requires the atomic mass and relative (natural) abundance of each isotope:

ISOTOPE	SYMBOL	ATOMIC MASS	ABUNDANCE
protium	^1H	1.0078 u	99.984%
deuterium	^2H	2.0141 u	1.54×10^{-2}%
tritium	^3H	3.016 u	1.00×10^{-15}%

$$\text{Relative atomic mass} = (1.0078\ \text{u} \times 0.99984) + (2.0141\ \text{u} \times 0.000154) + (3.016\ \text{u} \times 0.000000)$$
$$= 1.007949\ \text{u}$$

ATOMIC MASS UNITS

When John Dalton proposed a means of comparing atomic masses (Dalton used the term *weight*) in 1803, hydrogen was the central basis for comparison. Later the basis was changed to one-sixteenth the weight of oxygen, but the discovery of oxygen isotopes in 1929 resulted in atomic mass units (amu) being defined two ways. Physicists defined the amu (physical scale) as one-sixteenth the mass of an atom of oxygen-16. Chemists defined the amu (chemical scale) as one-sixteenth the mass of naturally occurring oxygen atoms, a definition more analogous to the current definition of average atomic mass. In 1961, to eliminate confusion, a common definition, the **unified atomic mass unit (u)**, was adopted based on one-twelfth the mass of carbon-12. However, a gradual movement has pressed to replace the use of the unified atomic mass unit with a unit called the **dalton (Da)** in honor of the concept's founder. The dalton has been officially recognized, but both the unified atomic mass unit and the dalton are in use today, with the dalton unit seeing more use in biochemistry. In fact, many texts still refer to the term atomic mass unit (amu).

Weight for the Masses

The relative atomic mass has been known historically as the **atomic weight** since the concept's inception in 1808. As modern science students learn, weight is the result of gravitational forces acting on a mass. Weight is not constant. Mass, however, is an inertial property of matter that factors out the gravitational effects. A given mass on Earth has the same mass on the moon. For scientific rigor, the historical terms *atomic weight* and *molecular weight* are now called *relative* (or *average*) *atomic mass* (A_r) and *relative molecular mass* (M_r), respectively. In practice, the term standard atomic weight is still used today, but the meaning is the same as average atomic mass.

Detailed Atomic Structure

The following section examines the structure of the atom.

Wave-Particle Duality

Aristotle hypothesized that light is a wave disturbance in air. Democritus hypothesized that light is in fact a type of solar atom particle. Isaac Newton determined that only particles could explain the behavior of light. Contemporaneously, Christian Huygens's wave equations for light explained phenomena that Newton's particle theory could not explain. The particle-versus-wave debate raged. During the 1860s, while studying electricity and magnetism, James Clerk Maxwell determined that visible light, ultraviolet (UV) light, and infrared (IR) light were all electromagnetic (EM) waves of differing frequencies, all traveling at the speed of light. The wave theory of electromagnetic radiation relates the **transverse wave velocity** (υ) to the **frequency** (f) of an EM wave (usually expressed in cycles per second [Hz]) and the wavelength (λ—lambda) of the EM wave (usually expressed in nanometers [nm]):

$$\upsilon = f\lambda \rightarrow \quad \text{In a vacuum this becomes} \rightarrow c = f\lambda$$

In a vacuum EM waves travel at the speed of light, c, or 2.998×10^8 m/sec. In other media, waves travel more slowly, but their frequencies remain constant. This is an important point. High-energy radiation (low wavelength, high frequency) can travel at different speeds up to and including the speed of light in a vacuum; it is the material that determines the extent to which the radiation is slowed.

While the wave theory of EM radiation explained some phenomena, it failed to explain other important phenomena. Applying wave theory to EM radiation from heated objects, so-called black-body radiation (an unfortunate choice of name, as the body being heated does not have to be colored black), resulted in a breakdown of the theory when the mathematics were applied to short wavelengths. This shortcoming became known as the ultraviolet catastrophe. Around 1900, the physicist Max Planck, while studying the radiation emitted from heated objects, found that the energy of emissions depended on the frequency of the oscillator and was not continuous. Rather, the energy was released in discrete bundles that he called **quanta**. The energy increment is known as **Planck's constant**, h, and has a value of 6.626×10^{-34} J · s.

In 1905, Albert Einstein applied Planck's quantum concept to explain the photoelectric effect, another phenomenon that the wave theory of EM radiation had failed to explain. The photoelectric effect refers to the emission of electrons from the surface of materials exposed to short wavelengths of EM radiation. Wave theory indicated that the energy of the emitted electrons should be a continuum proportional to the intensity of the EM radiation absorbed by a material. In fact, the energy of the emitted electrons depended on the frequency of the EM radiation, and *not* the intensity. Einstein saw the parallel with Planck's explanation of energy emissions from black bodies. Einstein theorized that the EM radiation (light) existed as discrete wave packets or light quanta, what we call **photons**, rather than as a continuous wave. The energy (E) in each quanta of light could be equated to the frequency (f) using Planck's constant (h). The resulting equation is known as the **Planck-Einstein equation**:

$E = hf \rightarrow$ Substituting for f using $c = f\lambda$ this becomes $\rightarrow E = \frac{hc}{\lambda}$

A photon can be symbolized as hf. Note that many texts now use ν for frequency, in which case the photon symbol would be $h\nu$.

Atomic Emission and Absorption Spectra

During the mid-1800s several scientists investigated the visible spectrum emissions and absorptions of elements. Robert Bunsen developed a gas burner that could be used to heat elements; this allowed the production of color spectra that were characteristic to each element. Another technique used glass tubes of elemental gases that were subjected to electric discharge, which again produced color spectra. These spectra were found to be unique to each element, a concept that underpins modern analytical spectroscopy. Gustav Kirchhoff developed three laws of spectroscopy:

1. A hot solid object or a hot, dense gas produces a continuous spectrum.
2. A hot, low-density gas produces spectral lines at discrete wavelengths that depend on the energy levels of the atoms in the gas (**atomic emission-line spectrum**).
3. A hot solid object viewed through a cool, low-density gas produces light with a nearly continuous spectrum that has gaps at discrete wavelengths depending on the energy levels of the atoms in the gas (known as an **atomic absorption-line spectrum**).

Hydrogen gas had been found to produce four distinct visible-spectrum emission lines, now known as the Balmer series of lines. In 1885 Johann Balmer developed a mathematical formula that related these emission wavelengths using integers. In 1888 Johannes Rydberg generalized and expanded the Balmer formula to relate the emission-line spectra to other atoms, specifically the alkali metals. Rydberg used the inverse of the wavelength, the **wavenumber** ($\frac{1}{\lambda}$), and an empirical constant, now known as the **Rydberg constant, *R***, to produce what we know as the **Rydberg formula**. Applying the formula to hydrogen yields this simplification where wavenumber ($\frac{1}{\lambda}$) relates to integers n_f, and n_i where $n_f < n_i$ (for emissions):

$$\frac{1}{\lambda} = R_\infty\left(\frac{1}{n_f^2} - \frac{1}{n_i^2}\right)$$

R_∞ represents the Rydberg constant where the mass of the atomic nucleus is considered infinite compared to the mass of the electron, an assumption that approximates the simple, single-electron conditions for hydrogen. Rydberg's formula not only related the known visible emission lines for hydrogen (Balmer series [$nf = 2$]) but also predicted the existence of nonvisible emission lines that were subsequently discovered (Lyman UV series [$n_f = 1$], Paschen IR series [$n_f = 3$], etc.). This validated the theory because it allowed for predictions that were later found experimentally to be correct.

Bohr Model of the Atom

In 1913 Niels Bohr published his model of atomic structure. Building on the Rutherford atom, Bohr applied Planck's quantum theory to classical mechanics and theorized that electrons orbit the nucleus in discrete orbits. In classical mechanics, an electron mass (m) orbiting a nucleus with constant angular momentum (L) could take on different speeds (ν) over a range of radii (r) as described by the formula $L = m_e\nu r$. Bohr asserted that an electron could orbit a nucleus without emitting radiation or losing energy, but the orbit would be quantized, limited to integral multiples of $\frac{h}{2\pi}$ where h is Planck's constant. The quantized angular momentum can be written as:

$$L = m_e v_n r_n = n\frac{h}{2\pi} = n\hbar$$

where $n = 1, 2, 3, \ldots$; it is called the **principal quantum number**. The minimum radius where $n = 1$ is known as the **Bohr radius.** Because many quantum equations involve $\frac{h}{2\pi}$, this constant is defined as the **reduced Planck constant,** $\hbar$, sometimes called "h bar."

Bohr derived the energy of the electron orbitals based on photon energies given by the Planck-Einstein equation. The assumption that electrons release energy in the form of photons when they drop from a higher orbital to a lower orbital allows us to derive the following equation:

$$E_{photon} = \Delta E_{atom} = E_{initial} - E_{final} = hc\frac{1}{\lambda}$$

Substituting the Rydberg formula into this equation allows us to derive the photon energy released when an electron moves from a high-energy orbital n_i to a lower energy orbital n_f:

$$E_{initial} - E_{final} = hcR_H\left(\frac{1}{n_f^2} - \frac{1}{n_i^2}\right) = -hcR_H\left(\frac{1}{n_i^2} - \frac{1}{n_f^2}\right)$$

Taking the Rydberg constant for hydrogen (R_H in m^{-1}), the Planck constant ($h = 6.626 \times 10^{-34}$J · s), and the speed of light ($c = 2.998 \times 10^8$ m/s), Bohr determined that hcR_H equaled 2.179×10^{-18}J · s. Thus Bohr was able to express the electron orbital energy levels as:

$$E_n = -hcR_H\left(\frac{1}{n^2}\right) = -2.179 \times 10^{-18} J\left(\frac{1}{n^2}\right)$$

When an electron moves from a higher orbital n_i to a lower orbital n_f, energy is conserved and the energy drop within the atom equals the energy of an emitted photon. Emissions are exothermic; the ΔE for the atom is negative and the photon energy is positive. Conversely, absorptions are endothermic; the ΔE for the atom is positive and equal to the energy of the absorbed photon. The two ΔE equations just presented were in terms of photon energy; the sign is reversed from the perspective of the atomic energy.

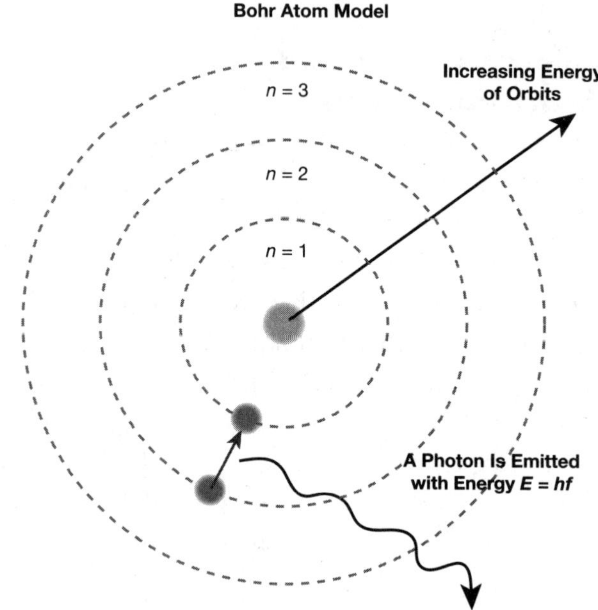

Bohr's model provided a theoretical framework that explained the observed emission-line spectra for hydrogen. The wavelength (λ) of the emitted photon can be determined as follows:

$$\lambda = hc\frac{1}{E_{photon}} = -hc\frac{1}{\Delta E_{atom}} = -\frac{1.986 \times 10^{-25 J \cdot m}}{\Delta E_{atom}}$$

Wavelengths of light in the (human) visible spectrum extend from 390 nm (ultraviolet end) to 750 nm (infrared end), but as with the Rydberg formula, this formula works for all EM radiation wavelengths observed for hydrogen.

Quantum Mechanical Model of the Atom

Bohr's model worked for single electron atoms (H, He^+, Li^{2+}) but failed when it was applied to multiple-electron atoms. His model failed to account for electron-electron interactions, primarily repulsion. In 1925 Werner Heisenberg, Max Born, and Pascual Jordan formulated a type of matrix mechanics, which came to be known as quantum mechanics. The old quantum theory represented by the Bohr model assumed an electron moved in a classical orbit, much like the moon around the earth. The new theory held that electrons moved within regions of space called orbitals (which were not necessarily circular). Within these orbitals, classical position and the momentum are no longer clearly defined. The **Heisenberg uncertainty principle** states that it is impossible to determine simultaneously both the position and momentum of a particle (e.g., an electron). Our experimental methods for determining the particle's position changes the momentum, and vice versa. This uncertainty principle is a fundamental limit to our knowledge of these quantum systems, but does not limit our understanding of everyday objects; it is only on the atomic scale that the uncertainty becomes appreciable.

In 1924 Louis de Broglie introduced the concept that any moving particle or object (such as an electron) has an associated wave. De Broglie's **matter-wave** is defined by a wavelength (λ) inversely proportional to momentum (p), and a frequency (f) proportional to energy (E), all related by Planck's constant (h):

$$\lambda = \frac{h}{p} = \frac{h}{mv} \quad \text{and} \quad f = \frac{E}{h} \quad \text{(Planck-Einstein)}$$

Expressing these relationships in terms of the reduced Planck constant, these become $p = \hbar k$ and $E = \hbar\omega$. At low velocities (v) and high mass (m), the associated wavelength approaches zero. However, with the negligible mass of the electron moving at high velocity, the associated wavelength becomes nontrivial. Experiments performed in 1928 proved the wave nature of electrons. Added to the particle nature of light, the wave-nature of matter completed the theory of wave particle duality. Electrons are neither particles nor waves; they have characteristics of both, and it is our failure of language and descriptive ability that introduces confusion when discussing the topic. Electrons are hybrids and can act as either a particle or a wave, depending on the circumstances.

In 1926 Erwin Schrödinger developed an equation based on the de Broglie wave theory that accurately reproduced the energy levels of the Bohr model. Schrödinger's matter-wave approach was found to be consistent with Heisenberg's matrix approach, and both approaches were found to be specific cases of a more general theory. However, for calculating the energy levels and other properties of atoms and molecules, Schrödinger's time-independent Schrödinger equation for a system in a stationary state usually suffices. Solving the Schrödinger equation yields **wavefunctions**, or state vectors, that describe a quantum state. These wavefunctions are colloquially called orbitals. Solutions to the equation describe the probability of finding electrons at a point in space. The probability of finding an electron is called the **electron density**. Orbitals are defined by wavefunctions, and are regions of space around an atom with set shapes and dimensions. Orbitals with high probabilities of finding an electron are said to have a high electron density. Due to the uncertainty principle, we cannot say precisely where the electron is located, but we can say that there is a high probability of electrons being located somewhere within the fuzzy clouds that are electron orbitals.

Quantum Numbers

Solutions to the Schrödinger equation require four values called **quantum numbers**; these numbers combine to completely describe an electron in an atom. Three of the quantum numbers are integers that describe the orbital: n describes the shell (energy level), ℓ describes the subshell, and m_ℓ describes the orbital within the subshell. The fourth quantum number, m_s, describes the electron spin.

Principal Quantum Number

The **principal quantum number, *n*,** is the same number used in the Bohr model. This number can be any positive integer and traditionally represents the electron shell, or energy level. Higher integers represent increasing shell distance from the nucleus. The Bohr model energy level equation applies; as with the Bohr model, increasing energy levels have decreasing energy differences. The maximum number of electrons in an energy-level, n, is $2n^2$. The outer-shell electrons constitute the valence electrons. Although higher values of n apply to atoms in excited energy states, elements in their ground state do not exceed $n = 7$, as can be seen in the Periodic Table of the Elements.

Azimuthal Quantum Number

The **azimuthal (angular momentum) quantum number, ℓ,** sometimes called the orbital shape quantum number, can have an integer value ranging from 0 to $n - 1$. These values are commonly known as the *s*-orbital ($\ell = 0$), *p*-orbital ($\ell = 1$), *d*-orbital ($\ell = 2$), *f*-orbital ($\ell = 3$), *g*-orbital ($\ell = 4$), etc. Each subshell can have a maximum of $4\ell + 2$ electrons. Higher values of ℓ represent higher energy levels.

Magnetic Quantum Number

The **magnetic quantum number, m_ℓ,** describes the spatial orientation of the orbital within the subshell. This quantum number is sometimes called the projection of angular momentum. Valid values for m_ℓ are the integers between $-\ell$ and $+\ell$. In the case of the *p*-orbital ($\ell = 1$), m_ℓ values can be –1, 0, or 1; these represent three dumbbell-shaped orbitals aligned on the *x*-, *y*-, and *z*-axes. For the *d*-orbital which has five different m_ℓ values, the visualization becomes rather complex, as shown in the diagram. Each orbital described by the magnetic quantum number can have no more than two electrons.

Orbitals

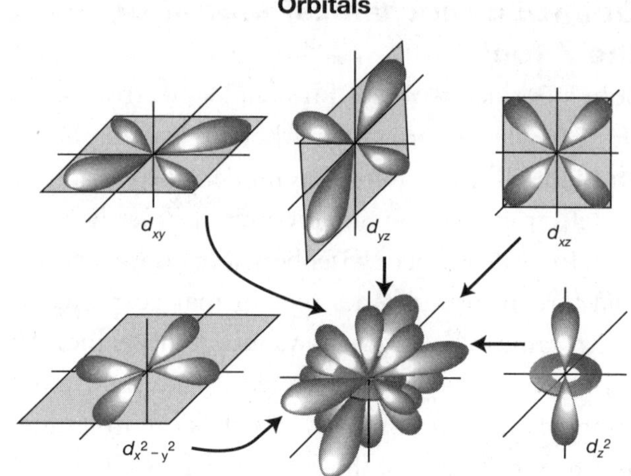

Spin Quantum Number

The spin quantum number, m_s, can have only two values, $+\frac{1}{2}$ and $-\frac{1}{2}$, each assigned to one of the two electrons allowed per subshell orbital. The spin quantum number is the intrinsic angular momentum of the particle. The Pauli exclusion principle and Hund's rule address spin restrictions when filling electron orbitals. The electrons don't spin in the sense that we normally envision an object spinning; it is simply a word used to describe a certain property (rotation) of the electron.

Electron Configurations and Orbital Filling

The rules of electron configuration dictate that electrons are added to the allowable orbitals for each atom starting from the lowest energy level and rising to the highest energy level as needed. The electron configuration of an atom or ion represents the filled orbitals using a notation that summarizes the three spatial quantum numbers n, ℓ, and m_ℓ. The shell, n, is represented by itself; the subshell is represented by its letter designation; and the orbital, m_ℓ, is represented by a superscript. Using this scheme, and as an example, the electron configuration of oxygen is written as $1s^22s^22p^2$. For higher-shell elements, an abbreviated notation allows using the preceding noble gas as a basis to avoid a lengthy notation. The electron scheme for calcium using the abbreviated notation would be

[Ar] $4s^2$. This indicates that calcium has the identical electron configuration as argon, with the addition of two more electrons in the 4*s* orbital. It should be emphasized that the outermost shell electrons, or **valence electrons**, are primarily responsible for determining an element's chemical reactivity.

Four rules govern the order of filling of the electron orbitals.

Aufbau Principle

The Aufbau principle, or "building up" principle, states that a maximum of two electrons are placed in orbitals, starting with the lowest-energy orbital and increasing in energy levels as necessary. As the shell number increases, the energy levels between orbitals decreases and overlap occurs. Madelung's rule extends this rule to resolve these orbital energy-level conflicts for atoms with more than 18 electrons.

Madelung's Rule

Madelung's rule states that

1. Orbitals are filled in order of increasing $n + \ell$.
2. Where two orbitals have the same value of $n + \ell$, the orbital with the lower n value fills first.

The first exception occurs between 3*p* ($n + \ell = 4$) and 3*d* ($n + \ell = 5$); the 4*s* subshell ($n + \ell = 4$) fills before the 3*d* subshell, but after the 3*p* subshell. The following chart shows the order of orbital filling with the principle (shell) quantum number on the left and the azimuthal quantum number (subshell) along the bottom.

Madelung's rule should be considered an approximation, as it starts to break down when dealing with the transition metals. For example, copper and chromium are exceptions in that the 3*d* level pulls electrons from the 4*s* level to yield electron configurations of [Ar]$3d^5 4s^1$ and [Ar]$3d^{10} 4s^1$, respectively. Further exceptions occur at even higher atomic numbers.

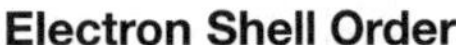

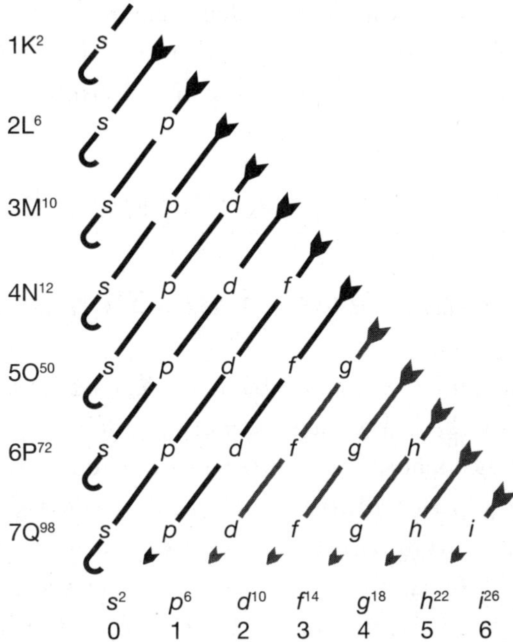

Pauli Exclusion Principle

This states that no two electrons in an atom may have the same four quantum number values. The practical implication of this is that while only two electrons can exist in any orbital, those electrons must also have opposite spin (known as **paired** electrons). This principle regarding paired spins applies to all half-integer-spin particles, including protons and neutrons.

Hund's Rule

Hund's rule, or the rule of maximum multiplicity, states that when equal energy orbitals are available, the electrons will fill the orbitals to produce the maximum number of half-filled orbitals with parallel (same spin value) spins. In the case of the *p* subshell, one electron will fill each of the p_x, p_y, and p_z orbitals, each with the same spin, before a fourth electron will pair up in one of the half-filled orbitals.

Hund's rule is manifest in the macroscopic world in the form of **paramagnetism**, a behavior exhibited by some materials. If a material has unpaired electrons, a magnetic field will align the electrons and cause a weak attraction. If the material has no unpaired electrons, then the material will be repelled by the magnet and is said to be **diamagnetic**.

The following lists the electron configuration for element 118 with the cumulative electron total in subscript below each subshell:

$$1s^2_{2}2s^2_{4}2p^6_{10}3s^2_{12}3p^6_{18}4s^2_{20}3d^{10}_{30}4p^6_{36}5s^2_{38}4d^{10}_{48}5p^6_{54}6s^2_{56}4f^{14}_{70}5d^{10}_{80}6p^6_{86}7s^2_{88}5f^{14}_{102}6d^{10}_{112}7p^6_{118}$$

Periodic Table of the Elements

The Russian chemist Dmitri Mendeleev noticed that elements had recurring patterns in their observed properties that seemed to correlate with their atomic weights. In 1869 Mendeleev refined the theories of his time and produced what is considered to be the first Periodic Table of the Elements. Over time, variations have developed, and Henry Moseley refined the order by using atomic number, but the concept, known as the periodic law, remains the same. The **periodic law** states generally that the physical and chemical properties of the elements tend to recur in a systematic way when ordered by their atomic numbers.

The current, generally accepted Periodic Table of the Elements is shown here. As of 2010, the Periodic Table lists 118 confirmed chemical elements. Only 94 of these elements occur naturally on Earth, and only 80 elements have stable isotopes. All the elements with atomic number of 84 or greater, along with elements 43 and 61, have no stable isotopes. The table lists each element with its name, symbol, atomic number, and relative (average) atomic mass as shown here.

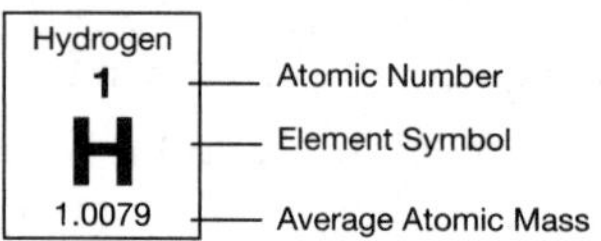

The Periodic Table summarizes a wealth of chemical information about each element over and above the simple listing of atomic number and average atomic mass. The 18 columns of the table are called **groups** (or families). The seven rows of the table are called **periods**. Blocks of elements can also be defined based on the electron subshells of the elements.

Periodic Table of the Elements

Decreasing Atomic Radii →
Increasing Ionization energy and electronegativity

Decreasing Ionization energy and electronegativity ↓
Increasing Atomic Radii

Group: IUPAC -	1	2		3	4	5	6	7	8	9	10	11	12	13	14	15	16	17	18
CAS -	IA	IIA		IIIB	IVB	VB	VIB	VIIB	VIIIB	VIIIB	VIIIB	IB	IIB	IIIA	IVA	VA	VIA	VIIA	VIIIA
Period 1	hydrogen 1 **H** 1.0079																		helium 2 **He** 4.0026
2	lithium 3 **Li** 6.941	beryllium 4 **Be** 9.0122												boron 5 **B** 10.811	carbon 6 **C** 12.011	nitrogen 7 **N** 14.007	oxygen 8 **O** 15.999	fluorine 9 **F** 18.998	neon 10 **Ne** 20.180
3	sodium 11 **Na** 22.990	magnesium 12 **Mg** 24.305												aluminium 13 **Al** 26.982	silicon 14 **Si** 28.086	phosphorus 15 **P** 30.974	sulfur 16 **S** 32.065	chlorine 17 **Cl** 35.453	argon 18 **Ar** 39.948
4	potassium 19 **K** 39.098	calcium 20 **Ca** 40.078		scandium 21 **Sc** 44.956	titanium 22 **Ti** 47.867	vanadium 23 **V** 50.942	chromium 24 **Cr** 51.996	manganese 25 **Mn** 54.938	iron 26 **Fe** 55.845	cobalt 27 **Co** 58.933	nickel 28 **Ni** 58.693	copper 29 **Cu** 63.546	zinc 30 **Zn** 65.39	gallium 31 **Ga** 69.723	germanium 32 **Ge** 72.61	arsenic 33 **As** 74.922	selenium 34 **Se** 78.96	bromine 35 **Br** 79.904	krypton 36 **Kr** 83.80
5	rubidium 37 **Rb** 85.468	strontium 38 **Sr** 87.62		yttrium 39 **Y** 88.906	zirconium 40 **Zr** 91.224	niobium 41 **Nb** 92.906	molybdenum 42 **Mo** 95.94	technetium 43 **Tc** [98]	ruthenium 44 **Ru** 101.07	rhodium 45 **Rh** 102.91	palladium 46 **Pd** 106.42	silver 47 **Ag** 107.87	cadmium 48 **Cd** 112.41	indium 49 **In** 114.82	tin 50 **Sn** 118.71	antimony 51 **Sb** 121.76	tellurium 52 **Te** 127.60	iodine 53 **I** 126.90	xenon 54 **Xe** 131.29
6	caesium 55 **Cs** 132.91	barium 56 **Ba** 137.33	57-70 *	lutetium 71 **Lu** 174.97	hafnium 72 **Hf** 178.49	tantalum 73 **Ta** 180.95	tungsten 74 **W** 183.84	rhenium 75 **Re** 186.21	osmium 76 **Os** 190.23	iridium 77 **Ir** 192.22	platinum 78 **Pt** 195.08	gold 79 **Au** 196.97	mercury 80 **Hg** 200.59	thallium 81 **Tl** 204.38	lead 82 **Pb** 207.2	bismuth 83 **Bi** 208.98	polonium 84 **Po** [209]	astatine 85 **At** [210]	radon 86 **Rn** [222]
7	francium 87 **Fr** [223]	radium 88 **Ra** [226]	89-102 **	lawrencium 103 **Lr** [262]	rutherfordium 104 **Rf** [261]	dubnium 105 **Db** [262]	seaborgium 106 **Sg** [266]	bohrium 107 **Bh** [264]	hassium 108 **Hs** [269]	meitnerium 109 **Mt** [268]	ununnilium 110 **Uun** [271]	unununium 111 **Uuu** [272]	ununbium 112 **Uub** [277]		ununquadium 114 **Uuq** [289]				

*Lanthanide Series	lanthanum 57 **La** 138.91	cerium 58 **Ce** 140.12	praseodymium 59 **Pr** 140.91	neodymium 60 **Nd** 144.24	promethium 61 **Pm** [145]	samarium 62 **Sm** 150.36	europium 63 **Eu** 151.96	gadolinium 64 **Gd** 157.25	terbium 65 **Tb** 158.93	dysprosium 66 **Dy** 162.50	holmium 67 **Ho** 164.93	erbium 68 **Er** 167.26	thulium 69 **Tm** 168.93	ytterbium 70 **Yb** 173.04
**Actinide Series	actinium 89 **Ac** [227]	thorium 90 **Th** 232.04	protactinium 91 **Pa** 231.04	uranium 92 **U** 238.03	neptunium 93 **Np** [237]	plutonium 94 **Pu** [244]	americium 95 **Am** [243]	curium 96 **Cm** [247]	berkelium 97 **Bk** [247]	californium 98 **Cf** [251]	einsteinium 99 **Es** [252]	fermium 100 **Fm** [257]	mendelevium 101 **Md** [258]	nobelium 102 **No** [259]

Groups

The columns of the Periodic Table are numbered 1 through 18 by the current IUPAC standard. An older Chemical Abstract Service (CAS) numbering scheme uses Roman numerals with letters; IA through VIIIA cover the main-group elements, and IB through VIIIB cover the transition elements. All elements in a group have the same valence electron configuration that largely determines the chemical reactivity of the elements. In the CAS numbering, the Roman numeral equals the number of valence electrons. The A groups (main-group elements) have only *s* and *p* subshells. The B groups (transition elements) also have *d* subshells.

Hydrogen

Hydrogen sits atop Group 1 (IA) and does not fit with the rest of the group. Hydrogen occurs naturally as a gas and in many respects behaves more like the Group 18 noble gases than the Group 1 alkali metals. Since hydrogen has only one valence electron in an *s*-orbital, it readily loses an electron like the alkali metals to form an H^+ ion, but it can also gain an electron to form a H^- ion more like the Group 17 halogens.

Alkali Metals

The Group 1 (IA) alkali metals, or lithium family, all have one valence electron in an *s*-orbital that is readily lost, making these metals highly reactive. These elements do not occur naturally in elemental form. When in elemental form, they are usually stored in mineral oil or kerosene to prevent reaction with moisture and oxygen in the air. All alkali metals have low melting points and low densities, making them relatively soft metals. All alkali metals react aggressively with the halogens to form ionic salts (e.g., NaCl). In water these metals form alkaline hydroxides (e.g., NaOH) in a vigorous reaction that also releases hydrogen gas; the heat evolved from the reaction can often ignite the hydrogen, resulting in an explosion.

Alkaline Earth Metals

The Group 2 (IIA) alkaline earth metals, or beryllium family, all have two valence electrons in an *s*-orbital, making them much less reactive than the alkali metals. All alkaline earth metals have high melting points; early chemists called these "earth metals" because they didn't melt in fires. Losing the outer two valence electrons, the elements react with halogens to form ionic salts (e.g., $CaCl_2$). The exception is Beryllium; due to its tightly held valence electrons, it does not form a Be^{2+} ion. Early chemists commonly found that the oxide form of these elements (e.g., CaO, or quicklime) form alkaline hydroxides when dissolved in water, thus explaining the first part of the group's name.

Halogens

The Group 17 (VIIA) halogens, or fluorine family, all have seven valence electrons (s^2p^5), making them highly reactive. Like the alkali metals on the opposite side of the table, these elements occur in nature only as compounds or ions, but can exist as a diatomic molecule bound to itself. Where the alkali metals readily lose an electron, the halogens readily gain an electron to complete their outer shell. In fact, fluorine is the most electronegative and most chemically reactive of all the elements. The halogens are the only group that collectively has elements naturally occurring in each of the three phases at room temperature and pressure; fluorine (F_2) and chlorine (Cl_2) are gases, bromine (Br_2) is a liquid, and iodine (I_2) and astatine are solids. Astatine is currently the rarest naturally occurring element and is highly radioactive.

Noble Gases

The Group 18 (VIIIA) noble gases, or helium/neon family, all have complete outer electron shells: two *s* electrons in the case of helium and eight valence electrons (s^2p^6) for the other elements in the group. The name *noble* refers to the extremely low reactivity of these gases, due to their already-filled valence shells. These gases were formerly considered inert gases and labeled Group 0 for their near zero electron affinity.

Although a few noble gas compounds have been formed, neutral compounds with neon or helium are not known. All noble gases are colorless, odorless, tasteless, and nonflammable under standard conditions. For most practical purposes, they can be considered as unreactive.

Periods

The period numbers correspond to the principal quantum number, *n*, and progression across each row corresponds to the progressive filling of the particular electron shell. In the main-group elements, most similarities correspond to the group. However, in the transition elements, and lanthanides and actinides, the similarities correspond more to the period.

Blocks

Blocks of the Periodic Table can be defined based on the subshell (*s*, *p*, *d*, or *f*) containing the outermost electron. The ***s*-block** covers hydrogen, helium, the alkali metals, and the alkaline earth metals. The ***p*-block** covers Group 13 (IIIA) through Group 17 (VIIA). Together the *s*-block and *p*-block make up the main-group elements. The ***d*-block** covers Group 3 (IIIB) through Group 12 (IIB), also known as the transition elements. The ***f*-block**, also known as the inner-transition elements, covers the lanthanides and actinides.

Transition Elements

The transition elements historically include all *d*-block elements, all of which are metals. Consequently, this block is often called the transition metals, although some people exclude Group 3 and Group 12 elements from that definition. These metals are hard, but very malleable. The five *d*-orbitals in the outer shell of these elements hold their electrons very loosely. Most of these elements are characterized by high melting points, high electrical conductivity, low ionization energies, and many possible oxidation states. These elements form complex ions, either in water or in combination with other nonmetals, that are often brightly colored due to *d*-orbital electron transitions.

Element Categories

The elements of the Periodic Table can generally be placed into three broad categories: metals, metalloids, and nonmetals.

Metals

Metals encompass the left-side elements and include the alkali metals, the alkaline earth metals, the transition elements, the inner-transition elements, and other metals. Aluminum (Al), gallium (Ga), indium (In), thallium (Tl), tin (Sn), lead (Pb), and bismuth (Bi) are considered other metals, although zinc (Zn), cadmium (Cd), and mercury (Hg) are sometimes included in this "other" category. Metals are all generally shiny solids at room temperature (with the exception of mercury [Hg]). Metals are ductile, malleable, and both thermally and electrically conductive.

Metalloids

Metalloids appear along a diagonal transition line on the right side of the Periodic Table and include the elements boron (B), silicon (Si), germanium (Ge), arsenic (As), antimony (Sb), tellurium (Te), and polonium (Po). These elements possess characteristics between those of metals and nonmetals, with a wide degree of variety within this category.

Nonmetals

Nonmetals include the rightmost elements, specifically the noble gases, the halogens, and other nonmetals. The other nonmetals are specifically hydrogen (H), carbon (C), nitrogen (N), oxygen (O), phosphorus (P), sulfur (S), and selenium (Se). Nonmetals tend to be dull, brittle, and nonconductive as solids.

Periodic Properties of the Elements

We have seen that the arrangement of the elements in the Periodic Table corresponds to the order of the filling of the electron shells. Moving across a period, the number of protons increase, adding to the nuclear charge, and electrons are added to existing shells. Moving down a group (up in principal quantum number) corresponds to electrons filling additional shells. The additional shells hold valence electrons further from the nuclear charge. The valence electrons also become more shielded from the nuclear charge by the inner shells. These changes alter the **effective nuclear charge** (Z_{eff}) experienced by the valence electrons. Changes in the effective nuclear charge have very definite effects on the elemental properties, especially in regard to their atomic radius, electron affinity, ionization energy, and electronegativity.

Atomic Radius

In general, the atomic radius is half the mean distance between the nuclei of two touching atoms of an element. As the nuclear charge increases across a period, the electrons are drawn tighter toward the nucleus. Consequently, the atomic radius decreases. The atomic radius of lithium can be nearly three times the radius of neon. Moving down the table (adding electron shells) adds to the atomic radius, but the increase due to additional electron shells is generally less than the contracting effect of the increased nuclear charge.

Electron Affinity

The **electron affinity** (**E_{ea}**) is the energy change when an electron is added to a neutral atom to form a negative ion. Conversely, the electron affinity represents the energy needed to pull an electron off a negatively charged ion. A positive electron affinity defines an electron acceptor, which is an atom that readily accepts an electron. This can only be measured for atoms in the gaseous state. The equation for electron affinity is as follows:

$$X_{(g)} + e^- \rightarrow X^-_{(g)} + E_{ea}$$

While electron affinities vary greatly across the Periodic Table, some generalizations apply. Electron affinity generally increases across a period and decreases going down a group. Nonmetals have greater electron affinity than metals, with chlorine attracting electrons most strongly and mercury most weakly. All the halogens exhibit strong electron affinities because the addition of an electron completes the outer shell (**octet rule**). The noble gases have near-zero electron affinity because they already have complete outer shells (a stable octet).

Ionization Energy

The **ionization energy** (**E_i**), formerly called ionization potential, is the minimum energy required to remove an electron from an atom in the gaseous state. Energy is always required to remove an electron from an atom, but some atoms donate electrons more readily than others. The closer and less shielded an electron is from the nucleus, the more readily it can be removed. The energy required to remove the first valence electron is called the **first ionization energy**. Once the atom is ionized, removal of additional electrons becomes increasingly difficult. Removal of a second valence electron is called the **second ionization energy**.

Ionization energies increase going across a period as the increased nuclear charge and reduced atomic radius act to hold electrons more tightly. Moving down a group, ionization energies decrease because the valence electrons are further from the nucleus and increasingly shielded by lower shells. The alkali metals have very low ionization energies and readily act as electron donors.

Electronegativity

Where ionization energy and electron affinity addressed free atoms (in the gaseous state), electronegativity measures the attraction an atom has for electrons in a chemical bond. Because electronegativity involves interaction with other atoms, this property cannot be directly measured and is not strictly an atomic property. Electronegativity is to an atom in a molecule as electron affinity is to a free atom. As with electron affinity, the smaller, higher-nuclear-charge atoms have higher electronegativity. Electronegativity generally increases across a period and decreases down a group. From the chart we can see that cesium has one of the lowest electronegativities, and fluorine has the highest.

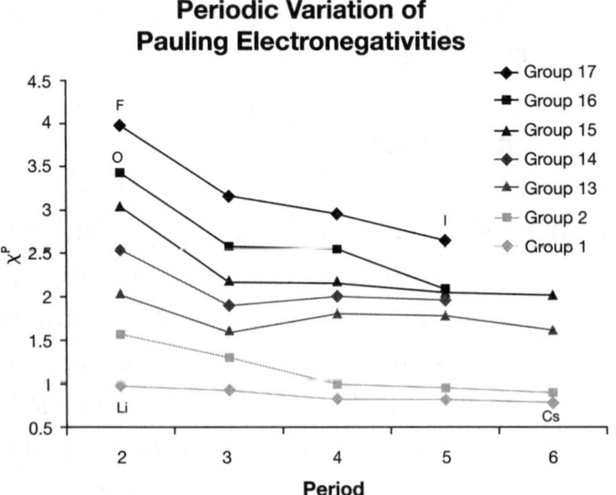

Chemical Bonding

Two or more different atoms can come together to form **chemical bonds**, which results in the formation of a **chemical compound**: a pure substance with distinct properties that differ from those of the constituent atoms. Atoms of pure elements may also form chemical bonds to combine into polyatomic molecules, but these molecules are still considered pure elements, not chemical compounds. In both cases the electrical properties of the valence-shell electrons will greatly affect the type of chemical bond formed.

Observation of the stability of the noble gases led to the development of the **octet rule**. Atoms tend to combine to achieve more stable electron configurations; there is a driving force for atoms to become more stable via adoption of these lower-energy states. Like the noble gases, main-group elements gain stability in ionic or molecular form when they have a complete valence shell (i.e., an outer shell s^2p^6 configuration). The octet rule is especially true for the main-group elements, in particularly the period 2 and period 3 elements. Group 1 and group 2 elements lose electrons to reach noble gas stability while nonmetals gain electrons to reach noble gas stability. Notable exceptions to the rule are:

- The two period 1 elements, hydrogen and helium, and two of the period 2 elements, lithium and beryllium, follow a **duet rule**. To achieve the stable He configuration, H must gain an electron, Li must lose an electron, and Be must lose two electrons. Note that H may also lose an electron yielding a proton.
- Period 2 element boron forms bonds such that it attains six valence electrons. These boron compounds act as Lewis acids (as they have a vacant p_z orbital that can accept electrons), reacting with Lewis bases to obtain a complete octet.
- Period 2 element nitrogen can form **radicals** with an odd number of electrons in the valence shell (e.g., NO and NO_3).
- Period 3 elements phosphorus, sulfur, and chlorine can all form **hypervalent molecules** with more than eight electrons in the valence shell.
- Transition elements with their *d*-orbitals have complex electron configurations, based around the **18-electron rule**; they are most stable with 18 valence electrons.

The electronegativities of the combining elements indicate how the combined atoms share their electron clouds. Chemical bonds are classified into three broad types based on how the components share the two electrons present in a bond.

- **Ionic bonding** occurs when one or more electrons from one atom transfer completely to the other atom in the bond. The electron transfer results in ions (one positive, one negative) held together by electrostatic forces. Component atoms having Pauling electronegativities that differ by approximately 2.0 or more generally form ionic bonds.

- **Covalent bonding** occurs when atoms share the two electrons from the bond, although the extent and direction of this electron sharing can vary greatly. Very uneven electron sharing that falls short of full ionization is called **polar covalent bonding.** Atoms having Pauling electronegativities that differ by less than 2.0 form a covalent bond, although only differences less than 0.4 are considered **nonpolar** (meaning that the electrons in the bond are almost exactly equally shared between the two atoms).
- **Metallic bonding** occurs among metal atoms that exist as cations surrounded by delocalized electrons. This type of bonding is not really atom to atom, but rather among atoms in a three-dimensional array called a lattice.

Ionic Bonding

Atoms with large differences in electronegativity ($\Delta_{\chi P} \geq$ 2.0 approx.) will not equally share electrons. Instead, one or more electrons will transfer from the atom with low electronegativity to the atom with the high electronegativity. The electron donor atom will become a positive ion, or **cation**. The electron acceptor (which now has an excess electron) will become a negative ion, or **anion**. The electrostatic attraction between the anion and cation form a bond called an **ionic**, or **electrovalent, bond.** Group 1 and group 2 elements (low electronegativity metals) form ionic compounds with Group 16 and 17 elements (high-electronegativity nonmetals), such as NaCl, $CaCl_2$, and CaO, as the difference in electronegativity values of the two component atoms are high.

Ionic compounds in the solid state form lattice structures with alternating ionic charges arranged to maximize ion packing. The **lattice energy** is a measure of the bond strength of the ionic solid. The bond strength will depend on these factors:

- **Ionic radius.** Ions with small ionic radii can pack closer together resulting in decreased charge separation and increased bond strength. Thus, LiF has a lattice energy approximately 33% greater (stronger) than the larger NaCl. Similarly, MgO has a lattice energy 24% greater than the larger BaO.
- **Ionic charge.** The more electrons transferred to the highly electronegative element, the higher the charge difference and the stronger the bond. Divalent ions have stronger attraction than monovalent ions. Thus, divalent BaO has a lattice energy over 3.8 times greater than monovalent NaCl. In fact, ionic charge has a vastly greater effect on bond energy than ionic radius. Both LiF and MgO have similar ionic radii (approximately 210 pm), but divalent MgO has a lattice energy 3.6 times greater than LiF.

Very ionic compounds will follow these rules closely, whereas marginally ionic (borderline bonds, aka partially covalent) compounds ($\Delta_{\chi P} \approx 2.0$) may deviate from these rules.

Ionic compounds exhibit similar characteristic properties including the following:

- **Solid at room temperature** with correspondingly high melting and boiling points due to the strong electrostatic bonds between ions
- **Soluble in polar solvents** such as water, alcohol, and acetone
- **Electrically conductive in molten or aqueous form**, but not in solid form
- **Low thermal conductivity**

Polyatomic Ions

While metals bonding with nonmetals form ionic compounds, either metals or nonmetals bonding with polyatomic ions can also possibly form ionic compounds. **Polyatomic ions**, or molecular ions, consist of two or more elements covalently bonded together such that the unit as a whole carries a positive or negative net charge. These polyatomic ions often act as conjugate acids or conjugate bases, a concept that will be discussed later under the review of acids and bases. Ammonium ion (NH_4^+), sulfate anion (SO_4^{2-}) and bicarbonate (HCO_3^-) are all examples of polyatomic ions that always exist as ionic compounds when bound with any other element.

Covalent Bonding

Atoms with small differences in electronegativity ($\Delta_{\chi P}$ < 2.0 approx.) will combine by sharing electrons to varying degrees in a **covalent bond.** Atoms in a covalent bond achieve a stable octet by sharing electrons in a fixed geometric structure called a **molecule**. Both polyatomic ions and molecules involve covalent bonds, so, generally speaking, both are molecules. However, molecules are generally electrically neutral (as a whole), and when they do carry a charge they are more specifically labeled molecular, or polyatomic, ions. Any **nonmetal** that combines with itself will form covalent bonds; the electronegativity difference is zero. Hydrogen and the halogens can form diatomic molecules (e.g., H_2, Cl_2, Br_2), as do other nonmetals such as oxygen (O_2) and nitrogen (N_2). Covalent bonding requires localized electron sharing. **Metals** bonding with themselves or other metals may have low or zero electronegativity difference; however, they share electrons in a delocalized lattice, not a fixed molecular structure. Consequently, metals bonding with themselves are said to form **metallic bonds**. Similarly, some nonmetals and metalloids form continuous networks of covalent bonds called **covalent network solids**. Network solids do not have individual molecules, but rather macromolecules that, like ionic compounds, have formulas representing the ratio of the elements in the structure. Carbon bonds with itself to form both three-dimensional (diamonds) and two-dimensional (graphite) network solids.

Covalent bond strength derives from the attraction of the shared electrons to the positive nuclei of the bound atoms. Atoms sharing one pair of electrons are said to have a **single bond**. Likewise, sharing of two and three pairs of electrons constitute **double bonds** and **triple bonds**, respectively. The number of bonds is called the **bond order**. Higher bond orders indicate stronger, more stable bonds. These covalent bonds are characterized by their bond length and bond dissociation energy:

- **Bond length.** The bond length is defined as the average distance between the nuclei of bound atoms. Higher bond orders result in shorter bond lengths. Bond lengths are typically given in picometers (pm) and can be approximated by adding the **covalent radii** of the two atoms in the bond for the applicable bond order. The covalent radius of an atom can be determined using x-ray diffraction.
- **Bond dissociation energy.** Bond dissociation energy (D_0) measures the energy (or more accurately, the enthalpy) required to break the covalent bond between two atoms. The energy required to break a bond is directly related to

ALLOTROPES

Diamond and graphite represent two network solid structures of the same element, carbon. These different forms are known as allotropes. Elements capable of different oxidation states, especially nonmetals and metalloids, tend to have allotropic forms. These different structural forms of the same element exhibit different properties. Although these structural changes often depend on the temperature and pressure during formation, these allotropes all represent the same phase of an element. Diamond and graphite are both solid-phase carbon. Oxygen, normally present as the diatomic molecule (O_2), has a very common allotrope, ozone (O_3). Both of these represent allotropes of oxygen in the gas phase.

bond order and inversely related to bond length. For diatomic molecules, this energy also equals the **bond energy**.

- **Bond energy.** Bond energy (E) is an aggregate measure of the strength of the bonds in a molecule. Bond energy measures the heat required to break a molecule into its individual atoms. For diatomic molecules, the energy equals the bond dissociation energy. Further discussion can be found under the review of thermochemistry.

Covalent compounds exhibit similar characteristic properties, including the following:

- State at room temperature varies with the compound—not typically a solid, like ionic compounds.
- Melting and boiling points vary with the compound—generally lower than for ionic compounds due to weak intermolecular forces.
- Solubility varies with the compound—usually less water soluble than ionic compounds.
- Covalent compounds are usually electrically nonconductive.
- They have low thermal conductivity.

Lewis Structures

In 1916 Gilbert Newton Lewis devised a notation to show the covalent bonding between atoms in molecules. Lewis discovered the covalent bond and developed the valence bond theory of electron sharing. **Lewis structures**, or **electron dot diagrams**, show the valence electrons involved in bonding and graphically represent the stable octet electron configuration of combined atoms. Lewis structures can be drawn for covalently bonded molecules and coordination compounds.

In a Lewis structure, the shared valence electrons, or **bonding electrons**, in the covalent bond appear as dots between the element symbols. The other valence electrons, or **nonbonding electrons**, appear as dots around the unbound sides of the element symbols. Each dot represents one electron. The nonbonding electrons are often drawn as electron pairs called **lone pairs**. Use the Periodic Table to determine the number of valence electrons for any given element. For the elements hydrogen and oxygen, the individual atoms and the diatomic molecular forms (H_2, O_2) are symbolized as follows:

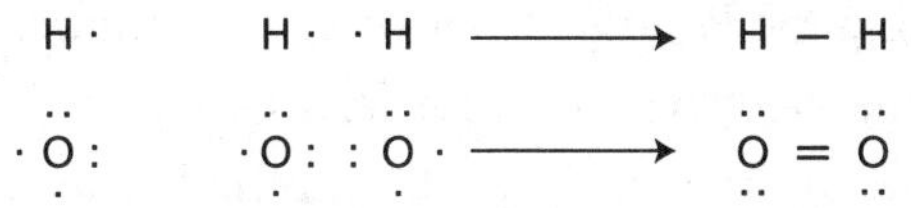

H·   H· ·H ⟶ H — H

·Ö: ·Ö: :Ö· ⟶ O = O

Hydrogen has only an *s* orbital with one valence electron. Two hydrogen atoms each contribute one electron to create a **single (electron pair) bond** as indicated by the single line between the hydrogen symbols on the right. Evaluating the stability of the molecule, consider the electrons in the bond as belonging to each atom, giving each shared use of a complete *s*-orbital pair, the configuration of the noble gas He. Oxygen has a $2s^2p^4$ valence electron configuration, or six valence electrons. To form the stable molecule, each oxygen atom contributes two electrons to create a **double bond** as indicated by the two lines between the oxygen symbols on the right. Counting the electrons around each oxygen, and counting each bond as two electrons, each oxygen now has eight valence electrons, creating a **stable octet** like the noble gas Ne. Each oxygen is left with two lone pairs. Sharing those to create more bonds would yield an electron count greater than eight and would exceed the capacity of the $2s^2p^6$ shell. Removing a bond, leaving a single bond, would add an electron dot to each oxygen, but the valence electron count would then be seven for each oxygen, less than the stable octet.

Creating Lewis structures for more complex molecules is best accomplished by following these four steps:

1. Write a preliminary structure by placing the least electronegative atom in the center of the

structure. Hydrogen is an exception and should never take a central position. Attach single bonds from the central atom to each of the other elements. To clarify the electron count, you may want to start by placing electron pairs between atoms as in the prior example; connect the electron pairs with a line when the bond structure has been finalized.

2. Using the Periodic Table, note the number of valence electrons for each element in the molecule. When in doubt, subtract the atomic number of the noble gas at the end of the prior period from the atomic number of the element in question to determine the valence electron count. Total the valence electrons contributed by the component elements and subtract 2 for each bond you drew in step 1. If the molecule has a charge, add electrons equal to the negative charge for anions or subtract electrons equal to the positive charge for cations. The net number tells you how many electrons need to be placed around the elements in the structure.
3. Use the octet rule to place the electrons tallied in step 2 around the elements in the structure. Start with the most electronegative element and work toward the least electronegative element, the central atom. Hydrogen needs only a single bond to stabilize its lone orbital and can accept no others. Remember that each bond pair counts toward the octet of each atom in the bond.
4. With all the electrons placed, determine whether all the atoms (excluding hydrogen) have a stable octet. If not, evaluate bond options to achieve stable octets.

By example, the Lewis structure for hydrogen cyanide, HCN, can be determined as follows using the same four steps:

1. Excluding hydrogen, carbon is positioned to the left of nitrogen in the periodic table, so carbon has a lower electronegativity than nitrogen. Our starting structure must be H··C··N.
2. From the Periodic Table we determine the following valence electron counts:

   H, 1 e^-; C, 4 e^-; N, 5 e^- Electrons to place $= 10\ e^- - (2 \text{ bonds} \times 2\ e^-) = 6\ e^-$

3. Starting from the outside and working to the center, we know that hydrogen is complete, so we add electrons to nitrogen. Adding all six electrons to nitrogen completes the octet for nitrogen.
4. Although we've placed all the electrons based on the octet rule, further inspection shows that carbon has only four valence electrons in the structure thus far. By moving two pair of lone pairs from nitrogen into a shared, bonding position with carbon, we find we can satisfy the octet rule for both carbon and nitrogen. The correct stable structure is shown on the right:

H··C··N —6e⁻→ H··C··N: ⟶ H··C::N: ⟶ H—C≡N:

For simple molecules, the following shortcut that starts with the valence electrons around each atom can quickly lead to the same result.

H··C··N: ⟶ H··C::N: ⟶ H—C≡N:

Resonance

In some cases a single correct Lewis structure cannot be drawn. Multiple possible Lewis structures often exist when multiple double and triple bonds can potentially exist depending on how one migrates lone pairs. Each of the possible structures is called a **resonance structure**. The actual molecule exists as a combination of all the possible structures and is called a **resonance hybrid**. The nitrate ion $[NO_3]^-$ provides a classic example of a resonance hybrid.

Following the four steps to create a Lewis structure we find:

1. Nitrogen is positioned to the left of oxygen in the periodic table and thus has the lower electronegativity. Our starting structure has nitrogen in the center with three bonds outward, one to each oxygen.
2. Nitrogen has five valence electrons and each oxygen has six valence electrons, plus we add an electron due to the anion charge for a total of 24 valence electrons. Six of those electrons go into our initial three single bonds.
3. Placing the remaining 18 electrons on the outer oxygen atoms completes our preliminary structure as shown here:

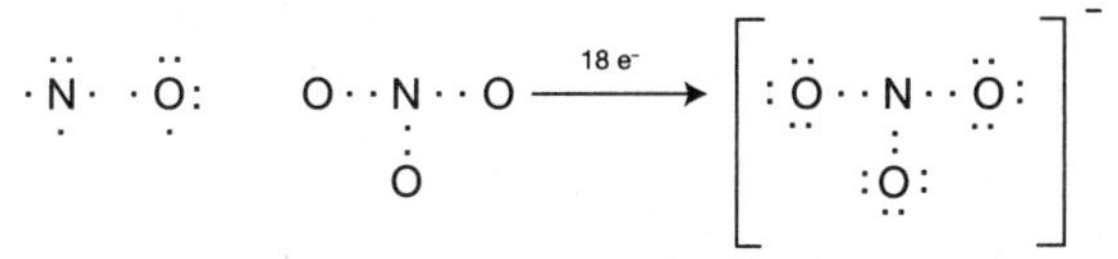

18 e⁻

4. Notice that nitrogen does not have a stable octet. Migrating a lone pair from one of the oxygen atoms will create one double bond and yield a stable octet for nitrogen. But which oxygen has the double bond with nitrogen? The answer is a combination of all of them. We can write three resonance structures with double-headed arrows to indicate the resonance:

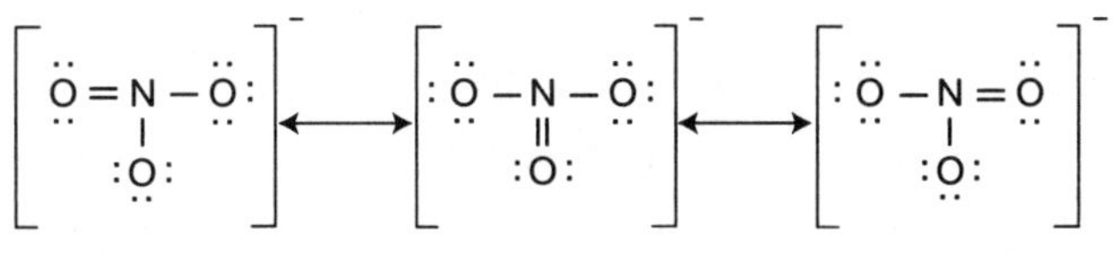

Spectral data indicate that all three of the nitrogen–oxygen bonds are the same. The actual molecular ion exists as a combination, a hybrid, of the resonance structures. To reinforce that concept we can represent the resonance hybrid as one structure using a dashed line as follows:

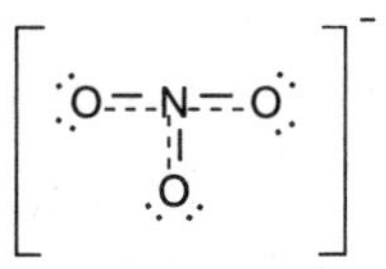

Formal Charge

In the previous example, the resonance structures for the nitrate ion (NO_3^-) changed only the position of the double bond, not the element involved in the bond. The resonance structures have the same energy and contribute equally to the composite resonance hybrid. Structures that are not so symmetrical do not contribute equally to the resonance hybrid. To evaluate relative energies of resonance structures requires a concept known as **formal charge**. Calculate the formal charge using the following formula:

$$C_f = V_e - N_e - \tfrac{B_e}{2} \quad \text{alternatively, substitute } B_n = \tfrac{B_e}{2}$$

where C_f is the formal charge, V_e is the number of valence electrons in the free atom, N_e is the number of nonbonding electrons on the atom, and B_e is the number of bonding electrons. As when counting electrons to determine a stable octet, both electrons in a bond count as bonding electrons, but this number is divided by half when calculating formal charge. Since each bond involves two electrons, an equivalent formula substitutes the bond order, B_n, for the halved bonding-electron number, B_e.

The following guidelines should be considered to determine the more stable resonance structure based on the calculated formal charges:

- For resonance structures of the same molecule, those structures with the fewest formal charges will be more stable and contribute more to the actual resonance hybrid.

- When formal charges are necessary, negative charges are more favored on more electronegative atoms, and, likewise, positive charges are more favored on the less electronegative atoms.

The calculation of formal charge assumes nonpolar covalent bonding. Highly polarized bonds may be less destabilized by a formal charge than would be figured based on this technique. The sum of the formal charges of the component atoms should equal the net molecular charge.

The cyanate ion $[NCO]^-$ provides an example of nonsymmetrical resonance structures. Following the steps to develop the Lewis structure, we determine two things:

1. The order of electronegativity from least to most follows the order C, N, O.
2. The valence electrons are C = 4, N = 5, and O = 6. Adding one electron for the anion charge gives us 16 electrons to distribute, of which four electrons go into our initial bonds.

Chemical Compounds and Nomenclature

This section reviews the representation of chemical compounds and nomenclature with which you should be familiar for the PCAT.

Molecular Mass, Moles, and Equivalents

To begin understanding how to represent simple compounds by formula and mass, the most important terms to start with are **molecular mass** and the definition of the **mole**. A mole is a unit of measurement (frequently abbreviated as mol), and a mole is equivalent to 6.022×10^{23} atoms. A simple analogy would be a dozen, meaning 12. This unit always refers to atoms. This number is called **Avogadro's number** (N_A). Regardless of the atom or molecule, the number of atoms in a mole never changes and is considered a constant, no matter what element is under consideration. The number of atoms in a mole of gold is equivalent to the number of atoms in a mole of lead.

Molecular masses are generally considered in grams of substance per mole (g mol^{-1}). The Periodic Table lists masses of atoms in grams per mole. The listed masses of each element are an average that takes into account the relative abundances of each atom's isotopes. So, in the case of the O_2 molecule, the mass can be determined by taking the masses from the Periodic Table for each atom and adding them together. Since one mole of O_2 contains two oxygen atoms, the mass of 15.999 g mol^{-1} added to another gives 31.988 g mol^{-1}. This means that 6.022×10^{23} atoms of O_2 would mass at about 32 grams.

Equivalent weight is based on the relative molar amounts that will (1) supply or react with one mole of H^+ ions in an acid-base reaction or (2) supply or react with one mole of electrons in a redox reaction. For example, H_3PO_4 has three hydrogens that can react in an acid-base reaction. So to calculate the equivalent weight, determine the molar mass of H_3PO_4 and divide by the reacting number of H^+. For example, 81.99 g mol^{-1} $\div$ 3 eq mol^{-1} = 27.33 g eq^{-1}. This gives the molar equivalent mass that will supply a reaction.

Representation of Compounds

The **Law of Constant Composition** states that a substance is always composed of the same components regardless of the process of its manufacture. For example, vitamin C is the same whether it is isolated from an orange or synthesized in a lab. Since the molecules are the same, they will have the same molecular formula. Another example would be carbon dioxide (CO_2) being generated from the combustion of wood compared to the intercellular breakdown of glucose by the body into H_2O and CO_2.

There are three common types of chemical formulas: empirical, molecular, and condensed. An empirical formula is the simplest whole-number ratio of atoms of each element in a molecule. A molecular formula identifies each atom in a molecule but not necessarily in the order of their structure. A condensed formula takes all atoms into account and is ordered to reflect structure. The following chart helps show how the formula types differ among molecule types.

SUBSTANCE	MOLECULAR FORMULA	EMPIRICAL FORMULA	CONDENSED FORMULA
water	H_2O	H_2O	H_2O
methane	CH_4	CH_4	CH_4
ethane	C_2H_6	CH_3	CH_3CH_3
sulfur	S_8	S	S_8
ethanol	C_2H_6O	C_2H_6O	CH_3CH_2OH
dimethyl ether	C_2H_6O	C_2H_6O	CH_3OCH_3

Each designation has its place depending on desired usage. Condensed formulas are important if structural isomers are common for a particular molecule, as they remove confusion regarding which molecule in particular is being discussed. This situation is often encountered in organic chemistry due to the large number of structural isomers that exist for even modestly sized molecules. Empirical formulas are useful when your focus is determining the ratios of the elements present in the molecule. Molecular formulas are the most common in small inorganic molecules and the common ionic anions.

To assist in describing molecular formulas of unknown compounds, the concept known as "percent composition" is very useful given the knowledge of the atoms contained in the sample along with the corresponding mass. Any sample of a pure molecule always consists of the same atoms combined in the same proportion by mass. This means that molecular composition can be shown in three ways:

1. In terms of number of atoms of each type per molecule or per formula unit, derived from the molecular formula
2. In terms of mass of each element per mole or per molecule of compound
3. In terms of the mass of each element in the compound relative to the mass of the overall compound (i.e., mass percent)

Determining Formulas of Compounds

Supposed you have 1.0 mol of BH_3 (mass 13.834 g mol^{-1}) and you want to determine the percentage compositions for the different atoms. The molecule consists of one boron atom (1.0 mol is 10.81 g mol^{-1}) and three hydrogen atoms (one mole equals mass 1.0079 g mol^{-1}, so three moles is 3.0237 g). To determine the percentage of mass made up from the boron, divide the boron's mass by the molecule's mass: $(10.810 \text{ g B} \div 13.834 \text{ g BH}_3) \times 100\% = 78.141\%$ boron. For completeness: $(3.0237 \text{ g H} \div 13.834 \text{ g BH}_3) \times 100\% = 21.883\%$ or 7.295% per hydrogen. Naturally, the total elemental composition for a given compound should always add to 100%.

Empirical and molecular formulas can be determined by percent composition. Given the elements in a sample, one can use this information along with the mass of the sample to derive the empirical formula. Given a 100 g sample of hydrazine, the percentage composition can be calculated to be 87.42% N and 12.58% H. Convert the percentages into grams: 87.42 g of N and 12.58 g of H. Next, convert each mass to moles by multiplying the mass by moles/grams. So, 87.42 g N × (1 mol N ÷ 14.01 g N) = 6.240 mol N. Hydrogen is treated the same way: 12.58 g H × (1 mol H ÷ 1.0079 g H) = 12.481 mol H. Finally, find the ratio by dividing 12.481 mol H by 6.240 mol N, giving a ratio of 2 mol H to 1 mol N. This gives the empirical formula of hydrazine, which is NH_2.

The empirical formula does not tell us everything; the molecular formular is also needed. To obtain this value, one needs experimental data. If experiments determine that the molecular weight of hydrazine is 30.04 g mol^{-1} and the empirical formula ratio is 2 mol H to 1 mol N, we can multiply the empirical formula NH_2 by the common factor of 2 to give the molecular formula $N_{(1 \times 2)}H_{(2 \times 2)}$. This gives the molecular formula N_2H_4, hydrazine.

Chemical Reactions and Stoichiometry

This section reviews the various types of chemical reactions that you should be familiar with for the PCAT exam, as well as net ionic equations, balancing equations, and stoichiometry.

Types of Chemical Reactions

A **combination reaction** is a chemical reaction in which two or more elements or molecules are combined to form products. The general form of this reaction is **A + B → AB**. Combination reactions are very common across all areas of chemistry. **Decomposition reactions** involve the chemical breakdown of one molecule into the two or more smaller products that together made up the larger molecule. This type of reaction is generally written as **AB → A + B**. Decomposition reactions happen naturally in unstable molecules and can be induced by heat or light. A **single-displacement reaction** exchanges an atom from one molecule with another. This is generally written as **A + BX → AX + B**. This type of reaction is common in ionic reactions. A **neutralization reaction** is an acid-base reaction that produces a salt and water as its products. A popular example is hydrochloric acid reacting with the base sodium hydroxide to form sodium chloride (table salt) and water. In full ionic form, $H^+ + Cl^- + Na^+ + OH^- \rightarrow H^+ + Cl^- + H_2O_{(l)}$.

Net Ionic Equations

Chemical equations are written with reactants (starting materials) on the left side of the reaction arrow and products on the right side. Ionic equations are used for reactions with ionic compounds reacting with one another. An example of a **chemical equation** would be $CaCl_{2(aq)} + 2\ AgNO_{3(aq)} \rightarrow Ca(NO_3)_{2(aq)} + 2\ AgCl_{(s)}$. The numbers before the molecules are called the stoichiometric coefficients, which are absolute values (they are always positive and can be fractions). The coefficients are used to balance equations. The ratios of reactants to products have to take into account all atoms and must be consistent with the **law of conservation of matter**. The lettered subscripts in parentheses reference the state that the molecule is in. Aqueous, dissociated into water solution, is represented by the subscript "aq." The regular states of matter are designated by "s" for solid, "g" for gas, and "l" for liquid. The reaction can also be written out in its **full ionic form**: $Ca^{2+} + 2\ Cl^- + 2\ Ag^+ + 2\ NO^{3-} \rightarrow Ca^{2+} + 2\ NO^{3-} + 2\ AgCl_{(s)}$. This shows all the separate ions; however, the $AgCl_{(s)}$ is still written together because it is not in aqueous solution. Silver chloride is insoluble in water, and forms a precipitate during this reaction. In **reduced balanced form** (also called the net ionic equation) only the ions forming nonaqueous product are shown. For example: $Ag^+ + Cl^- \rightarrow AgCl_{(s)}$.

Balancing Equations

Balanced chemical equations are starting points for quantifications of chemical reactions. Consider the reaction $Al_{(s)} + Cl_{2(g)} \rightarrow AlCl_3$. The components are there but the equation is not balanced because the number of atoms on the reactant side do not equal the atoms on the right. If the **stoichiometric coefficients** are included, the equation becomes $2\ Al_{(s)} + 3\ Cl_{2(g)} \rightarrow 2\ AlCl_3$, which accounts for all atoms. The stoichiometric coefficients are ratio amounts that can be read as: Two moles of Al plus three moles of chlorine gas produces two moles of aluminum chloride. A handy trick to balancing an equation is to set the coefficient of the diatomic chlorine equal to what is needed for the product side (3 Cl_2 is six chloride atoms; 2 $AlCl_3$ contains six chloride atoms) and the coefficient needed to finish balancing is usually obvious. Of course, increasing the number of reactants and products increases the challenge of correctly balancing the equation.

Stoichiometry

Stoichiometry deals with quantifiable relationships in chemistry. Balanced equations contain information, such as reactant/product ratios, that aid in determining mass relationships, determining the limiting reactant in a reaction, and finding product yields. Using the equation from the previous section, we see two moles of aluminum reacting with three moles of chlorine to form two moles of aluminum chloride. If only 3.0 g of aluminum are available, the amount of chlorine needed to consume all the aluminum can be determined. First, convert mass to moles: 3.0 g Al × (1 mol Al ÷ 26.98 g Al) = 0.1112 mol Al. Now that we have the molar amount of the aluminum we use the stoichiometric factor from the balanced equation. 0.1112 mol Al × (3 mol Cl_2 required ÷ 2 mol Al available) = 0.1668 mol Cl_2 required for the reaction to proceed to completion with all of the aluminum consumed. Last, simply convert the moles of Cl_2 to grams: 0.1668 mol Cl_2 × (70.90g Cl_2 ÷ 1 mol Cl_2) = 11.83g Cl_2, and the mass of chlorine gas needed for the reaction is determined.

Having the masses of reactants allows for the determination of mass of products. For example, if you had 3.0 g of Al and 11.83 g of Cl_2, you can again use the stoichiometric factor from the balanced equation to quantify a possible amount of product. 0.11 mol Al × (2 mol $AlCl_3$ produced ÷ 2 mol Al available) = 0.11 mol $AlCl_3$ produced. Converting to grams, 0.11 mol $AlCl_3$ × (133.33 g $AlCl_3$ ÷ 1 mol $AlCl_3$) = 14.83 g $AlCl_3$. Remembering the law of conservation of matter, 3.0 g of Al + 11.83 g Cl_2 = 14.83 g. This can also be called the theoretical yield of the reaction—theoretical because it is mathematically derived and doesn't reflect the reality of actually performing lab work: accidents, spills, incomplete reactions, and so on. To determine the actual percent yield of a reaction, the formula Percent yield = (Actual yield ÷ Theoretical yield) × 100 is used. The theoretical yield is the mathematical maximum that a reaction can produce. The actual yield is the mass of product divided by the mathematically derived theoretical yield. If the massed product of $AlCl_3$ was 9.94 g, then (9.94 g $AlCl_3$ ÷ 14.83 g $AlCl_3$) × 100 = 67.03% actual (product) yield. Any experimental yield above 90% is generally considered acceptable.

There are instances when a reaction has a limited supply of one reactant. In a reaction such as burning magnesium metal to form magnesium oxide, the metal burns until all of it is converted to oxide ($Mg_{(s)} + O_{2(g)} \rightarrow 2\ MgO_{(s)}$). If the magnesium is ignited in open air, the magnesium is the limiting reactant due to the fact that there is plenty of oxygen in the surroundings. If we take the reaction $2\ Al_{(s)} + 3\ Cl_{2(g)} \rightarrow 2\ AlCl_3$, and we're given 75 g Al and 50 g Cl_2 as starting materials, we can use stoichiometry to determine which reactant limits the reaction (i.e., is exhausted first) and which is in excess. Converting mass to moles, 75 g Al × (1 mol Al ÷ 26.98 g Al) = 2.78 moles Al available and 50 g Cl_2 × (1 mol Cl_2 ÷ 79.90 g Cl_2) = 0.63 moles Cl_2 available. The stoichiometric ratio of reactants required by the balanced equation is 3 mol Cl_2 ÷ 2 mol Al = 1.5 mol Cl_2 ÷ 1 mol Al. The ratio of reactants available is 0.63 mol Cl_2 ÷ 2.78 mol Al = 0.23 mol Cl_2 ÷ 1 mol Al. The chlorine required is 1.5 mol, but only 0.23 mol are available, so chlorine is the limiting reactant for this particular example. If the molar amount of chlorine was higher, the aluminum would be the limiting reactant.

Kinetics and Equilibrium

This section reviews reaction rates, reaction orders and the rate law, equilibrium and equilibrium constants, the law of mass action, and Le Chatelier's principle.

Reaction Rates

Chemical kinetics deals with the rates of chemical reactions (how fast they occur), which in turn depends on the reaction mechanism—how the reaction works at the molecular level. A **rate** is simply a unit of space over a unit of time, like a car that measures its rate of travel by looking at the change in distance over change in time. The **rate of a chemical reaction** is the change in concentration over the change in time (Rate of reaction = Change in concentration ÷ Change in time). Chemical rates are determined experimentally by measuring changes in concentrations of various chemical species. When a chemical reaction proceeds, the concentrations of the reactants decrease over time, with the concentrations of the products increase. Consider the decomposition of hydrogen peroxide, with the equation $2\ H_2O_2 \rightarrow 2\ H_2O + O_2$. As the reaction proceeds, the concentration of H_2O_2 decreases and this is measured along with the time until the concentration ceases to change. The concentration decrease could be measured by increased O_2 pressure or the overall pH change in the solution. To relate this mathematically: Rate of reaction = Change in concentration ÷ Change in time = $-\Delta[H_2O_2] \div \Delta t$, with concentration in mol L^{-1} and t in minutes. Say the concentration of H_2O_2 decreases to 1.4 moles from 2.5 moles over 45 seconds, which is 0.75 minutes. $-\Delta[H_2O_2] \div \Delta t = -(1.4\text{ mol L}^{-1}) - (2.5\text{ mol L}^{-1}) \div 0.75\text{ min.} = 1.47$ (mol H_2O_2 consumed ÷ L min.). This rate is in respect to change of H_2O_2, and can be performed in respect to products as well by the same method to determine rate of formation.

Reaction Orders and the Rate Law

The **rate law** is given by the general equation $r = k[A]^x[B]^y$, where A and B are concentrations of reactants in molarity (M with units moles L^{-1}) and k is the rate constant for the reaction. The exponents have to do with the order of the reaction and must be determined experimentally. If a catalyst is involved, it is included in the reactants even though it does not appear in the balanced equation. The **reaction order** is determined by the exponents of the rate equation. The reaction order is the sum of the exponents of the concentrations. So, in the reaction $r = k[H_2O_2]$, there is not an exponent so it is understood to be 1, making this is a first-order reaction. If MnO_2 was introduced as a catalyst, the rate would be $r = k[H_2O_2][MnO_2]$. Both are first-order reactions in respect to themselves but the overall order is 2. Doubling the concentration of one or the other would increase the rate by a factor of 2. To determine these exponents, several experiments are done with concentrations varied to determine the rate.

EXPERIMENT	$[H_2O_2]$ mol L^{-1}	$[MNO_2]$ mol L^{-1}	RATE mol L^{-1} s^{-1}
1	0.4	0.3	0.004
2	0.8	0.3	0.016
3	0.4	0.6	0.016
4	0.8	0.6	0.004

This comparison chart is an example of how to set up a concentration scheme to determine reaction order.

The **rate constant, *k*,** is a constant that relates rate and concentrations at a specific temperature. With the decomposition of H_2O_2, if the rate constant is 0.035 s^{-1} at 25°C, then Rate = (0.035 s^{-1}) × $[H_2O_2]$ at any concentration at the same temperature. Rate constants have different units depending on the order. The decomposition reaction is first-order, and k has units of time^{-1}. In second-order reactions, k has units of L mol^{-1} time^{-1}; in zero-order reactions, k has units of mol L^{-1} time^{-1}. To determine a rate equation, determine your rate as before and determine the order. Solving the equation for k supplies the rate constant for the temperature at which the reaction was performed.

Equilibrium and the Equilibrium Constant

Equilibrium can be thought of as a stable point where nothing changes; that is, there is no net change over time. It can also mean that the forward reaction and the reverse reaction are happening at the same rate with no noticeable change; this is called dynamic equilibrium. Equilibrium illustrates the reversibility of chemical reactions. **Equilibrium constants (*k*)** are determined at equilibrium point of a reaction by the general equation, $k = [C]^c \div [A]^a [B]^b$ (products over reactants). In the production of hydrochloric acid, with a balanced equation of $H_{2(g)} + Cl_{2(g)} \rightarrow 2\ HCl_{(g)}$, the equilibrium constant can be determined from $k = [HCl]^2 \div [H_2][Cl_2]$, with concentrations in molarity. If concentrations are given (i.e., $k = [0.0276]^2 \div [0.0037]\ [0.0037]$), then $k = 56$ at the specific temperature, volume, and pressure of the reaction. A chart referred to as the ICE table can assist in keeping track of molarities and changes in concentration.

EQUATION	$H_{2(g)}$	+	$Cl_{2(g)}$	$2HCl_{(g)}$
I = Initial concentration	0.0175		0.0175	0
C = Change in concentration as reaction proceeds to equilibrium	–0.0138		–0.0138	+0.0276
E = Equilibrium concentration	0.0037		0.0037	0.0276

Law of Mass Action

The **law of mass action** predicts behaviors of solutions. There are two areas: equilibrium, which is concerned with reaction mixture composition, and kinetics, which is concerned with rate equations for reactions. When two reactants A and B react together at a given temperature in a reaction, the affinity is proportional to the masses, [A] and [B], each raised to a particular power. The equation resembles the rate equation and is expressed by: Affinity = $\alpha\ [A]^x[B]^y$.

Le Chatelier's Principle

Le Chatelier's principle is stated as: "If a chemical system at equilibrium experiences a change in concentration, volume, or temperature, then there is an equilibrium shift to counteract that change and a new equilibrium is established." In a chemical system, if the concentration changes, it can affect the yield of products. Addition of more reactants will increase the equilibrium toward products since more reactants are available to collide and react. If more products are added, the equilibrium shifts toward reactants (removing products as they are formed can help control this). A change in volume can affect the equilibrium of a system. Since the basis of chemical reactions is molecules colliding, it should not be surprising that the larger the space, the less the chance for collisions, meaning reactant-favored equilibrium, while smaller volumes would shift the equilibrium toward products. This is especially true with gases. Changing temperature has two primary effects: alteration of solubility and energy supplied to the system. Many molecules are more soluble at higher temperatures. If solubility increases, there are more reactants in solution to react, shifting equilibrium toward products; if solubility decreases, less reactant will be in solution, meaning less product will be formed. If the temperature is increased, more energy is supplied to the system, and activation energy requirements are increasingly met. In an endothermic reaction the addition of heat will shift the equilibrium toward products. In an exothermic reaction (where heat is released and can be seen as a product), the equilibrium shifts toward products. Lowering the temperature has opposite effects.

Thermochemistry

Thermochemistry is the study of energy associated with chemical reactions. Energy can be released in the form of heat, light, electricity, or sound. Thermochemistry is useful for predicting and determining both the spontaneity and the favorability of a reaction, and is used in the calculations for heat capacity, enthalpy, and free energy. Thermochemistry is closely related to thermodynamics. The SI (International System of Units) energy unit is the joule (J), with 1 J = 1 kg m^2 s^{-2}. The kilojoule (kJ) is generally more convenient and is equivalent to 1,000 J.

Heat

Heat is a form of energy and should not be confused with temperature. Temperature is a measurement of heat content. Thermal energy is the sum of an object's individual energies of all its components. In thermochemistry it is helpful to view your reaction as the system, and the environment around your reaction as the surroundings. Heat transfer is unidirectional; heat will transfer only from a hotter body to a colder body until both are at the same temperature. Processes can be **endothermic**, which absorb energy from the surroundings, or **exothermic**, which release energy into the surroundings. Every object has a **specific heat capacity** (*C*) that is dependent on the quantity and chemical makeup of the material; it has units of J $g^{-1}K^{-1}$. It is the amount of energy required to raise one milligram of the substance by one degree Celsius. The quantity of the amount of heat gained or lost when a substance undergoes a temperature change is given by the equation $q = C \times m \times \Delta T$ (q = heat transferred in J, m = mass of substance, and ΔT = temperature change). Heat capacities of various substances can usually be found in reference books. The specific heat capacity of water is 4.184 J $g^{-1}K^{-1}$ and has a large impact on our planet. For example, it takes a large amount of energy to change the temperature of a lake. By contrast, aluminum has a very low specific heat capacity of only 0.897 J $g^{-1}K^{-1}$, so it transfers only a small amount of heat to another object at a time.

States and State Functions

The states of matter are solid, liquid, and gas. Every substance can exist in any of the states depending on the heat and pressure of the surroundings. A sample of ice kept in a freezer at 0°C does not have enough energy to keep the water molecules apart, so it exists as a solid. The amount of heat required to melt the ice is called the **heat of fusion**. As more heat is added, the liquid water heats to 100°C. At that point, the amount of energy required to completely evaporate the liquid water into steam (the gas state) is called the **heat of vaporization**. For water, these quantities are well known. The heat of fusion for water at 0°C is 333 J g^{-1} and the heat of vaporization at 100°C is 2,256 J g^{-1}. It is a simple task to calculate the amount of heat required to cause a phase change in, for example, 400 g of ice. To melt that much ice at 0°C requires (333 J g^{-1}) × (400 g) = 133,200 J or 133.2 kJ. To convert that same amount of water to gas at 100°C requires (2,256 J g^{-1}) × (400 g) = 902,400 J or 9,024 kJ. It is important to note that temperature remains constant during a phase change. Boiling water is always 100°C (at standard pressures), and the temperature of the liquid does not rise, no matter how much heat is applied, until all the water has evaporated.

A **state function** is a property of a system that depends only on the current state of the system, and it is independent of the path taken to get there. Enthalpy, entropy, and the Gibbs free energy are all state functions.

Enthalpy is the heat content of a substance at constant pressure. The enthalpy change (ΔH) in a reaction is the difference between the final and the initial heat content. Enthalpy measurements focus on the changes rather than overall value of heat. Enthalpy has sign conventions; a negative ΔH specifies that energy transfers from system to surroundings (exothermic), and a positive ΔH specifies that energy transfers from the surroundings to the system (endothermic). The enthalpy of a system can be calculated with the equation $H = U + pV$. In this equation, U is internal energy, p is pressure, and V is volume. Chemical reactions involve enthalpy changes. For example, the reaction of one mole of water in the equation $H_2O_{(g)} \rightarrow H_{2(g)} + \frac{1}{2} O_{2(g)}$ has a enthalpy change of $\Delta H = +241.8$ kJ. The value is positive, indicating that energy is being transferred from surroundings to system (endothermic). The reverse of the reaction $H_{2(g)} + \frac{1}{2} O_{2(g)} \rightarrow H_2O_{(g)}$ has an enthalpy change of –241.8 kJ. A negative value shows that energy is released from the system into the surroundings (exothermic; the reaction gives off heat). **Hess's law** states that if the overall reaction process is the sum of two or more reactions, then the overall ΔH is the sum of the ΔH values of all the reactions. A good example is combustion reactions in which the oxidation of $C_{(s)}$ to $CO_{2(g)}$ can be viewed as a two-step reaction. The first step is oxidation of $C_{(s)}$ to CO and the second step is the oxidation of CO to CO_2.

$C_{(s)}$	+	$\frac{1}{2} O_{2(g)}$	→	$CO_{(g)}$	$\Delta H_1 = ?$
$CO_{(g)}$	+	$\frac{1}{2} O_{2(g)}$	→	$CO_{2(g)}$	$\Delta H_2 = -283.0$ kJ
$C_{(s)}$	+	$O_{2(g)}$	→	$CO_{2(g)}$	$\Delta H_3 = -395.5$ kJ

Since the enthalpy of the second step and the overall reaction are known, enthalpy for the first step is a simple calculation. Since $\Delta H_3 = \Delta H_1 + \Delta H_2$, –393.5 kJ $= \Delta H_1 + (-283.0$ kJ), and therefore $\Delta H_1 = -110.5$ kJ. The enthalpy of a reaction can be calculated from the equation $\Delta H = \Sigma \Delta H_f$ (products) $- \Sigma \Delta H_f$ (reactants), or the sum of all products minus the sum of all reactants. The values for the enthalpies of the reactants and products for many reactions can be found in standard reference tables.

Another property of thermodynamics is **entropy**, which, like enthalpy, is a state function. It is defined in the third law of thermodynamics, which states that in a spontaneous process, entropy always increases. It is easier to think of entropy as a measure of disorder in a system. Mathematically it is expressed with the equation $\Delta S = q_{rev} \div T$, where q_{rev} is the heat absorbed and T is the temperature in Kelvin. The entropy S ends with units of J K^{-1} mol^{-1}. The reference point for entropy is defined at 0 K, where in a perfect crystal, $S = 0$. Conceptually with the idea of disorder, it helps to think about phases. Ice is in a crystal lattice with molecules in fixed locations and is definitely not as disordered as liquid water, where the molecules have more freedom of movement. Likewise, liquid water is not as disordered as water vapor since in a gas almost all intramolecular forces are nonexistent. The entropy of a reaction can be calculated by the equation $\Delta S = \Sigma \Delta S_f$ (products) $- \Sigma \Delta S_f$ (reactants).

Gibbs free energy is defined as the amount of free energy in a system. Free energy is the amount of energy available to do work. It is defined mathematically as $G = H - TS$, where H is enthalpy, T is temperature in

Kelvin, S is entropy, and G is the Gibbs energy with units of Joules. Gibbs energy is used to determine if a reaction is spontaneous (favored), not spontaneous (unfavored), or at equilibrium.

Note that spontaneity has nothing to do with the rate of a reaction! Many reactions are very slow but at the same time thermodynamically favored. A negative value of ΔG defines the reaction as spontaneous; a positive value of ΔG means it is not spontaneous; and if ΔG is 0, then the reaction is at equilibrium. Calculating the free energy of a reaction is done the same way as earlier: $\Delta G = \Sigma \Delta G_f$ (products) $- \Sigma \Delta G_f$ (reactants). This calculation is performed at a specific temperature.

Gas Phase and Gas Laws

This section reviews the gas phase and various gas laws and theories.

Ideal Gases

Only four quantities are required to describe the behavior of gases: pressure (P), temperature (T in units of Kelvin), volume (V), and amount of gas present (n, moles). Several gas laws help us fully understand the behavior of gases. **Boyle's law** deals with the compressibility of gases. This law states that for a fixed amount of gas at a given temperature, the volume is inversely proportional to the pressure. Mathematically, this can be written as $P \propto \frac{1}{V}$. If another term, the proportionality constant, C_B, is introduced into the equation, then $P = CB \times \frac{1}{V}$ where $PV = C_B$ when n (the number of moles of the particular gas) and T are both constant. Another form of Boyle's law is the equation $P_1V_1 = P_2V_2$, which again holds true when both n and T are constant. This equation is helpful when computing the volume change of a gas when the pressure is changed, as the equation can be rearranged to solve for any of the four variables. **Charles's law** states that the volume of a constant quantity of gas at constant pressure decreases with lowering of temperature. This volume-temperature relationship can be mathematically represented by $V = C_c \times T$, where C_c is the proportionality constant dependent on gas quantity and pressure. Boyle's law and Charles's law can be combined to make the general gas law. This is a useful merger because it eases calculation when two of the three parameters (P, V, and T) change but specifically the amount of gas does not change. Mathematically they can be combined into the equation $P_1V_1 \div T_1 = P_2V_2 \div T_2$ for a given amount of gas, n (measured in moles).

Gay-Lussac's law deals with combining volumes and states that the ratio of the volumes of reactant gases and the product gas can be expressed as whole numbers. Under standard temperature and pressure, three cubic meters of hydrogen (H_2) and one cubic meter of nitrogen (N_2) produce two cubic meters of ammonia (NH_3). In the balanced equation, $3\ H_2 + N_2 \rightarrow 2\ NH_3$, the coefficients show the volume change of the reaction without any needed calculation. **Avogadro's principle** states that equal volumes of gases under likewise conditions of temperature and pressure have an equal number of particles.

The **ideal gas law** gives rise to one of the most popular equations in science, the ideal gas equation: $pV = nRT$. The R is a constant equal to 0.082057 L atm K^{-1} mol^{-1}. The ideal gas law is the mathematical combination of the other gas laws. The law describes the behavior of ideal gases under standard conditions of temperature and pressure (STP, sometimes called STD). STP gives standard temperature and pressure, which are 273.15 K and 1 atmosphere (atm). Under those conditions, 1 mole of gas (behaving ideally) occupies 22.4 L. Real gases under standard pressure around one atmosphere and standard temperature behave closely enough to ideal gases for close approximations. Reorganization of the ideal gas equation to $d = m \div V = PM \div RT$, where d is density and M is molar mass, allows for calculation of gas density.

Dalton's Law of Partial Pressures

The air in Earth's atmosphere is a mixture of nitrogen, oxygen, carbon dioxide, water, and other trace gases such as argon and carbon monoxide. Each gas exerts part of the total pressure of the air; to account for this, chemists turn to **Dalton's law of partial pressure.** The partial pressure of one gas in the mixture exerts the pressure it would exert if it occupied the same volume by itself, so it is a sum of different pressures. Mathematically this is shown as $P_{total} = P_1 + P_2 + P_3 \ldots$, where P_1, P_2, and P_3 are the different pressures arising from the different gas components in the mixture. Since each gas acts independently, the ideal gas equation can be calculated for each gas separately and as a system. For a mixture of gases, it is useful to use **mole fractions** (x), which relate the moles of a particular substance to the total number of moles present. The equation for a three-component mixture would read $x_A = n_A \div (n_A + n_B + n_C) = n_A \div n_{total}$. The equation $P_A = x_A P_{total}$ gives the pressure that the single gas contributes to the whole. An example for determining mole fractions is as follows: Consider a container with a total pressure of 1.30 atm, holding 27 g of O_2 and 12 g of Cl_2. Convert the masses to moles: 27.0 g $O_2 \times$ (1 mol $O_2 \div$ 31.998 g O_2) = 0.844 mol, 12 g $Cl_2 \times$ (1 mol $Cl_2 \div$ 70.90 g Cl_2) = 0.169 mol. The second step is to convert to mole fraction: x_{Cl2} = 0.169 mol $Cl_2 \div$ 1.01 total moles = 0.167. Since there are only two gases, you can simply subtract the mole fraction for one gas from the total fraction to find the mole fraction for O_2: 1 – 0.167 = 0.833. As a final calculation, the partial pressures can be calculated via the equation $P_{Cl2} = x_{Cl2} \times P_{total}$. P_{Cl2} = 0.167 × 1.3 atm = 0.217 atm. P_{O2} = 1.30 atm – 0.217 = 1.08 atm.

Real Gases

As stated before, at STP real gases do not act much differently than ideal gases. To take into account the small differences encountered with real gases, the van der Waals equation was derived: $(P + a[n \div V]^2)(V - bn) = nRT$. The a is the correction for intermolecular forces. These forces are weak in gases but not nonexistent. The b is the correction for molecular volume. These are the van der Waals constants for different gases, and can be obtained from various reference sources.

Kinetic Molecular Theory of Gases

Our atmosphere is made up of particles, each of which has mass, and their movements are governed by the rules of physics. In gases, intermolecular forces that keep substances together are largely negated. The kinetic molecular theory of gases contains three central parts. First, gases are particles whose separation distance is much greater than the size of the particles themselves. Second, the average kinetic energy of particles in gas is proportional to the temperature. Last, the particles that make up gas are in random motion. As they move, they collide between themselves and the vessel walls without losing energy—a so-called elastic collision. Gas particles do not all travel at the same speed, but instead have a distribution of speeds. The kinetic energy of a molecule is given by the equation KE $- \frac{1}{2} \times$ Mass of molecule $\times$ Speed$^2 = \frac{1}{2} mv^2$ (v is velocity), and this is an average speed, so it is not uncommon to see a bar over KE and v. The average kinetic energy can also be given by KE $= \frac{3}{2} RT$, where R is the gas constant in SU (8.314 J K^{-1} mol^{-1}) showing the proportionality to temperature. When averages are used, it is not uncommon to use the root mean square of the speed $(u^2)^{\frac{1}{2}} = (3\ RT \div M)^{\frac{1}{2}}$, with M being molar mass. Gas pressure is caused by the force of collisions over a given area; envision a car tire, pressurized to 30 pounds per square inch.

Diffusion is the mixing of two or more gases due to random molecular motions. **Effusion** is movement of a gas from an area of higher pressure to an area of lower pressure.

Phases and Phase Changes

A **phase transition** is when a material changes from one phase (solid, liquid, gas), to another phase. Energy is what determines the state of a particular type of matter. These energies include **intermolecular forces**, which are forces that keep materials together; these forces are directly related to boiling points and melting points, and to solubility. To understand intermolecular forces, it is helpful to think of electron density as a cloud around an atom. Water is a common example of a **permanent dipole**. The oxygen has a higher **electronegativity** than the hydrogens, which causes electrons shared between the oxygen and the hydrogens to spend more time near the oxygen. This creates a partial negative charge on the oxygen and a partial positive charge on the hydrogens, causing the dipole. Molecules with dipoles are referred to as **polar**. When two water molecules approach each other, the electron cloud becomes distorted and the two molecules become attracted to each other in an electrostatic interaction called a dipole-dipole interaction.

Water has a high boiling point compared to many other molecules, and most of this is due to another type of intermolecular force called **hydrogen bonding**. This can happen when a hydrogen is bonded to a highly electronegative atom (oxygen, nitrogen). The leaves the hydrogen has a high positive partial charge that is fairly attractive to another highly electronegative atom. Water has two hydrogens that carry a partial positive charge and offers two hydrogen bonding sites for the oxygen in other water molecules. This type of intramolecular hydrogen bonding is quite strong, and raises the boiling point of molecules capable of this behavior, as the molecules stick together more efficiently in the liquid state.

Nonpolar molecules do not have permanent dipoles and are mostly insoluble in a polar medium; the principle "like dissolves like" is applied. Another interaction with a permanent dipole is a **dipole/induced-dipole interaction**, where a dipole is induced in a nonpermanent dipole by interactions of partial charge onto the nonpolar molecule. This process is called polarization and is generally easier to induce with larger electron clouds. In other words, the higher the mass, the more easily the molecule can be polarized. I_2 is a large nonpolar molecule that can be polarized by water and hence be made soluble. Without this induced dipole, I_2 would be insoluble.

London dispersion forces are induced-dipole/induced-dipole forces between two nonpolar molecules. These dually induced dipoles allow for nonpolar molecules to be soluble with each other.

Solids

Solids are the lowest entropy phase of matter. Solids can melt to a liquid or sublime to a gas (the gas-to-solid process is called deposition). The heat energy required to melt a solid at its melting point is the **enthalpy of fusion** (ΔH_{fusion}). The reverse of this process is the **enthalpy of crystallization**, defined by $-\Delta H_{fusion}$. If enough heat energy is applied fast enough, solids can sublime straight to the gas phase; this is governed by the $\Delta H_{sublimation}$. The atoms and molecules that make up solids are packed together more closely than in other phases. Common solids include ionic solids such as table salt that are held together by the ionic attraction of cations and anions. Metallic atoms, such as iron, pack together by electrostatic attraction. Molecular solids such as ice water hold together by hydrogen bonds, dipole forces, and London dispersion. Network solids like diamond are held together by a network of covalent bonds in three dimensions. Many solids for crystal lattices are made up of three-dimensional unit cells. A **unit cell** is a cross section of the molecular packing—how they are stacked together. Unit cells come in four types: simple cubic (sc), body-centered cubic (bcc), and face-centered cubic (fcc).

Liquids

Vaporization (or evaporation) is the change from the liquid state to the gas state (the gas-to-liquid transformation is called condensation). Liquids share some characteristics with gases, such as having an average kinetic energy. When a molecule in the liquid has enough kinetic energy to overcome the intermolecular forces between molecules, it can enter the gas phase. This process is endothermic, because energy is added to the system to gain the kinetic energy necessary to escape the surface of the liquid. The amount of heat energy needed to cause this vaporization for one mole of material is the **standard molar enthalpy of vaporization, ΔH_{vap}**. The reverse of this process is **condensation (ΔH_{con})**. When the gas phase loses heat energy, it can return to the liquid phase in an exothermic process. The enthalpy changes for vaporization and condensation are the same except that they differ by sign. Vaporization is positive since it is gaining energy and condensation is negative because it is losing energy. The amount of energy required is heavily influenced by both intermolecular and intramolecular forces.

In a closed container, liquid evaporates until the free space is saturated. At this point the rate of vaporization is the same as the rate of condensation, so the process is in equilibrium. Once the equilibrium is established, the vapor pressure of the liquid can be measured. **Volatility** is the tendency of a molecule to leave the liquid phase for gas. Organic liquids have many species that are volatile and evaporate very quickly, fast enough to see it happening.

The **Clausius-Clapeyron equation**, $\ln(P_2 \div P_1) = \Delta H_{vap} \div R[(1 \div T_1) - (1 - T_2)]$ ($R = 8.3145 \text{ J K}^{-1}$), provides a method for determining values of ΔH_{vap}. To use the equation with experimental data, the same substance would be set at a series of different temperatures and the resulting pressures recorded. If a sample of water was subjected to temperatures of 300 K (T_1) that measured 34.5 mmHg of pressure and then raised to 350 K (T_2) that measured 43.7 mmHg of pressure, the resulting ΔH_{vap} would be: $\ln(43.7 \text{ mmHg} \div 34.5 \text{ mmHg}) = \Delta H_{vap} \div 0.0083145 \text{ kJ K}^{-1}[1 \div 300 \text{ K} - 1 \div 350 \text{ K}]$, resulting in a $\Delta H_{vap} = 4.13 \text{ kJ mol}^{-1}$. Notice the ideal gas constant was converted to kJ in this problem.

Phase Diagrams

Phase diagrams are charts that can be used to reference the phases of a substance between two quantities. A simple phase diagram would be a plot of pressure on the *y*-axis and temperature on the *x*-axis. The temperature/pressure relationship between phase changes is quite laid-out on these charts.

Three particular areas of the chart are interesting, and those are the triple point, the critical point, and the phase boundaries. A **phase boundary** is the line between two phases, and along this line the two phases exist in equilibrium. In the case of a boundary between ice water and liquid water, some liquid and some ice would exist in the same space. The **triple point** is at an exact temperature and pressure where all three phases exist at one space. So in water, one space would have all three phases in equilibrium. Above the **critical point** the liquid and gas phases become indistinguishable and the combined material is called a supercritical fluid.

Colligative Properties

Colligative properties are properties of solutions and depend on concentrations of the different species. These properties include changes in vapor pressure, changes in phase change temperature, and osmotic pressure. **Raoult's law** states that the vapor pressure of a solution is the sum of the pressure created by its parts. It is not much different from the partial pressure seen with gas laws and is expressed mathematically as: $P_{solvent} = X_{solvent} \times P_{solvent}$. When liquids are mixed together, the boiling point of the resultant mixture can be elevated or depressed. To calculate this change, the equation $\Delta T_{BP} = K_{BP} \times$ (Moles of compound added $\div$ Mass of solution) is used. K_{BP} is the molar boiling point elevation constant from reference. Freezing point depression follows a similar equation: $\Delta T_{FP} = K_{FP} \times$ (Moles of compound added $\div$ Mass of solution). A common example is seen in the winter when salt is put on ice to get it to melt. Addition of the salt lowers the freezing point of the water.

Osmosis is the migration of solvent molecules from an area of high concentration to one of low concentration via semipermeable membranes (a lining with very small holes that allow small molecules to pass through). This phenomenon is how our cells control their water content. If a solution of charged ions is placed in a semipermeable bag and then placed in water, water molecules will migrate into the bag. The driving force is the **osmotic pressure**, which pushes water from the more dilute area into the more ionically concentrated area. The osmotic pressure can be calculated by the equation $\Pi = cRT$, where c is the molar concentration in moles per liter, R is the gas constant, and T is temperature.

Solutions

This section reviews various information with respect to solutions that you should be familiar with for the PCAT exam.

Nature of Solutions

A **solution** is a homogeneous mixture of more than one substance in a single phase. Solutions commonly are liquids in the laboratory. The **solvent** is the compound in which the other component, the **solute**, is dissolved. Sugar dissolved in a glass of water is a solution; solder is a solid solution of lead and tin. When a soluble solid is placed in solution, the solid dissolves. With ionic substances, the molecule dissociates into cation and anion components that are surrounded and stabilized by molecules in the solution. The equation for the dissolution of table salt is: $NaCl_{(s)} \rightarrow Na^{+}_{(ag)} + Cl^{-}_{(ag)}$. **Solubility** is defined as the mass of solute that will dissolve in a mass of solvent, and is dependent on intermolecular forces and temperature. Liquids mix to different extents just as solids do. If a liquid is soluble in another liquid, it is called *miscible*. If liquids do not mix, they are referred to as *immiscible*. Liquid-liquid mixtures follow the "like prefers like" principle. Ethanol is miscible with water. Both molecules are polar due to OH groups that they contain. Two nonpolar compounds are miscible with each other (wax and oil), but a nonpolar compound will not be miscible with a polar compound (oil and water do not mix). In this case one liquid will sit on top of the other. The liquid with the greater density will be below the one with less density. A **supersaturated** solution contains as much solute as the solvent can dissolve or mix with. If you put too much sugar in water, it will eventually stop dissolving and the extra solid sugar will sit at the bottom of the vessel. Heat can change the solubility of a solute.

Ions

Liquids can contain many ions that cannot be seen with the naked eye. Water is generally successful at dissolving ionic solids since water has a partial negative charge on the oxygen and partial positive charges on the hydrogens. In solution, water molecules surround both cations and anions, with the oxygen in water pointing toward the cation and the hydrogens pointed toward the anion. If electrodes are put into the solution, the normal evenly distributed dissociation is disturbed, and the anions move to the positive electrode and the cations move toward the negative electrode. Ions in solution make good conductors for electricity and in this sense are termed **electrolytes**, since they make possible the passage of electrical current. Those compounds that dissolve but do not ionize are called nonelectrolytes.

SOLUBLE MOLECULES	EXCEPTIONS
most ionic molecules with Na^+, K^+, NH_4^+	halides (Cl^-, Br^-, I^-) of Pb^{2+}, Hg^{2+}, Ag^+
most nitrates $(NO_3)^-$	group 2 metals with fluoride
most chlorates, $(ClO_3)^-$	group 2 metals with sulfate
acetate $(CH_3CO_2)^-$	carbonate, phosphate, chromate with NH_4^+, and group 1 cations
most ionic molecules with halogens, F^-, Cl^-, Br^-, I^-	
most sulfates, SO_4^{2-}	

INSOLUBLE MOLECULES	EXCEPTIONS
most carbonates, CO_3^{2-}	
most phosphates, PO_4^{3-}	
most chromate, CrO_4^{2-}	
most sulfides, S^{2-}	
most oxides, hydroxides	

The chart shows some of the trends of ionic molecules in water. The exceptions can be useful for certain reactions since products that form may be insoluble.

In **net ionic equations** only ions that form products of different phase are included. For example, the total reaction $Na^+_{(aq)} + Cl^-_{(aq)} + Ag^+_{(aq)} + NO^-_{3(aq)} \rightarrow AgCl_{(s)} + Na_{(aq)} + NO^-_{3(aq)}$ lists every ion in solution. In the net ionic equation, only the reactant ions that are part of the product and the nonaqueous products are listed; for example, $Cl^-_{(aq)} + Ag^+_{(aq)} \rightarrow AgCl_{(s)}$. The other ions are called spectator ions because they do not take the part in the reaction to form products.

Concentration

Concentrations in liquid solutions can be measured as **molarity (uppercase M)** and as **molality (lowercase m)**. Molarity is defined as: Molar concentration of a specific solute = Moles of specific solute ÷ Volume of overall solution in liters. Molarity is the commonly used measurement used in the laboratory setting but does have the drawback that the exact amount of solvent used to make the solution is unknown. Since the common technique for making a solution is solvent added after solutes are added, in a 1-liter vessel one only knows that the amount is close to a liter. Molality is defined as: Molality of solute = Amount of solute (mol) ÷ Mass of solvent (kg). In this type of measurement, the exact amounts of both solute and solvent are known.

Weight percent is the mass of one compound divided by the total mass of the mixture: Weight % of compound (g) = Mass of specific compound ÷ Total mass mixture (g). Mole fraction of a liquid is performed in the same fashion as gases: Mole fraction of specific compound $(X_A) = n_A \div n_A + n_B + n_C$; $X_A + X_B = 1.0$.

Solution Equilibriums

Several factors in solution can change the amount of solute that dissolves in a given solvent. Temperature is a large factor in solubility. Generally speaking, liquids and solids experience an increase in solubility with rising temperature. Gases do not necessarily follow this trend; carbon dioxide is more soluble in cold water than in hot water. The energetics of gas solubility in liquid does follow Le Chatelier's principle, which was seen before in reactions. When heat is added to solution, the equilibrium shifts in response to the incoming energy. In the reaction Gas + Liquid $\rightleftarrows$ Saturated solution + Heat, adding energy shifts the equilibrium to the left, giving free gas and solvent. The energy of a solution is mathematically determined by: $\Delta H_{hydration} - \Delta H_{lattice} = \Delta H_{solution}$. The enthalpy of the crystal lattice (the solid structure of ionic solids) is always negative if it is stable. For heat of solution, a simple chart assists calculation.

formation of ionic molecule	$Na_{(s)} + \frac{1}{2} Cl_2 \rightarrow NaCl_{(s)}$	$\Delta H_f = -411.12$ kJ mol^{-1}
dissolving ionic molecule	$NaCl_{(s)} \rightarrow NaCl_{(aq)}$	$\Delta H_{soln} = +3.88$ kJ mol^{-1}
net process	$Na_{(s)} + \frac{1}{2} Cl_2 \rightarrow NaCl_{(aq)}$	$\Delta H_f = -407.24$ kJ mol^{-1}

The energy is calculated by the equation $\Delta H_{soln} = \Sigma\ [\Delta H_f\ (\text{products})] - \Sigma\ [\Delta H_f\ (\text{reactants})]$, with each enthalpy available in references.

Acid-Base Reactions

This section reviews acid-base reactions.

Definitions of Acid-Base Concepts

There are four major acid-base concepts of behavior. The **Arrhenius concept** states that acids produce hydrogen cations (hydronium) in aqueous solution (water). The equation for an Arrhenius acid-base reaction can be written as Acid + Base → Salt + Water. A simple example is hydrochloric acid reacting with sodium hydroxide and forming aqueous sodium chloride and water. The drawback of the Arrhenius concept is that it is suitable for use only in aqueous liquid solutions and a small group of molecules.

Other systems improved upon this acid-base concept. The **Bronsted-Lowry concept** of acid-base chemistry defines an acid as a donator of hydrogen cations and a base as an acceptor of hydrogen cations. This idea encompasses the Arrhenius theory and can include gas reactions. This is where the idea of **conjugate acids and bases** comes from. Conjugate acids and bases generally differ from each other by only a hydrogen atom. A strong acid has a weak conjugate base and a strong base has a weak conjugate acid. Hydronium (H_3O^+) and water (H_2O) is a conjugate acid-base pair.

The **solvent system concept** states that ions dissociate from the solvent and can be anions or cations; it is a base if anions are present and it is an acid if cations are present. Water is the classic example: 2 $H_2O \Leftrightarrow H_3O^+ + OH^-$, with H_3O^+ being the acid and OH^- being the base.

The **Lewis acid-base concept** defines an acid as an electron pair acceptor and a base as an electron pair donor. Lewis acid-base theory is very useful when discussing the behavior of transition metals. The classic example of a Lewis acid-base reaction is the reaction of BF_3 and NH_3. In the reaction an **adduct** forms between the lone pair on the nitrogen in the NH_3 and the empty *p*-orbital on the boron atom in BF_3. Due to the fluorines, the boron carries a partial positive charge and is therefore an attractive target for the electron pair.

Properties of Acids and Bases

One of the most commonly encountered properties of acids and bases is pH. The pH is defined mathematically by: $pH = -\log_{10}[H_3O^+]$, with $[H_3O^+]$ being the concentration of hydronium ion in solution. You can calculate the pOH in a similar way: $pOH = -\log_{10}[OH^-]$). The pH and pOH add to 14. The common range of pH values is from 0 to 14. High hydronium concentrations mean a lower pH and a stronger acid; inversely, high pH values mean a stronger base. Pure water is pH 7.00, or neutral in terms of acidity.

An equilibrium constant for acids and bases (K_a) is the procedure of quantitatively representing strengths of acids and bases. To calculate this value: $K_a = [H^+][A^-] \div [HA]$, which are the concentrations of hydronium multiplied by the concentration of anion, divided by the nondissociated concentration of acid. K_b for bases can be calculated in the same fashion. Large values of K_a correlate with high acid strength, higher percentage of dissociation, and lower pH. High values of K_b correlate to higher base strength and higher pH. pK_a is the logarithmic scale of relative acid strength.

Salt Formation

A **salt** is an ionic compound formed from an acid-base reaction. Salts are ionic substances containing both a cation and an anion and are overall electrically neutral. They are acidic or basic depending on the ions released when dissolved in solution. If hydronium is produced, the salt is considered acidic; and if hydroxide is produced, it is considered basic. It is important not to confuse a salt with zwitterions (molecules containing both anionic and cationic parts yet bound together with covalent bonds). The most common salt encountered in everyday life is table salt, NaCl.

Polyvalence and Normality

Polyvalence refers to the number of bonds an atom can form. *Poly-* refers to more than one. Group 1 metals are univalent, forming only one bond to another atom, as do halogens in most cases. Oxygen is divalent, and carbon is tetravalent. Organometallics tend to be either tetravalent or hexavalent.

Normality is a type of concentration measurement that is useful when dealing with salts in solution. Since salts dissolve into different species, normality takes into account ratios of cations and anions. Group 2 metals generally carry +2 charges in ionic compounds. For $Ca(OH)_2$ there is one Ca^{2+} for two OH^-, so the OH^- is called 2*N* in respect to Ca^{2+}. Acids that can give off more than one proton have to count each acidic hydrogen. A monoprotic acid like HNO_3 equates 1 mol = 1 gram equivalent. The mathematical expression is N = Gram equivalent ÷ Liters solution.

Amphoteric Species

An **amphoteric species** is a molecule that can react as both an acid and a base. This is common in biological molecules such as amino acids. Metalloids such as boron and metals such as aluminum and tin have oxides or hydroxides with amphoteric characteristics and are generally zwitterions. These species commonly follow Bronsted-Lowry acid-base behavior. Water is the most common amphoteric molecule. It acts as a base when reacting with HCl but acts like an acid when reacting with ammonia (NH_3).

Titrations and Buffers

Titrations are an important laboratory technique for quantifying the amount of acid, base, or another compound in a solution. The classic strong acid/strong base reaction is between HCl and NaOH in equal concentrations. When a strong base is added to a weak acid, the pH rises slowly until it reaches a smaller interval between 49% and 51% base. The pH at 50% strong acid/50% strong base is 7. From 0% base to 49% base the pH changes only from 1 to 3. This is a common pH behavior. Any acid and base mixed at a 1:1 ratio will have a particular pH called the **equivalence point**. Within 1% of that point there is a rapid change in pH. A titration curve is a two-dimensional graph with pH on the *y*-axis and volume of added compound on the *x*-axis. During a titration an indicator can be used to show when the equivalence point is reached. There are several indicators that show a color change at the equivalence point, each with its own pH range. Here is an example titration between a weak acid and a strong base: acetic acid and NaOH. The balanced equation is $CH_3CO_2H + {}^-OH \rightarrow H_2O + CH_3CO^-_{2(aq)}$. If we have 0.2 mol of CH_3CO_2H and 0.15 mol of NaOH, we can compute the pH with the help of a chart.

initial	0.2 mol CH_3CO_2H	0.15 mol NaOH	0 mol $CH_3CO_2^-$
change	–0.15 mol CH_3CO_2H	–0.15 mol NaOH	+0.15 mol $CH_3CO_2^-$
after reaction	0.05 mol CH_3CO_2H	0 mol NaOH	0.15 mol $CH_3CO_2^-$

So pH = pK_a + log(Conjugate base produced ÷ Weak acid remaining). The pH = 4.78 + log(0.15 ÷ 0.05) = 5.26. In this equation you can see the relationship between concentrations and pH change.

Titrating weak acids with strong bases is a different case. A weak acid will not have a very low pH compared to a strong acid. A **buffer** resists change in pH. Take acetic acid (a weak acid) and sodium acetate, good for a 3.8 to 5.5 pH range, as an example. If a solution of acctic acid has a base introduced, such as NaOH, sodium acetate is formed, which is the conjugate base of acetic acid. The equation for determining pH between the start and the equivalence point is pH = pK_a + log(Conjugate base produced ÷ Weak acid remaining). At the equivalence point, pH = pK_a. A buffer can resist pH change only so far. Sticking with acetic acid as an example, setting up an ICE chart (see the following) can assist in determining pH changes. We have to know the concentrations of weak acid and its conjugate base; for the given example, we're going to adopt the values of 0.450M and 0.375M, respectively. The solvent in this case is water. $CH_3CO_2H + H_2O \rightarrow H_3O^+ + CH_3CO_2^-$

CONCENTRATION (IN MOLARITY)			
initial	CH_3CO_2H	$\rightarrow H_3O^+$	$+CH_3CO_2^-$
change	0.450	0	0.375
equilibrium	–x	+x	+x
	0	x	0.375 + x
	0.450 – x		

Using this chart, solve for x from the equation K_a = $(x)(0.375 + x) \div 0.450 - x$. The interactive K_a value of acetic acid is 1.75×10^{-5}. Due to the small sizes of x, it can be assumed that it has a negligible effect on the large values of 0.375 and 0.450. So, an easier approximation is $K_a = (x)(0.375) \div 0.450$. The variable x (which is the concentration of hydronium ion) = 2.10×10^{-5}, so the pH = $-\log(2.10 \times 10^{-5}) = 4.68$.

Redox Reactions and Electrochemistry

This section reviews redox reactions and electrochemistry concepts that you should be familiar with for the PCAT exam.

Oxidation and Reduction Reactions

Oxidation-reduction (redox) reactions are reactions that involve electron transfer between two species. Oxidation is the loss of electrons, and reduction is the gaining of electrons. In this type of reaction, one species is the oxidizing agent; it oxidizes the other species and is itself reduced. A reducing agent reduces the other species and is itself oxidized. In redox equations, the number of electrons, as well as the atoms, must balance on both sides of the equation. The **oxidation number** can assist in determining whether a species has been oxidized or reduced. Oxidation numbers can be seen in a similar way as charge in some cases, and this works well for metals. Pure elements have an oxidation number of 0. Monoatomic ions have the same oxidation number as charge; for example, Ca^{2+} is oxidation number 2. Oxygen has an oxidation number of –2, except when bonded to another oxygen or a halogen. Halogens (F, Cl, Br, I) have an oxidation number of –1. The sum of oxidation numbers must be equal to the overall charge of the molecule.

It is important to understand that an oxidation reaction requires a corresponding reduction reaction to occur; one requires the other. *Redox* is often the term for this type of reaction since both happen at the same time. When balancing oxidation-reduction equations, it is helpful to first write them as half-reactions (see chart). One reaction describes the reduction part of the reaction and the other the oxidation part. The half-reactions are then combined for the overall balanced ionic equation.

reduction half-reaction	$2Cu^{+}_{(aq)} + 2e^{-} \rightarrow 2Cu_{(s)}$
oxidation half-reaction	$Zn_{(s)} \rightarrow ZN^{2+}_{(aq)} + 2e^{-}$
overall balanced ionic equation	$2Cu^{+}_{(aq)} + Zn_{(s)} + \cancel{2e^{-}} \rightarrow 2Cu_{(s)} + ZN^{2+}_{(aq)} + \cancel{2e^{-}}$

The number of electrons should balance and cancel out in a properly balanced equation. These equations have to be balanced differently if in acidic or basic solution. In acidic solution, balance for all atoms except oxygen and hydrogen. Balance oxygen by adding water molecules to the side of the equation that requires oxygen atoms. Balance water hydrogens by adding hydrogens to the opposite side. In basic solution OH^{-} is added to the side lacking oxygen. Water is added to the other side to balance OH^{-}. Just as with electrons, H^{+}, OH^{-}, and H_2O subtract from the opposite side.

Electrochemical and Electrolytic Cells

The transfer of electrons from one species to another (the flow of electrons) causes an electrical current. If a strip of copper metal (Cu) is placed into an $NaNO_3$ solution in one beaker and a zinc (Zn) strip is placed into an $NaNO_3$ solution in another beaker, then two half-cells are made. Connecting the two with a salt bridge ($NaNO_3$ is common) and a wire (electrode) from one strip to another makes a simple voltaic cell. A salt bridge is an ionic compound dissolved in solution that is itself an electrolyte to assist in the flow of current. The **anode** is the electrode (metal strip) where oxidation occurs; the **cathode** (other metal strip) is where reduction occurs. In this case using the $2\ Cu^{+}_{(aq)} + Zn_{(s)} \rightarrow 2\ Cu_{(s)} + ZN^{2+}_{(aq)}$ reaction, Cu is the cathode (+ charge, like on a 9-volt battery) and Zn is the anode (– charge). In the salt bridge, NO_3^{-} anions move toward the ZN^{2+} being produced in the anode and Na^{+} moves toward the anode, and current flows from the anode to the cathode. As ZN^{2+} cations are produced, Na^{+} leaves the cell; in the other half-reaction, NO_3^{-} leaves as Cu is reduced. The current produced can easily be measured by a voltmeter. Each half-reaction carries with it a voltage associated with it, all based on hydrogen, which is zero volts. The potential of the $Cu^{+}_{(aq)} \rightarrow Cu_{(s)}$ half-reaction is 0.521 V. For the half-reaction $Zn_{(s)} \rightarrow ZN^{2+}_{(aq)}$, the potential is 0.763 V. The total cell potential is given by $E^{o}_{cell} = E^{o}_{cathode} - E^{o}_{anode}$, which in this case comes to 0.242 V. Cells under nonstandard conditions, like most batteries in real life, can be understood with the **Nernst equation**, $E = E^{o} - (RT \div nF) \ln Q$. F is the Faraday constant of $9.645 \times 10^{4}\ C\ mol^{-1}$, R is the gas constant, T is temperature, n is number of moles, and Q is the reaction quotient. If the temperature remains constant at 25°C, the equation can be simplified to $E = E^{o} - (0.0257 \div n) \ln Q$. The purpose of this equation is to correct for nonstandard conditions or concentrations. The equation can also be used to determine an unknown concentration if the cell potential is already known by solving for n; $n = [(E^{o} - 0.0257) \div E] \ln Q$.

Reductive Potentials and Electromotive Force

We've just seen voltages used as a way to determine a voltaic cell's voltage. The voltages for a half-reaction by themselves indicate favorability of the reduction happening. Positive voltages are favored reactions, while negative voltages are not favored. For example, $ZN^{2+} \rightarrow Zn$ has a reduction potential of –0.763 V, which is not favorable. The opposite reaction, $Zn \rightarrow ZN^{2+}$, is +0.763 V. This shows you that the reduction of ZN^{2+} is not favored but the oxidation of Zn is. The **electromotive force (emf)** is the work per unit charge to produce electrical current. Emf is in units of volts ($1V = 1J \div 1C$). The electric potential difference is created by opposing positive and negative charges, which creates an electrical field. This electrical field pushes current flow. Voltaic cells generate emf because the current is generated from the spontaneous chemical reactions taking place inside them.

Thermodynamics of Redox Reactions

Thermodynamics states that internal energy (U or ΔE) is related to heat (q) and work (w), $\Delta E = q + w$. In a voltaic cell, the internal energy decreases with electrical work performed on the surroundings. The maximum work done by a voltaic cell is given by $w_{max} = nFE$, where E is cell voltage, F is Faraday's constant, and n is moles. Free energy, ΔG, is related to w_{max}, and for the system, $\Delta G^o = -nFE^o$. Since the energy content of the surroundings increases with work, nFE is positive in the max work equation. The system is negative, as shown in the ΔG^o, due to the energy decreasing. Batteries don't really die; the reaction just reaches equilibrium. Concentrations of reactants decrease, lowering the amount of maximum work that can be done. E^o can be related to the equilibrium constant K mathematically by the expression, $\ln K = nE^o \div 0.0257$ at 25°C.

Nuclear Chemistry

Nuclear chemistry is an area of chemistry where the actual nuclei of atoms undergo a change. The reactions that we have seen previously deal with electrons and formation or breaking of bonds that are themselves sharing of electrons. Radioactivity is a natural process in which unstable nuclei give off radiation in the form of α (alpha) radiation, β (beta) radiation, and γ (gamma) radiation. When a nucleus gives off an alpha particle, the nucleus ejects a particle containing two neutrons and two protons, a helium atom. The atom loses two atomic numbers due to the loss of two protons. The equation for an alpha particle is $^{238}_{92}U \rightarrow {}^{4}_{2}\alpha + {}^{234}_{90}Th$. Alpha particles are the least penetrating of radioactive radiation and can be blocked by any matter even as thin as a sheet of paper. Another form of emission from decay is β particles; a neutron ejects an electron, becoming a proton. In β decay the atomic number goes up by one: $^{223}_{87}Fr \rightarrow {}^{0}_{-1}e + {}^{223}_{88}Ra$. β decay can be stopped by a thin sheet of lead. γ radiation does not change the mass of the an atom but is by far the highest energy. γ radiation is the same as gamma rays in the electromagnetic spectrum. Radioactive decay of an element can undergo a series of alpha and beta decay to become stable. There are other types of radioactive decay that follow along the mass changes of alpha and beta decay. Two of these are positron emission ($^{0}_{1}\beta$) and electron capture ($^{0}_{-1}e$). In positron emission, a positron (antimatter version of an electron) is emitted. In electron capture, an electron is pulled into the nucleus and goes into a proton, rendering its charge zero and converting it to a neutron.

The **half-life** of a radioactive atom is the amount of time it takes for half of the nuclei in a sample to undergo a nuclear reaction and change. Half-lives can vary from milliseconds to thousands of years depending on the element. The stability of atomic nuclei is highest at low atomic numbers (<20) with a neutron-to-proton ratio of 1:1. As the atomic number grows, stable nuclei have more neutrons than protons. After atomic number 83 (bismuth), all isotopes are unstable and undergo decay. If a radioactive atom has too many neutrons, it tends to undergo alpha emission to lose neutrons. If it has too few protons, it will undergo beta emission to increase atomic number. The **band of stability** graphs neutrons on the *y*-axis and protons on the *x*-axis. The further from the center, the shorter the half-life for decay.

Nuclear binding energy is the amount of energy required to separate a nucleus into the components of the nucleus, protons, and neutrons. The H_2 bond energy is 437 kJ mol^{-1}, but the energy needed to separate the proton and neutron in deuterium (hydrogen isotope with a neutron) is 2.14×10^8 kJ mol^{-1}. There is an observation that the mass of an actual nucleus is always less than the sum of the masses of protons and neutrons called the **mass defect (Δ*m*)**. It is thought that the missing mass could be explained by equating it to the energy that holds the nucleus together. The loss of mass can be calculated by determining the change in mass of reacting particles. A deuterium (^2_1D) masses 2.0141 g mol^{-1} and comes from ^1_1H, at 1.007825 g mol^{-1} and a neutron, 1.008665 g mol^{-1}. By subtracting the mass of reactants from the mass of products the mass defect can be seen, in this case 0.00240 g mol^{-1}. The mass defect can be put into the equation $E = \Delta mc^2$, giving a binding energy per mole of 2.157×10^{14}. Dividing the energy by the number of particles (protons or neutrons) in the nucleus, termed nucleons, gives the binding energy associated with each nucleon in the nucleus. This energy can be used to show which atoms have the most stable nuclei. Atoms with mass number between 50 and 80 (vanadium to bromine) have the most stable nuclei.

Nuclear chemistry can be applied in several ways. One example is carbon-14 (^{14}C) dating, which measures age by comparing the amount of the isotope in the object of interest to the relative amount in the atmosphere. Carbon makes up a high proportion of all living matter. Carbon-14 is created when high-energy photons from our sun strike the upper atmosphere and cause an electron capture reaction that converts ^{14}N to ^{14}C. This is then taken up by CO_2 respiration in plants and can pass on to animals that consume the plants. When something dies, it ceases to take up ^{14}C. The drawback of carbon dating is that it cannot be used on something that is either too young, where not enough decay has happened (less than 100 years), or too old, where too much decay has happened (over 40,000 years).

Inside nuclear reactors, neutrons are fired at ^{235}U, creating ^{236}U that is very unstable, and the atom fission breaks apart into ^{141}Ba, ^{92}Kr, and 3^1_n simultaneously and releases a larger amount of energy (2×10^{10} kJ mol^{-1}) in the form of heat. The heat transfers water running into the system into steam, which turns a turbine. This is a chain reaction because the particles that come from fission of uranium can go on to strike other uranium atoms and cause fission in them. If the supply for neutrons is stopped, the reaction will die down. To control the rate of fission, cadmium rods are used because they can absorb neutrons. Twenty percent of the world's electricity comes from this type of generation.

Nuclear chemistry also has medicinal uses. Everyone is exposed to a certain amount of radiation from natural decay of radioactive elements in the enviroment. The unit for biological radiation is the rem. Some other natural sources of radiation other than ^{14}C and ^{235}U are ^{40}K, ^{232}Th, ^{238}U, and ^{86}Rn. The average human in the United States receives less than 200 mrem a year, much from natural sources. A single large dose can cause damage. A typically performed diagnostic X-ray accounts for about 50 mrem per year for the average person. Medical imaging uses radioactive isotopes injected into areas of the body. The isotope that is used is dependent on the tissue. Positron-emission tomography (PET) scanners create images from emitted positrons. Radiation therapy relies on gamma radiation from ^{60}Co to destroy tumors, but it also harms healthy tissue. Research into other radiation treatments to decrease the drawbacks is continually being pursued. Food irradiation is a technique that can be useful to increase the lifetime of foodstuffs, by using low doses of gamma radiation to kill bacteria that can lead to the food spoiling. This process can easily damage bacterial DNA and kill them but does not cause the food to admit any more radiation than it already would.

Organic Chemistry

Organic chemistry is the study of carbon-containing molecules. Therefore, understanding the structure and physical properties of the carbon atom is the fundamental basis of organic chemistry.

Atomic Structure and Bonding

In a molecule, atoms can be bound together either ionically or covalently. An ionic bond forms between atoms held together by electrostatic forces. An example of an ionic bond would be table salt: NaCl or sodium chloride. There is an ionic bond between a sodium ion and a chloride ion. In this case, the unpaired valence electron on Cl^- (which gives it the negative charge) is *accepted* by the positively charged Na^+.

In a covalent bond, the two valence electrons that make up the bond are *shared* between atoms. They may not be equally shared—one atom may have more than its fair share of electron density—but not all of the electron density rests solely on one partner of the bond, which is the characteristic of ionic bonds. This electron sharing tightly binds the atoms because the electrons are associated with the nuclei of both atoms simultaneously. The electrons are drawn to the positively charged protons of the other nuclei but also repelled by the atom's electrons. At a certain distance between atoms these opposing forces—the attractive and repulsive tendencies—reach an equilibrium of sorts, and the two atoms are said to be covalently bound.

Whereas carbon atoms can participate in ionic bonds only in certain circumstances, they almost always can form covalent bonds. When compared to ionic compounds, covalent compounds have lower melting and boiling points. This is because a large amount of energy is required to overcome the strong attraction between a full positive charge and a full negative charge, as in the example of table salt. Table salt (an ionic compound) is very difficult to melt, while table sugar (a covalent compound) can be melted at a much lower temperature. Also, being largely nonpolar, most organic compounds are poor conductors of electricity.

If one could separate a single carbon atom, it would have four valence electrons—that is, four electrons in its outermost energy shell. In order for carbon to be most stable (at its lowest-energy state) it must find four other valence electrons with which to pair or share. This is because carbon follows the octet rule. The octet rule states that each atom is in its most favorable (most stable, lowest-energy) configuration when it has eight valence electrons. It is for this reason that in a stable, nonionic, organic molecule, every carbon atom will have four covalent bonds.

Other atoms follow the octet rule as well. Again, if you could isolate an atom of fluorine, it would naturally have seven valence electrons, as it is in Group VII from the Periodic Table. According to the octet rule, it seeks one more valence electron to form eight. Thus fluorine usually forms only one covalent bond (one shared valence electron), and then is satisfied, as it has reached an octet of electons. In their natural states,

- Nitrogen has five valence electrons and seeks three shared electrons (bonds).
- Oxygen has six valence electrons and seeks two shared electrons (bonds).
- Chlorine, fluorine, bromine, and iodine each have seven valence electrons and seek one shared electron (bond).

The octet rule can be broken under certain circumstances. Carbon occasionally breaks the octet rule when it forms a carbocation (CH_3^+), which can happen after the molecule somehow loses an electron. The positively charged carbon atom is unstable, however, and usually finds another electron to share almost immediately (to once again reach a filled octet of valence electrons). Nitrogen, sulfur, boron, and other elements that appear in organic molecules can be seen bending or breaking the octet rule. When they do, these atoms form relatively reactive chemical species. For the most part and especially for carbon atoms, the octet rule holds.

In order to understand how carbon atoms covalently bind to one another, it is important to understand the electron orbitals of a carbon atom. According to the Heisenberg uncertainty principle, you cannot simultaneously know the exact location and the exact momentum of any single electron. Nevertheless, if one is to learn about the behavior of electrons around nuclei, one needs to establish a reasonable approximation. For carbon molecules this approximation is done through electron orbitals that provide an approximate location for electrons in an atom. While there are other, higher-order orbitals, most organic molecules (and those on standardized exams) can be described by *s*, *p*, and *sp* hybrid orbitals. An orbital is simply a certain region of space surrounding an atom, defined by a particular shape and size, in which there is a high probability of finding an electron.

The easiest way to think of an *s*-orbital is by considering hydrogen. Hydrogen has a 1*s* orbital that is simply a spherical cloud containing a single electron. The spherical cloud is symmetrical and does not possess an inherent directionality. Where, precisely, is the electron around the hydrogen atom? We cannot say; we simply say that there is a very high probability that it is somewhere within the spherical 1*s* orbital.

Few electrons actually reside in pure *s*-orbitals. More often, electrons are found in *p*-orbitals. These *p*-orbitals have a roughly dumbbell or figure eight shape that is centered around the nucleus (with a lobe going in one direction over the atom, and another lobe extending in the opposite direction, with the atom at the skinny center). An atom can have three *p*-orbitals at one time at a given energy level. These three orbitals can be visualized as existing at right angles to one another, much like the *x*, *y*, and *z* coordinates of a three-dimensional graph. Organic chemists sometimes designate these as p_x, p_y, and p_z, in cases where it is necessary to indicate which particular *p*-orbital is under discussion.

Carbon contains a combination of both *s*- and *p*-orbitals. They are hybrids of both *s* and *p*, and their name depends on how many *p*-orbitals were included in the mix: there are *sp* orbitals, sp^2, and sp^3 orbitals. An *sp* hybrid orbital is roughly the same shape as a *p*-orbital except for being slightly rounded, accounting for the spherical *s*-orbital. According to the valence-shell electron-pair repulsion (VSEPR) theory, electrons—even valence electrons within the same atom—repel each other as much as possible (electrons are negatively charged, and like charges repel each other). Thus, when carbon participates in four single bonds with other atoms, the four sp^3 orbitals in carbon are 109.5° from each other, which is the farthest apart they can be. This VSEPR property explains carbon's tetrahedral structure. Think of the carbon atom as being at the center of a pyramid with a triangular base; the four sp^3 orbitals would point toward the three bottom corners and also toward the top of the pyramid.

Carbon is in a tetrahedral shape, however, only when it has four sp^3 orbitals. When a carbon atom participates in a double or triple bond with another atom, the orbitals are indicated as sp^2 and *sp*, respectively. Following VSEPR theory, sp^2 hybrid orbitals take the trigonal planar shape (atoms are 120° from each other; envision a flat two-dimensional triangle, with the carbon at the center; the sp^2 orbitals point toward the corners of the triangle). Finally, *sp* hybrid orbitals take a linear shape (atoms are 180° from each other).

We have been discussing single, double, and triple bonds, but what does that mean? Simply put, the single, double, and triple bonds correspond to the number of times an atom is bonded to any other atom. More specifically, it denotes how many valence electrons are shared between atoms. For each bond, one valence electron pair (two electrons total) is shared between two atoms.

Let us consider the simplest organic molecule, methane or CH_4. Carbon has four valence electrons and shares a single valence electron with each of four hydrogen atoms. Thus in methane, carbon forms four single bonds, one with each atom of hydrogen. These single bonds are referred to as sigma (σ) bonds. A σ bond is formed by overlapping orbitals directly between the nuclei of two atoms. In the case of methane, the σ bonds exist between carbon and hydrogen. For each of the C-H bonds, the carbon shares one electron in the form of a filled sp^3 orbital, and the hydrogen shares its' single electron in a 1*s* orbital. The orbitals overlap, forming a covalent bond. The atoms attached by a σ bond can rotate freely about the axis of the bond.

The simplest organic molecule with a double bond is ethene (C_2H_4). Recall that the carbon atoms in a double bond have sp^2 hybrid orbitals. In the case of a double bond between the two carbon atoms in ethane, one C-C bond is a σ bond and the other is a pi (π) bond. The σ bond is created by overlapping sp^2 orbitals between the two carbon atoms. Each carbon atom is left with an electron in a π orbital; the C-C π bond is created by the overlap of these two adjacent π orbitals (perpendicular to the σ bond). Likewise, ethyne, the simplest organic molecule with a triple bond, has one σ bond and two π bonds. Because of the π bonding, double and triple bonded atoms are fixed and cannot rotate about the bond. Trying to rotate around the bond would break the alignment of the π-orbital overlap (which would take a lot of energy) and therefore is usually not possible.

Up until this point, we have discussed the electron sharing that occurs in covalent bonds as if it were done equally across any two pairs of atoms. This is not entirely accurate. Covalent bonds can be classified as either polar covalent or nonpolar covalent bonds, depending on the physical properties of the atoms on either side of the bond. If the atoms share electrons more or less equally, the bond is considered nonpolar. However, if the shared electrons are closer to one atom than another (meaning that atom has a higher appetite for electron density), the covalent bond is considered polar. While the terms may seem dichotomous, in actuality the polarity of a covalent bond follows a continuum from nonpolar (equally shared) to highly polar (electrons resting quite close to one of the two atoms), with examples all along the way.

Why would shared electrons be found closer to one atom over another? The relative position is based on the electronegativity of the atom. Electronegativity is a physical property of an atom that describes its propensity to attract shared electrons. This is directly related to the atom's desire to form a fully filled octet. If an atom such as fluorine (which has seven valence electrons) can somehow attract another electron, it will; such action will gain it a filled octet. Fluorine is electron-greedy, or electronegative.

ELECTRONEGATIVITY VALUES OF ATOMS COMMONLY FOUND IN ORGANIC MOLECULES

ATOM	ELECTRONEGATIVITY VALUE
C	2.6
H	2.2
N	3.0
O	3.4
F	4.0
P	2.2
S	2.6
Cl	3.2
Br	3.0
I	2.7

While fluorine has the highest electronegativity value listed and is the most electronegative atom on the Periodic Table, the polarity of a covalent bond depends on the two atoms involved in the covalent bond. Hydrogen fluoride (HF) contains a highly polar covalent bond because the difference between the electronegativity of H (2.6) and F (4.0) is large. This difference in electronegativity creates what is known as a dipole (unequal distribution of electric charge) between the two atoms, with relative negativity (more electron density) on the fluorine atom and relative positivity (less electron density) at the hydrogen atom. Fluorine occurs naturally as a diatomic molecule of two fluorine atoms (F_2). As a diatomic molecule, the covalent bond in F_2 is nonpolar since the electronegativity of each fluorine atom is the same. Each partner in the covalent bond has the same propensity to attract electron density, so the overall *net* result is zero; both fluorine atoms end up with the same amount of electron density. Therefore, there is no dipole created between these two atoms.

Nomenclature and Functional Groups

We have already touched on the basic nomenclature of carbon molecules with terms such as methane, ethane, and ethyne. Rules exist to make the naming of more complex molecules easier for chemists. Hydrocarbons (chains of hydrogen and carbon molecules) are named by finding the highest number of carbon-carbon bonds (longest uninterrupted chain of C-C bonds) in the molecule. If a hydrocarbon chain has only single bonds between carbon atoms, its name ends in *-ane*. If there is even one double bond in the molecule, the name of that molecule ends in *-ene*. A carbon-carbon triple bond in a hydrocarbon means the name ends in *-yne*. Triple bonds take precedence over double bonds, which take precedence over single bonds. Even if you had a molecule with 12 single bonds, four double bonds, and just one triple bond between carbon atoms, the molecular name would end in *-yne*.

That takes care of hydrocarbon suffixes, but what about the prefixes? Hydrocarbons are named by the number of carbon atoms in the chain. The prefixes for hydrocarbons of carbon lengths 1 through 10 should be committed to memory.

PREFIXES OF HYDROCARBONS ACCORDING TO NUMBER OF CARBONS

NUMBER OF CARBONS	PREFIX
1	meth-
2	eth-
3	prop-
4	but-
5	pent-
6	hex-
7	hept-
8	oct-
9	non-
10	dec-

Organic molecules also contain a number of functional groups that determine the reactivity and chemical properties of that molecule (hence the name—these groups of atoms determine the function of the molecule). While single, double, and triple bonds are useful for naming hydrocarbons, they lose priority when the molecule contains a different functional group. In fact, the functional groups have a hierarchy that dictates the overall name of the organic molecule. In other words, the final suffix of the molecule is determined by the group with the highest naming priority. For example, if a compound has an alcohol and a carboxylic acid, the molecule would end in *-oic acid* (the suffix for carboxylic acid) and not *-ol* (the suffix for alcohol). Since alkanes are of the lowest priority, the presence of even a single functional group will mean the *-ane* can no longer be used.

STRUCTURE OF FUNCTIONAL GROUPS IN ORGANIC CHEMISTRY (FROM LOWEST TO HIGHEST PRIORITY)		
FUNCTIONAL GROUP NAME	**STRUCTURE**	**PREFIX OR SUFFIX**
halide	Cl—H Br—H	halo-
ether	R–O–R	alkoxy-
amine	$R{-}NH_2$	-amine
alcohol	R—OH	-ol
ketone	R–C(=O)–R	-one
aldehyde	R–C(=O)–H	-al
amide	$R{-}C(=O){-}NH_2$	-amide
carboxylic acid	R–C(=O)–OH	-oic acid
ester	R–C(=O)–O–R	-oate

The naming of organic molecules can be complex. The International Union of Pure and Applied Chemistry (IUPAC) naming conventions have been accepted as the standard way to name all molecules—the IUPAC book on organic compounds alone is over 500 pages long. The basic naming conventions that cover most organic molecules are reasonably straightforward, however. The two basic things to look for are: (1) the longest carbon chain in the molecule and (2) the highest-priority functional group. Organic molecule nomenclature hinges on those two things.

1. Find the longest hydrocarbon chain. If the compound contains a ring, this is often the longest chain (though not always). If there are two chains of equal length, the one with more substituents or the one with the highest-priority functional group prevails.
2. The first substituent or highest-priority functional group is the lowest number. Each carbon is numbered in sequence away from carbon 1.
3. Every substituent other than a carbon-carbon or carbon-hydrogen bond is named using a prefix. If a single carbon has multiple, identical substituents, name them as *di-*, *tri-*, or *tetra-*. Ringed compounds without resonance (a special property involving a particular number of alternating single and double bonds) have the prefix *cyclo-*. Substituents are placed in alphabetical order within the name.

PREFIXES OF ORGANIC FUNCTIONAL GROUPS	
FUNCTIONAL GROUP NAME	**PREFIX**
halide	halo-
nitro	nitro-
thiol	mercapto-
ether	alkoxy-
amine	amino-
alcohol	hydroxy-
ketone	oxo-
aldehyde	oxo-
nitrile	cyano-
amide	(none)
carboxylic acid	carboxy-

For the PCAT exam it is important to be very comfortable with naming rules and conventions of organic compounds.

Resonance and Cyclic Compounds

Organic molecules that are rings take two forms: those with resonance and those without. Let us compare two different ringed molecules with six carbons, cyclohexane (C_6H_{12}) and benzene (C_6H_6). By knowing that carbon forms four bonds (shares four valence electrons), you can predict the structure of each of these molecules from their chemical formulas.

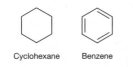

Cyclohexane Benzene

Because benzene has alternating single and double bonds, the molecule is flat. In contrast, cyclohexane is joined only by single bonds and can be found in either boat or chair conformations.

Benzene is said to be resonance-stabilized because the electrons that are participating in the covalent bonds are delocalized across the molecule. The molecule exists *simultaneously* in two forms.

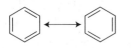

That is not to say that the molecule flips back and forth between these two configurations; the manner in which the molecule is drawn is simply a convention that is used to help visualize the structure. In actuality, the molecule is in a conformation that is halfway between these two states. Imagine a mule—it's not a donkey; it's not a horse; it's a hybrid of the two. It doesn't become a horse one second and a donkey the next; it's a mule. Benzene is the same way; we simply don't have an easy way to represent resonance stabilization when writing down the structure using pencil and paper. Each carbon is sp^2 hybridized—not alternating sp^3 and sp^2 bonds in sequence. Such molecules have stabilities that are far greater than an analogous molecule of cyclohexane—so-called resonance stabilization.

Benzene is just one an example of an aromatic compound. An aromatic compound is an unsaturated, cyclic hydrocarbon that obeys Hückel's rule. Simply put, Hückel's rule states that an aromatic compound must have precisely $4n + 2$ number of π electrons (where $n = 0, 1, 2, 3, \ldots$) in an alternating sequence of single and double bonds. Benzene obeys the rule because there are 6π electrons. Other examples of aromatic compounds obeying Hückel's rule are naphthalene, anthracene, furan, and thiophene. Note that furan and thiophene have oxygen and sulfur atoms in their rings, respectively, yet qualify as aromatic.

The concept of resonance stabilization is not just important to cyclic compounds; it also helps explain the chemical properties of other molecules with adjacent single and double bonds. One example is the carboxylic acid functional group.

Carboxylic Acid with Resonance

O R OH R O O

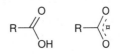

The adjacent single and double bonds stabilize the molecule through resonance. Resonance stabilization explains the acidity of a carboxylic acid, at least in part. The two oxygen molecules are stable even without the hydrogen atom attached. Molecules with multiple double bonds can make mildly acidic protons out of some unlikely hydrogens (e.g., a hydrogen covalently bound to a carbon). This is an intriguing feature of resonance that underlies certain reactions in organic chemistry.

You may encounter a rather specific nomenclature for six member rings that contain substituents (though it is occasionally used in other cyclic molecules). It is sometimes referred to as the "arene substitution rules," though more familiarly it is known as the *ortho-*, *meta-*, *para-* system. In this naming system, the highest-priority substituent is placed in the 12 o'clock position and the other substituents are described relative to it. If the substituent is adjacent to the priority substituent, it receives an ortho- prefix. If it is two carbons away, it is the meta- substituent, and if the substituent is directly across or three carbons away, it is in the para- position.

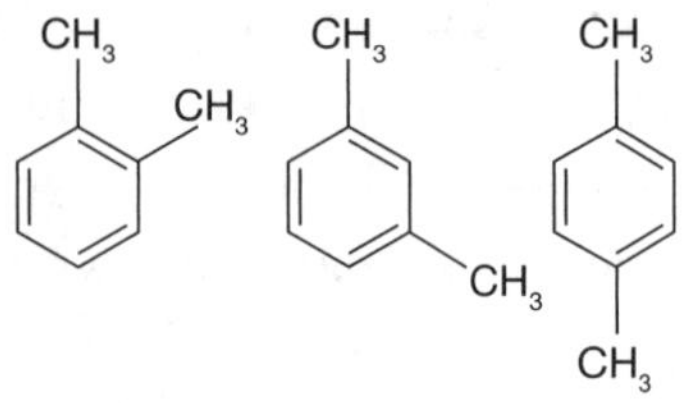

CH_3 CH_3 CH_3 CH_3 CH_3 CH_3

Ortho- Meta- Para-

Physical Properties

Recall that atoms can be bound by either ionic or covalent bonds—covalent bonds being the primary form found in organic molecules. However, there are a number of intermolecular forces that can exist between the atoms of different molecules. In organic chemistry, two important intermolecular forces are London dispersion forces (sometimes called van der Waals interactions) and hydrogen bonding.

When any two molecules come together, they create London dispersion forces. These London dispersion forces form fleeting, temporary dipoles between atoms. In contrast to a permanent dipole that exists between two atoms of differing electronegativity, London dispersion forces create dipoles that are only temporary. In pure nonpolar molecules, London dispersion forces are the only intermolecular forces at work, and are quite weak compared to other intermolecular interactions that exist, such as hydrogen bonding. As an example, candle wax is held together primarily by these London dispersion forces; the resulting structure is soft, low-melting, and lacking in physical strength.

The other important intermolecular force in organic chemistry is hydrogen bonding. Hydrogen bonding takes place between two relatively electronegative atoms that have a hydrogen atom covalently bonded to one of them. The simplest example of hydrogen bonding is what takes place between molecules of water. A molecule of water can participate in three hydrogen bonds at once. The two hydrogen atoms can be hydrogen-bonded to the oxygen atoms in other water molecules while the oxygen can participate in a hydrogen bond with an O-H of yet another water molecule. Carbon does not have enough electronegativity to participate in hydrogen bonding under normal circumstances. However, if the hydrocarbon has a hydroxyl group or carboxylic acid group, for example, hydrogen bonding forces may exert an effect, depending on the local environment (other electronegative atoms).

Hydrogen bonds are quite strong, relatively speaking. The principle behind them relies on the fact that an H-O bond has most of the electron density drawn toward the oxygen, due to the higher electronegativity on the oxygen (polar covalent bond). This leaves that hydrogen with a partial positive charge (lack of electron density); it's relatively exposed. A lone pair of electrons on another oxygen atom (which is negatively charged, don't forget) is attracted to this partially positive hydrogen atom, and the hydrogen bond is formed. In the diagram, hydrogen bonds are shown as dashed lines.

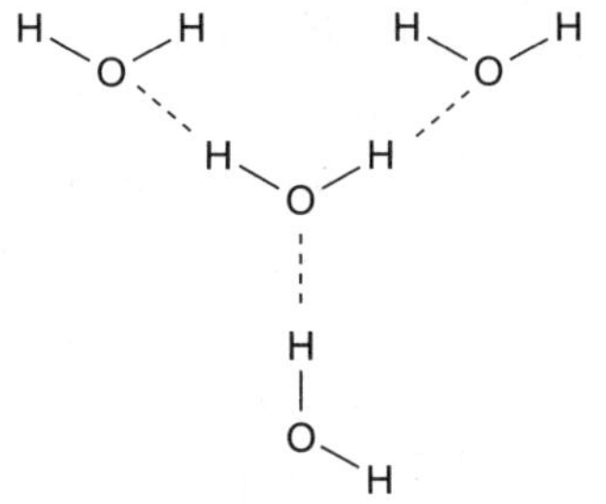

The boiling point of a substance is determined by the forces acting on that substance to keep it in a liquid state. If the intermolecular forces are strong, the boiling point will be high, as a lot of energy will be required to overcome these intermolecular forces and force the molecules to separate (going into the gas phase). This is exemplified in alkanes of increasing length. The longer the number of carbons in an alkane chain, the higher the boiling point of the compound. That is because larger molecules have a greater number of atoms with which to participate in London dispersion forces.

If an alkane has a substituent that is polar, the boiling point is higher than it would be if it were a simple hydrocarbon with the same number of carbons. Take ethane and ethanol, for example. The hydroxyl group in ethanol can participate in hydrogen bonding with other ethanol molecules. Ethane, on the other hand, participates only in London dispersion forces. Therefore, it is not surprising that the boiling point of ethane is –89°C but ethanol's boiling point is 78°C. This is another example of how hydrogen bonds are much stronger intermolecular interactions than London dispersion forces.

Pure hydrocarbons are nonpolar compounds and have low solubility or miscibility in water. As such they are sometimes referred to as hydrophobic (water-fearing). Hydrocarbons will form a layer that is distinct from water because of this. While in common experience oil forms on top of water (e.g., in a salad dressing) this is not always the case. If the hydrocarbon (organic phase) is more dense than water (the aqueous phase), then it will settle at the bottom in a discrete layer. The longer the hydrocarbon chain, the less soluble the molecule will be in water.

What if the hydrocarbon has a polar substituent, such as a hydroxyl group? Because the hydroxyl group is polar and hydrophilic (water-loving), it makes the compound more soluble in water, as it can engage in hydrogen bonding with the water-solvent molecules. However, the length of the hydrocarbon chain and the number of hydrophilic substituents are working in opposite directions in terms of water solubility. A long hydrocarbon with a single hydrophilic substituent is less soluble in water than a short hydrocarbon with the same substituent. Likewise, multiple polar groups on a hydrocarbon will increase the water solubility of that molecule. It's a tug-of-war of sorts, and it can sometimes be difficult to predict the solubility of an organic compound, but by following the general principles listed earlier you should do well.

These same properties exist for solubility in organic solvents, though more care must be taken in their application. Organic solvents can be either polar or nonpolar, depending on their functional groups. Methanol (CH_3OH) behaves quite similiarly to water in terms of what it can and cannot dissolve; we can say that very polar organic solvents behave somewhat like water in their solubility characteristics. However, most organic solvents are nonpolar, as they contain mostly hydrocarbons and maybe only one to two polar functional groups. In these cases, these nonpolar organic solvents would dissolve nonpolar compounds easily, but have trouble dissolving polar compounds.

Organic Reactions

Understanding how substrates (reactants, starting materials) form products when exposed to a particular catalyst and in a particular solvent is at the core of the study of organic chemistry. Knowledge of organic chemistry reactions allows one to predict products and create novel compounds. Memorizing organic chemistry reactions, however, has traditionally been the most feared and loathed component of an organic chemistry course. This need not be the case if one simply learns the basic reactions very well. All of these basic reactions rely on even more fundamental rules regarding electron flow, polarity/nonpolarity, valence, and electronegativity. These are all fundamental skills that you should master, as doing so will increase your success in organic chemistry.

There are two important terms that need to be defined before one can interpret almost any organic reaction: nucleophile and electrophile. A nucleophile is an attacker. It's either a negative ion or an uncharged atom that has a relatively high density of electrons (e.g., a lone pair). An electrophile, in contrast, is a target, an atom that has either a positive charge (cation) or a relative lack of electron density. As their name suggests, nucleophiles are attracted to areas of relative positivity and positively charged entities, such as electrophiles. Nucleophiles attack electrophiles, not the other way around; bonds are formed by electrons, and the electrons reside on the nucleophiles. Most organic reactions that you will encounter involve the interaction between a nucleophile and an electrophile.

Substitution

One of the most common and fundamental reactions in organic chemistry is the substitution reaction. In a substitution reaction, a nucleophile reacts with an electrophile, a process known as a nucleophilic attack. There are two main types of nucleophilic substitution reactions, namely SN1 and S_N2. For ease of explanation, we will consider the S_N2 reaction first.

In an S_N2 reaction, a nucleophile attacks an electrophile and forms a new covalent bond. This attack forces a leaving group (some part of the electrophilic target molecule) to be displaced and depart from the molecule. These steps—the attack of the nucleophile and the loss of the leaving group—*happen at the same time*; it is a concerted reaction. In the process, the orientation of the three remaining substituents changes around the carbon atom. In the given example, the lone pair on the oxygen is the nucleophile and the carbon is the electrophile. It is important to note that the nucleophile attacks from the rear of the molecule—the side opposite that of the leaving group, which is chlorine in this example. This happens in all S_N2 reactions; this rearside attack is characteristic.

S_N2 Reaction

H–Ö:–H + R^1, R^2, R–C–Cl ⟶ HO–C(R^1)(R^2)R + HCl

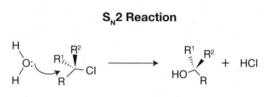

The carbon is electrophilic in this case because the chlorine atom is more highly electronegative (versus carbon) and draws electron density away from the carbon to which it is attached. The chlorine atom is the leaving group, that is, the atom that is inclined to depart from the molecule. Chlorines are good leaving groups, as once they leave with the electron they were sharing in the C-Cl covalent bond, they have filled their octet of valence electrons, which (if you remember) is very stable and preferable. If the electrophilic carbon is a stereocenter, the carbon will still be chiral after the S_N2, but the substituents will have flipped due to the rearside attack of the nucleophile pushing all of the substituents forward. It is important to reassign the correct *R* or *S* nomenclature anew after S_N2 reaction products have been determined.

The "1" in an S_N1 reaction means that it obeys first-order kinetics. In an S_N1 reaction, the leaving group is not forced off the molecule at the same time as the nucleophile attack, as it is in an S_N2 reaction. The leaving group departs first, which leaves behind a carbocation. This is *always* the slow, rate-determining step in an S_N1 reaction. A carbocation is a positively charged carbon atom and, as such, is quite electrophilic (a good target for electron-rich nucleophiles). A carbocation can be considered to have a trigonal planar geometry (bond angle of 120°; i.e., flat). Thus, when the nucleophile attacks the carbocation, it may do so from either side—from above or from below. Therefore, if the original molecule was an enantiomerically pure stereoisomer, the products will be roughly racemic after the S_N1 reaction. This is because the nucleophilic attack will occur at random from either side (just as successive coin flips will sort into roughly 50% heads and 50% tails).

From the discussion on covalent versus ionic bonding it should be no surprise that the formation of carbocation through an S_N1 reaction requires the carbocation to be relatively stable and the leaving group to be very naturally inclined to leave. Otherwise, the reaction's activation energy will be too high, and the reaction rate will be so slow that it will take years to complete. Excellent leaving groups include molecules such as tosylates and mesylates, as they are quite stable in their ionic form due to resonance stabilization of the resulting negative charge on the leaving group. Even with a stable leaving group and relatively stable carbocation, the carbocation exists for a very short time in the presence of a nucleophile. The movement of an S_N1 reaction through the carbocation form is a fleeting event known as a transition state.

S_N2 reactions are affected by a physical property of some tetrahedral molecules called steric hindrance. Since a nucleophile must physically interact with an electrophile for this substitution reaction to occur, if the substituents are large and/or bulky (in terms of size), the attacking nucleophile cannot readily access the electrophile. This steric hindrance will often slow down or even prevent the reaction from proceeding. Steric hindrance is not a factor in S_N1 reactions since the trigonal planar shape of the carbocation makes plenty of room for the nucleophile to attack the carbon.

In a free radical substitution, a free radical acts as the nucleophile. The mechanism is not as simple as S_N1 and S_N2 reactions since free radicals can propagate into secondary reactions. The mechanism is characterized by three components: initiation, propagation, and termination phases. In the initiation phase it is common to see ultraviolet light used to create a free radical from a halogen diatom. For example, molecular bromine, or Br-Br, with its two electrons in that covalent single bond, will split up and the result is two bromine radicals, which are bromines with one electron each. Once created, the free radical can interact with most other atoms in the local environment. The reaction is said to propagate because the free radical will be transferred between molecules until it interacts with another free radical, which terminates the reaction. Stereocenters are not preserved in free radical substitution.

Elimination

As the name implies, an elimination reaction is one in which an atom or functional group is eliminated (removed) from a molecule, and usually results in an increase in the number of double or triple bonds in the final product. Like substitution reactions, elimination reactions generally fall into two categories, E1 and E2. Like S_N1 reactions, E1 reactions require an excellent leaving group that will be stable once it leaves with its (new) negative charge. E2 reactions involve two compounds, one of which strips an atom or group from the other.

Let us consider an E2 reaction first. In the illustrated case, the sodium hydroxide reacts with a hydrogen atom on the carbon adjacent to the carbon containing the chlorine. The two electrons that were in that C-H covalent bond flow over to the chlorine-containing carbone, which kicks off the leaving group, which in this case is the chlorine. This is another example of a concerted reaction: Everything happens in one step. The proton is removed by the base; the electrons flow over (creating the double bond), and the chlorine leaves, all in one step. Instead of leaving a hydroxyl group on the molecule—which would be the result of an S_N2 reaction—here, the reaction forms salt, water, and a double bond on the organic molecule.

E2 Reaction

$$R\text{-}CH(Cl)\text{-}CH_3 \xrightarrow{NaOH} R\text{-}CH{=}CH_2 + H_2O + Na^+Cl^-$$

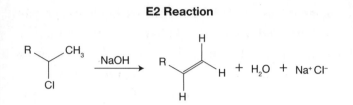

As you may have noticed, there is a fine line between substitution and elimination reactions. There are certain conditions that determine whether a reaction is likely to proceed through one mechanism or the other. A reaction is more likely to proceed by elimination over substitution if the nucleophile is weak (relatively low electron density), if the reaction takes place at high temperature or in the presence of a strong base (especially a bulky base), or if there is a significant amount of steric hindrance on the electrophile. Also, elimination is more likely if the solvent is a small alcohol, such as ethanol. The presence of water, by contrast, favors substitution.

Condensation

In organic chemistry, condensation is a reaction in which two molecules are united as they expel a smaller molecule (e.g., water or methanol). Condensations occur through various mechanisms. Most, however, proceed through an addition and elimination reaction in sequence. The mechanism of an aldol condensation is illustrative of most condensations.

Dehydration

Dehydration reactions can be thought of as a specific type of elimination reaction in which water is always the leaving group. Dehydrations are sometimes referred to as a type of condensation reaction, but this is not always true. While a condensation requires that two molecules unite, this is not true of dehydration reactions. The base molecule involved in a dehydration must contain a hydroxyl group that can leave the molecule. For instance, a dehydrated alcohol becomes an alkene and a dehydrated carboxylic acid can become an acid anhydride or a nitrile; there are several possibilities. Just remember that dehydration reactions mean that water is lost during the reaction.

Before an organic reactant can undergo dehydration, the hydroxyl group must pick up an additional proton (a hydrogen ion is a proton). This additional hydrogen may come from the solvent, from another reactant, or from within the same molecule. Most often, though, an acid catalyst is used to facilitate the dehydration. The lone pair of the hydroxyl's oxygen picks up a proton from a strong acid such as sulfuric acid. This is necessary as the molecular fragment ^-OH is a very poor leaving group; it already has a negative charge, and when it acts as a leaving group, it's going to have to take on even more negative charge. By becoming protonated, it is transformed into a good leaving group, as it can leave as a neutral molecule (water).

Oxidation and Reduction

In organic chemistry, the terms *oxidation* and *reduction* have slightly different usages than they do in general chemistry or inorganic chemistry, although the strict meanings are the same. For this discussion, oxidation is a reaction in which an oxygen atom is added to a molecule or hydrogen(s) is/are removed. Reduction is just the opposite. A reduction takes place when hydrogen(s) is/are added to a molecule or an oxygen atom is removed.

Perhaps the most straightforward example of organic oxidation and reduction is the conversion between an aldehyde and a carboxylic acid.

$$R\text{-}C(=O)\text{-}H \underset{\text{Reduction}}{\overset{\text{Oxidation}}{\rightleftarrows}} R\text{-}C(=O)\text{-}OH$$

Alternatively, if an alkane is converted to an alkene it is a reduction reaction because hydrogen atoms are added to the molecule. Likewise, the conversion from an alkene to an alkane is an oxidation. If two hydrogen atoms and one oxygen atom join or leave the molecule, it is no longer considered an oxidation or reduction reaction. These reactions would be referred to as hydration or dehydration reactions, respectively.

There are a number of reagents that will lead to oxidations and reductions, but certain reactants or catalysts are traditionally used (and appear on tests). Common organic oxidizing agents are chromic acid or its sodium or potassium salt (usually with sulfuric acid). Potassium permanganate is also an organic oxidizing agent. Common reducing agents include nickel/hydrogen gas mixtures, lithium aluminum hydride, and sodium tetrahydridoborate (commonly called sodium borohydride [$NaBH_4$]).

Esterification

Esterification refers to the creation of an ester from an alcohol and a carboxylic acid. It occurs in the presence of an acid catalyst and is reversible, which means the product (an ester) may revert to the reagents (alcohol and acid) under certain conditions. In general, esterification is a slow process. The larger the resulting ester molecule, the longer the reaction will take. It is common for esterification reactions to be shown with the term *reflux* on the reaction arrow (note a reversible reaction arrow). This is because the ester will usually have a lower boiling point than either the carboxylic acid or the alcohol. Therefore, once the ester is formed, it volatilizes and is distilled out of the sample. Removing the product drives the equilibrium toward the right and prevents the reaction from occurring in the reverse direction.

Depending on how you draw the steps of the reaction, an esterification takes place in five or six steps—complex when compared to other mechanisms. The net result of this complex reaction is that the oxygen atom on the alcohol is the nucleophile and the carbon of the carboxylic acid is the electrophile. The oxygen that is expelled from the molecule is the one in the hydroxyl group of the carboxylic acid.

Addition

When two molecules unite to form a larger molecule, it is called an addition reaction. It can be thought of as the opposite of an elimination reaction. Addition reactions involve molecules with double- and triple-bonded atoms, including alkenes, alkynes, carbonyl groups, and imine groups (C=N). In essence, a π bond is broken to form two new σ bonds, one with each previously double-bonded atom.

Addition reactions can be classified as electrophilic, nucleophilic, or free radical additions. Since we have discussed several reactions in which the nucleophile attacks, nucleophilic addition is a reasonable place to start. As with other mechanisms, nucleophiles such as the oxygen in water or alcohol or the nitrogen in an amine attack atoms with low electron density (electrophiles). Examples of electrophiles that participate in nucleophilic addition are carbons on either side of a π bond (alkene) or a carbonyl carbon. The nucleophilic attack on the carbon opens the double bond. Thus there is an unbound valance electron that can be shared. This negative charge draws a proton or other positively charged species from the local environment.

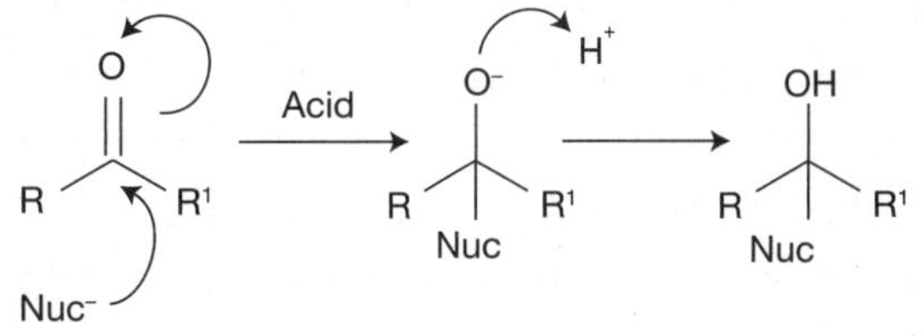

In a π bond, the electrons are not as closely associated with the carbon atom as they are in a σ bond. Thus in an electrophilic addition, the electrons in the π bond find a suitable electrophile with which to bind. This leaves a carbocation after the π bond is broken. The carbocation then covalently binds with a nucleophile or positively charged species involved in the reaction. A useful example of an electrophilic addition is the reaction of a hydrogen halide with an alkene.

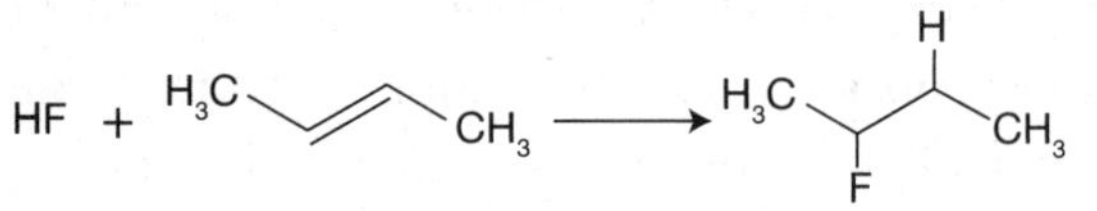

Since most mechanisms in organic chemistry focus on nucleophilic attack, we must reverse the process a bit for electrophilic addition. Do not be confused by the name; the electrophile does not add to anything; bonds are formed by the flow of electrons, which come from nucleophiles. Since we are still pushing electrons in our mechanisms, we use the electrons in the π bond to interact with the hydrogen atom, which is both a proton and an electrophile. The fluoride ion that remains after the disruption of hydrogen fluoride is now the nucleophile and covalently binds to the carbocation.

Electrophilic addition is subject to Markovnikov's rule. Markovnikov's rule states that when a protic acid (HX) is combined with an asymmetric alkene, the hydrogen will bond on the side of the double bond that has the most hydrogen atoms already bonded (or fewer alkyl substituents). Markovnikov's rule is not a physical or chemical principle, but rather a means of predicting products in an organic reaction. What determines the final orientation is the mechanism that creates the most stable carbocation intermediate. The carbocation will form on the carbon with the most electron-donating substituents (more alkyl substituents). Therefore, the hydrogen is left to bond to the other carbon. This can be understood if you consider the intermediate state (the carbocation); the reaction that proceeds is the one in which the most stable carbocation is formed.

Some free radical addition reactions do not abide by Markovnikov's rule. In fact, they follow the anti-Markovnikov's rule. In most cases, hydrogen halides and alkenes will react through the electrophilic addition mechanism. However, when hydrogen bromide is reacted with an alkene in the presence of an organic peroxide, it adds to the opposite carbon that would be predicted by Markovnikov's rule. This is mostly due to the fact that the free radical addition reaction rate of hydrogen bromide is very high compared to its electrophilic addition reaction rate (in the presence of peroxide).

Free Radical Addition

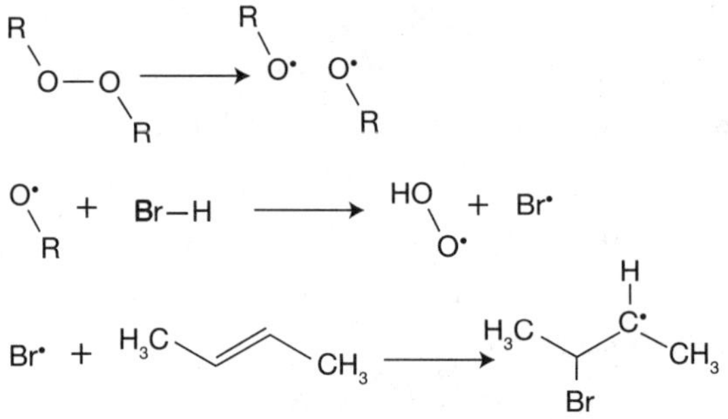

The free radical on carbon can go on to form new radicals with the organic peroxide, HBr, or form a longer organic polymer, until the reaction terminates.

Structure of Biomolecules

The study of organic chemistry is of vital importance to the study of biology. Every organism is comprised of organic molecules, and most require organic molecules for survival.

Lipids

Lipids perform a number of important biological functions. They are the primary long-term energy storage molecule, they are the main component of cell membranes, and they act as vitamins and hormones. The prototypical lipid, a fatty acid, has a carboxylic acid head with a long hydrocarbon tail. The carboxylic acid head is relatively hydrophilic, whereas the hydrocarbon tail is hydrophobic. This means that one end is relatively soluble in water while the other end is not. Compounds that possess both hydrophilic and hydrophobic components long enough to influence solubility independently are called amphiphilic molecules.

The nomenclature of fats that is used on food nutrition labels is drawn directly from organic chemistry nomenclature. A lipid is saturated if each carbon in the hydrocarbon tail is bonded only with single bonds. Monounsaturated fats (lipids) have one double bond in the hydrocarbon chain, whereas polyunsaturated fats (lipids) have more than one double bond.

It should be mentioned that oils and fats are both lipids and are chemically identical; the only distinction between oils and fats is whether they are a liquid or a solid at room temperature. A lipid's melting point can be predicted by the structure and degree of substitution in the carbon chain. As you would expect, saturated fatty acids form close intermolecular associations in the solid form because their shape packs together quite well. Thus it requires more heat energy to separate the molecules and cause a change of phase (melt the substance). The more carbons in the hydrocarbon tail, the higher the melting point of that compound because there is a greater number of places for intermolecular forces to operate between molecules.

Since the double bonds of mono- and polyunsaturated fats do not permit free rotation, these molecules are not flat and have fewer sites for intermolecular forces to hold them together. Thus the melting point of these compounds is lower (less energy is required to change their phase). By the same principle, the presence of additional double bonds in the molecule decreases the melting point. This means that, carbon for carbon, polyunsaturated fats have lower melting points than monounsaturated fats. Taken one step further, transunsaturated fats can form molecules that stack together nearly as tightly as saturated fats. Unsaturated fats in the cis- configuration have a bend in the molecule that prevents them from stacking tightly. This loose stacking limits the intermolecular forces at work on the molecules and means that cisunsaturated fats have a lower melting point than trans fats.

If one were to take pure fatty acids and place them in water, the hydrophobic tails would seek out each other while the hydrophilic heads would partially dissolve (become stabilized) by the water. What results is a sphere of fatty acids with the hydrophobic tails facing inward and the hydrophilic heads facing outward toward the water molecules. This spontaneously formed sphere is called a micelle.

Three other biologically important amphiphilic lipids are triglycerides, phospholipids, and glycolipids. Each of these lipids has a three-carbon molecule of glycerol at its core. For each of these lipids, two of the three carbons are attached to a fatty acid through an ester bond. When the third glycerol carbon forms an ester with a fatty acid, it is a triacylglycerol (triglyceride). If the third carbon is a polar phosphate group, it forms a phospoholipid; and if it is a carbohydrate (sugar), it forms a glycolipid.

Lipids

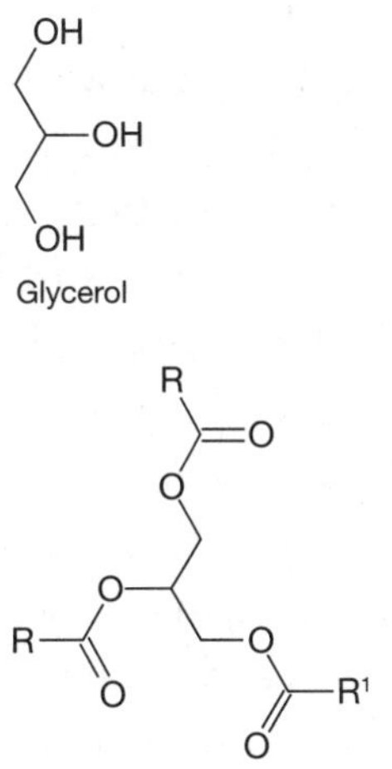

Glycerol

R^1 = Fatty acid—Triglyceride

R^1 = Phosphate—Phospholipid

R^1 = Carbohydrate—Glycolipid

As before, if one were to take pure phospholipids and place them in water, the hydrophobic tails would point toward each other, leaving the water-loving phosphate heads exposed to the water. However, instead of forming a micelle, the phospholipids actually organize into two layers. The hydrophobic tails face each other as they are sandwiched between hydrophilic heads. This configuration is known as a phospholipid bilayer. Since the phospholipid bilayer has two hydrophilic surfaces, it can form a sphere with water on the outside and in its core. In fact, a phospholipid bilayer is the basic structure of animal cell membranes. Alternatively, a glycolipid bilayer is the major structure of plant cell membranes.

Carbohydrates

In their simplest form, carbohydrates have the common formula of $C_n(H_2O)_n$ such that for every carbon there is also a hydroxyl group and a hydrogen. Carbohydrates range widely in their complexity, from three-carbon sugars, such as glyceraldehydes, to complex polymers of carbohydrates, such as glycogen. The most abundant carbohydrate is the six-carbon sugar called glucose. Glucose is the molecule that provides energy to animal cells through metabolism via glycolysis, the tricarboxylic acid cycle, and the electron transport chain.

Glucose is called a monosaccharide because it has a single polyhydroxyl ketone or aldehyde. Two molecules of glucose (or any two monosaccharides) linked by an O-glycosidic bond form a disaccharide. An O-glycosidic bond is created through a condensation reaction known as a Fischer glycosidation. The hydroxyl group of one sugar reacts with an anomeric carbon of another sugar, releasing a molecule of water. Alternatively, when glycosylation occurs between an anomeric carbon of a sugar and a nitrogen atom, it creates an N-glycosyl bond, which is found in RNA and DNA nucleosides.

Fischer glycosidations can occur many times to a carbohydrate, adding another monosaccharide each time. This long and likely branched polymer of monosaccharides is called a polysaccharide. In animals, carbohydrates are stored as large polymers of glucose called glycogen. In plant cells, the storage molecules are known as starches, specifically amylopectin and amylose. The primary difference between these large polysaccharides is which two carbons are united with an O-glycosidic bond. Amylose molecules form long, unbranched polymers, whereas amylopectin is highly branched. Glycogen is even more highly branched than amylopectin, and is thus more compact (more glucose molecules in a given space).

Aside from their role in energy, carbohydrates have structural roles in biological organisms. Cellulose is a polysaccharide found in the cell walls of plants. Chitin is a carbohydrate that makes up the exoskeleton of insects and crustaceans. Hyaluronic acid and glycosaminoglycan are important components of the extracellular matrix and connective tissues.

Proteins

Proteins are involved in virtually every biological process in the human body in one form or another. They act as enzymes that catalyze countless organic chemical reactions in the body, provide physical structure within and between cells, serve as signaling molecules within and between cells, act as the cell's gatekeeper (as cell membrane channels) to ions and other molecules, and participate in muscle contraction.

Proteins are polymers made up of monomers called amino acids. Amino acids share a common structure with an amino group, carboxylic acid, and a variable side chain indicated as R.

```
 O       R
  \\    /
   C—C—H
  /     \
HO       NH2
```

There are 20 standard amino acids found in the proteins of eukaryotic cells, each with a unique side chain; however, hundreds of amino acids have been synthesized. While more modern techniques have been developed to synthesize amino acids, the classic reaction is the Strecker synthesis.

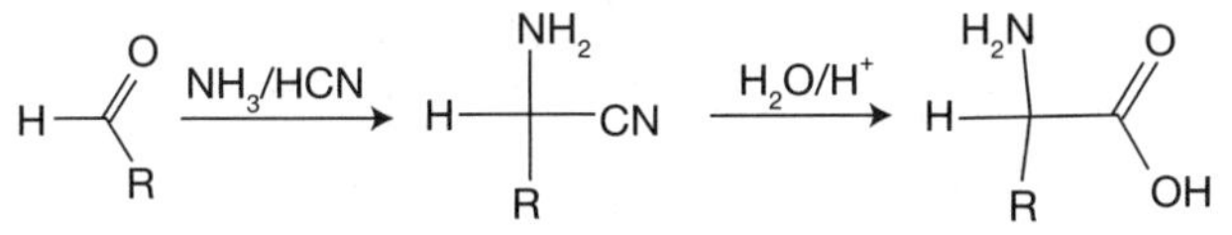

$$\text{H–C(=O)–R} \xrightarrow{NH_3/HCN} \text{H–C(NH}_2\text{)(R)–CN} \xrightarrow{H_2O/H^+} \text{H–C(H}_2\text{N)(R)–C(=O)OH}$$

When forming peptides (short amino acid polymers) and proteins (long amino acid polymers), amino acid monomers are linked by a peptide bond. Like glycosylation, the formation of a peptide bond between two amino acids occurs through a condensation reaction in which a molecule of H_2O is released.

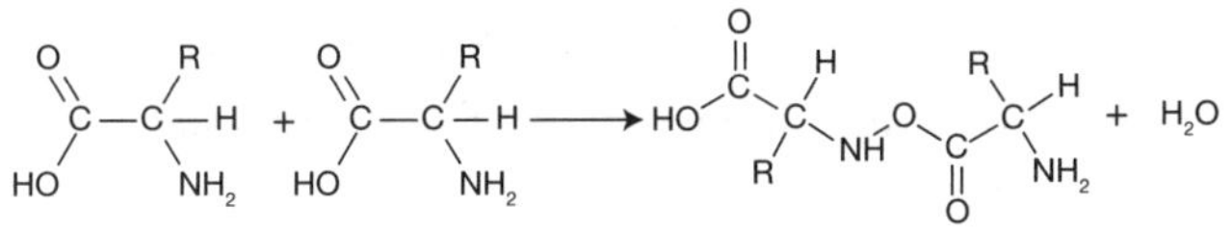

$$\text{HO–C(=O)–C(R)(H)–NH}_2 + \text{HO–C(=O)–C(R)(H)–NH}_2 \longrightarrow \text{HO–C(=O)–C(R)(H)–NH–C(=O)–C(R)(H)–NH}_2 + H_2O$$

In an aqueous solution, each amino acid monomer has the potential to form a zwitterion. A zwitterion is a molecule that has two charged atoms with different polarities. Depending on the pH of the aqueous solution, the carboxylic acid and the amine group may or may not carry an electric charge. For example, in a highly acidic environment, the carboxylic acid group may have a hydrogen atom associated with it and the amine group may also have an additional proton. This gives the amino acid a net charge of +1. By contrast, in a basic solution the carboxylic acid may be deprotonated along with the amine group. However, at an intermediate pH the amino acid may possess both positive and negative charge, making it a zwitterion. This pH is called the isoelectric point. The pH at which a particular functional group is 50% protonated (the functional group is equal parts protonated and unprotonated) is called its pKa. The amino group and the carboxylic acid group each have their own pKa value.

Moreover, the order in which the amino acids are present in a protein predict its overall three-dimensional structure and often its biological function.

AMINO ACID SEQUENCE DETERMINES OVERALL STRUCTURE	
primary	covalent bonds between amino acid monomers
secondary	recurring shapes that appear within proteins such as α-helices and β-pleated sheets
tertiary	three-dimensional shape of the protein
quaternary	structure of multiple proteins interacting (e.g., four subunits of hemoglobin)

Practice Questions

1. A sealed aluminum bottle filled with an unknown gas is heated from room temperature (25°C) to a temperature of 325°C. Assuming no changes in the volume of the bottle or the amount of gas in the bottle, what will be the approximate change in pressure inside the bottle?

a. The pressure increases by a factor of 12.
b. It increases by a factor of 2.
c. It decreases by a factor of 2.
d. It decreases by a factor of 12.

2. $CO_{2(g)} + H_2O_{(l)} \rightleftharpoons H_2CO_{3(aq)}$

The figure describes one of the equilibrium reactions involved in the dissolution of carbon dioxide gas into the bloodstream. Which of the following conditions is most likely to favor increased production of H_2CO_3?

a. increased blood pressure
b. decreased blood pressure
c. increased blood oxygen concentration
d. decreased blood oxygen concentration

3. Sodium bicarbonate ($NaHCO_3$) is often used by pharmacists as a buffering agent. What product is formed when an excess of sodium bicarbonate is added to a solution of sulfuric acid (H_2SO_4)?

a. a strongly acidic solution
b. a weakly acidic solution
c. a neutral solution
d. a weakly basic solution

4. Which of the following species is most likely to accept an electron during the course of a chemical reaction?

a. chlorine atom
b. iodine atom
c. chloride ion
d. iodide ion

5. Which of the following has the largest atomic/ionic radius?

a. chlorine atom
b. iodine atom
c. chloride ion
d. iodide ion

6. Tyrosine, one of the 20 amino acids commonly found in proteins, contains several different functional groups. The molecular structure of tyrosine is depicted here:

HO
H_2N
O
OH

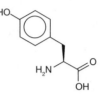

Which of the following functional groups is *least* responsible for the acidic nature of tyrosine?

a. alkane
b. carboxylic acid
c. amine
d. phenol

7. The molecular structure of a water molecule is depicted here:

H—Ö—H

What is the *electron* geometry around the oxygen atom in a water molecule?

a. linear
b. bent
c. trigonal planar
d. tetrahedral

8. When 5 g of sodium chloride is added to a glass containing an unknown amount of water (normal freezing point of 0°C), the freezing point of the resultant solution is –2°C. What would be the freezing point of a solution of an equal mass of magnesium chloride in the same glass?

a. –1°C
b. –2°C
c. –3°C
d. –4°C

9. The following diagram depicts the change in the temperature of a pure substance as heat is added uniformly:

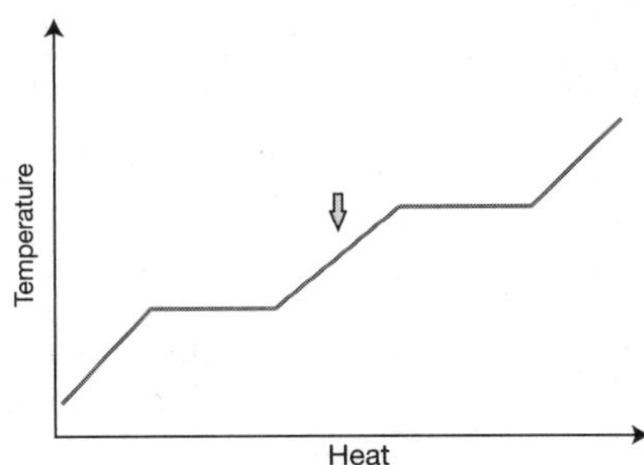

Which process is the substance undergoing at the point designated by the arrow?

a. heating of a solid
b. melting transition
c. heating of a liquid
d. boiling transition

10. Which of the following terms best describes a reaction with one reactant and multiple products?

a. decomposition
b. combination
c. single replacement
d. double replacement

11. A radioisotope undergoes one α decay, one γ decay, and one β^+ decay. What is the difference between the atomic number of the parent nucleus and the daughter nucleus?

a. 1
b. 2
c. 3
d. 4

12. The two most common isotopes of chlorine by far are ^{35}Cl and ^{37}Cl. Considering that chlorine has an atomic mass of approximately 35.5, what is the ratio of ^{35}Cl to ^{37}Cl in a sample of naturally occurring chlorine gas (as would be found in the environment)?

a. 4:1
b. 3:1
c. 2:1
d. 1:1

13. Halogen-based automotive headlamps function at a variety of different temperature ranges. Assuming that all other factors are held constant, which of the following best describes the apparent color of the light emitted by lamps functioning at different temperatures?

a. Higher-temperature lamps will emit more yellow or red light, while lower-temperature lamps will emit more blue or violet light.
b. Higher-temperature lamps will emit more blue or violet light, while lower-temperature lamps will emit more yellow or red light.
c. Higher-temperature lamps will emit more yellow or violet light, while lower-temperature lamps will emit more red or blue light.
d. Higher-temperature lamps will emit more red or violet light, while lower-temperature lamps will emit more yellow or blue light.

14. In an electrolytic cell containing pure water with no solutes, which of the following will migrate toward the anode?

I. Free electrons
II. O^{2-} ions
III. H^+ ions

a. I only
b. II only
c. I and II only
d. I and III only

15. $Al(OH)_3$ is a common ingredient in many over-the-counter antacid formulations. Which of the following is NOT a correct name for $Al(OH)_3$?
- **a.** aluminum hydroxide
- **b.** aluminum (III) hydroxide
- **c.** aluminic hydroxide
- **d.** aluminum hydride

16. Which of the following organic compounds represents the molecular formula of a carboxylic acid?
- **a.** $CH_3CH_2OCH_2CH_2CH_2CH_3$
- **b.** CH_3CH_2Cl
- **c.** $CH_3CH_2CH_2COOH$
- **d.** $CH_3CH_2CH_2CONH_2$

17. Which of the following organic compounds contains the highest boiling point?
- **a.** n-butyl alcohol, $CH_3CH_2CH_2CH_2OH$
- **b.** pentane, $CH_3CH_2CH_2CH_2CH_3$
- **c.** 1-nonene, $CH_2{=}CHCH_2CH_2CH_2CH_2CH_2CH_2CH_3$
- **d.** trifluoroacetic acid, CF_3COOH

18. When an alkane reacts with Br_2 in the presence of untraviolet (UV) light, what is true?
- **a.** Peroxides attack bromine, and an alcohol is formed.
- **b.** The alkyl bromide that forms started from the most stable carbocation.
- **c.** A Markovnikov addition of bromine occurs.
- **d.** A free radical mechanism is involved. Molecular bromine equally divides into two bromine radicals, with one electron each. One bromine radical abstracts hydrogen from the alkane. An alkyl radical intermediate is then formed.

19. A tertiary alkyl halide reacts with a strong base. The base is not sterically hindered. What would be the major products?
- **a.** At lower temperatures, a tertiary alcohol forms.
- **b.** At higher temperatures, a tertiary alcohol forms.
- **c.** At lower temperatures, a trisubstituted alkene forms.
- **d.** At higher temperatures, an ether forms.

20. Predict the major product of the chemical reaction:

$$CH_3(CH_2)_7CH{=}CH(CH_2)_7COOH + LiAlH_4 \rightarrow + H_3O^+ \rightarrow$$

- **a.** $CH_3(CH_2)_7CH_2CH_2(CH_2)_7COOH$
- **b.** $CH_3(CH_2)_7CH{=}CH(CH_2)_7CH_2OH$
- **c.** $CH_3(CH_2)_7CH{=}CH_2(CH_2)_7COO(CH_2)_7CH{=}CH(CH_2)_7CH_3$
- **d.** $CH_3(CH_2)_7CH_2CH_2(CH_2)_7CH_3$

21. For this reaction, what products are most likely to be synthesized?

$$CH_3CH_2CO(CH_2)_3CH_3 + CH_3OH + H_3O^+ \rightarrow \text{Product 1} + CH_3OH \rightarrow \text{Product 2} - H_2O$$

- **a.** product 1: $CH_3CH_2COH(OCH_3)CH_2(CH_2)_2CH_3$; product 2: $CH_3CH_2C(OCH_3)_2CH_2(CH_2)_2CH_3$
- **b.** product 1: $CH_3CH_2COH(OCH_3)CH_2(CH_2)_2CH_3$; product 2: $CH_3CH_2C(OH)_2CH_2(CH_2)_2CH_3$
- **c.** product 1: $CH_3CH_2C(OH)_2CH_2(CH_2)_2CH_3$; product 2: $CH_3CH_2C(OCH_3O)CH_2(CH_2)_2CH_3$
- **d.** product 1: $CH_3CH_2COH(OCH_3)CH_2(CH_2)_2CH_3$; product 2: $CH_3CH_2C(OOCH_3O)CH_2(CH_2)_2CH_3$

22. What is the product of a reaction of phenol with chromate in acidic solution?

a. benzaldehyde
b. benzoic acid
c. para-benzoquinone
d. benzyl benzoate

23. Methyl bromide is first treated with magnesium in ether. This product is then treated with oxirane, an epoxide, and the following product is acidified. What is the final product?

a. methanoic acid
b. dimethyl ether
c. 1-propanol
d. methanoate

24. Pyridinium chlorochromate (PCC) is commonly utilized for oxidation of organic compounds. In a dichlormethane solvent, what is the major product for this reaction?

$CH_3\ CH_2\ CH_2CH_2CH_2OH + PCC \rightarrow$

a. $CH_3\ CH_2\ CH_2CH_2CH_2Cl$, pentyl chloride
b. $CH_3\ CH_2\ CH_2CH_2COCH_3$, hexanone
c. $CH_3\ CH_2\ CH_2CH_2COOH$, pentanoic acid
d. $CH_3\ CH_2\ CH_2CH_2COH$, pentanal

25. Treating 2-butanone with sodium borohydride yields

a. 1-butanol, upon final acidification.
b. 2-butanol, upon final acidification.
c. butanal, upon final addition of base.
d. butanoic acid, upon final acidification.

Answers and Explanations

1. b. According to the ideal gas law ($PV = nRT$), the pressure in a closed container is directly proportional to the temperature of the container (in Kelvin temperature units). This statement assumes no changes in the volume of the container or the number of gas molecules in the container (moles, designated by *n* in the equation). Conversion of Celsius temperature units to Kelvin units is accomplished by adding 273.15 to the temperature in Celsius; in this problem, the temperature of the container is increased from 298°K (25°C) to 598°K (325°C). Since the temperature (in Kelvins) is approximately doubled, the pressure will also double. Note that the ideal gas law can be simplified in this case, as the question states that the volume does not change, and neither does the amount of gas present; *R* is a constant, so the equation collapses to $P_1T_1 = P_2T_2$, where 1 signifies the initial state and 2 represents the container after heating to the new temperature. It therefore becomes easy to see that a doubling of reaction temperature (in Kelvins, as that is the temperature unit required by the constant *R*) must result in a doubling of the pressure.

2. a. Several factors can affect an equilibrium process. According to LeChatelier's principle, an increase in pressure will shift the equilibrium toward the side with fewer gas molecules. In this problem, the left side of the equation ($H_2O + CO_2$) contains one molecule of carbon dioxide gas, while the right side contains no gas. Therefore, increased pressure will shift the equilibrium to the right and lead to increased production of H_2CO_3. Options **c** and **d** are incorrect because the oxygen concentration will have no direct effect on the amounts of any of the molecules involved in this reaction; oxygen does not appear in the reaction under discussion. While oxygen concentrations may affect carbon dioxide concentrations in the body in various ways, an increase in pressure will always push the reaction toward the right side.

3. d. A buffer is a compound that resists changes in pH. $NaHCO_3$ is a weak base (in aqueous solutions it dissociates into Na^+, a neutral cation, and HCO_3^-, a weakly basic anion), so when present in adequate quantities, it will neutralize any strong acid completely. In this question, $NaHCO_3$ is present in excess quantities; this means that even after it neutralizes all of the acid, there are still $NaHCO_3$ molecules present, which (being basic) make the solution slightly basic. ($NaHCO_3$ is only a weak base, so despite the quantity of excess used, the solution becomes only slightly basic.)

4. a. An atom's tendency to accept electrons is measured by its electron affinity, which is the change in energy when an electron is added to a neutral atom of an element in order to form a negative ion. This property is closely related to electronegativity, which is the tendency of atoms to draw electrons toward themselves (forming anions). In general, both electronegativity and electron affinity are higher for elements that are farther up and/or to the right on the Periodic Table. This is a result of the desire of those elements to obtain a filled outer (valence) shell of electrons. Chlorine has the highest electron affinity of all elements, while fluorine has the highest electronegativity (chlorine has the second-highest electronegativity). While iodine is also fairly electronegative, it is not as strongly electronegative as chlorine, due to the atomic size of iodine; the positive charge of the nucleus is further removed from the outer shell of electrons, so there is less attractive force for incoming electrons. Chloride ions and iodide ions, meanwhile, exhibit a very low electronegativity. This is because they have already accepted an electron, which fills their outer (valence) shell, and they therefore exhibit noble gas behavior, having little to no desire to accept any more electrons.

5. d. Atomic radius is higher for elements that are farther down and/or to the left on the Periodic Table. This comes about due to increasing positive charge of the atoms going to the right along the Periodic Table; this results in a stronger electronic attraction between the positively charged protons and the surrounding electrons, which shrinks the overall radius of the atom. Also, the anion of any atom will have a larger radius than the neutral atom because the added electron decreases the force with which the nucleus can pull on each individual electron, thereby allowing the entire ion to expand. For the same reason, cations are generally smaller than their corresponding atoms.

6. c. Of the four functional groups mentioned, an amine group is the most strongly basic; therefore, it is least likely to contribute to the acidic properties of a molecule. Carboxylic acids are acidic due to the resulting carboxylate anion (upon deprotonation) residing on an electronegative atom (oxygen) as well as being resonance stabilized. Phenol groups are slightly acidic (but less acidic than a carboxylic acid) for similar reasons; the phenolate anion has the negative charge concentrated on the electronegative oxygen, resonance stabilized over the benzene ring. Alkane groups are relatively neutral, as once deprotonated, the negative charge is stuck on a nonelectronegative atom (carbon) with no resonance stabilization possible.

7. d. The electron geometry around an atom is determined by the number of electron pairs, paired and unpaired, around the atom. In this question, the oxygen is surrounded by two free electron pairs and two electron pairs that are shared with the hydrogen atoms. When four electron pairs surround an atom, the electron geometry is marked as tetrahedral. Do not be confused about the difference between electronic and molecular geometry. The water molecule actually possesses bent molecular geometry, as the two lone pairs of electrons do not form visible covalent bonds to other atoms. The Lewis structure of water appears at first glance to be linear (a straight line, H-O-H), until the electronic repulsion of the two sets of lone pairs is taken into consideration. They push the covalent bonds slightly backward, creating a bent molecular geometry. The electron geometry, however, is tetrahedral.

8. c. According to the colligative properties of water, the decrease in freezing point of an ionic solution is equal to the product of the solution's molality (mass of solute divided by moles of solvent), the number of ions in solution, and a standard freezing point depression constant. In this case, the molality of the sodium chloride (NaCl) solution is identical to the molality of the magnesium chloride ($MgCl_2$) solution, as the mass of the solute and the moles of solvent remain the same in both cases. However, $MgCl_2$ dissociates into three ions (one Mg^{++} ion and two Cl^- ions), while NaCl dissociates into only two ions (one Na^+ ion and one Cl^- ion). Since the number of ions in the $MgCl_2$ solution is 1.5 times the number of ions in the NaCl solution, the $MgCl_2$ solution will cause 1.5 times the freezing point depression; therefore, if the NaCl solution lowers the freezing point of water by 2°C, the $MgCl_2$ solution will lower the freezing point by 3°C.

9. c. A heat transfer diagram depicts the nonuniform change in temperature as a substance is heated. (1) The first upward diagonal line segment represents the increase in temperature of the substance as its solid form is heated. (2) The first horizontal line segment represents the heat that is absorbed by the solid as it gathers the energy required to melt into a liquid (a value specific to each chemical compound, related to its heat of fusion). During this period, there is no change in temperature as heat is applied. When the substance has completely melted into its liquid form, the temperature will then continue to increase as long as the application of heat is continued. (3) The second diagonal line segment represents the increase in temperature as the liquid form is heated. The arrow in the question stem refers to a point along this phase. (4) The second horizontal line segment represents the heat that is absorbed by the liquid as it gathers the energy required to vaporize into a gas (a value specific to each chemical compound, related to its heat of vaporization). (5) The final diagonal line segment represents the increase in temperature as the gas form is heated.

10. a. When a single reactant forms multiple products, it has undergone a *decomposition* reaction; in other words, one substance has *decomposed* into several other substances. When multiple reactants *combine* to *synthesize* a single product, the reaction is termed a *synthesis* or a *combination. Single replacement* and *double replacement* reactions both involve at least two reactants and two products.

11. c. In an α decay, a nucleus loses two protons (alpha particles are forms of helium atoms, with an atomic number of 2), thereby decreasing the atomic number of a radioisotope by 2. In β^+ decay, one proton is converted to one neutron (along with a positron and an electron neutrino), thereby decreasing the atomic number of the radioisotope by an additional 1. In γ decay, the atom only emits energy (in the form of a high-energy photon), but there is no change in atomic number as there is no change in the number of protons present in the radioisotope under this type of process. The overall reaction therefore constitutes a loss of three protons from the parent nucleus. The atomic number decreases by 3.

12. b. The atomic mass of an element tells us the average mass of a sample of that element as it is found in its natural form in the environment. Chlorine gas exists naturally as a mixture of several isotopes. The *average* atomic mass (from the Periodic Table) of chlorine (35.5) is about 0.5 amu (atomic mass units) more than the mass of ^{35}Cl and 1.5 amu less than the mass of ^{37}Cl. Since $\frac{1.5 \text{ amu}}{0.5 \text{ amu}} = 3$, we can see that on average there must be three atoms of ^{35}Cl for every atom of ^{37}Cl in order to have this effect. By contrast, if the two isotopes were present in equal quantities, the atomic mass of chlorine would be equal to the average of the masses of the two isotopes (in this case, 36 amu).

13. b. As heat energy is added to a system, the energy of the system increases. Consequently, lamps functioning at higher temperatures (assuming that all other factors are equal) will emit higher-energy light. According to Planck's law ($E = h\nu = \frac{hc}{\lambda}$), where h is the Planck constant, the energy of a photon is directly proportional to its frequency; this means that the higher-energy lamps will emit light at higher frequencies (lower wavelengths). On the visible electromagnetic spectrum, higher frequencies correspond with blue and violet light, whereas lower frequencies (higher wavelengths) correspond with red, orange, and yellow light. An easy way to remember the spectrum is to keep in mind that it follows the same trend as the colors of the rainbow—red, orange, yellow, green, blue, violet (in order of increasing frequency and decreasing wavelength).

14. b. An electrolytic cell uses an electric current to provide the energy required to break a compound into its constituent elements (water, in this case, which breaks down ultimately into hydrogen gas and oxygen gas). In such a cell, cations (positively charged ions) migrate to the cathode (hence the name *cat*hode) and anions (negatively charged ions) migrate to the anode (hence the name *an*ode). Free electrons always migrate to the cathode to balance the positive charge from the cations, where they normally reduce the positively charged ions to neutral atoms (such as in the case of the electrolysis of molten sodium chloride, which produces sodium metal). Since this cell contains only water, the anion (O^{2-}) will always migrate to the anode, while the cation (H^+) will migrate to the cathode along with free electrons.

15. d. Aluminum's main oxidation state is +3, while hydroxide ions carry a –1 charge. When aluminum and hydroxide form a stable compound, three OH^- ions will form ionic bonds with one Al^{3+} ion, thereby producing $Al(OH)_3$. Since this is the major (most common) ionic salt of aluminum and hydroxide, we can call it by the common name *aluminum hydroxide* without indicating any numbers. It is also acceptable to call it aluminum (III) hydroxide, which is slightly more correct as it leaves no confusion regarding the charge on the central aluminum ion. Aluminic hydroxide is another acceptable name because +3 is aluminum's highest oxidation state, although this is a much less common name for this compound and might be unfamiliar to numerous chemists. Aluminum hydride, however, refers to AlH_3, since the term *hydride* refers to the H^- anion.

16. c. A carboxylic acid contains the –COOH functional group.

17. c. Pentane is a moderately low molecular weight alkane with only the small-scale dispersion forces such as van der Waals interactions and London forces that influence its boiling point. Trifluoroacetic acid experiences a high electron withdrawing inductive effect from the presence of the three fluorine atoms, which pull electron density further away from the –COOH group. This strong inductive effect observed in trifluoroacetic acid reduces the ability to form intramolecular acid dimers, which would raise the boiling point. Butanol has a polar group for dipole interactions, yet it is still quite low in molecular weight. The organic compound with the highest boiling point is actually nonene. Even though nonene illustrates mild van der Waals intermolecular interactions, its molecular weight is sufficient to win out versus the polarity and electron withdrawing effects of its competitors. The literature values for the boiling points (T_b) are as follows: for pentane, $T_b = 36°C$; for trifluoroacetic acid, $T_b = 72°C$; for butanol, $T_b = 117°C$; and for 1-nonene, $T_b = 147°C$.

18. d. In the presence of UV light and/or heat, an alkane can replace a hydrogen with a halogen through a free radical mechanism. The UV light first breaks the bond of the diatomic bromine molecule, causing a bromine radical to form that then abstracts hydrogen from the alkane. The most stable alkyl radical intermediate forms. Rearrangement of the carbon skeleton may occur to obtain optimal stability. Termination steps then follow, in order to combine the bromine radical with the alkyl radical.

19. a. At low temperatures, a strong base that is not sterically hindered can act as a good nucleophile. This nucleophile then reacts with the tertiary alkyl halide to generate a tertiary alcohol.

20. b. The carboxylic acid group is reduced to an alcohol in the presence of the powerful reducing agent $LiAlH_4$.

21. a. Hemiketals and ketals form when an alcohol and water add to a ketone. Product 1 is a hemiketal, for only one mole of methanol has added. Product 2 is a ketal, for two moles of methanol have added.

22. c. Chromate is a strong oxidizing agent. Para-benzoquinone forms when chromate oxidizes phenol.

23. c. This Grignard reagent generates an alcohol. No additional alkyl group is added to the product, for there is no alkyl group first bonded to the magnesium reagent.

24. d. The primary alcohol is oxidized to an aldehyde.

25. b. Sodium borohydride is a reducing agent. Following acidification, the ketone intermediate is reduced to an alcohol.

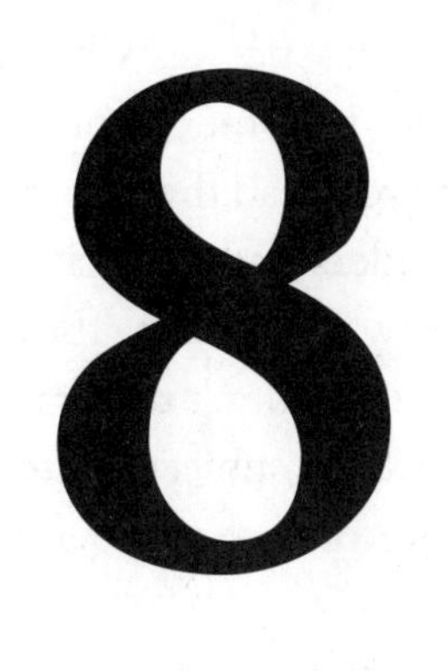

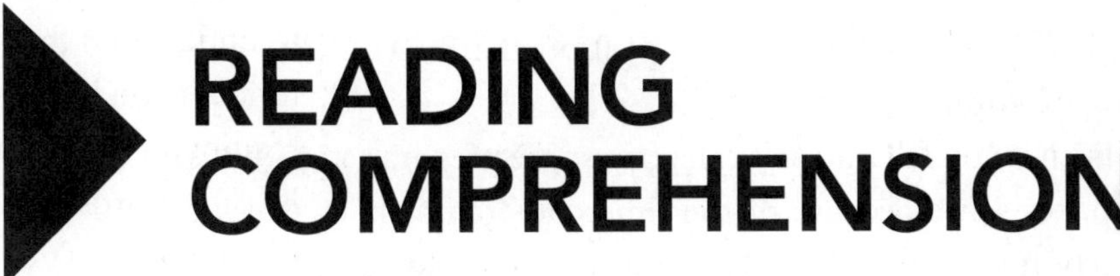

CHAPTER 8 READING COMPREHENSION

The Reading Comprehension section of the PCAT, in which you will have 50 minutes to read six passages and answer 48 multiple-choice questions related to those passages, is a little bit like the essays. Unlike the biology, chemistry, and quantitative sections, there isn't a set of information that you can attempt to memorize to help you get the correct answers. Instead, reading comprehension tests your ability to understand, analyze, and evaluate information from passages that are likely to be unfamiliar to you.

Unlike the essays, this section is scored like the other multiple-choice portions of the test using a scale of 200 to 600.

While you can't memorize specific facts and equations in order to study for the Reading Comprehension section, there are things you can—and should—do to prepare for this portion of the PCAT.

The reading passages are usually between 300 and 400 words and will always be nonfiction. Most of them will be science-related. In many cases, the specific concept or idea will be something that is unfamiliar to you.

How to Prepare

To prepare for the Reading Comprehension test, start with an honest assessment of your own abilities. You can do this by looking at how you have performed on tests you've taken before that have similar reading comprehension sections. If you have done well on them, it is likely that you will do well on the PCAT Reading Comprehension.

Even if you fall into this category, some preparation makes sense because of the time constraint on this section of the PCAT. Fifty minutes is not a long time to read and analyze six passages, and then correctly answer 48 multiple-choice questions about those passages. This is especially true when you are unfamiliar with the subject matter within the passages. For you, practice tests are a good approach, so you can make sure you're moving through the passages and questions quickly enough to finish.

Read, Read, Read

For those of you who have struggled more with reading comprehension, and for those of you for whom English may not be your first language, the more preparation you do for this section, the better your results will be. One of the best ways to prepare is to read. In particular, start making it a habit to read the science section or science articles in your local newspaper. The *New York Times* publishes a Science section every Tuesday, so if your local paper doesn't have many science articles, go to the *Times*'s website and read the articles there.

You should also try reading articles from medical journals such as *Science*, *Nature*, *The Lancet*, and the *Journal of the American Medical Association*. Selected articles from these publications are available online. These articles begin with what's called an abstract, which is a summary of the article's findings. Read the abstract first and see if you understand it. Then read the article and see if your understanding was correct. It may seem tedious, but after a while you will find that your ability to understand and analyze complex material you have not seen before will improve.

Practice Reading Comprehension Passages

As you read passages from practice tests or articles just like those mentioned, see how much you are able to understand the first time you read through the material. If you have trouble understanding what you are reading, try to figure out why. Is it because the author is using words or jargon that you don't understand, is it that you don't comprehend the subject matter, or is it that you can't quite figure out what the author is trying to say?

Then go back and reread the passage slowly, breaking it down into bite-size pieces by looking at each paragraph separately. Make notes to help you work through each passage. When you do this with practice tests, answer the multiple-choice questions at the end of each passage after you've read it once; then go back and read it more carefully and answer the questions again before you check to see how you did.

Know What to Expect

Just like most other sections of the PCAT, the more you practice and the more aware you are of what to expect, the less anxious you will be on test day, and the more prepared you will be to get good scores on all of the sections of the test.

There are three basic types of reading comprehension questions that you will find on the PCAT: comprehension, analysis, and evaluation.

Comprehension

Approximately one-third of the questions will be to see whether you understand the passage. They will include questions similar to the following:

- What is the main idea of the passage?
- Are you able to identify details and evidence from the passage that support the main idea?

- Do you understand the meaning of specific vocabulary words that are underlined in the passage?

What do you do if you don't know what an underlined word means? You can try to figure out the meaning by reading the words and sentences around it. Then you can look at the choices and go through them one by one, replacing the underlined word with each choice, reading the sentence, and trying to figure out which one works best. Even if you aren't sure, this method should help you eliminate some of the wrong answers. This is a good time to remember that on the PCAT there is no guessing penalty, so it's better to try to eliminate a couple of wrong choices and then make your best guess than it is to leave an answer blank.

Analysis

Approximately 40% of the questions will be based on your ability to analyze the passage. These questions will ask you to interpret the passage in a number of different ways.

- What is the purpose of the passage?
- How is the passage structured?
- What does the passage mean?
- What predictions could you make based on the passage?
- What conclusions can you draw based on the passage?
- What is the author's purpose in writing the passage?
- What does the passage imply about the author's view of the subject?

Since these analysis questions will appear throughout the Reading Comprehension section, it's helpful to develop your own strategy for answering them. The paragraphs of each passage are numbered, so you might consider making some notes on each paragraph. Alternatively, as you do your practice tests and read other articles, keep notes on the structure, meaning, and purpose of each passage you read. Once you get into the habit of reading passages this way, your ability to answer the analysis questions will improve.

Evaluation

The final 30% of questions will ask you to analyze things such as the evidence presented in the passage and the tone of the passage.

- Is the argument effective?
- Is the argument credible?
- Does the evidence provided support the main idea of the passage?
- Can you distinguish fact from opinion in the passage?
- Can you evaluate the tone of the passage?

Looking at the author's choice of words will help you evaluate the tone of each passage. The words will tell you how the author feels about the subject matter. The tone can be optimistic or pessimistic. It can be humorous, serious, cynical, or even angry. Using the same method described for addressing the analysis questions, as you read practice passages, make notes about the author's tone, and then see how it compares to the correct answers to the questions related to that passage.

Use Your Time Wisely

The passages on the Reading Comprehension section are likely to be challenging to understand the first time through. But don't get stuck if you miss something the first time you read each passage. Start by reading the passage from beginning to end, and reading the associated questions for that passage. If there are one or two you can answer right away, do so, but don't worry if you need a second read-through before you tackle the questions. On your second reading of the passages, look for the sections that will help you answer the questions. Answer the questions and move on to the next section. If you have time at the end, you can go back over questions where you made educated guesses to see if you can narrow your choices down further.

Practice under PCAT Time Constraints

The most effective way to put to use the information about the types of questions you will be faced with in the PCAT Reading Comprehension section is to practice as if you are actually taking the test. While most of you could get the questions right if you had enough time to read and reread the passages, 50 minutes goes by quickly, so it's more than just learning about the questions and reading practice passages.

With 50 minutes, six passages, and 48 questions, you'll have approximately eight minutes for each passage and associated questions. So time yourself even if you're only reading and answering the questions one passage at a time. In other words, use all of the information in this chapter, approach the passages as described earlier, and do it under test conditions so that when test day arrives, you won't spend so much of your time on the first four passages that you have to rush and guess on the final two.

Practice Passages

Following are four practice reading comprehension passages with multiple-choice questions. Following each passage are detailed explanations of the answers. Again, remember that although you may not always be familiar with the subject matter of the passages, you should still be able to use your reading skills to figure out the right answers.

Passage 1

(1) After the discovery of penicillin, the first antibiotic, in 1929 by Alexander Fleming, the world entered an era in which diseases that had previously been deadly or debilitating became curable. Optimism reigned as new drugs were discovered or synthesized in laboratories around the world.

(2) Today, there are very few new antibiotics in the pipeline, and government officials in the United States are discussing the possibility of offering financial incentives, such as tax breaks and patent extensions, to pharmaceutical companies to spur the development of vitally needed drugs to fight bacterial infections.

(3) What happened to the age of optimism? Over time, bacteria developed resistance to the drugs created to cure the infections they cause. There are multiple reasons for this, some of them man-made. For example, when a physician prescribes a course of 10 days of antibiotics to cure an infection and the patient feels better after six days and stops taking the medication, it is likely that the infection has not, in fact, been cleared or cured. Some bacteria may remain. This could mean that if the patient gets the same infection again, it will be resistant. Or worse, it could mean the patient is still infectious and can spread disease to others.

(4) There's more to the story. For the pharmaceutical industry, the incentives to develop and market medications to treat chronic conditions such as high cholesterol and diabetes are obvious. Not only do these medications help patients, but also patients need to take these medications for months, years, or even lifetimes, so the potential profits, which are part of why drug companies are in business, are large. Antibiotics, in contrast, are usually taken for only 10 days or two weeks, and then in many cases the patient is cured. The better the drug, the shorter the duration

of treatment. While that's good for patients, it's not so lucrative for drug companies.

(5) To make the situation worse, today there is so much drug resistance, the best way to use a new antibiotic would be to save it and use it very judiciously to keep it effective and prevent resistance to it from arising for as long as possible.

(6) Although this idea is new and controversial, it may ultimately be the best way to combat the overwhelming rise in antibiotic resistance that can make it challenging, if not impossible, to cure disease in patients who 25 years ago would have been better after a short course of medication.

Questions for Passage 1

1. The word *synthesized* in the first paragraph means which of the following?
a. occurring in nature
b. man-made
c. created
d. natural

2. The purpose of the third paragraph is to
a. discuss the end of the age of optimism.
b. define antibiotic resistance.
c. explain one of the ways antibiotic resistance occurs.
d. describe how antibiotics work.

3. Which of the following assertions does the author support?
a. New antibiotics are no longer necessary.
b. Antibiotics are no longer useful.
c. Antibiotic resistance is a problem that can easily be overcome.
d. New antibiotics must be used judiciously in order for them to remain effective.

4. Which of the following would be the best title of this passage?
a. "Incentives for Development of New Antibiotics"
b. "Antibiotics Don't Work Anymore"
c. "New Approaches to Drug Development"
d. "Antibiotic Resistance in Today's World"

5. The tone of the passage is
a. negative.
b. cautiously optimistic.
c. scared.
d. angry.

6. The main point of the passage is which of the following?
a. It is time to consider alternative approaches to encouraging pharmaceutical companies to develop new antibiotics.
b. Antibiotic resistance has become an intractable problem.
c. Drug companies aren't making antibiotics anymore.
d. Without incentives, there will be no new antibiotics.

Answers and Explanations for Passage 1

1. b. Questions that ask about the meaning of a particular word are one type of comprehension question. Synthesized antibiotics are man-made, as opposed to those found in nature. Although choice **c**, created, is close, it is not as good an answer as choice **b** because it does not fit the context of the rest of the paragraph. The passage discusses drugs that were discovered or synthesized, which implies that if people didn't discover them, they had to produce or make them. Choice **d**, natural, is the opposite, and therefore not correct.

2. c. Questions that ask about the purpose of a particular paragraph are analysis questions. The third paragraph includes a specific example of one of the ways that antibiotic resistance may develop: when a patient doesn't comply with the doctor's instructions for taking medication. While choices **b** and **d** may seem like correct answers, they refer to the overall tone and meaning of the passage, and are therefore too general to be correct. While the paragraph mentions the age of optimism, it is only as a lead-in to the discussion about antibiotic resistance.

3. d. This is an example of an evaluation question. One of the main points of the passage is that for new antibiotics to be effective, they must be used very carefully and in a limited manner; otherwise, bacteria will develop resistance to them and they will be rendered ineffective. Choices **a**, **b**, and **c** are all false statements.

4. a. Questions that ask about the best title for a passage are a type of comprehension question. Here, choice **a**, "Incentives for Development of New Antibiotics," is the correct answer. Choice **b** is false. Choice **c** is too general—this passage refers specifically to antibiotics, not all drug development. Choice **d** is also too general.

5. b. Questions that ask about the tone of a passage are evaluation questions. While the author of this passage does not say that incentives will solve the problem, the tone is cautiously optimistic because there are options being discussed that may help to address the problem of antibiotic resistance. Although the author is discussing serious issues and gaps in drug development, the tone is not negative, nor does the author express overriding fear or anger.

6. a. Questions that ask about the main point of a passage are yet another type of comprehension question. Here, the main point of this passage is that it is time to consider new options so that pharmaceutical companies continue to attempt to discover new antibiotics to treat bacterial infections. The author never states that the problem is intractable or unsolvable. While choices **c** and **d** may seem like possible answers, the author does not state that development of new antibiotics has stopped, or that incentives for pharmaceutical companies are the only possible approach to address the problem.

Passage 2

This passage is adapted from an article by the environmental protection organization Greenpeace regarding Finland's destruction of old-growth forests.

(1) Time is running out for the old-growth forests of Finland. The vast majority of Finland's valuable old-growth forest is owned by the state and logged by the state-owned company Metsähallitus. Metsähallitus's logging practices include clear-cutting, logging in habitats of threatened and vulnerable species, and logging in areas of special scenic or cultural value—including in areas that are critical for the reindeer herding of the indigenous Sami people.

(2) Despite being involved in a "dialogue process" with two environmental organizations (World Wildlife Fund and the Finnish Association for Nature Conservation) to try to reach agreement regarding additional protection for old-growth forests, Metsähallitus is now logging sites that should be subject to negotiation. In June 2003, Greenpeace and the Finnish Association for Nature Conservation (FANC) presented comprehensive maps of the

old-growth areas that they felt should be subject to moratorium, pending discussion and additional protection, to all those involved in the dialogue process. Metsähallitus then announced a halt to new logging operations in these mapped areas. Sadly, the halt in logging was short-lived. In August and September logging took place in at least six old-growth forest areas in northern Finland.

(3) It seems Metsähallitus wants to have its cake and eat it, too—friendly talks with environmental groups at the same time as they keep logging critical habitat. To be blunt, their commitment to the dialogue process has proven untrustworthy. The new logging has been without consensus from the dialogue process or proper consultation with the Sami reindeer herders. Now there's a risk the logging will expand to include other old-growth areas.

(4) Greenpeace investigations have revealed a number of companies buying old-growth timber from Metsähallitus, but the great majority goes to Finland's three international paper manufacturers, Stora Enso, UPM-Kymmene, and M-Real. Greenpeace recommends that companies ask for written guarantees that no material from any of the recently mapped old-growth areas is entering or will enter their supply chain, pending the switch to only timber that has been independently certified to the standards of the Forest Stewardship Council in order to stop this risk to protected forests.

Questions for Passage 2

1. To help protect forests in Finland, Greenpeace recommends
- **a.** written guarantees for companies preventing the use of old-growth materials.
- **b.** stopping logging in Finland.
- **c.** not buying timber from Metsähallitus.
- **d.** regulating paper manufacturers.

2. As used in paragraph 3, *consensus* most nearly means which of the following?
- **a.** oral presentation
- **b.** concurrence
- **c.** dispute
- **d.** concession

3. According to the passage, all of the following are logging practices engaged in by Metsähallitus EXCEPT
- **a.** employing the clear-cutting method.
- **b.** logging in the habitat of reindeer.
- **c.** logging within the boundaries of the indigenous Sami.
- **d.** logging in traditional Norwegian fjords.

4. The author's tone may best be classified as
- **a.** sarcastic.
- **b.** urgent.
- **c.** indifferent.
- **d.** panicked.

5. The main purpose of this passage is to
- **a.** alert citizens that their forests may be in danger.
- **b.** agitate for change in Finland's logging practices.
- **c.** encourage consumers to boycott Finnish wood products.
- **d.** rally support for Greenpeace's international causes.

Answers and Explanations for Passage 2

1. **a.** This is an analysis question. The last paragraph of the passage states that Greenpeace recommends that paper companies secure written guarantees to ensure that old-growth materials are not used. Greenpeace does not suggest a halt to logging or that companies refuse to buy from Metsähallitus. Although Greenpeace would probably favor some regulation, this idea is not discussed in the passage.
2. **b.** This is a comprehension question. The word *consensus* means general agreement, thus the correct answer is choice **b**, concurrence, which also means agreement. You could eliminate choice **c**, dispute, based on the context of the paragraph and the reference to Metsähallitus's commitment to the dialogue process proving untrustworthy, in the immediately preceding sentence. Don't confuse the word *concession* (choice **d**) with *consensus*. Even though they sound somewhat similar, they are not synonyms.
3. **d.** This is also a comprehension question. Choice **d** is the correct answer because the Norwegian fjords are not part of Finland. All of the other choices are logging practices that the passage states that Metsähallitus has engaged in.
4. **b.** Questions that ask about tone are evaluation questions. The passage focuses on practices that the author believes threaten to destroy forests in Finland. The author's genuine concern for the subject rules out choices **a** and **c**. There is no tone of panic in the passage, so that rules out choice **d**. The answer is therefore choice **b**, urgent.
5. **b.** Questions that ask about purpose are analysis questions. The purpose of the passage is to promote awareness and change. Choice **c** does not appear in the passage, choice **a** is false (not all forests are in danger), and there is no discussion in the passage of other Greenpeace international causes (choice **d**).

Passage 3

(1) Molecular epidemiology is a relatively new field of scientific research that applies the tools and techniques of molecular biology to the study of the distribution and determinants of infections and communicable diseases. While traditional epidemiology focuses on <u>retrospective</u> studies, the addition of molecular techniques enables clinicians and researchers to track, analyze, slow, or stop current disease outbreaks in real time.

(2) Specific applications of molecular epidemiology help researchers to correlate risk factors and disease transmission, detect and confirm disease outbreaks in hospitals and other institutional settings, distinguish between new infections and reactivation of disease, understand the virulence and resistance mechanisms of different strains, track the global spread of specific diseases, improve knowledge regarding transmission dynamics and dissemination pathways of infectious diseases, and develop strategies for the treatment and prevention of disease.

(3) One of the most practical components of molecular epidemiology is to address nosocomial infections that spread in hospitals. Microbiologists can help determine whether multiple cases in a unit or hospital are caused by the same bacterial strain spreading from patient to patient, by multiple strains, by a strain that is most commonly found in the community, or by a combination of these factors.

(4) This is a two-step process that begins with the identification of bacterial strains, which is usually insufficient for discriminating among isolates. A second step that utilizes molecular typing techniques (i.e., DNA fingerprinting) helps to answer the specific questions about whether strains that are spreading are genetically related.

(5) These techniques were used successfully in the 1990s to evaluate the transmission of tuberculosis during outbreaks of multidrug-resistant disease in the United States. They were able to help researchers and clinicians distinguish transmission, relapse, and exogenous reinfection. They were also useful in finding cases of laboratory cross-contamination, particularly important since the most common strain was highly resistant to first-line antibiotics, and was therefore treated with less effective and more toxic second-line drugs. Knowing which drugs each patient needed or didn't need as quickly as possible helped to save lives.

(6) This work helped to identify one strain of disease, called the W strain based on an alphabetic system of nomenclature. This strain caused disease in more than 500 patients, was always resistant to the four first-line tuberculosis drugs, and was especially dangerous for HIV-positive patients, who were more susceptible to disease due to their compromised immune systems.

(7) These techniques are currently being applied to the study of the spread of methicillin-resistant *Staphylococcus aureus* (MRSA). MRSA can spread rapidly in a hospital or in the community and the arsenal of useful drugs is rapidly shrinking, so an understanding of how the bacterium is spreading in real time should be useful in developing effective policies for hospitals and nursing homes, as well as appropriate public health interventions.

Questions for Passage 3

1. In the first paragraph, the author uses the word *retrospective*. In this context, *retrospective* means
a. complete.
b. past.
c. future.
d. later.

2. According to this passage,
a. DNA fingerprinting cannot identify like strains of bacteria.
b. molecular epidemiology has not yet been used effectively.
c. molecular epidemiology is a useful tool in analyzing disease outbreaks as they happen.
d. molecular epidemiology is most useful for identifying tuberculosis strains.

3. Which of the following cannot be accomplished using molecular epidemiology?
a. detection of outbreaks in hospitals
b. information regarding virulence of organisms and strains
c. patterns of disease transmission
d. curing diseases

4. The word *exogenous* in paragraph 5 refers to infections that
a. are caused by reactivation of a previous infection.
b. are caused by a different strain of an organism.
c. are caused by a patient not taking medication properly.
d. are caused by the same strain that had previously infected a patient.

5. According to the passage, the W strain of tuberculosis
   a. infected patients all over the world.
   b. was highly infectious in HIV-positive patients.
   c. did not spread rapidly.
   d. was easily curable with antibiotics.

Answers and Explanations for Passage 3

1. b. In this context, *retrospective studies* refer to analysis of events that occurred in the past. *Future* and *later* are the opposite of the correct answer. While *complete* comes close, it does not make sense in the context of the rest of the paragraph.

2. c. One of the main points of the passage is that molecular epidemiology enables clinicians and researchers to work in real time, analyzing outbreaks as they happen and in some cases using the information to intervene or to change interventions so they are more effective. Choices **a** and **b** are false. Choice **d** refers to one specific example in the passage and therefore it does not represent the entire passage.

3. d. As indicated in paragraph 2, molecular epidemiology helps doctors and scientists understand disease outbreaks, virulence, and patterns of transmission. While it may inform treatment decisions doctors make for their patients, it is not in and of itself a method to cure disease.

4. b. In this context, the word *exogenous* means an infection caused by a different, or new strain. By looking at the words around it you can determine that it is not transmission or relapse, and there is no reference in the paragraph to medication being related to exogenous reinfection.

5. b. According to the passage, the W strain was highly infectious among HIV-positive patients. Be careful: Although you may assume that it may also have infected patients all over the world (choice **a**), that fact is not stated within the passage. You must base your answer only on what is contained in the passage, not outside knowledge. The other two choices, **c** and **d**, are false.

Passage 4

(1) For centuries time was measured by the position of the sun with the use of sundials. Noon was recognized when the sun was the highest in the sky, and cities would set their clock by this apparent solar time, even though some cities would often be on a slightly different time. "Summer time" or daylight saving time (DST) was instituted to make better use of daylight. Thus, clocks are set forward one hour in the spring to move an hour of daylight from the morning to the evening and then set back one hour in the fall to return to normal daylight.

(2) The United States Congress passed the Standard Time Act of 1918 to establish standard time and preserve and set daylight saving time across the country. This act also devised five time zones throughout the United States: Eastern, Central, Mountain, Pacific, and Alaska. The first time zone was set on "the mean astronomical time of the seventy-fifth degree of longitude west from Greenwich" (England). In 1919 this act was repealed. President Roosevelt established year-round daylight saving time (also called "War Time") from 1942 to 1945. However, after this period each state adopted their own DST, which proved to be <u>disconcerting</u> to television and radio broadcasting and transportation.

(3) In 1966, President Lyndon Johnson created the Department of Transportation and signed the Uniform Time Act. As a result, the Department of Transportation was given the responsibility for the time laws. During the oil embargo and energy crisis of the 1970s, President Richard Nixon extended DST through the Daylight Saving Time Energy Act of 1973 to conserve energy further. This law was modified in 1986, and daylight saving time was set for beginning on the first Sunday in April (to "spring ahead") and ending on the last Sunday in October (to "fall back"). It has since been extended, currently lasting from March to November.

(4) Through the years, the U.S. Department of Transportation conducted polls concerning daylight saving time and found that many Americans were in favor of it because of the extended hours of daylight and the freedom to do more in the evening hours. In further studies the U.S. Department of Transportation also found that DST conserves energy by cutting the electricity usage in the evening for lights and particular appliances.

(5) During the darkest winter months (November through February), the advantage of conserving energy in late-afternoon daylight saving time is outweighed by the need for more light in the morning because of late sunrise. In Britain, studies showed that there were fewer accidents on the road because of the increased visibility resulting from additional hours of daylight.

(6) Despite these advantages, there is still opposition to DST. One perpetual complaint is the inconvenience of changing many clocks, and adjusting to a new sleep schedule is another common complaint. Farmers often wake at sunrise and find that their animals do not adjust to the changing of time until weeks after the clock is either moved forward or back. Many places around the globe still do not observe daylight saving time—such as Arizona (excluding Navajo reservations), five counties in Indiana, Hawaii, Puerto Rico, Japan, and Saskatchewan, Canada. Countries located near the equator have equal hours of day and night and do not participate in daylight saving time.

Questions for Passage 4

1. In paragraph 2 the word *disconcerting* most nearly means
a. useful.
b. functional.
c. confusing.
d. enlightening.

2. According to the passage, all of the following are beneficial effects of DST EXCEPT
a. changing sleeping patterns.
b. fewer car accidents.
c. conservation of energy.
d. additional time for family outings.

3. According to the passage, in which area of the world is DST least useful?
a. the tropics
b. Indiana
c. Navajo reservations
d. Canada

4. Which of the following statements is true of the U.S. Department of Transportation?
a. It was created by President Richard Nixon.
b. It set the standards for DST throughout the world.
c. It oversees all time laws in the United States.
d. It established the standard railway time laws.

5. Which of the following statements is the best title for this passage?

a. "The History and Rationale of Daylight Saving Time"

b. "Lyndon Johnson and the Uniform Time Act"

c. "The U.S. Department of Transportation and Daylight Saving Time"

d. "Daylight Saving Time around the World"

6. Which of the following does the passage cite as a rationale for not extending daylight saving time year-round?

a. During November through February, the need for light in the morning is more important than the advantage of conserving energy.

b. During November through February, there are more accidents on the road in the evening than in the morning.

c. During March through October, it is easier to adjust to a new sleep schedule.

d. During March through October, it is easier for animals to adjust to the changing of time.

Answers and Explanations for Passage 4

1. c. *Disconcerting* most nearly means confusing. If you didn't know the meaning of *disconcerting*, you might still be able to identify that the prefix *dis-* likely indicates a word that has a negative connotation. Of all the choices, only choice **c**, confusing, has such a connotation. All of the other choices have positive connotations. Choices **a** and **b**, useful and functional, also have very similar meanings, and since both can't be correct, this indicates that neither is likely to be correct. Finally, just because the passage involves daylight saving time, don't get suckered into choosing a word like choice **d**, enlightening, which makes no sense in the context of the sentence.

2. a. Changing sleeping patterns is cited in the passage as a negative effect, not a beneficial one. All of the other choices are discussed within the passage as beneficial effects.

3. a. The tropics are near the equator, and thus already experience equal amounts of day and night all year-round; therefore there is no need in that part of the world to extend the hours of daylight. The other choices are incorrect because the Navajos have DST, and parts of Indiana and Canada do observe DST.

4. c. The Department of Transportation oversees all time laws in the United States. Richard Nixon did not create it, and it controls time laws only in the United States, not throughout the world.

5. a. Choices **b**, **c**, and **d** are incorrect because they each refer to specific points raised in the passage, but not throughout the entire passage. Choice **a** best describes the point of the entire passage, and therefore is the best title.

6. a. The article states, "During the darkest winter months (November through February), the advantage of conserving energy in late-afternoon daylight saving time is outweighed by the need for more light in the morning because of late sunrise." None of the rationales stated in choices **b**, **c**, or **d** are supported by the passage.

CHAPTER 9

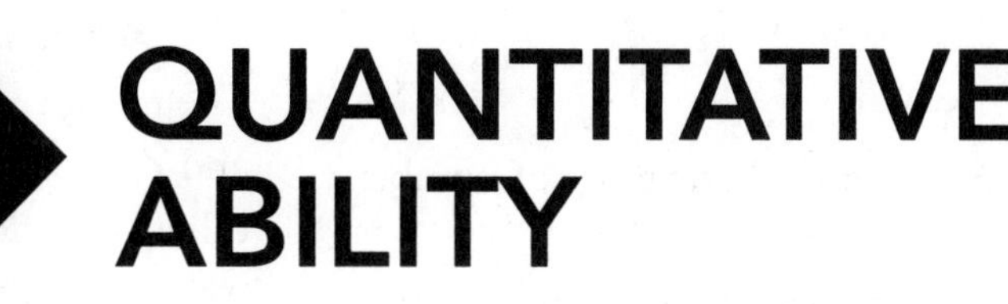

QUANTITATIVE ABILITY

The Quantitative Ability section of the PCAT contains 48 questions covering the following topics:

- Basic math: approximately 15% of the questions
- Algebra: approximately 20% of the questions
- Probability and statistics: approximately 20% of the questions
- Precalculus: approximately 23% of the questions
- Calculus: approximately 22% of the questions

This section must be completed within 40 minutes, which can be a challenge for those for whom math is not the strongest subject. You can't use a calculator on the exam, so it is particularly important to be able to perform basic calculations quickly and accurately. To prepare, review the material that follows and practice completing the practice questions in a timed environment.

Basic Math

The basic math questions on the PCAT test your knowledge of math techniques you'll need for the entire Quantitative Ability section. You'll need to know about numbers, operators, and basic math properties.

Numbers

Understand the names for the basic types of numbers:

- **Natural numbers.** Also called counting numbers, these include numbers you use to count things, starting with 1. Natural numbers are: 1, 2, 3, . . .
- **Whole numbers.** These are all the natural numbers, and zero, too. Whole numbers are: 0, 1, 2, . . .
- **Integers.** Integers are all whole numbers and all negative natural numbers. Integers are: . . . , –2, –1, 0, 1, 2, . . .
- **Real numbers.** Real numbers are all integers and all numbers between any two integers. In other words, real numbers include numbers with fractional or decimal parts. Real numbers include numbers such as: –2.47, 0.12, 1.5, . . .

We use the placement system to express number values. In any number, such as 423, the placement of each digit has a meaning. The rightmost digit, 3, represents the ones place. The next digit to the left, 2, represents the number of 10s. Each digit place represents 10 times the digit to the right. So, the number 423 really means:

$$(4 \times 100) + (2 \times 10) + (3 \times 1) = 400 + 20 + 3 = 423$$

The same rule applies as you continue to the right across the decimal point. Each place to the right is one-tenth the value of the previous place. Once you cross over the decimal point, you divide by 10 for each place to the right. The number 317.43 means:

$$(3 \times 100) + (1 \times 10) + (7 \times 1) + (4 \div 10) + (3 \div 100) = 300 + 10 + 7 + 0.4 + 0.03 = 317.43$$

The Number Line

The number line is a valuable tool for understanding and describing numbers, how they relate to one another, and how math operations work. Understand what the number line is and how to use it to represent numbers. The number line is a straight line, normally horizontal, with markings that represent number values. You represent individual numbers on the line using points or hash marks.

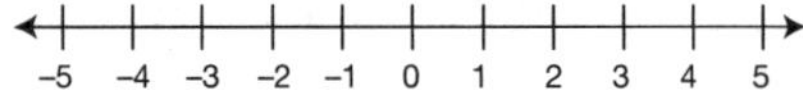

Larger numbers are toward the right side of the number line and smaller numbers are to the left. You can easily tell how numbers relate by placing them on a number line. It is easy to tell that negative 4.2 (–4.2) is less than negative 2.4 (–2.4) by looking where each number appears on the number line: –4.2 is farther left than –2.4. The number zero is generally the center of a number line and is called the origin. All negative numbers are to the left of the origin and all positive numbers are to the right of the origin.

Operations

There are four basic arithmetic operations: addition, subtraction, multiplication, and division. There are also two more operations and symbols you'll see: parentheses and exponents.

Operations and Signs

The sign of a number can change how you evaluate expressions and can be confusing. Know how signs affect basic operations.

SIGNS AND BASIC ARITHMETIC OPERATIONS		
OPERATION	NOTE	EXAMPLE
addition	Addition generally means to increase in value (move to the right on the number line). Adding a negative number means to decrease in value (move to the left on the number line). Adding a negative number is the same as subtracting a number.	7 + –3 = 4
subtraction	Subtraction generally means to decrease in value (move to the left on the number line). Subtracting a negative number means to increase in value (move to the right on the number line). Subtracting a negative number is the same as adding a number.	7 – –2 = 9
multiplication and division	Multiplying or dividing two numbers with the same sign results in a positive number. If the signs are different from each other in a multiplication or division problem, the result is negative.	3 × –2 = –6 and –3 × –2 = 6

Use the number line to help keep adding and subtracting numbers easy. Just pick the starting point (the first number), and then move to the left or right depending on the operation and the sign. Remember, adding a positive number (or subtracting a negative number) moves to the right. Adding a negative number (or subtracting a positive number) moves to the left.

Order of Operations

When you solve any mathematics problem, always pay attention to the order of operations. You must apply each operation in the correct order to get the correct answer. Use the phrase "**P**lease **E**xcuse **M**y **D**ear **A**unt **S**ally" to help you remember the correct order of operations. Solve all math problems in this order:

- parentheses
- exponents
- multiplication and division
- addition and subtraction

If you ever have multiple operations of the same type, such as several addition operations, evaluate them from left to right.

Properties of Arithmetic

Arithmetic operations have several basic properties:

PROPERTIES OF ARITHMETIC OPERATIONS			
NAME	DESCRIPTION	PROPERTY	EXAMPLE
commutative property of addition	Changing the order of any two numbers when adding them does not change the result	$a + b = b + a$	3 + 6 = 6 + 3
commutative property of multiplication	Changing the order of any two numbers when multiplying them does not change the result.	$a \times b = b \times a$	3 × 6 = 6 × 3
associative property of addition	Changing the way numbers are grouped when adding them does not change the result.	$(a + b) + c = a + (b + c)$	(2 + 5) + 3 = 2 + (5 + 3)

(continued)

PROPERTIES OF ARITHMETIC OPERATIONS (*continued*)			
NAME	DESCRIPTION	PROPERTY	EXAMPLE
associative property of multiplication	Changing the way numbers are grouped when multiplying them does not change the result.	$(a \times b) \times c =$ $a \times (b \times c)$	$(2 \times -5) \times 3 =$ $2 \times (5 \times 3)$
distributive property of multiplication	Multiplying a number, *a*, by the sum of two numbers, *b* and *c*, is the same as multiplying *a* by *b* and *c* first, and then adding the two results.	$a \times (b + c) =$ $a \times b + a \times c$	$3 \times (5 + 4) =$ $(3 \times 5) + (3 \times 4)$
identity property of addition	Adding zero to any number does not change the number.	$a + 0 = a$	$3 + 0 = 3$
inverse property of addition	Adding any number and its opposite results in zero.	$a + -a = 0$	$4 + -4 = 0$
identity property of multiplication	Multiplying any number by 1 does not change the number.	$a \times 1 = a$	$6 \times 1 = 6$
inverse property of multiplication	Multiplying any number by its multiplicative inverse (reciprocal) results in 1.	$a \times \frac{1}{a} = 1$	$2 \times \frac{1}{2} = 1$

Fractions

Simple fractions are represented by one integer divided by another integer. For example, $\frac{1}{2}$ or $\frac{3}{4}$.

The top number is the numerator and the bottom number is the denominator.

Operations with Fractions

Understand how each of the basic operations work with fractions.

OPERATIONS WITH FRACTIONS		
OPERATION	DESCRIPTION	EXAMPLE
multiplication	To multiply fractions, multiply the numerators and then multiply the denominators.	$\frac{2}{3} \times \frac{1}{5} = \frac{2}{15}$
division	To divide fractions, invert the second fraction (turn it upside down) and then multiply the fractions.	$\frac{1}{4} \div \frac{2}{3} = \frac{1}{4} \times \frac{3}{2} = \frac{3}{8}$
addition (same denominator)	You can add only fractions that have the same denominator. If the fractions have the same denominator, just add the numerators and keep the same denominator.	$\frac{2}{7} + \frac{3}{7} = \frac{5}{7}$
addition (different denominator)	If the fractions have different denominators, you have to find a common denominator. Use the quickest method for the exam. Multiply each fraction by a new fraction whose numerator and denominator are both the same as the denominator of the other fraction. (Remember that any fraction with the same numerator and denominator is equal to 1.) After multiplying both fractions by the two new fractions, you can add the numerators.	$\frac{1}{4} + \frac{2}{3} = (\frac{1}{4} \times \frac{3}{3}) + (\frac{2}{3} \times \frac{4}{4}) =$ $\frac{3}{12} + \frac{8}{12} = \frac{11}{12}$

OPERATIONS WITH FRACTIONS *(continued)*		
OPERATION	**DESCRIPTION**	**EXAMPLE**
subtraction	Subtracting fractions follows the same rules as adding fractions. If the denominators are the same, subtract the numerators. If the denominators are different, follow the same procedure as when finding a common denominator for adding fractions.	$\frac{5}{7}-\frac{2}{7}=\frac{3}{7}$
reduction	Reducing fractions is the process of dividing both the numerator and the denominator by the same value. Keep dividing by common factors until there are no common factors left.	$\frac{8}{12}=\frac{8\div 4}{12\div 4}=\frac{2}{3}$

Comparing Fractions

Some questions on the exam may ask you to determine which fraction is larger than another fraction. The easiest way to compare fractions is to ensure they have the same denominator. Then you can just compare the numerators to see which one is larger. Consider the two fractions $\frac{7}{10}$ and $\frac{3}{5}$. Which one is larger? The first step in answering this question is to find a common denominator. Use the same procedure you use when adding or subtracting fractions. (Multiply each fraction by a new fraction. The new fraction has both the numerator and denominator that are the same as the denominator of the other fraction.)

$\frac{7}{10}\times\frac{5}{5}=\frac{35}{50}$

$\frac{3}{5}\times\frac{10}{10}=\frac{30}{50}$

$\frac{35}{50}>\frac{30}{50}$; therefore $\frac{7}{10}>\frac{3}{5}$

(This method is generally the fastest, but it doesn't always give you the *smallest* common denominator. Use the fastest method to avoid wasting time on the exam.)

Mixed Numbers

A mixed number is an integer and a fraction. The two numbers are added together to form a single value. For example, $4+\frac{1}{2}=4\frac{1}{2}$. If you need to combine a mixed number with another number, you should convert it to an improper fraction first.

An improper fraction is any fraction where the numerator is larger than the denominator. To convert a mixed number into an improper fraction, multiply the denominator by the integer and add the sum to the numerator.

Convert $4\frac{1}{2}$ into an improper fraction:

$$4\tfrac{1}{2}=\frac{(4\times 2)+1}{2}=\frac{8+1}{2}=\frac{9}{2}$$

To convert an improper fraction to a mixed number, divide the numerator by the denominator to find the integer part; then leave the remainder in the numerator.

Convert $\frac{9}{2}$ into a mixed number:

$(9\div 2)=4$ with a remainder of 1

$4+\frac{1}{2}=4\frac{1}{2}$

To add mixed numbers you add the integer parts, and then add the fractional parts. If the denominators are different, you have to find a common denominator first. Once you're done, reduce the fraction if possible.

$$2\tfrac{2}{3}+3\tfrac{2}{3}=(2+3)+(\tfrac{2}{3}+\tfrac{2}{3})=5+\tfrac{4}{3}=5+\tfrac{3}{3}+\tfrac{1}{3}=5+1+\tfrac{1}{3}=6\tfrac{1}{3}$$

Subtracting mixed numbers can be a little more difficult. First, ensure that the denominators are the same. If the second numerator is larger, you must borrow 1 from the first integer to make the first numerator larger.

$2\frac{3}{7} - 1\frac{5}{7}$

Borrow 1, or $\frac{7}{7}$ from the first integer (2):

$(1 + \frac{7}{7} + \frac{3}{7}) - 1\frac{5}{7} = 1\frac{10}{7} - 1\frac{5}{7} = (1 - 1) + (\frac{10}{7} - \frac{5}{7}) = \frac{5}{7}$

Decimals

Another way to express a number that contains an integer part and a fractional part is to use decimal notation. Decimal notation separates the integer from the fractional part with a decimal point (.). You can express numbers that contain integers and fractional parts either as mixed numbers or as decimals.

COMMON FRACTIONS AND DECIMAL VALUES

FRACTION	DECIMAL VALUE
1	1.0
$2\frac{1}{2}$	2.5
$4\frac{3}{4}$	4.75
$5\frac{1}{3}$	$5.\overline{33}$ (The bar over the decimal value indicates the value repeats without ever ending.)

Converting between Fractions and Decimals

You convert a fraction to a decimal by dividing the numerator of the fraction by the denominator. If you start with a mixed number, convert it to an improper fraction first.

Converting a decimal value to a fraction is easier and quicker in most cases. You know that the fractional part (the part of the number to the right of the decimal point) is a fraction with the denominator that is a multiple of 10. Just count the number of places to the right of the decimal point and write the same number of zeros after 1 for the denominator. The numerator is just all the digits to the right of the decimal point. The number to the left of the decimal point stays the same—the integer value of the mixed number. For example, 12.138 has three digits to the right of the decimal point. That means the denominator will be 1,000 (1 followed by three zeros). The final number is: $12\frac{138}{1,000}$. Here's another example: $4.5 = 4\frac{5}{10}$. However, notice that both 5 and 10 are divisible by 5. So, we can (and should) reduce the fraction. $\frac{5}{10} = \frac{5 \div 5}{10 \div 5} = \frac{1}{2}$. So, $4.5 = 4\frac{1}{2}$

Operations with Decimals

Understand how each of the basic operations work with decimal numbers.

OPERATIONS WITH DECIMALS			
OPERATION	DESCRIPTION	EXAMPLE	
addition	Adding decimal values is easy—as long as you keep the decimal points lined up. The fastest and easiest way to add decimal numbers is to write them in a column with the decimal points lined up. Then, just add them like you would add integers. If one or more numbers have fewer digits to the right of the decimal point, you can just add zeros to make them all even. The decimal point in the answer should line up, too.	213.105 + 633.4	213.105 + 633.400 846.505
subtraction	Subtracting decimals is easy, too. Line up the decimal points and ensure all the numbers have the same number of digits to the right of the decimal point (you can add zeros to the end of shorter numbers) and then subtract. As with addition, the decimal point in the answer should line up, too.	348.31 – 208.457	348.310 – 208.457 139.853
multiplication	Multiplying decimal numbers is a little different. The process involves two steps. In the first step, just multiply the numbers as if they were integers (ignore the decimal points). Once you have an answer, place the decimal point in the correct location by counting the number of digits to the right of the decimal point in *both* numbers you are multiplying. Starting at the rightmost digit of your answer, move the decimal point to the left the same number of places as the digits you just counted.	12.48 × 17.9	12.48 (2 digits to the right of the decimal point) × 17.9 (1 digit to the right of the decimal point) 223.392 (3 digits to the right of the decimal point)
division	The easy way to divide decimals is to convert them into integers first. Count the number of digits to the right of the decimal point in *each* number in the division problem. Don't add the number of digits; just pick the larger number of digits. Multiply both numbers from your division problem by 1 followed by the same number of zeros as the number you just counted. This will give you two integers. Just divide the integers to find your answer.	17.5 ÷ 8.75	(17.5 × 100) ÷ (8.75 × 100) = 1,750 ÷ 875 = 2

Scientific Notation

Some numbers are so large or so small they are difficult to express using regular notation. Scientific notation is a method of expressing numbers in a more compact form. A number in scientific notation is in the form $a \times 10^b$ and has two parts. The first part, a, is the coefficient, and the second part is the number 10 raised to some power, b. The coefficient is some number between –10 and 10. To convert any decimal number into scientific notation, move the decimal point right or left until there is only one digit to the left of the decimal point. The number of positions you moved the decimal point is the power of 10, or b. If you had to move the decimal point left, b is positive. If you had to move the decimal point to the right, b is negative.

OPERATIONS WITH DECIMALS	
DECIMAL VALUE	SCIENTIFIC NOTATION
423	4.23×10^2
1,023,415	1.023415×10^6
0.000165	1.65×10^{-4}
0.75	7.5×10^{-1}

Operations with numbers in scientific notation are easy. To add or subtract, first make sure the exponents are the same. If they are not, you have to move the decimal point to change the exponent. Moving the decimal point in the coefficient to the right decreases the exponent. Moving it to the left increases the exponent. For example,

$(2.5 \times 10^3) + (3 \times 10^2)$ Need to change one exponent

$(2.5 \times 10^3) + (0.3 \times 10^3)$ Moved the decimal point to the left one place in the second number

2.8×10^3

Multiplying and dividing numbers in scientific notation is even easier. Multiply or divide the coefficients just like they were regular numbers; then add the exponents for multiplication or subtract the coefficients for division.

$$(2.3 \times 10^3) \times (2 \times 10^4) = (4.6 \times 10^7)$$
$$(3.75 \times 10^3) \div (3 \times 10^5) = (1.25 \times 10^{-2})$$

Percents

A percent is a decimal value that represents a fraction with a denominator of 100. The word *percent* means per 100. Any time you see a number represented as a percent, such as 75%, you can also think of the number as $\frac{75}{100}$ or 0.75. Converting between the three representations is easy.

CONVERTING BETWEEN PERCENTS, DECIMALS, AND FRACTIONS		
CONVERSION	PROCESS	EXAMPLE
percent to decimal	Drop the percent sign and move the decimal point two places to the left.	46% = 0.46
percent to fraction	Drop the percent sign and express as a fraction with a denominator of 100. Reduce the fraction if possible.	$46\% = \frac{46}{100} = \frac{46 \div 2}{100 \div 2} = \frac{23}{50}$
decimal to percent	Multiply by 100 and add the percent sign.	0.78 = 78%
fraction to percent	There are multiple methods. For the exam, convert the fraction to a decimal (divide the numerator by the denominator); then multiply by 100 and add the percent sign.	$\frac{3}{4} = 3 \div 4 = 0.75 = 75\%$

You may be asked to use common percents on the exam. Memorize the most common percents and their corresponding fraction and decimal values.

COMMON PERCENTS, DECIMALS, AND FRACTIONS		
PERCENT	DECIMAL	FRACTION
10%	0.1	$\frac{1}{10}$
$12\frac{1}{2}$%	0.125	$\frac{1}{8}$
20%	0.2	$\frac{1}{5}$
25%	0.25	$\frac{1}{4}$
$33\frac{1}{3}$%	$0.\overline{3}$	$\frac{1}{3}$
$37\frac{1}{2}$%	0.375	$\frac{3}{8}$
50%	0.5	$\frac{1}{2}$
$62\frac{1}{2}$%	0.625	$\frac{5}{8}$
$66\frac{2}{3}$%	$0.\overline{6}$	$\frac{2}{3}$
75%	0.75	$\frac{3}{4}$
$87\frac{1}{2}$%	0.875	$\frac{7}{8}$
100%	1.0	$\frac{1}{1}$

Algebra

Algebra is the first mathematics study that focuses on using variables to represent numbers. You'll need to demonstrate that you understand how to solve problems to find the value of one or more variables. Remember that variables are just ways of representing generic values for numbers.

Exponents

Many algebra problems include exponents. Exponents provide a convenient way to repeat multiplication operations. Raising any number (base) to a power (exponent) simply means multiplying the number by itself a certain number of times. Working with exponents follows these rules:

EXPONENT RULES		
RULE	EXPLANATION	EXAMPLE
multiplying the same base with exponents	Use the same base and add the exponents.	$x^2 \times x^4 = x^{(2+4)} = x^6$
dividing the same base with exponents	Use the same base and subtract the exponents.	$x^5 \div x^3 = x^{(5-3)} = x^2$
composite exponents	Use the same base and multiply the exponents.	$(x^3)^2 = x^{(3\times2)} = x^6$
multiplying different bases with the same exponent	Multiply the bases and use the same exponent.	$2^x \times 5^x = (2 \times 5)^x = 10^x$
dividing different bases with the same exponent	Divide the bases and use the same exponent.	$10^x \div 5^x = 2^x$

Using these simple rules, exponents are easy to evaluate. Remember two additional exponent rules: Negative exponents mean the base is in the denominator of a fraction. For example, x^{-2} is the same as $\frac{1}{x^2}$. The other rule applies to fractional exponents. An exponent that is expressed as a fraction means you take the root of the exponent's denominator. For example, $x^{\frac{1}{2}} = \sqrt{x}$, and $x^{\frac{3}{2}} = \sqrt{x^3}$.

Polynomials

You'll encounter questions that require you to demonstrate how to work with polynomials. A polynomial is an expression that contains constants and variables, and only addition, subtraction, multiplication, and positive integer exponent operations. You'll need to know how to combine polynomials using the four basic operations.

POLYNOMIAL OPERATIONS		
OPERATION	DESCRIPTION	EXAMPLE
addition	To add polynomials you combine like terms by adding their coefficients.	$(2x^2 + 3x + 4) + (3x^2 + 5) = (2x^2 + 3x^2) + 3x + (4 + 5) = 5x^2 + 3x + 9$
subtraction	To subtract polynomials you combine like terms by subtracting their coefficients.	$(4x^2 + 3x + 4) - (3x^2 + x + 5) = (4x^2 - 3x^2) + (3x - x) + (4 - 5) = x^2 + 2x - 1$
multiplication	To multiply polynomials you multiply each term by every other term. Use the FOIL method to keep track of the steps (see below for more information).	$(x + 2)(x + 3) = x^2 + 3x + 2x + 6 = x^2 + 5x + 6$ (see FOIL description that follows)
division	Dividing polynomials requires that you use long division.	$(3x^3 + 15x^2 + 16x - 6) \div (x + 3) = 3x^2 + 6x - 2$

The FOIL Method

Always use the FOIL method to multiply binomials (expressions consisting of two terms). It helps you keep track of the steps. FOIL stands for: first, outside, inside, last. This is the order you should use when multiplying each of the terms. For polynomial multiplication (more than two terms each), you can't use FOIL but you should use the same strategy to ensure that you multiply each term by every other term. Here's an example of using FOIL with binomials:

$$(3x - 2)(x + 5) = 3x^2 + 15x - 2x - 10$$
$$= 3x^2 + 13x - 10$$

first: $3x \times x$
outside: $3x \times 5$
inside: $-2 \times x$
last: -2×5

Polynomial Division

Using long division for polynomials is the same as using long division for numbers. The only difference is that you have to keep track of multiple terms. At each step, multiply a term of the quotient by the divisor, and then subtract that value from the dividend.

Factoring

Factoring polynomials is the opposite of multiplying them. Factoring is the process of finding which two polynomials will produce a specific result when multiplied together. The process involves two main strategies. First, learn to recognize common polynomial forms. Second, apply the FOIL method in reverse for other polynomials.

Common Polynomial Forms

Look for any of the following common polynomial forms when solving factoring problems. If you recognize these, you can save yourself time on the exam.

COMMON POLYNOMIAL FORMS		
POLYNOMIAL FORM	**STRATEGY**	**EXAMPLE**
common factor	If you can identify a factor that is common to all terms, remove it, and place it outside parentheses.	$6x^3 + 3x^2 + 9x = 3x(2x^2 + x + 3)$
difference of squares	The difference of two squares, *a* and *b*, is always the product of the sum and difference of the terms: $a^2 - b^2 = (a + b)(a - b)$	$16x^2 - 9 = (4x + 3)(4x - 3)$
binomial squares	The square of any binomial, *a* and *b*, is the square of the first term, plus or minus two times the product of the terms, plus the square of the second term. Any time you see this pattern, think of the square of a binomial: $a^2 + 2ab + b^2 = (a + b)^2$, and $a^2 - 2ab + b^2 = (a - b)^2$	$9x^2 + 12x + 4 = (3x + 2)^2$

Reverse FOIL

If you don't recognize any of the common polynomial forms, you'll have to factor using a reverse FOIL method. First, reduce any terms as much as possible. Factor out any common factors first. Then, factor the first term. Since the FOIL method starts with the first term, that's the best place to start factoring. If the first term in the problem is $6x^2$, you know the first terms in your answer will be either x and $6x$ or $2x$ and $3x$. Pick one pair and see if you can select the other terms to correspond with the last product value. For example, if the last term in the problem is 8, the last terms will be either 1 and 8 or 2 and 4.

For example, to factor $6x^2 + 2x - 8$, first write two sets of empty parentheses: ( ) ( ). Try each of the options for the first and last terms to see which values result in the polynomial you are factoring. In this example, $(2x - 2)(3x + 4)$ is the correct answer. Always factor your answer to make sure it produces the polynomial you started with.

Finding Unknowns

One of the main goals in algebra problems is to find the value of one or more variables. You do this by solving a problem. You solve an algebra problem by moving the variable to one side of the equal sign and everything else to the other side. You can do pretty much anything to an equation as long as you do the same thing to both sides. In short, just get rid of everything except the variable, and whatever is left is your answer.

TECHNIQUES FOR FINDING VALUES FOR VARIABLES

TECHNIQUE	DESCRIPTION	EXAMPLE	
Remove terms using subtraction.	If the variable is connected to other values with addition, subtract a value from both sides of the equation to isolate the variable.	$x + 10 = 12$	Subtract 10 from both sides: $x + 10 - 10 = 12 - 10$; $x = 2$
Remove terms using addition.	If the variable is connected to other values with subtraction, add a value to both sides of the equation to isolate the variable.	$x - 4 = 7$	Add 4 to both sides: $x - 4 + 4 = 7 + 4$; $x = 11$
Remove terms using division.	If the variable is connected to other values with multiplication, divide both sides of the equation by some value to isolate the variable.	$7x = 21$	Divide both sides by 7: $7x \div 7 = 21 \div 7$; $x = 3$
Remove terms using multiplication.	If the variable is connected to other values with division (the variable is in the denominator), multiply both sides of the equation by some value to isolate the variable.	$\frac{x}{6} = 4$	Multiply both sides by 6: $\frac{x}{6} \times 6 = 4 \times 6$; $x = 24$
Cross multiply.	If you encounter fractions with variables, you can maintain equality by multiplying one numerator by the other denominator, and setting that value equal to the product of the remaining denominator and numerator. Then just solve the problem using other techniques.	$\frac{4}{x} = \frac{6}{x+1}$	Cross multiply: $4 \times (x + 1) = x \times 6$; $4x + 4 = 6x$; $4 = 2x$; $2 = x$
Variables in exponents	Express the terms using a common base. Then you can ignore the base and solve the problem as if the exponents were the only terms.	$9^x = 27^{x+1}$	Convert to the same base ($9 = 3^2$ and $27 = 3^3$): $(3^2)^x = (3^3)^{x+1}$; $3^{2x} = 3^{3x+3}$. With same base, you can just evaluate the exponents: $2x = 3x + 3$; $x = -3$

Ratios

A ratio expresses how two values relate to one another. For example, if a computer manufacturer builds five laptop computers for every three desktop computers, the ratio of laptops to desktops is 5 to 3. This ratio is often expressed as 5:3 or as a fraction, $\frac{5}{3}$. You will see some problems that require you to solve ratio problems. To solve ratio problems, you need to read the problem carefully and then set up an equation with a variable. For example, suppose you are asked to use the previous ratio of desktops to laptops to determine how many computers are manufactured on a day in which 75 laptops are manufactured. The first step is to determine the number of desktops. Set up ratio problems as equivalent fractions: $\frac{5}{3} = \frac{75}{x}$, where x is the number of desktops.

Solve by cross multiplying: $5x = 75 \times 3$; $x = \frac{75 \times 3}{5} = \frac{225}{5} = 45$.

Since the question asked for the number of computers, add 75 and 45 (laptops + desktops) to find the answer: 120.

Solving Percents

There are two main types of percentage problems you might see on the exam. You may be asked to determine the percentage of some quantity or determine the percentage of some change.

Determining the percentage of a quantity is straightforward. The percentage of any quantity as it relates to a total is the ratio of the portion to the total. For example, what percentage of a fruit basket are oranges if you have 3 oranges and 12 total pieces of fruit? The percentage of oranges is $\frac{3}{12}$, or 25%.

The other type of problem is a change problem. To solve this type of problem, divide the amount of change (increase or decrease) by the original value. For example, what is the percentage increase if you added 5 gallons of water to an existing 20 gallons of water in a 30-gallon aquarium? The answer is: $\frac{5}{20} = 0.25 = 25\%$ (the 30-gallon capacity is useless information in this problem).

Quadatric Equations

There are two ways to solve quadratic equations. Factoring is generally faster, but you can't easily use factoring for all problems. Know how to use both methods for the exam.

Factoring to Solve Quadratic Equations

For simple problems, set the equation to zero and factor the left side. Then, set each factor equal to 0 and solve. The solution should generally produce two answers. For example, solve $x^2 + x = 6$.

First, express the equation with 0 on the right side: $x^2 + x - 6 = 0$

Next, factor the left side: $(x - 2)(x + 3) = 0$

Set each factor equal to 0: $x - 2 = 0$ or $x + 3 = 0$

Solution: $x = 2$ or $x = -3$

The Quadratic Formula

If the left side isn't easy to factor, use the quadratic formula. First, express the equation in the standard form: $ax^2 + bx + c = 0$. Then, substitute a, b, and c into the quadratic formula:

$$x = \frac{-b \pm \sqrt{b^2 - 4ac}}{2a}$$

Multiple Unknowns

Some problems include more than one variable. If you have only a single equation, you can solve for only one variable. That means your answer may still have a variable left in it. That's okay if you have only a single equation. Use the same rules as before to solve for any variable. Use techniques to put everything else (including the other variable) on the opposite side of the equal sign. For example, solve for x: $2x - 4y = 6$.

Add $4y$ to both sides: $2x = 4y + 6$

Divide both sides by 2: $x = \frac{4y + 6}{2} = 2y + 3$

Simultaneous Equations

If you have two or more different equations and two or more variables, you can solve for each variable. One way is to solve for one variable using one equation. Then, substitute the result into the other equation. For example, suppose you have two equations: $x + y = 6$ and $2x + \frac{y}{4} = 5$. Although this one is easy to figure out, use the first equation to solve for x: $x = 6 - y$.

Now substitute this value into the other equation:

$$2(6 - y) + \frac{y}{4} = 5$$
$$12 - 2y + \frac{y}{4} = 5$$
$$(-\tfrac{7}{4})y = -7$$
$$y = 4$$

Now that you know y, go back to the first equation and find x.

$$x + 4 = 6$$
$$x = 2$$

You can also add or subtract equations in some cases to solve them simultaneously. Consider these two equations:

$$2x + 3y = 10$$
$$x - 3y = 20$$

You can add the two equations to get $3x = 30$; $x = 10$.

Now use the value of x in either original equation to solve for y.

$$2(10) + 3y = 10$$
$$20 + 3y = 10$$
$$3y = -10$$
$$y = -\tfrac{10}{3}$$

Inequalities

Solving inequalities is similar to solving equalities, with one important exception. Any time you multiply or divide both sides of an inequality by a negative number, you have to reverse the sign. Don't forget this important step!

Solve the inequality:

$12 - \frac{x}{3} < 18$

$-\frac{x}{3} < 6$

Multiply both sides by –3 (change the sign from $<$ to $>$): $x > -18$.

You'll also see inequalities when working with absolute value problems. Absolute value problems generally have two answers. For example, $|x| = 4$ has two solutions: $x = 4$ and $x = -4$. Combining absolute value and inequalities results in multiple ranges of answers. Remember this mnemonic when solving inequalities with absolute values: GOAL. That stands for: "Greater than = Or, And is for Less than." Here are a few examples:

$|x + 3| < 4$ (less than means the result uses multiple terms combined with the AND operator)

$x + 3 > -4$ AND $x + 3 < 4$

$x > -7$ AND $x < 1$ (another way to express this is: $-7 < x < 1$)

Here's another example: $|x - 2| > 5$ (greater than = use OR for the solution)

$x - 2 < -5$ OR $x - 2 > 5$

$x < -3$ OR $x > 7$

Logarithms

Logarithms are closely related to exponents. In one sense, a logarithm is the inverse of an exponent. Recall that raising a base, b, to an exponent, a, produces a result, x: $b^a = x$. The value x is the result. Suppose you wanted to find the exponent you would have to raise b in order to obtain x. The answer is the logarithm to the base b of x. We write this equation as: $\log_b(x) = a$.

So, for any $\log_b(x) = a$, $b^a = x$. Keep this relationship in mind when solving logarithm problems. You can often rewrite simple problems in the alternate format to solve them quickly. For example, solve for x: $\log_4(x) = 3$. Rewriting the equation, we get: 43 = x, so $x = 64$.

Remember the basic properties of logarithms for the exam.

PROPERTIES OF LOGARITHMS		
PROPERTY	DESCRIPTION	EXAMPLE
product property	The logarithm of the product of two numbers is the same as the sum of the logarithms of the two numbers: $\log_b(xy) = \log_b(x) + \log_b(y)$	$\log_4(16 \times 64) = \log_4(16) + \log_4(64)$ $\log_4(1{,}024) = 2 + 3$ $5 = 5$
quotient property	The logarithm of the quotient of two numbers is the same as the difference of the logarithms of the two numbers: $\log_b(\frac{x}{y}) = \log_b(x) - \log_b(y)$	$\log_5(\frac{125}{25}) = \log_5(125) - \log_5(25)$ log5(5) = 3 – 2 1 = 1
power property	The logarithm of the one number raised to a power is the same as the value of the exponent times the logarithm of the base: $\log_b(x^y) = y \log_b(x)$	$\log_8(64^2) = 2 \log_8(64)$ $\log_8(4{,}096) = 2 \times 2$ $4 = 4$

If you ever see a logarithm expressed without a base, the base of 10 is assumed. For example, log(x) is the same as $\log_{10}(x)$.

Probability and Statistics

Probability is the study of the likelihood that some event will occur, and statistics is the process of collecting, organizing, and interpreting data. The two topics often occur together since they share many basic concepts.

Probability

Although many common probabilities are percentages, you can express them as percentages, fractions, or decimals. For example, you could say that there is a 60% chance it may rain tomorrow, or a 6 in 10 chance, or a 0.60 probability. Each representation means the same thing.

The probability of any event occurring is the ratio of the number of desired outcomes to the total number of possible outcomes. For example, what is the probability you will roll an odd number on a six-sided die? Since there are three odd numbers, the ratio of desired outcomes (3) to total possible outcomes (6) is: $\frac{3}{6} = \frac{1}{2}$. There is a $\frac{1}{2}$ or 50% chance you will roll an odd number any time you roll a die.

Here's another example: Suppose you purchase 10 tickets for a raffle. There were a total of 10,000 tickets sold in the raffle. What are your chances of holding the winning ticket? The probability of your winning is $\frac{10}{10{,}000}$, or $\frac{1}{1{,}000}$.

Sometimes you need to calculate the probability of multiple events. Solving this type of problem requires a little more work. First, understand the difference between independent and dependent events. Independent events do not affect one another. Rolling a die is a good example. Each time you roll a die the probability of rolling any number is the same. To calculate the probability of multiple independent events, you multiply the individual probabilities. For example, what is the probability of rolling a 1 twice on a six-sided die? Since the probability of rolling a 1 is $\frac{1}{6}$, rolling a 1 twice is $\frac{1}{6} \times \frac{1}{6}$, or $\frac{1}{36}$. Some questions require you to do a little work to set up the problem. For example, suppose you are asked what the probability is of rolling an odd number on a six-sided die three times in a row. First, you must calculate the probability of rolling an odd number. That probability is $\frac{3}{6}$, or 0.5. Then, multiply each of the three probabilities together: $0.5 \times 0.5 \times 0.5 = 0.125$, or 12.5%.

If you are asked to calculate the probability of mutually exclusive events, you add the individual probabilities. Mutual exclusive events are events that can occur individually, but not at the same time. For example, the probability that you roll a 1 or a 5 on a six-sided die is the sum of the individual probabilities, or $\frac{1}{6} + \frac{1}{6} = \frac{2}{6} = \frac{1}{3}$.

One type of common exam problem is one that includes independent events that affect the total number of possible outcomes. For example, assume you have a bag of marbles that contains five clear marbles and five blue marbles. What is the probability that you will select two blue marbles if you randomly choose two marbles one at a time? The probability of the first selection is $\frac{5}{10}$, or $\frac{1}{2}$. But now there are only nine marbles left. If you selected a blue marble the first time, there are four blue and five clear marbles left. So the probability of selecting a blue marble the second time is $\frac{4}{9}$. The probability of selecting two blue marbles is $\frac{1}{2} \times \frac{4}{9} = \frac{4}{18} = \frac{2}{9}$.

Another common problem is one in which you must really think about the meaning of the events. Suppose you must calculate the probabilities that there will be snow tomorrow in one of two cities. If the probability of snow for city A is 60%, the probability of snow in city B is 45%, and the probability it will snow in both cities is 30%, what is the probability that it will snow in just one of the two cities? To solve this problem you add the individual probabilities, 60% + 45% = 105%, and then subtract the joint probability, 30%. So the probability that it will snow in one of the two cities is (60% + 45%) – 30% = 75%.

Statistics

You won't see any advanced statistics on the exam, but you should be comfortable with the absolute basics. Understand how to describe collections of data.

Mean, Range, Median, and Mode

Four of the most common values that describe collections of data are the mean, range, median, and mode. The *mean*, also called the average, is the sum of all values divided by the number of items. The mean describes a value that is closest to the center of a set of data. The *range* of a data set describes how the largest and smallest values differ. You calculate the range by subtracting the smallest value from the largest value. The *median* is the center value between the largest value and the smallest value. If the data have two center values, the median is the mean of the two values. If data are uniformly distributed, the median and the mean are equal. The *mode* is the data value that occurs the most times in a set.

Consider the following set of values: 1, 2, 2, 2, 3, 4, 4, 5, 7, 7, 8, 10, 10. The mean of the set is $\frac{65}{13} = 5$. To calculate the mean, add all the numbers and divide the sum by 13. The range of the data set is 10 – 1 = 9. The median of the set is $\frac{10-1}{2} = 4.5$. The mode is 2 since there are more 2s than any other number.

What are the mean, range, median, and mode for the set of numbers: 2, 2, 3, 4, 4, 5, 6, 6, 7, 7, 7, 8, 10? The mean of the set is $\frac{71}{13} = 5.46$. The range of the numbers is 10 – 2 = 8. The median of the numbers is $\frac{10-2}{2} = 4$. The mode is 7.

Precalculus

Precalculus is the bridge between previous math topics and calculus. Make sure you are comfortable with the content in this section before you tackle the calculus section. It is important to recognize and be comfortable with the basic ideas presented in precalculus.

Functions

A function is a mathematical statement that takes a value as input and produces another value. Since the output value depends on the input value you provide, we say that the output is dependent on the input. It is common to represent functions using x and y. For example, $y = 2x - 2$ is a function. The value of y depends in the value of x you provide to the function. When x is 3, y is 4. If x is a different value, y will be a different value. Another common way to represent a function is to use the notation $f(x) = 2x - 2$. In the previous example, $f(3) = 4$. Just replace x with 3 and solve the equation.

You can solve functions using a set of values and even combine functions. For example, if $f(x) = 2x + 2$, what are the solutions for the input set A = {1, 3, 4, 6}? To solve this problem, evaluate the function for each member of A. You can express answers as a collection of ordered pairs, $(x,f(x))$. The solution is the set of ordered pairs: {(1,4), (3,8), (4,10), (6,14)}.

What is the solution set of the function $f(x) = (\frac{1}{2})x^2 + 3x + 4$ for the input set A = {2, 3, 6, 8}? Again, just substitute each value in the input set for x and evaluate the function. The solution set is the set of ordered pairs: {(2,12), $(3,\frac{35}{2})$, (6,40), (8,60)}.

Suppose you have a new function, $g(x) = x - 2$. You may be asked to evaluate combined functions. For example, what is $f(g(x))$ when x is 8? First, find $g(8)$. $g(8) = 8 - 2 = 6$. Then, evaluate $f(6)$. $f(6) = 2(6) + 2 = 14$. So, $f(g(8)) = 14$.

Graphs

A basic math skill is the ability to create visual images of functions. You do this by recording points that represent the x and $f(x)$ values on a standard grid. Then you connect the points to represent the function. This is called graphing a function. The most common grid when graphing functions is a coordinate plane with a horizontal axis used to represent x values and a vertical axis to represent y values.

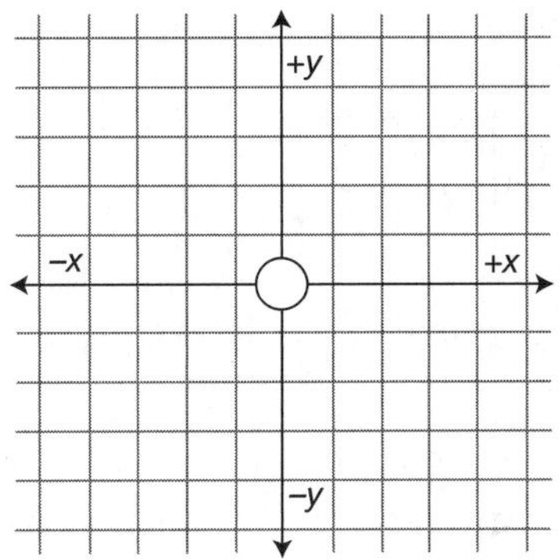

You represent points on the graph using ordered pairs, $(x,f(x))$, or $(x,-y)$. Graphs of functions have general shapes based on their order. The order of a function is the highest exponent of x.

ORDER OF A FUNCTION

ORDER	EXPONENT OF X	EXAMPLE
first	x	$f(x) = 2x + 3$
second	x^2	$f(x) = x^2 + 4x + 6$
third	x^3	$f(x) = x^3 + 8$

For the exam, make sure you recognize common graphs and their order.

$y = x$ Graph

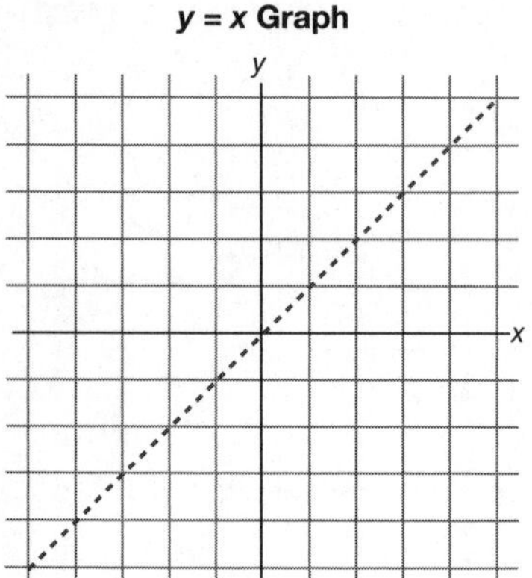

$y = |x|$ Graph

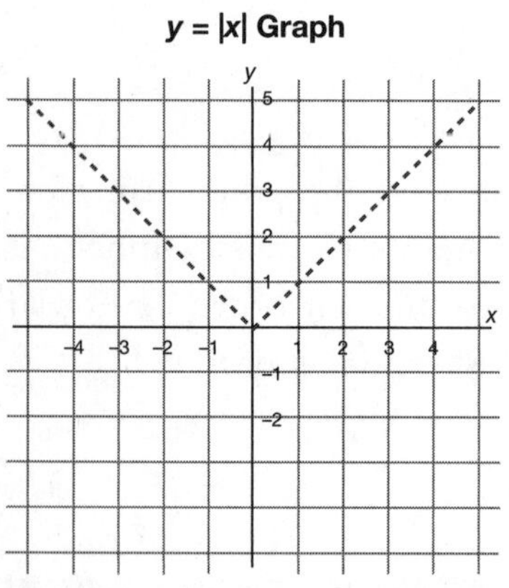

$y = \sqrt{x}$ Graph

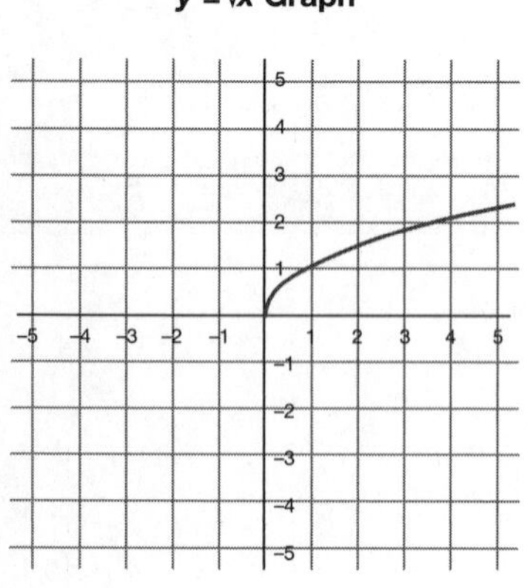

$y = x^2$ Graph

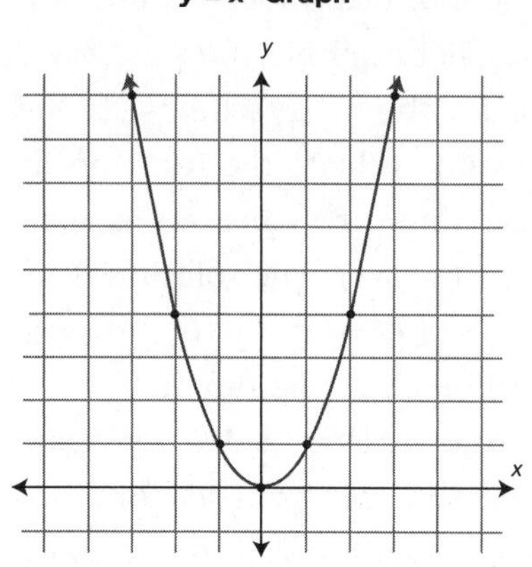

$y = x^3$ Graph

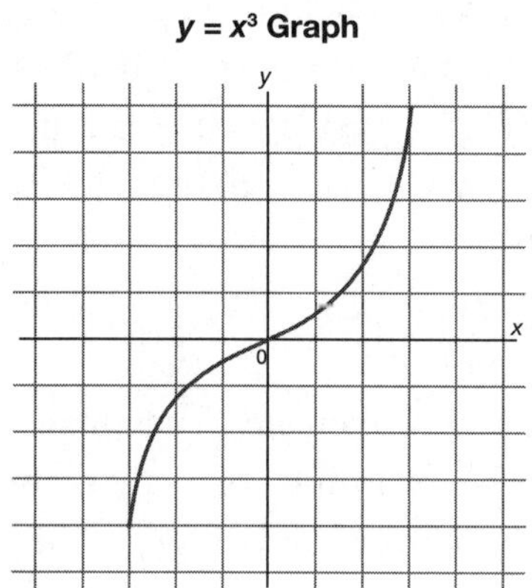

Lines

Before getting into more advanced topics, it is important to understand the basics of lines and slope. A line is a simple type of graph in which all points lie along a straight line. A line is a first-order function. The slope of a line indicates the rate of change between points on the line. The slope is expressed as "rise over run."

The symbolic representation of slope is $\frac{\Delta y}{\Delta x}$ or $\frac{y_2 - y_1}{x_2 - x_1}$.

Another common formula for finding slope is the slope intercept form of a line. In this form, $y = mx + b$, m is the slope and b is the y-intercept, or the point at which the line crosses the y-axis. For example, when given the function $y = 3x - 4$, the slope of the line is 3. What is the slope of the line $2y - x = 6$? First, solve for y. Add x to each side and divide all terms by 2. You should end up with $y = (\frac{1}{2})x + 3$. The slope is $\frac{1}{2}$.

Remember a few facts about slope:

- The slope of any horizontal line is zero.
- The slope of any vertical line is undefined.
- The slopes of any two parallel lines are equal.
- The slopes of any two perpendicular lines are multiplicative and additive inverses of one another. For example, two lines with slopes of 4 and $-\frac{1}{4}$ are perpendicular.

A line with a positive slope is said to be increasing (left to right). A line with a negative slope is said to be decreasing, and a line with a slope of zero is said to be constant.

What is the slope of the line that passes through the points (–2,–4) and (1,3)? The *rise over run* rule states that the slope of a line is $\frac{y_2 - y_1}{x_2 - x_1}$. The slope of the line is $\frac{3-(-4)}{1-(-2)} = \frac{7}{3}$.

For another example, what is the equation of the line that passes through the points (0,4) and (2,2)? First, the slope of the line is $\frac{4-2}{2-0} = 1$. Since you know the y-intercept, you can use the slope-intercept form of a line, $y = mx + b$. Thus, $m = 1$ and $b = 4$, since the point (0,4) is the y-intercept, and the equation of the line is $y = x + 4$.

Calculus

Calculus is the study of change. You don't have to know the highest-level details of calculus for the exam, but you will have to understand the fundamentals of calculus and be able to solve differentiation and integration problems.

Derivatives

The derivative of any function is a measurement of how the value of the function changes as its inputs change. The derivative of a function $f(x)$ is $f'(x)$ (f prime of x). The formula for the derivative of a function, $f(x) = -x^n$, is: $f'(x) = nx^{n-1}$. For example, if $f(x) = 3x^3$, $f'(x) = 6x^2$.

You may also see the dx notation for the derivative. The notations $f'(x)$ and $\frac{dy}{dx}$ are used interchangeably.

What is the derivative of $f(x) = 2x^4$? The answer is: $f'(x) = 8x^3$.

You may be asked to calculate the derivative at a point, or $f'(b)$. The derivative at a point is the slope of the line that is tangent to the curve at that point. To solve derivatives at a specific point, just calculate the derivative of the function and substitute the supplied value for the variable. For example, find the slope of $f(x) = 3x^2 + 2$ when x is 3. First, find $f'(x)$, and then evaluate $f'(3)$. $f'(x) = 6x$, so $f'(x) = 18$.

Derivatives of Polynomials

You will likely see a derivative question involving polynomials on the exam. These questions aren't much more difficult than simple derivatives. Just find the derivative of each term of the polynomial separately. For example, find $f'(x)$ for:

$$f(x) = 3x^2 + 12x - 8$$
$$f'(x) = (2)3x^{2-1} + 12 - 0$$
$$f'(x) = 6x + 12$$

Find the $f'(x)$ for:

$$f(x) = 2x^4 - 3x^3 + 5x^2 - 2x - 3$$
$$f'(x) = (4)2x^3 - (3)3x^2 + 5x - 2$$
$$f'(x) = 8x^3 - 9x^2 + 5x - 2$$

Derivatives and Slope

Recall that the derivative is the slope of a line that is tangent to a curve at a specific point. You can calculate that slope by evaluating the derivative at some value of x. The slope tells you how the function (or the curve on the graph) is changing at the point. If the slope ($f'(x)$) is greater than zero (> 0) the function is increasing. If the slope ($f'(x)$) is less than zero

(< 0) the function is decreasing. And if the slope ($f'(x)$) is equal to zero (= 0), the function is constant.

For example, what is the slope of a line tangent to the curve $f(x) = x^2 + 4x + 1$ at the point (1,6)? First, find the derivative. $f'(x) = 2x + 4$. Then, evaluate the derivative for $x = 1$. $f'(1) = 2(1) + 4 = 6$. Thus, the slope of the line tangent to the curve $f(x) = x^2 + 4x + 1$ as the point (1,6) is 6.

Second Derivative

The derivatives you have seen so far are called first derivatives. You can also take the derivative of the first derivative to get the second derivative. The first derivative is $f'(x)$, and the second derivative is $f''(x)$. The second derivative describes the concavity of a function. In other words, the second derivative tells you how the slope of a function changes over different values of the function. A U shaped graph of the second derivative (called "concave up") means that the slope is increasing. An upside-down U (called "concave down") means the slope is decreasing.

You can tell what the graph looks like at any point using the second derivative. Like the first derivative, the value of the second derivative at a specific point tells you whether slope is increasing, decreasing, or constant. If $f''(x)$ is greater than zero (> 0) the slope is increasing. If $f''(x)$ is less than zero (< 0) the slope is decreasing. And, if $f''(x)$ is equal to zero (= 0) the slope is constant.

Local Minima and Maxima

So, why do we care about the second derivative? The second derivative is a convenient method to find the local minimum and local maximum of a function. You can find the minimum and maximum values of a function for a specific range of a graph (local values). The local minimum is the lowest point in a section of a graph, and the local maximum is the highest point in a section of a graph.

To find the local minimum and local maximum of a function, you want to find the points at which $f'(x) = 0$. Then, find $f''(x)$ at these points to determine the sign of the second derivatives. If the second derivative is negative at a point (the slope is decreasing), the point is a local maximum. If the second derivative is positive at a point (the slope is increasing), the point is a local minimum.

For example, find the local minimum of $f'(x) = 2x^2 - 12x$.

First, find $f'(x)$ and solve for $f'(x) = 0$.

$f'(x) = 4x - 12$
$4x - 12 = 0$
$x = 3$

Find $f''(x)$, and evaluate the sign.

$f''(x) = 4$

Since $f''(x)$ is positive (4), the slope is increasing and the point is a local minimum.

Now evaluate $f(3)$ to find the local minimum.

$f(3) = 2(3)^2 - 12(3) = -18$

The local minimum is (3,–18).

Integrals

An integral is the reverse of a derivative. In fact, you can generally consider integrals to be antiderivatives. There are two main notations for integration (the process of finding integrals). The integral of $f(x)$ is sometimes referred to with a capital letter: $F(x)$. The other, more common notation uses the integral symbol: $\int$. Integrals with no bounds are called indefinite integrals.

The process of integration is simply the opposite of derivation. To calculate the integral of a function, increase the exponent of the term and divide the term by the new exponent. For example, what is $\int 9x^2dx$? (The dx term is necessary for integration, but a discussion of why it is needed is beyond the scope of the PCAT exam requirements.)

$\int 9x^2dx = \frac{9x^3}{3} = 3x^3$ (Note that if you reverse the process and take the derivative of $3x^3$ you end up with $9x^2$.)

Calculating integrals of polynomials is also similar to calculating derivatives of polynomials. Just reverse the process for each term. In other words, just calculate the integral for each term to integrate the entire polynomial. For example, what is $\int (2x^2 - 3x + 7)dx$?

$\int (2x^2 - 3x + 7)dx$
$\int 2x^2\,dx + \int -3xdx + \int 7dx$
$(\frac{2}{3})x^3 - (\frac{3}{2})x^2 + 7x$

Constants in Integrals

Although an integral is the opposite of a derivative, you can't always get back to a starting point by calculating a derivative and then calculating an integral on the result. The problem is that constants in the original functions are consumed by the derivation process. In other words, constants go away when you differentiate a function. For that reason, integrals always contain an arbitrary constant, C, that represent any lost constants. For example, if $f(x) = 3x^2 + 2x + 4$, then $f'(x) = 6x + 2$. If you calculate the integral on the result, $\int 6x + 2dx = (\frac{6}{2})x2 + 2x = 3x^2 + 2x$. Although this is close, it is not exact. That is why integration solutions should always include the constant C. The real solution is: $3x^2 + 2x + C$.

Definite Integrals

A definite integral is calculating the value of an integral over a range of values. Unlike taking the derivative at a point, we evaluate integrals over a range. We specify the lower limit, a, and the upper limit, b, of the definite integral using the standard notation: $\int_a^b$. The process of finding the definite integral is: find the integral of the function, calculate the integral at a and at b, then subtract the value of the integral at a from the value of the integral at b. For example,

Find $\int_{-1}^{3}(8x^3 + 3x)dx$
$\int_{-1}^{3}(8x^3 + 3x)dx = \int_{-1}^{3}(8x^3)dx + \int_{-1}^{3}(3x)dx = (\frac{8}{4})x^4 + (\frac{3}{2})x^2 = 2x^4 + \frac{3}{2}x^2$

Next, evaluate at 3 and –1

$[2(3)^4 + \frac{3}{2}(3)^2] - [2(-1)^4 + \frac{3}{2}(-1)^2]$
$[2(81) + \frac{27}{2}] - (2 + \frac{3}{2})$
$162 + \frac{27}{2} - 2 - \frac{3}{2}$
$160 + \frac{24}{2} = 160 + 12 = 172$

Definite integrals are extremely helpful for finding the area under curves. Although finding the area under a line is easy, calculating the area under a curve is very difficult without calculus. To calculate the area under any curve between two points, simply calculate the definite integral over the range between the points.

For example, calculate the area under the curve represented by $f(x) = 2x^3 + 4x + 8$, from $x = 1$ to $x = 3$.

$\int_1^3 (2x^3 + 4x + 8)dx = \int_1^3 (2x^3)dx + \int_1^3 (4x)dx + \int_1^3 (8)dx$
$(\frac{2}{4})x^4 + (\frac{4}{2})x^2 + 8x$
$\frac{1}{2}x^4 + 2x^2 + 8x$

Now calculate the definite integral:

$[(\frac{1}{2})(3)^4 + 2(3)^2 + 8(3)] - [(\frac{1}{2})(1)^4 + 2(1)^2 + 8(1)]$
$(8\frac{1}{2} + 18 + 24) - (\frac{1}{2} + 2 + 8)$
$\frac{165}{2} - \frac{21}{2} = 72$

Here's another example: Calculate the area under the curve represented by $f(x) = 4x^4 + 5x^3 - 2x + 7$, from $x = 0$ to $x = 2$.

$\int_0^2 (4x^4 + 5x^3 - 2x + 7)dx = \int_0^2 (4x^4)dx + \int_0^2 (5x^3)dx - \int_0^2 (2x)dx + \int_0^2 (7)dx$
$(\frac{4}{5})x^5 + (\frac{5}{4})x^4 - (\frac{2}{2})x^2 + 7x$
$(\frac{4}{5})x^5 + (\frac{5}{4})x^4 - x^2 + 7x$

Now calculate the definite integral:

$[(\frac{4}{5})(2)^5 + (\frac{5}{4})(2)^4 - 2^2 + 7(2)] - [(\frac{4}{5})(0)^5 + (\frac{5}{4})(0)^4 - 0^2 + 7(0)]$
$(\frac{128}{5} + 20 - 4 + 14) - 0$
$\frac{128}{5} + 30 = 55\frac{3}{5} = 55.6$

Summing It Up

As you have seen, the PCAT tests your mastery of concepts and skills in arithmetic, algebra, probability and statistics, precalculus, and calculus. If you didn't keep track of the skills that you had difficulty with and need to practice more as you went through this chapter, do so now. Go back and solve the equations and problems within the chapter until you feel you have mastered each part of the quantitative test. Once you are comfortable with the knowledge and skills you need in all five of the quantitative categories, time yourself as you work on the questions within the chapter. The Quantitative Ability section is often cited as the part of the PCAT that many students don't finish. So time is of the essence!

Proceed to the practice questions that follow when you have fully reviewed everything from whole numbers to polynomial integration. Remember to answer the questions you know best before spending extra time on the ones with which you have more difficulty. Keep an eye on the clock, especially when you are solving the problems or equations that initially stumped you. The more you practice and time yourself, the less stressed you will feel come test day!

Practice Questions

1. $\frac{3}{4} \times \frac{36}{30} \times \frac{9}{0}$

Write as a mixed number and convert to a decimal.

a. $8\frac{1}{10}$, 8.1
b. 36, 36.0
c. $7\frac{1}{5}$, 7.2
d. $\frac{81}{10}$, 8.1

2. There are 14 boys and 18 girls in a second-grade class. What percentage of the class are girls? (Round to the nearest hundredth.)
a. 77.78%
b. 43.75%
c. 36.56%
d. 56.25%

3. $(2.7 \times 10^{13}) \div (7.8 \times 10^{-27}) =$
a. -5.1×10^{39}
b. 3.5×10^{-39}
c. -3.5×10^{39}
d. 3.5×10^{39}

4. Evaluate $(x^3 + 8x^2 + 4x + 16) \div (x + 4)$.
a. $x^2 + 4x - 12$ R. 64
b. $x^3 + 4x^2 + 12$
c. $x^2 - 4x - 12$
d. $x^2 + 4x + 12$

5. $\frac{x}{12} = \frac{5}{7}$

Solve for x. Round to the nearest thousandth.

a. 8
b. 8.58
c. 8.571
d. 8.6

6. $-3x + 4 \geq 13$

Solve for x.

a. $x \geq -3$
b. $x \leq -3$
c. $x \leq -5$
d. $x \geq -5$

7. $3x + 2y + z = 12$
$x - y - z = 2$
$y + z = 6$

Solve for x, y, and z.

a. $x = -4, y = 9, z = 12$
b. $x = -8, y = 18, z = -24$
c. $x = 8, y = -18, z = 24$
d. $x = 4, y = -9, z = 12$

8. If $\log_8 x = 3$, then
a. $x = 512$
b. $x = 2$
c. $x = 6{,}561$
d. $x = \frac{8}{3}$

9. A bag contains 50 identical balls numbered 1 through 50. If a ball is drawn randomly, what is the probability (as a percentage) that it will have a number between 19 and 31 (including 19 and 31)?
a. 26%
b. 2.6%
c. 13%
d. 1.3%

10. Two dice are in a bag. One die has the numbers 1 through 10 on its sides, and the other has sides numbered 11 through 20. What is the probability (as a percentage) that both dice, when thrown, will be odd?
a. 50%
b. 25%
c. 33%
d. 75%

11. Sixty dimes, 40 quarters, and 100 pennies are in a box. Half of the dimes, quarters, and pennies were minted in 1990, and half were minted in 2000. If a coin is drawn from the box at random, what is the probability (as a percentage) that it will be a dime or minted in 2000?
a. 40%
b. 20%
c. 65%
d. 30%

12. There is a forecast of a 50% chance of snow in Baltimore and a 20% chance of snow in Atlanta. What is the probability (as a percentage) that it will snow in both cities? What is the probability of it snowing in either city?
a. both = 70%, either = 10%
b. both = 30%, either = 60%
c. both = 60%, either = 30%
d. both = 10%, either = 60%

13. Two regular six-sided dice are thrown. What is the probability (given as percentage) that their results will add up to 10?
a. 11.1%
b. 5.6%
c. 40%
d. 15%

14. $f(x) = 2x + 9$

What are the solutions of the function f for the input set A, where A = {1, 3, 7, 11}?

a. (11,1), (15,3), (23,7), (31,11)
b. 11, 15, 23, 31
c. 80
d. (1,11), (3,15), (7,23), (11,31)

15. Calculate the slope of the following line.

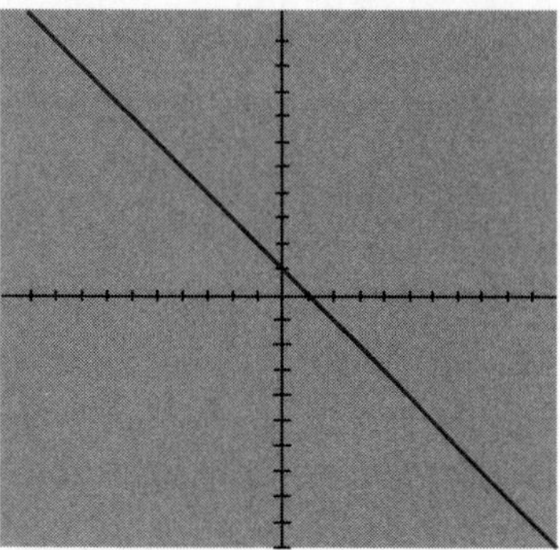

a. −1
b. 1
c. $\frac{1}{2}$
d. 2

16. Which graph most closely resembles the function $f(x) = x^2 - 3$?

a.

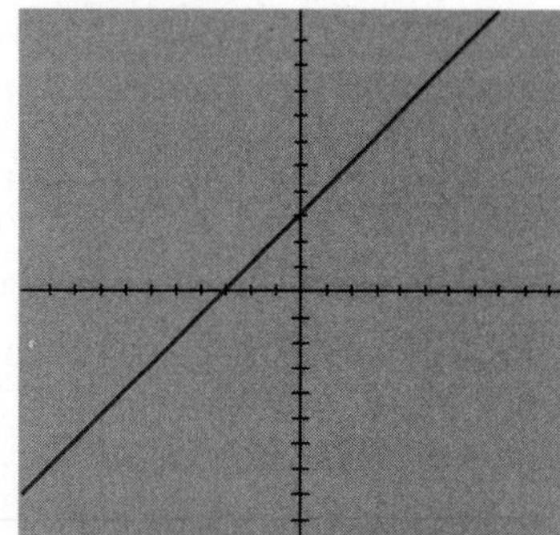

b.

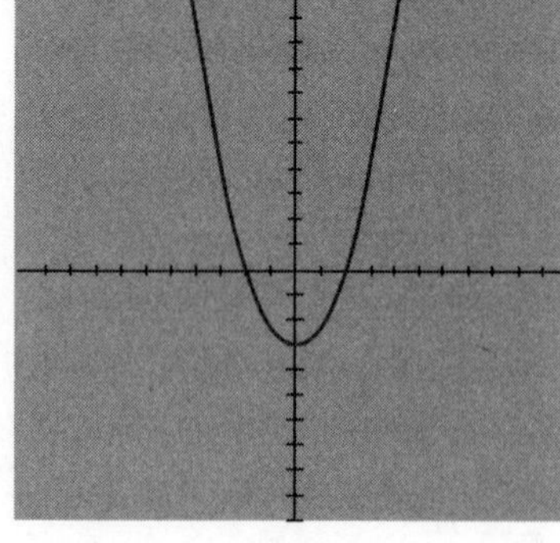

c.

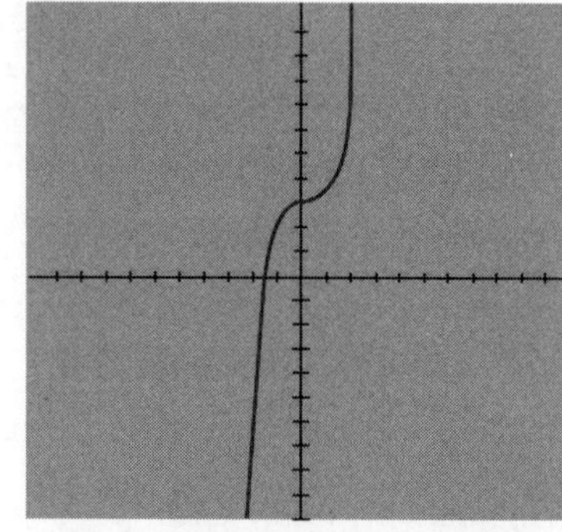

d.

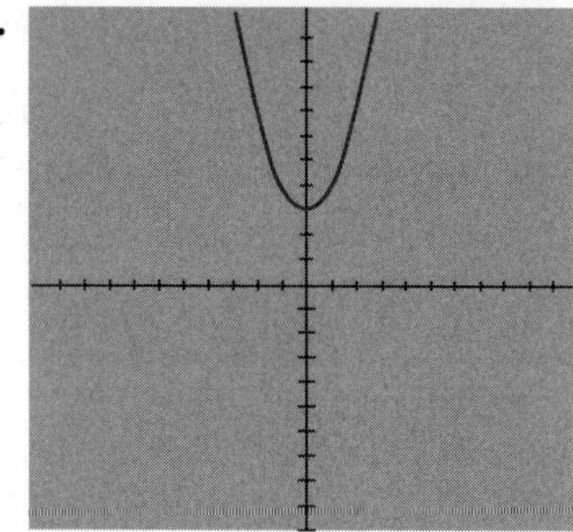

17. $f(x) = 4x^2 - 3x + 11$

Define the function for domain A, where A = {3, 9, 27, 81}.

a. (38,3), (308,9), (2846,27), (26012,81)
b. 38, 308, 2846, 26012
c. (3,38), (9,308), (27,2846), (81,26012)
d. 29204

18. Which graph most closely resembles the function $f(x) = \sqrt{x} + 4$?

a.

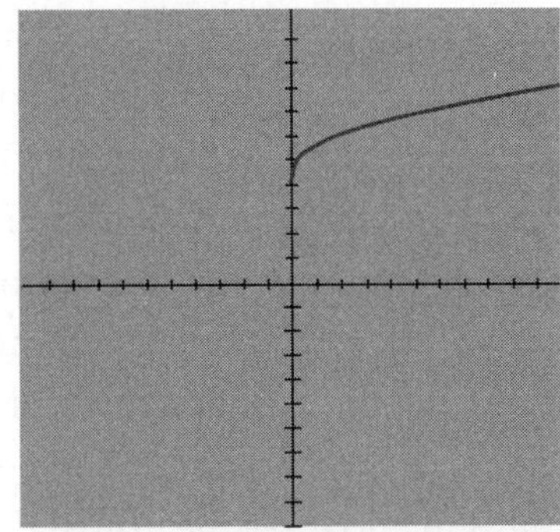

b.

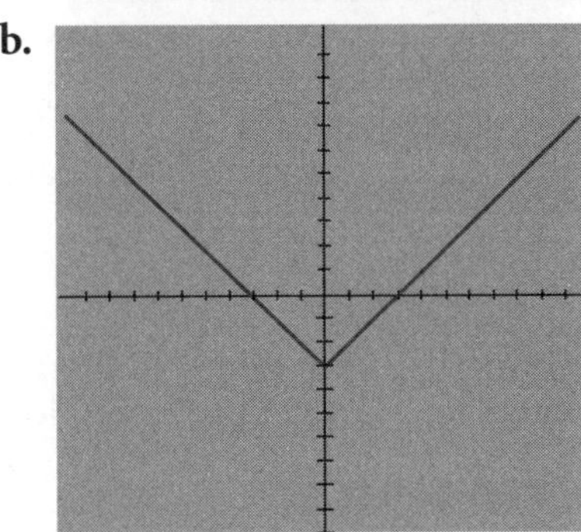

c.

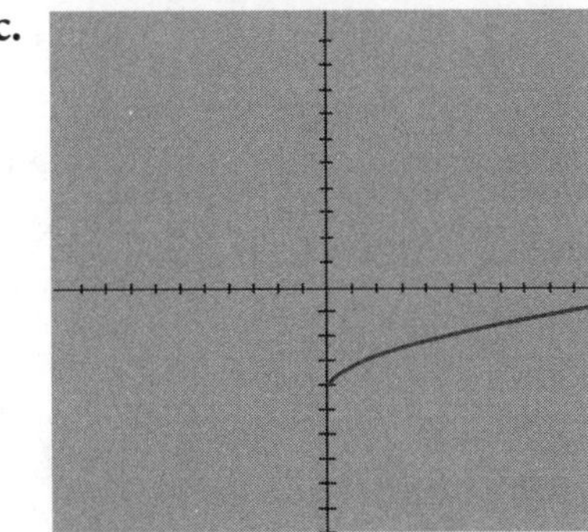

d.

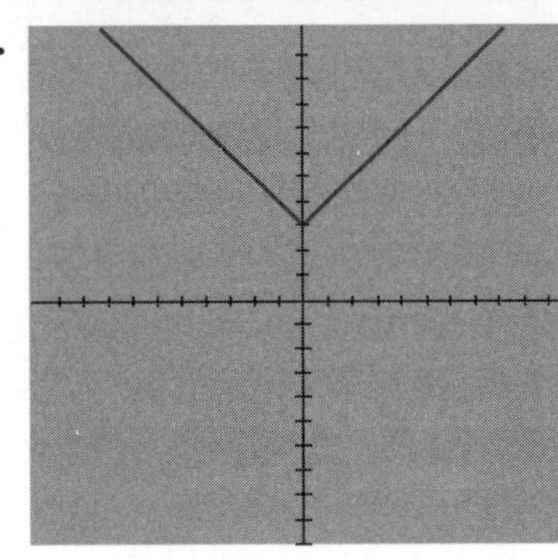

19. Calculate the slope of the following line.

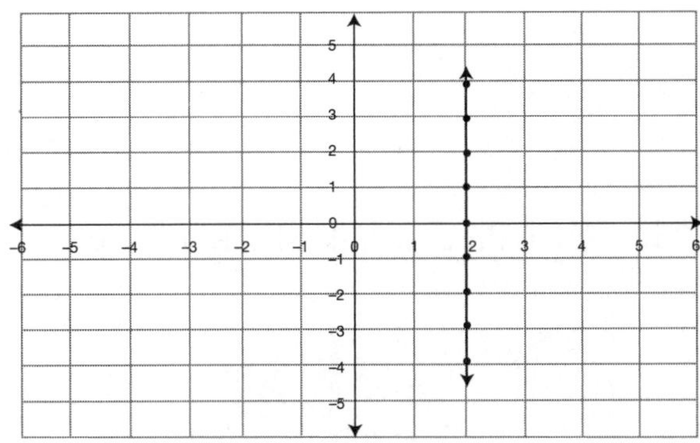

a. undefined
b. 0
c. 1
d. 2

20. Find the first derivative of the function $f(x) = x^3 + 2x^2 + 5x + 2$.
a. $f'(x) = 3x + 4$
b. $f'(x) = x^2 + 2x + 5$
c. $f'(x) = 3x^2 + 4x + 7$
d. $f'(x) = 3x^2 + 4x + 5$

21. Find the second derivative of the function $f(x) = 5x^4 - 12x^2 + 5$.
a. $5x^3 + 5$
b. $60x^2 - 24$
c. $20x^3 - 24x$
d. $5x^2 - 5$

22. Find the minimum or maximum point on the graph of the function $f(x) = x^2 - x - 12$.
a. minimum at the point $(\frac{1}{2}, -\frac{51}{4})$
b. maximum at the point $(\frac{1}{2}, \frac{51}{4})$
c. minimum at the point $(\frac{1}{2}, -\frac{49}{4})$
d. maximum at the point $(\frac{1}{2}, \frac{49}{4})$

23. Solve the indefinite integral $\int x^2 + 3x + 4dx$.
a. $(\frac{1}{3})x^3 + (\frac{3}{2})x^2 + 4x + C$
b. $2x + 3$
c. $x^3 + 3x^2 + 4x$
d. $x + 3$

24. Solve $\int_2^4 \frac{1}{4}x^3 + 3x^2 - 2x + 7$.

a. 73
b. 85
c. –85
d. 97

25. What is the area of the shaded region?

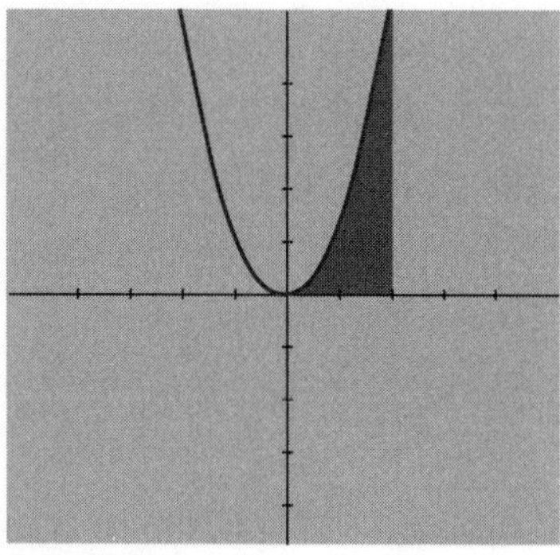

$f(x) = x^2$ with the area shaded above the x-axis, below the curve, between $x = 0$ and $x = 2$

a. $\frac{8}{3}$
b. $-\frac{8}{3}$
c. 0
d. 1

Answers and Explanations

1. a. Before multiplying the three fractions together, reduce them as much as possible. The second fraction, $\frac{36}{30}$, becomes $\frac{6}{5}$. The first and third fractions cannot be simplified. Now you can multiply the three numerators together as well as the three denominators. After reducing the product, this will result in $\frac{81}{10}$. To reach the mixed number, perform long division and leave the remainder as a fraction. This gives you $8\frac{1}{10}$. Divide 1 by 10 to get the decimal (.1).

2. d. Divide the number of girls in the class by the total number of students. The answer is $\frac{18}{14+18} = \frac{18}{32} = 56.25\%$.

3. d. For this problem, you must divide the entire expression. This is done by first dividing 2.7 by 7.8, giving you $2.7 \div 7.8 = 0.35$, when rounded to the nearest hundredth. Then, you must determine the sign of the scientific notation by evaluating $10^{13} \div 10^{-27}$. This can be evaluated by subtracting the second exponent from the first, as follows: $10^{13-(-27)} = 10^{13+27} = 10^{40}$. Then you simply write the entire new expression out as follows: 0.35×10^{40}. However, we want a number greater than or equal to 1, so we move the decimal one place to the right and subtract 1 from the exponent, giving us 3.5×10^{39}.

4. a. To solve this problem, we must perform long division with the polynomials. Set it up like this: $x^3 + 8x^2 + 4x + 16 \div x + 4$. Start by dividing $x^3 + 8x^2$ by $x + 4$. The goal is to get the first term of each expression to cancel. In order to do this, we multiply $x + 4$ by x^2, which gives us $x^3 + 4x^2$. We then evaluate $(x^3 + 8x^2) - (x^3 + 4x^2)$, which results in $4x^2$. Now we bring down the second term of the expression.

$$
\begin{array}{r|l}
 & x^2 + 4x - 12 \quad \text{R. } 64 \\
x + 4 & x^3 + 8x^2 + 4x + 16 \\
 & -x^3 + 4x^2 \\
 & \quad 4x^2 + 4x \\
 & \quad -4x^2 + 16x \\
 & \qquad -12x + 16 \\
 & \qquad -12x - 48 \\
 & \qquad\qquad 64
\end{array}
$$

5. c. The easiest way to solve this equation is by cross multiplying (multiplying the numerator of each side with the denominator of the opposite side). By doing this, we get $7x = 60$. In order to solve for x, we must now divide, giving us $x = 60 \div 7$ or $x = 8.571$, when rounded to the thousandths place.

6. b. This inequality is solved just like a normal equation, with one exception at the end. First, subtract 4 from both sides, giving you $-3x + 4 - 4 \geq 13 - 4$ or $-3x \geq 9$. Then, divide both sides by -3 but remember that you must reverse the sign of the inequality, as you are dividing by a negative. Thus, the answer is $x \leq -3$.

7. c. To solve this equation, first add $y + x = 6$ and $x - y - z = 2$. This will give you $x = 8$. Now subtract $y + z = 6$ from $3x + 2y + z = 12$. This evaluates to $3x + y = 6$. Since we know $x = 8$, this can now be written as $3(8) + y = 6$. Evaluate to find that $y = -18$. Now simply substitute -18 for y in $y + z = 6$, giving you $-18 + z = 6$. Thus, z is 24.

8. a. Since $\log_x y = z$ means that $y = x^z$, we know that $\log_8 x = 3$ means $x = 8^3$ or 512.

9. a. To determine the probability of a single event occurring, determine the number of possible occurrences (in this problem, 50, as the balls are numbered 1 through 50) and the number of desired occurrences (numbers 19 through 31, so 13). Then divide: $\frac{13}{50} = 0.26$. As a percentage, 0.26 can be rewritten as 26% by multiplying the decimal by 100.

10. b. To determine the probability of two events occurring at once, take the probability of each event occurring individually and multiply them together. Since there are ten sides on each die and five sides of each die are odd, each die has a five in ten chance to land on an odd number: $\frac{5}{10}$ or $\frac{1}{2}$. Thus, multiplied together, you would get $\frac{1}{2} \times \frac{1}{2} = \frac{1}{4}$ or 0.25. Multiply by 100 to get the percentage: 25%.

11. c. To determine the probability of either of two distinct events occurring, take the probability of each one and add them together. Then, subtract the probability that they both occur. For this problem, there are 60 dimes in a box of 200 coins, and 100 of the coins were minted in 2000. Thus, the probability of picking out a dime will be $\frac{60}{200}$ and the probability of picking a coin minted in 2000 is $\frac{100}{200}$. To find the probability of both events occurring, multiply the two together to get $\frac{3}{20}$ after simplification. Thus, the answer is $\frac{60}{200} + \frac{100}{200} - \frac{30}{200} = \frac{130}{200} = \frac{13}{20} = 0.65$. Multiply by 100 to get the percentage: 65%.

12. d. This problem simply combines the concepts of the previous two problems. To determine the probability of snow in both cities, convert the percentages into decimals, multiply them together, and convert back into a percentage: $0.2 \times 0.5 = 0.1 = 10\%$. To determine the probability of snow in either city, convert the percentages into decimals, add them together, subtract the probability that it snows in both cities and convert back into a percentage: $0.2 + 0.5 - 0.1 = 0.6 = 60\%$.

13. a. For this problem, first determine how many events would fit the desired profile and how many possible events there are. For the results to add up to 10, there are $6 + 4$, $4 + 6$, $5 + 5$, $5 + 5$, so four possible solutions. There are 36 total events, so there is a $\frac{4}{36}$, or $\frac{1}{9}$ (11.1%) chance any roll of two dice will add up to 10.

14. d. For this problem, all you have to do is plug each of the numbers given in domain (input set) A into the x variable in the given function $f(x) = 2x + 9$. Then give the answer in ordered pairs of numbers, with the initial value given in domain A first and the number produced by the equation after substitution second. Thus, you get (1,11), (3,15), (7,23), (11,31).

15. a. To calculate the slope of the given line, take two points on the line—for example, (0,1) and (1,0)—and determine the difference in y divided by the difference in x: $\frac{y_1 - y_2}{x_1 - x_2}$. This evaluates to $\frac{1-0}{0-1} = -1$.

16. b. For this problem, you must determine which graph most closely corresponds to the equation given. We know that a parabola is the graph given for $f(x) = x^2$, so the parabola is the best choice, which eliminates choices **a** and **c**. To find the correct answer, look at the second part of the equation. The parabola should be 3 points below the x-axis, which makes **b** the correct answer.

17. c. Again, for this problem, all you must do is plug each of the numbers given in domain A into the x variable in the given function $f(x) = 4x^2 - 3x + 11$. Then give the answer in ordered pairs of numbers, with the initial value given in domain A first and the number produced by the equation after substitution second. Thus, you get (3,38), (9,308), (27,2846), (81,26012).

18. a. For this problem, you must determine which graph most closely corresponds to the equation given. We know the graph given for $f(x) = \sqrt{x} + 4$, so choices **b** and **c** are eliminated. To find the correct answer, look at the second part of the equation. The graph should be four units above the y-axis, which makes **a** the correct answer choice.

19. a. Since this is a vertical line, the slope is undefined.

20. d. The first derivative for the function $f(x) = x^3 + 2x^2 + 5x + 2$ is $f'(x) = 3x^2 + 4x + 5 + 0$, or simply $f' = 3x^2 + 4x + 5$.

21. b. The first derivative for the function $5x^4 - 12x^2 + 5$ is $f'(x) = 20x^3 - 24x$. To find the second derivative, simply take the derivative of $f'(x) = 20x^3 - 24x$, which becomes $f''(x) = 60x^2 - 24$.

22. c. To find relative extrema of a function, find where the first derivative is equal to zero. First take the first derivative of $f(x) = x^2 - x - 12$, which is $2x - 1$. Set the derivative equal to zero and solve for x. The solution for x is $\frac{1}{2}$. Next, plug $\frac{1}{2}$ into our original equation to find the y-value of the extrema, $-\frac{49}{4}$. In order to decide whether the point is a minimum or maximum, find the second derivative of the function and plug in $\frac{1}{2}$. The second derivative is 2, which is positive. This shows we have a minimum at the point $(\frac{1}{2}, -\frac{49}{4})$.

23. a. To find the indefinite integral of $x^2 + 3x + 4$, you take the integral of each term separately. For each integral, you will add 1 to the exponent and divide the whole term by the new exponent. In the case of x^2 the exponent becomes a 3 and the whole term is divided by 3, resulting in $\frac{x^3}{3}$. Repeat the same process with the other two terms. Then add the constant of integration C at the end of the answer to account for the unknown constant.

24. a. To find the definite integral, you must first find the indefinite integral. Split the terms up and find the integral of each term. For each integral, you will add 1 to the exponent and divide the whole term by the new exponent. In this case, the result should be $f(x) = \frac{1}{16}x^4 + x^3 - x^2 + 7x$. Next, compute $f(4) - f(2)$. The result should be $92 - 19 = 73$.

25. a. To find the area of the shaded region, take the definite integral from 0 to 2 of the function $f(x) = x^2$. Add one to the exponent and divide by the new exponent, giving you $\frac{x^3}{3}$. To evaluate the definite integral, plug 2 into the result of the derivative, which evaluates to $\frac{8}{3}$. Then subtract the result of plugging 0 into the result of the derivative, which evaluates to 0, as well. The result is $\frac{8}{3} - 0 = \frac{8}{3}$.

CHAPTER

10 PCAT PRACTICE TEST

This practice exam should be taken after completing the practice questions at the end of each chapter and studying the subject areas you have identified as those in which you need more review. Because the format mimics that of the PCAT, taking it will familiarize you with the exam format. You will be able to practice answering the types of questions that are on the exam as you review the content areas.

One of the main reasons for taking this practice exam, in addition to getting more practice in answering the kinds of questions on the PCAT, is to identify your strengths and weaknesses. Make a note of the types of questions you miss and the topics on which you need to further concentrate your study time. Do not neglect any subject area unless you have an almost perfect score in that area. Develop a study plan, and after studying your textbook, start reviewing the individual topics in Chapters 4 to 9.

Section 2: Verbal Ability

1.	ⓐ	ⓑ	ⓒ	ⓓ
2.	ⓐ	ⓑ	ⓒ	ⓓ
3.	ⓐ	ⓑ	ⓒ	ⓓ
4.	ⓐ	ⓑ	ⓒ	ⓓ
5.	ⓐ	ⓑ	ⓒ	ⓓ
6.	ⓐ	ⓑ	ⓒ	ⓓ
7.	ⓐ	ⓑ	ⓒ	ⓓ
8.	ⓐ	ⓑ	ⓒ	ⓓ
9.	ⓐ	ⓑ	ⓒ	ⓓ
10.	ⓐ	ⓑ	ⓒ	ⓓ
11.	ⓐ	ⓑ	ⓒ	ⓓ
12.	ⓐ	ⓑ	ⓒ	ⓓ
13.	ⓐ	ⓑ	ⓒ	ⓓ
14.	ⓐ	ⓑ	ⓒ	ⓓ
15.	ⓐ	ⓑ	ⓒ	ⓓ
16.	ⓐ	ⓑ	ⓒ	ⓓ
17.	ⓐ	ⓑ	ⓒ	ⓓ
18.	ⓐ	ⓑ	ⓒ	ⓓ
19.	ⓐ	ⓑ	ⓒ	ⓓ
20.	ⓐ	ⓑ	ⓒ	ⓓ
21.	ⓐ	ⓑ	ⓒ	ⓓ
22.	ⓐ	ⓑ	ⓒ	ⓓ
23.	ⓐ	ⓑ	ⓒ	ⓓ
24.	ⓐ	ⓑ	ⓒ	ⓓ
25.	ⓐ	ⓑ	ⓒ	ⓓ
26.	ⓐ	ⓑ	ⓒ	ⓓ
27.	ⓐ	ⓑ	ⓒ	ⓓ
28.	ⓐ	ⓑ	ⓒ	ⓓ
29.	ⓐ	ⓑ	ⓒ	ⓓ
30.	ⓐ	ⓑ	ⓒ	ⓓ
31.	ⓐ	ⓑ	ⓒ	ⓓ
32.	ⓐ	ⓑ	ⓒ	ⓓ
33.	ⓐ	ⓑ	ⓒ	ⓓ
34.	ⓐ	ⓑ	ⓒ	ⓓ
35.	ⓐ	ⓑ	ⓒ	ⓓ
36.	ⓐ	ⓑ	ⓒ	ⓓ
37.	ⓐ	ⓑ	ⓒ	ⓓ
38.	ⓐ	ⓑ	ⓒ	ⓓ
39.	ⓐ	ⓑ	ⓒ	ⓓ
40.	ⓐ	ⓑ	ⓒ	ⓓ
41.	ⓐ	ⓑ	ⓒ	ⓓ
42.	ⓐ	ⓑ	ⓒ	ⓓ
43.	ⓐ	ⓑ	ⓒ	ⓓ
44.	ⓐ	ⓑ	ⓒ	ⓓ
45.	ⓐ	ⓑ	ⓒ	ⓓ
46.	ⓐ	ⓑ	ⓒ	ⓓ
47.	ⓐ	ⓑ	ⓒ	ⓓ
48.	ⓐ	ⓑ	ⓒ	ⓓ

Section 3: Biology

1.	ⓐ	ⓑ	ⓒ	ⓓ
2.	ⓐ	ⓑ	ⓒ	ⓓ
3.	ⓐ	ⓑ	ⓒ	ⓓ
4.	ⓐ	ⓑ	ⓒ	ⓓ
5.	ⓐ	ⓑ	ⓒ	ⓓ
6.	ⓐ	ⓑ	ⓒ	ⓓ
7.	ⓐ	ⓑ	ⓒ	ⓓ
8.	ⓐ	ⓑ	ⓒ	ⓓ
9.	ⓐ	ⓑ	ⓒ	ⓓ
10.	ⓐ	ⓑ	ⓒ	ⓓ
11.	ⓐ	ⓑ	ⓒ	ⓓ
12.	ⓐ	ⓑ	ⓒ	ⓓ
13.	ⓐ	ⓑ	ⓒ	ⓓ
14.	ⓐ	ⓑ	ⓒ	ⓓ
15.	ⓐ	ⓑ	ⓒ	ⓓ
16.	ⓐ	ⓑ	ⓒ	ⓓ
17.	ⓐ	ⓑ	ⓒ	ⓓ
18.	ⓐ	ⓑ	ⓒ	ⓓ
19.	ⓐ	ⓑ	ⓒ	ⓓ
20.	ⓐ	ⓑ	ⓒ	ⓓ
21.	ⓐ	ⓑ	ⓒ	ⓓ
22.	ⓐ	ⓑ	ⓒ	ⓓ
23.	ⓐ	ⓑ	ⓒ	ⓓ
24.	ⓐ	ⓑ	ⓒ	ⓓ
25.	ⓐ	ⓑ	ⓒ	ⓓ
26.	ⓐ	ⓑ	ⓒ	ⓓ
27.	ⓐ	ⓑ	ⓒ	ⓓ
28.	ⓐ	ⓑ	ⓒ	ⓓ
29.	ⓐ	ⓑ	ⓒ	ⓓ
30.	ⓐ	ⓑ	ⓒ	ⓓ
31.	ⓐ	ⓑ	ⓒ	ⓓ
32.	ⓐ	ⓑ	ⓒ	ⓓ
33.	ⓐ	ⓑ	ⓒ	ⓓ
34.	ⓐ	ⓑ	ⓒ	ⓓ
35.	ⓐ	ⓑ	ⓒ	ⓓ
36.	ⓐ	ⓑ	ⓒ	ⓓ
37.	ⓐ	ⓑ	ⓒ	ⓓ
38.	ⓐ	ⓑ	ⓒ	ⓓ
39.	ⓐ	ⓑ	ⓒ	ⓓ
40.	ⓐ	ⓑ	ⓒ	ⓓ
41.	ⓐ	ⓑ	ⓒ	ⓓ
42.	ⓐ	ⓑ	ⓒ	ⓓ
43.	ⓐ	ⓑ	ⓒ	ⓓ
44.	ⓐ	ⓑ	ⓒ	ⓓ
45.	ⓐ	ⓑ	ⓒ	ⓓ
46.	ⓐ	ⓑ	ⓒ	ⓓ
47.	ⓐ	ⓑ	ⓒ	ⓓ
48.	ⓐ	ⓑ	ⓒ	ⓓ

Section 4: Chemistry

1.	ⓐ	ⓑ	ⓒ	ⓓ
2.	ⓐ	ⓑ	ⓒ	ⓓ
3.	ⓐ	ⓑ	ⓒ	ⓓ
4.	ⓐ	ⓑ	ⓒ	ⓓ
5.	ⓐ	ⓑ	ⓒ	ⓓ
6.	ⓐ	ⓑ	ⓒ	ⓓ
7.	ⓐ	ⓑ	ⓒ	ⓓ
8.	ⓐ	ⓑ	ⓒ	ⓓ
9.	ⓐ	ⓑ	ⓒ	ⓓ
10.	ⓐ	ⓑ	ⓒ	ⓓ
11.	ⓐ	ⓑ	ⓒ	ⓓ
12.	ⓐ	ⓑ	ⓒ	ⓓ
13.	ⓐ	ⓑ	ⓒ	ⓓ
14.	ⓐ	ⓑ	ⓒ	ⓓ
15.	ⓐ	ⓑ	ⓒ	ⓓ
16.	ⓐ	ⓑ	ⓒ	ⓓ
17.	ⓐ	ⓑ	ⓒ	ⓓ
18.	ⓐ	ⓑ	ⓒ	ⓓ
19.	ⓐ	ⓑ	ⓒ	ⓓ
20.	ⓐ	ⓑ	ⓒ	ⓓ
21.	ⓐ	ⓑ	ⓒ	ⓓ
22.	ⓐ	ⓑ	ⓒ	ⓓ
23.	ⓐ	ⓑ	ⓒ	ⓓ
24.	ⓐ	ⓑ	ⓒ	ⓓ
25.	ⓐ	ⓑ	ⓒ	ⓓ
26.	ⓐ	ⓑ	ⓒ	ⓓ
27.	ⓐ	ⓑ	ⓒ	ⓓ
28.	ⓐ	ⓑ	ⓒ	ⓓ
29.	ⓐ	ⓑ	ⓒ	ⓓ
30.	ⓐ	ⓑ	ⓒ	ⓓ
31.	ⓐ	ⓑ	ⓒ	ⓓ
32.	ⓐ	ⓑ	ⓒ	ⓓ
33.	ⓐ	ⓑ	ⓒ	ⓓ
34.	ⓐ	ⓑ	ⓒ	ⓓ
35.	ⓐ	ⓑ	ⓒ	ⓓ
36.	ⓐ	ⓑ	ⓒ	ⓓ
37.	ⓐ	ⓑ	ⓒ	ⓓ
38.	ⓐ	ⓑ	ⓒ	ⓓ
39.	ⓐ	ⓑ	ⓒ	ⓓ
40.	ⓐ	ⓑ	ⓒ	ⓓ
41.	ⓐ	ⓑ	ⓒ	ⓓ
42.	ⓐ	ⓑ	ⓒ	ⓓ
43.	ⓐ	ⓑ	ⓒ	ⓓ
44.	ⓐ	ⓑ	ⓒ	ⓓ
45.	ⓐ	ⓑ	ⓒ	ⓓ
46.	ⓐ	ⓑ	ⓒ	ⓓ
47.	ⓐ	ⓑ	ⓒ	ⓓ
48.	ⓐ	ⓑ	ⓒ	ⓓ

Section 6: Reading Comprehension

Passage 1

1.	ⓐ	ⓑ	ⓒ	ⓓ
2.	ⓐ	ⓑ	ⓒ	ⓓ
3.	ⓐ	ⓑ	ⓒ	ⓓ
4.	ⓐ	ⓑ	ⓒ	ⓓ
5.	ⓐ	ⓑ	ⓒ	ⓓ
6.	ⓐ	ⓑ	ⓒ	ⓓ

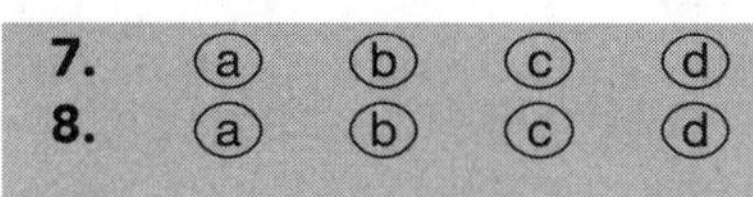

7.	ⓐ	ⓑ	ⓒ	ⓓ
8.	ⓐ	ⓑ	ⓒ	ⓓ

Passage 2

9.	ⓐ	ⓑ	ⓒ	ⓓ
10.	ⓐ	ⓑ	ⓒ	ⓓ
11.	ⓐ	ⓑ	ⓒ	ⓓ
12.	ⓐ	ⓑ	ⓒ	ⓓ
13.	ⓐ	ⓑ	ⓒ	ⓓ
14.	ⓐ	ⓑ	ⓒ	ⓓ
15.	ⓐ	ⓑ	ⓒ	ⓓ
16.	ⓐ	ⓑ	ⓒ	ⓓ

Passage 3

17.	ⓐ	ⓑ	ⓒ	ⓓ
18.	ⓐ	ⓑ	ⓒ	ⓓ
19.	ⓐ	ⓑ	ⓒ	ⓓ
20.	ⓐ	ⓑ	ⓒ	ⓓ
21.	ⓐ	ⓑ	ⓒ	ⓓ
22.	ⓐ	ⓑ	ⓒ	ⓓ
23.	ⓐ	ⓑ	ⓒ	ⓓ
24.	ⓐ	ⓑ	ⓒ	ⓓ

Passage 4

25.	ⓐ	ⓑ	ⓒ	ⓓ
26.	ⓐ	ⓑ	ⓒ	ⓓ
27.	ⓐ	ⓑ	ⓒ	ⓓ
28.	ⓐ	ⓑ	ⓒ	ⓓ
29.	ⓐ	ⓑ	ⓒ	ⓓ
30.	ⓐ	ⓑ	ⓒ	ⓓ
31.	ⓐ	ⓑ	ⓒ	ⓓ
32.	ⓐ	ⓑ	ⓒ	ⓓ

Passage 5

33.	ⓐ	ⓑ	ⓒ	ⓓ	36.	ⓐ	ⓑ	ⓒ	ⓓ	39.	ⓐ	ⓑ	ⓒ	ⓓ
34.	ⓐ	ⓑ	ⓒ	ⓓ	37.	ⓐ	ⓑ	ⓒ	ⓓ	40.	ⓐ	ⓑ	ⓒ	ⓓ
35.	ⓐ	ⓑ	ⓒ	ⓓ	38.	ⓐ	ⓑ	ⓒ	ⓓ					

Passage 6

41.	ⓐ	ⓑ	ⓒ	ⓓ	44.	ⓐ	ⓑ	ⓒ	ⓓ	47.	ⓐ	ⓑ	ⓒ	ⓓ
42.	ⓐ	ⓑ	ⓒ	ⓓ	45.	ⓐ	ⓑ	ⓒ	ⓓ	48.	ⓐ	ⓑ	ⓒ	ⓓ
43.	ⓐ	ⓑ	ⓒ	ⓓ	46.	ⓐ	ⓑ	ⓒ	ⓓ					

Section 7: Quantitative Ability

1.	ⓐ	ⓑ	ⓒ	ⓓ	17.	ⓐ	ⓑ	ⓒ	ⓓ	33.	ⓐ	ⓑ	ⓒ	ⓓ
2.	ⓐ	ⓑ	ⓒ	ⓓ	18.	ⓐ	ⓑ	ⓒ	ⓓ	34.	ⓐ	ⓑ	ⓒ	ⓓ
3.	ⓐ	ⓑ	ⓒ	ⓓ	19.	ⓐ	ⓑ	ⓒ	ⓓ	35.	ⓐ	ⓑ	ⓒ	ⓓ
4.	ⓐ	ⓑ	ⓒ	ⓓ	20.	ⓐ	ⓑ	ⓒ	ⓓ	36.	ⓐ	ⓑ	ⓒ	ⓓ
5.	ⓐ	ⓑ	ⓒ	ⓓ	21.	ⓐ	ⓑ	ⓒ	ⓓ	37.	ⓐ	ⓑ	ⓒ	ⓓ
6.	ⓐ	ⓑ	ⓒ	ⓓ	22.	ⓐ	ⓑ	ⓒ	ⓓ	38.	ⓐ	ⓑ	ⓒ	ⓓ
7.	ⓐ	ⓑ	ⓒ	ⓓ	23.	ⓐ	ⓑ	ⓒ	ⓓ	39.	ⓐ	ⓑ	ⓒ	ⓓ
8.	ⓐ	ⓑ	ⓒ	ⓓ	24.	ⓐ	ⓑ	ⓒ	ⓓ	40.	ⓐ	ⓑ	ⓒ	ⓓ
9.	ⓐ	ⓑ	ⓒ	ⓓ	25.	ⓐ	ⓑ	ⓒ	ⓓ	41.	ⓐ	ⓑ	ⓒ	ⓓ
10.	ⓐ	ⓑ	ⓒ	ⓓ	26.	ⓐ	ⓑ	ⓒ	ⓓ	42.	ⓐ	ⓑ	ⓒ	ⓓ
11.	ⓐ	ⓑ	ⓒ	ⓓ	27.	ⓐ	ⓑ	ⓒ	ⓓ	43.	ⓐ	ⓑ	ⓒ	ⓓ
12.	ⓐ	ⓑ	ⓒ	ⓓ	28.	ⓐ	ⓑ	ⓒ	ⓓ	44.	ⓐ	ⓑ	ⓒ	ⓓ
13.	ⓐ	ⓑ	ⓒ	ⓓ	29.	ⓐ	ⓑ	ⓒ	ⓓ	45.	ⓐ	ⓑ	ⓒ	ⓓ
14.	ⓐ	ⓑ	ⓒ	ⓓ	30.	ⓐ	ⓑ	ⓒ	ⓓ	46.	ⓐ	ⓑ	ⓒ	ⓓ
15.	ⓐ	ⓑ	ⓒ	ⓓ	31.	ⓐ	ⓑ	ⓒ	ⓓ	47.	ⓐ	ⓑ	ⓒ	ⓓ
16.	ⓐ	ⓑ	ⓒ	ⓓ	32.	ⓐ	ⓑ	ⓒ	ⓓ	48.	ⓐ	ⓑ	ⓒ	ⓓ

Section 1: Writing

1 Essay Prompt
Time: 30 minutes

Essay 1

Prompt: Discuss solutions to the problem of food safety in the United States.

Section 2: Verbal Ability

48 Questions
Time: 30 minutes (for the entire Verbal Ability section)

Analogies

Directions: For questions 1 through 29, select the word that best fits the analogy.

1. SHOWER : DELUGE :: PEBBLE : ______
- **a.** walkway
- **b.** boulder
- **c.** pond
- **d.** sand

2. SNOUT : DOG :: BEAK : ______
- **a.** anteater
- **b.** rostrum
- **c.** human
- **d.** dolphin

3. LUNGS : RESPIRATORY SYSTEM :: BONES : ______
- **a.** anatomy
- **b.** skeletal system
- **c.** muscular system
- **d.** musculoskeletal

4. CALENDAR : MONTHS :: BOOK : ______
- **a.** chapters
- **b.** pages
- **c.** titles
- **d.** index

5. TRAPEZOID : QUADRILATERAL :: OCTAGON : ______
- **a.** cubes
- **b.** parallelogram
- **c.** polygon
- **d.** rhombus

6. ERASER : MISTAKES :: DETERGENT : ______
- **a.** purity
- **b.** grime
- **c.** composites
- **d.** cleanliness

7. PAUCITY : DEARTH :: DUPLICITY : ______
- **a.** implication
- **b.** frankness
- **c.** honest
- **d.** guile

8. USHER : THEATER :: PROVOST : ______
- **a.** university
- **b.** studio
- **c.** library
- **d.** kindergarten

9. WARM : OVERHEATED :: ANXIOUS : ______
- **a.** placated
- **b.** disparaged
- **c.** attenuated
- **d.** petrified

10. SHEEP : EWE :: PIG : ______
- **a.** hog
- **b.** sow
- **c.** boar
- **d.** sty

11. SUGAR : CUBE :: BUTTER : ______
- **a.** pat
- **b.** margarine
- **c.** churn
- **d.** rectangle

12. FURTIVE : SURREPTITIOUS :: INCHOATE : ______
- **a.** quiescent
- **b.** plenary
- **c.** insidious
- **d.** nascent

13. GLARE : SQUINT :: DUST : ______
   a. squelch
   b. waver
   c. cough
   d. descry

14. AMBIGUOUS : CLARITY :: OBDURATE : ______
   a. sense
   b. intelligence
   c. compassion
   d. pragmatism

15. HAUGHTY : MODEST :: SEDULOUS : ______
   a. inactive
   b. impudent
   c. honest
   d. sagacious

16. INSTIGATE : CONFLICT :: FOSTER : ______
   a. volatility
   b. talent
   c. controversy
   d. disdain

17. DOGGED : INTRANSIGENT :: PLAINTIVE : ______
   a. magnanimous
   b. buoyant
   c. doleful
   d. austere

18. MISANTHROPE : CYNICAL :: PHILANTHROPIST : ______
   a. altruistic
   b. egoistic
   c. equivocal
   d. skeptical

19. SOB : BLUBBER :: STATE : ______
   a. whisper
   b. express
   c. depict
   d. exclaim

20. EXOTHERMIC : COMBUSTION :: ENDOTHERMIC : ______
   a. temperature
   b. photosynthesis
   c. explosion
   d. molecules

21. HACKSAW : KNIFE :: CALIPER : ______
   a. hammer
   b. crowbar
   c. chisel
   d. protractor

22. INSULT : CONTEMPTUOUS :: STENCH : ______
   a. noisome
   b. offend
   c. pleasing
   d. nosy

23. CASPIAN SEA : LAKE SUPERIOR :: ANGEL FALLS : ______
   a. Niagara
   b. Lake Tahoe
   c. Yosemite Falls
   d. Baltic Sea

24. HYDROMETER : DENSITY :: SEISMOGRAPH : ______
   a. water
   b. movements
   c. shape
   d. waves

25. LEAVE : ABSCOND :: CALM : ______
   a. sated
   b. negotiate
   c. remain
   d. placate

26. PHLEGMATIC : STOLID :: BILIOUS : ______
   a. fervid
   b. apathetic
   c. cantankerous
   d. laconic

27. QUADRATIC : EQUATION :: LABOR : ______
   a. toil
   b. law
   c. equalization
   d. holiday

28. LION : VALOR :: DOG : ______
   a. steadfastness
   b. dogmatism
   c. fickleness
   d. artifice

29. CAPITULATE : RESIST :: BLANDISH : ______
   a. feign
   b. yield
   c. rescind
   d. intimidate

Sentence Completions

Directions: For questions 30 through 48, select the word or word set that best fits the meaning and sense of the sentence. All sentences have either one blank for a word or two blanks for a word set.

30. Even though they still had a lot of studying to accomplish, they _____ their better judgment and went out with friends instead.
   a. embraced
   b. ignored
   c. faulted
   d. targeted

31. Here was grown the most bounteous, _____, and finest wheat in the entire world.
   a. craven
   b. dullest
   c. loquacious
   d. richest

32. It is the general aim of the biological sciences to _____ something of the order of _____ in the living world.
   a. disprove . . . animals
   b. falsify . . . plants
   c. infer . . . anatomy
   d. learn . . . nature

33. Families in the region often are large. This means that in many families there is _____ a period of _____ before the children become old enough to work.
   a. inevitably . . . poverty
   b. scarcely . . . scarcity
   c. often . . . wealth
   d. inexcusably . . . mockery

34. The man, who felt desperate, sprang from his chair and paced across the room in a state of _____.
   a. felicity
   b. agitation
   c. efficacy
   d. languish

35. The woman often _____ on the matter, as she generally was swayed by the person with whom she was speaking at the moment.
   a. conversed
   b. shouted
   c. vacillated
   d. gossiped

36. The father and son liked to hyperbolize, so when they told stories of the small events of their daily lives, the events sounded _____ and _____.
a. innocuous . . . guileless
b. romanticized . . . exalted
c. dispassionate . . . insipid
d. elongated . . . mollified

37. Algorism is distinguished from abacist computation by recognizing seven rules, including addition and subtraction. It is further _____ by the use of zero.
a. characterized
b. confounded
c. obviated
d. tempered

38. The first known domestication of the horse was not done in the work of a day, but, like other great accomplishments, was brought about by a _____ process of _____ and discoveries.
a. quick . . . chicanery
b. wretched . . . ropes
c. gradual . . . experiments
d. prodigal . . . books

39. The children likely were in _____ danger from exposure to a night of cold and wet in an open boat without _____ clothing and food.
a. trivial . . . copious
b. limited . . . ample
c. neutral . . . suitable
d. grave . . . sufficient

40. The week had gone by without one customer, so when, at last, three people entered the store, the owner greeted them _____ and talked incessantly.
a. sullenly
b. pusillanimously
c. jubilantly
d. demurely

41. Many people regard the practice of serving several dishes at a meal as _____ and _____, when, in fact, it can be easy and inexpensive.
a. hapless . . . cheap
b. onerous . . . costly
c. facile . . . exorbitant
d. burdensome . . . reasonable

42. It was not until after the Revolutionary War period that the spinet and harpsichord were _____ in this country by the piano.
a. conceded
b. renounced
c. subsidized
d. superseded

43. The earth lodges of the Omaha tribe were made by the women, and were intended _____ for summer use, when the people were not migrating or going on the hunt.
a. principally
b. arbitrarily
c. fervently
d. allegorically

44. Oregon is a word derived from the Spanish, and means "wild thyme"; the early explorers found the _____ growing there in great _____.
a. sustenance . . . colors
b. shrubs . . . meagerness
c. herb . . . profusion
d. economy . . . strides

45. In his book *Elements of Chemistry*, the author says he makes it his own law to advance only from what is known to what is unknown, and never to form any _____ that is not an immediate _____ from observation and experiment.
a. opinion . . . reconciliation
b. consideration . . . precursor
c. permutation . . . conjecture
d. conclusion . . . consequence

46. He had seen shell games at circuses and fairgrounds when he was much younger, but he supposed they had long since been abandoned in favor of more _____ and less discreditable methods of robbery.
a. derisive
b. ingenious
c. ingenuous
d. inept

47. The arterial pressure of man is not lowered by the ordinary fatigue of daily life. It is only in extreme states of _____ that the pressure may be found _____ when the subject is in the standing position.
a. exercise . . . mitigated
b. activity . . . increased
c. exhaustion . . . decreased
d. turpitude . . . erratic

48. Miss Polly did not usually make hurried movements; she specially prided herself on her _____ of manner.
a. repose
b. verbosity
c. petulance
d. agitation

Section 3: Biology

48 Questions
Time: 30 minutes (for the entire Biology section)

Directions: Choose the best answer to each of the following questions.

1. When homologous structures with a common evolutionary origin evolve different variations over time it is called
a. microevolution.
b. divergent evolution.
c. convergent evolution.
d. parallel evolution.

2. A relationship between two organisms in which one organism benefits and the other is unharmed is called
a. pleiotropy.
b. parasitic.
c. mutualistic.
d. commensalism.

3. The migration of individuals out of or into a population, either taking their contribution to the gene pool with them or adding it to the gene pool of a population, is referred to as
a. genetic drift.
b. natural selection.
c. gene flow.
d. adaptation.

4. What is the order of the taxonomic ranks in the classification system?
a. kingdom, domain, phylum, class, order, family, genus, species
b. domain, kingdom, phylum, class, order, family, genus, species
c. kingdom, domain, order, phylum, class, family, genus, species
d. phylum, order, domain, kingdom, class, family, genus, species

5. Members of this kingdom are unicellular prokaryotes, most of which do NOT have peptidoglycan in their cell walls. They can be either autotrophs or heterotrophs.
   a. Fungi
   b. Archaeabacteria
   c. Eubacteria
   d. Protista

6. Which type of organism is NOT a consumer that must get its food (energy source) from consuming other organisms?
   a. decomposer
   b. detritivore
   c. autotroph
   d. heterotroph

7. Members of this kingdom are either unicellular or multicellular eukaryotic heterotrophs that have a cell wall composed of chitin.
   a. Fungi
   b. Archaeabacteria
   c. Eubacteria
   d. Protista

8. Which of the following is a taxonomic grouping that includes the most recent common ancestor of all of the organisms, but does NOT include all of the descendants of the most recent common ancestor?
   a. monophyletic taxon
   b. polyphyletic taxon
   c. natural group
   d. paraphyletic taxon

9. The function of this prokaryotic organelle is to house the genes that code for the proteins needed by the cell.
   a. flagella
   b. ribosome
   c. nucleoid
   d. cell wall

10. Which of the following is a protein in the plasma membrane that plays a role in signal transduction?
   a. channel protein
   b. receptor protein
   c. recognition protein
   d. carrier protein

11. Which of the following is the organelle in eukaryotic cells responsible for sorting and modifying proteins and lipids, folding polypeptides, and sorting and packaging molecules into vacuoles and vesicles?
   a. Golgi apparatus
   b. endoplasmic reticulum
   c. lysosome
   d. centriole

12. Which of the following organelles in eukaryotic cells is responsible for the production of adenosine triphosphate (ATP)?
   a. vesicles
   b. cytoskeleton
   c. peroxisome
   d. mitochondria

13. Of which protein are microtubules and flagella and cilia in eukaryotes composed?
   a. actin
   b. cohesin
   c. tubulin
   d. flagellin

14. Which of the following joins cells together at transportation and communication channels formed by proteins deposited in the plasma membrane of the adjoining cells?
   a. occluding junctions
   b. spot desmosomes
   c. gap junctions
   d. plasmodesmata

15. Which of the following is a protein in the plasma membrane that transports attached molecules and ions via facilitated diffusion and active transport?
a. channel protein
b. receptor protein
c. recognition protein
d. carrier protein

16. Of which protein are microfilaments composed?
a. actin
b. cohesin
c. tubulin
d. flagellin

17. Which of the following is the process by which sperm and eggs are produced?
a. gastrulation
b. spermiogenesis
c. gametogenesis
d. blastulation

18. The germ cell layer that develops into the bone, blood, cartilage, extracellular matrix, collagen, and muscles, including the heart muscle, is the
a. endoderm.
b. ectoderm.
c. archenteron.
d. mesoderm.

19. This egg membrane develops from the posterior of the gastrointestinal (GI) tract of the embryo and forms a sac that is instrumental in gas exchange (O_2 and CO_2), water and salt exchange, and nitrogenous waste removal.
a. chorion
b. allantois
c. amnion
d. yolk sac

20. The bacterial shape that looks like a rod and can have a flagellum is
a. spirillum
b. cocci
c. bacilli
d. vibrio

21. This type of bacteria has optimum growth temperatures between 25°C and 45°C.
a. psychrophile
b. hyperthermophile
c. thermophile
d. mesophile

22. Which of the following specifically refers to the type of sweat gland that releases its product into an associated hair follicle?
a. apocrine sweat gland
b. ceruminous gland
c. sudoriferous gland
d. eccrine sweat gland

23. Which term describes joints that are freely movable?
a. synarthroses
b. diarthroses
c. synostoses
d. amphiarthroses

24. The hormones released from the adrenal cortex of the adrenal glands include all of the following EXCEPT
a. cortisol.
b. epinephrine.
c. aldosterone.
d. androgens.

25. Which of the following is a specialized fibrous joint between the teeth and the mandible and maxilla?
a. syndesmoses
b. synchondroses
c. gomphoses
d. suture

26. Which of the following sets of movements of synovial joints describes the up-and-down movements of the foot?
a. flexion/extension
b. plantar flexion/dorsiflexion
c. inversion/eversion
d. pronation/supination

27. Which of the following are channels that transmit blood vessels from the periosteum into the bone?
a. lacunae
b. Haversian canals
c. lamellae
d. Volkmann's canals

28. When the environment is hypertonic to a cell, which of the following does NOT occur?
a. Crenation occurs in eukaryotic animal cells.
b. Osmotic lysis or cytolysis occurs in eukaryotic animal cells.
c. Eukaryotic plant cells become turgid, or swollen and distended.
d. Water enters the cell from the exterior where there are fewer solutes relative to water.

29. From which of the following glands is melatonin is released?
a. thyroid
b. anterior pituitary
c. pineal
d. thymus

30. Which of the following is the time period in the bacterial growth cycle in which there is an equal rate of reproduction and death?
a. decline period
b. logarithmic period
c. stationary period
d. lag time

31. Which of the following is the connective tissue layer that covers a fascicle or bundle of muscle fibers?
a. periosteum
b. endomysium
c. perimysium
d. epimysium

32. Why are penicillin and its derivatives ineffective against pneumonia caused by bacteria in the genus *Mycoplasma*?
a. *Mycoplasma* are Gram-negative bacteria and do not have a thick layer of peptidoglycan in their cell walls.
b. *Mycoplasma* do not have a cell wall.
c. *Mycoplasma* produce a capsule that is impenetrable to antibiotics.
d. *Mycoplasma* is a fungus and penicillin and its derivatives do not kill fungus.

33. Which of the following is a yeast infection contracted by inhaling the dust of soil contaminated with certain types of bird droppings, particularly pigeons?
a. cryptococcosis
b. coccidioidomycosis
c. blastomycosis
d. histoplasmosis

34. In the pyramid diagram that depicts the flow of energy through an ecosystem, the least energy is available to the
a. producers.
b. tertiary consumers.
c. primary consumers.
d. herbivores.

35. Which of the following is the contractile muscle tissue of the heart?
a. epicardium
b. myocardium
c. interventricular sulci
d. endocardium

36. Which of the following are the three vessels of the right atrium?
a. superior vena cava, inferior vena cava, right pulmonary vein
b. superior vena cava, inferior vena cava, brachiocephalic artery
c. coronary sinus, right pulmonary vein, superior vena cava
d. superior vena cava, inferior vena cava, coronary sinus

37. Which of the following red blood cell (RBC) precursors is an indication in the blood count of how well the red bone marrow is producing new RBCs?
a. reticulocytes
b. normoblasts
c. hemocytoblasts
d. proerythroblasts

38. Which of the following are obligate intracellular parasites?
a. *Mycoplasma* and *Rickettsia*
b. *Bacillus* and *Clostridium*
c. *Chlamydia* and *Mycoplasma*
d. *Chlamydia* and *Rickettsia*

39. These least abundant WBCs are granulocytes with dark-staining, purplish-black granules and an S- or U-shaped nucleus that release histamine to stimulate vasodilation during the inflammatory response.
a. neutrophils
b. eosinophils
c. basophils
d. monocytes

40. Where do the light-dependent reactions of photosynthesis occur?
a. thylakoid membrane
b. thylakoid compartment or lumen
c. stroma
d. grana

41. Which of the following is an example of pleiotropy and incomplete dominance?
a. Tay-Sachs disease
b. Marfan syndrome
c. sickle-cell anemia
d. Huntington's disease

42. Which of the following is the genetic occurrence in which one or more genes inhibit the expression of another gene?
a. hypostasis
b. polygenic inheritance
c. pleiotropy
d. epistasis

43. If a heterozygous blood type A female is crossed with a heterozygous blood type B male, the probability of producing a child with type AB blood is
a. 50%.
b. 100%.
c. 25%.
d. 0%.

44. Select the disease caused by a spore-forming bacterium.
a. anthrax
b. lymphogranuloma venereum
c. giardiasis
d. trachoma

45. When blood is centrifuged to perform a complete blood count, the top layer after centrifugation is the
a. red blood cells (RBCs).
b. plasma.
c. white blood cells (WBCs).
d. buffy coat.

46. The type of bond that forms between the complementary nitrogenous bases on the double-stranded DNA molecule are
a. phosphodiester bonds.
b. covalent carbon-hydrogen bonds.
c. high-energy phosphate bonds.
d. hydrogen bonds.

47. Mutations are caused by
a. changes in the sequence of nitrogen bases on a DNA strand.
b. disruption of the deoxyribose sugar on the sugar-phosphate backbone of DNA.
c. loss of a phosphate group on a DNA molecule.
d. changes in the sequence of nitrogen bases on a RNA strand.

48. Glycolysis produces
a. six molecules of CO_2, six molecules of water, and 36 to 38 molecules of adenosine triphosphate (ATP).
b. two pyruvate molecules and two molecules of ATP.
c. two acetyl CoA molecules and two molecules of CO_2.
d. two lactate molecules and two molecules of ATP.

Section 4: Chemistry

48 Questions
Time: 30 minutes (for the entire Chemistry section)

Directions: Choose the best answer to each of the following questions.

1. As part of an attempt to identify a 100 g sample of an unknown liquid, a scientist applies a known quantity of heat and measures the resulting change in temperature. Assuming that the liquid does not begin to vaporize during the heating process, which of the following properties of the element may be calculated from these three values (mass, amount of heat applied, and temperature change)?
a. heat capacity
b. heat of fusion
c. heat of vaporization
d. heat conductivity

2. The activation energy of an exothermic reaction is
a. greater than the activation energy of the reverse reaction.
b. less than the activation energy of the reverse reaction.
c. equal to the activation energy of the reverse reaction.
d. equal to zero.

3. As a result of the first steps of acid rain formation, solid sulfur combines with oxygen gas to form gaseous sulfur trioxide. For this simplified overall reaction, how many moles of oxygen are used up by each mole of sulfur?
a. 1
b. 1.5
c. 2
d. 3

4. What is the smallest element with a full-valence electron shell?
a. hydrogen
b. helium
c. lithium
d. beryllium

5. Which of the following substances has the highest density at room temperature and atmospheric pressure?
a. xenon
b. krypton
c. iodine
d. bromine

6. Which of the following carbon-carbon bonds is the shortest?
a. C–C
b. C=C
c. C≡C
d. impossible to determine

7. An unknown substance is found to be able to form compounds with at least two different oxidation states. Which of the following is *least* likely to describe this unknown substance?
a. alkali metal
b. nonmetal
c. transition metal
d. metalloid

8. In the following reaction, how many electrons are consumed for every Cr^{2+} ion produced?

$$Cr_2O_7^{2-} + H^+ + e^- \longrightarrow Cr^{2+} + H_2O$$

a. two
b. four
c. seven
d. eight

9. Each of the following electron configurations represents an electrically neutral atom; which of these is most likely to act as a reducing agent?
a. $1s^2 2s^2 2p^6 3s^2 3p^4$
b. $1s^2 2s^2 2p^6 3s^2 3p^5$
c. $1s^2 2s^2 2p^6 3s^2 3p^6 4s^1$
d. $1s^2 2s^2 2p^6 3s^2 3p^6 4s^2$

10. Which of the following types of radioactive decay will increase the atomic number of the daughter nucleus?
a. α decay
b. β^+ decay
c. β^- decay
d. γ decay

11. In a slow multistep reaction, a catalyst may be added to speed the reaction progress. The most useful purpose of a catalyst in such a situation would be to increase
a. the net change in enthalpy.
b. the activation energy.
c. the rate of the slow step.
d. the rate of the fast step.

12. To help identify an unknown metal, a student dissolves it in a solution of hydrochloric acid (HCl). The reaction gives off bubbles of a gas and the resulting solution turns green in color. Which of the following is the most likely identity of the unknown metal?

a. copper
b. sodium
c. magnesium
d. aluminum

13. A 4 g sample of NaOH is added to 100 mL of a 0.1 M HCl solution. What is the concentration of NaCl in the resulting mixture?

a. 10 M
b. 1 M
c. 0.1 M
d. 0.01 M

14. Which of the following acids has the lowest K_a value?

a. HF
b. HCl
c. HBr
d. HI

15. The ideal gas law approximates the behavior of a gas based on its volume, temperature, pressure, and quantity. Which of the following additional properties can help to make a more precise calculation?

a. total potential energy stored by the gas
b. total kinetic energy of the gas particles
c. molecular mass of individual gas particles
d. intermolecular forces between gas particles

16. On a pressure-temperature phase diagram of water, the temperature at the triple point (the point at which the water coexists in its gas, liquid, and solid phases) is approximately 273 K. For water to exist as a gas at this temperature, the pressure must be

a. far greater than 1 atm.
b. near 1 atm.
c. far less than 1 atm.
d. exactly 1 atm.

17. What is the most electronegative element on the Periodic Table?

a. fluorine
b. helium
c. neon
d. hydrogen

18. At which of the following temperatures does water have the highest density?

a. –20°C
b. 1°C
c. 20°C
d. 100°C

19. Which of the following phenomena best explains the state in the diagram below?

$$S{=}C{=}N^{\ominus} \longleftrightarrow {}^{\ominus}S{-}C{\equiv}N$$

a. equilibrium
b. resonance
c. isomerism
d. tautomerism

20. What is the molecular formula for aluminum carbonate?

a. $AlCO_3$
b. Al_2CO_3
c. $Al_3(CO_3)_2$
d. $Al_2(CO_3)_3$

21. Which of the following compounds contains only covalent bonds?
a. Na_2O
b. MgO
c. CH_2O
d. B_2O_3

22. What is the molecular geometry around the carbon atom in a methane (CH_4) molecule?
a. bent
b. tetrahedral
c. trigonal bipyramidal
d. trigonal planar

23. Supose 100 g of a liquid with a specific heat of 2.09 J/(g K) is heated to a temperature of 400 K and mixed with water (specific heat of 4.18 J/(g K)) at 300 K. After the mixture is stirred to a homogeneous consistency, the temperature is found to be 350 K. Assuming no heat is lost to the environment, how much water was in the original container?
a. 200 g
b. 100 g
c. 50 g
d. 33 g

24. Which of the following forms of electromagnetic radiation carries the least energy?
a. microwave
b. infrared
c. violet
d. ultraviolet

25. In a galvanic cell, the cathode and anode are connected by a bridge. Which of the following is most likely to be found in the bridge?
a. $CuSO_4$
b. Cu
c. Br_2
d. CH_2O

26. On an expedition to a distant planet, a space probe finds several new elements with high atomic numbers, including a few with a *g* subshell in its fifth energy level. How many electrons will this subshell hold?
a. 7
b. 9
c. 14
d. 18

27. How many pi bonds are found in a C=C bond?
a. zero
b. one
c. two
d. three

28. Chlorous acid ($HClO_2$) has a K_a of approximately 10^{-2}. What percentage of chlorous acid will dissociate in solution?
a. 0.1%
b. 1%
c. 10%
d. 100%

Organic Chemistry Questions

29. What is the relationship between these two structures?

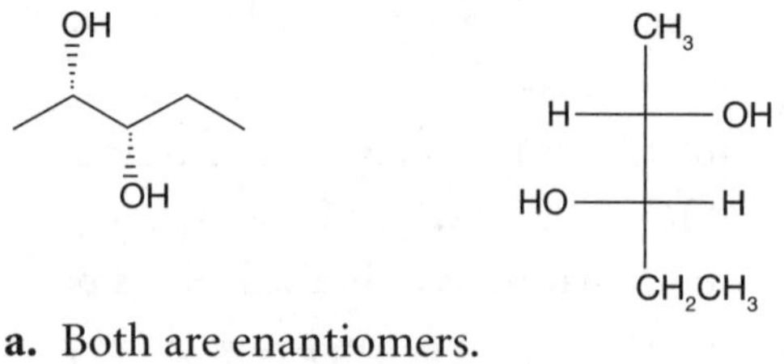

OH
OH

CH$_3$
H — — OH
HO — — H
CH$_2$CH$_3$

a. Both are enantiomers.
b. Both are diastereomers.
c. They are exactly identical.
d. They are completely different compounds.

30. What product is produced by the following reaction?

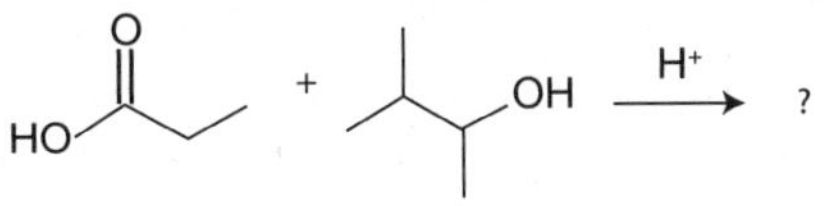

HO OH H+ ?

a. HO HO O

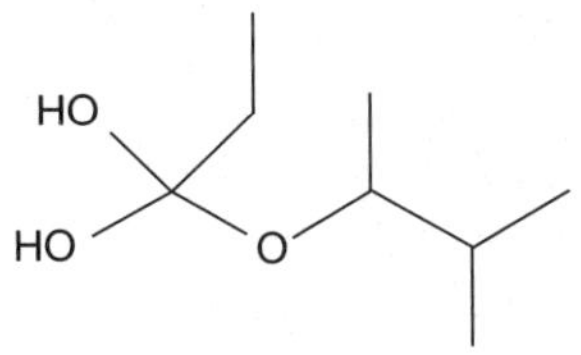

b.

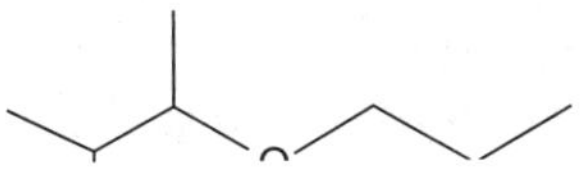

c. O O

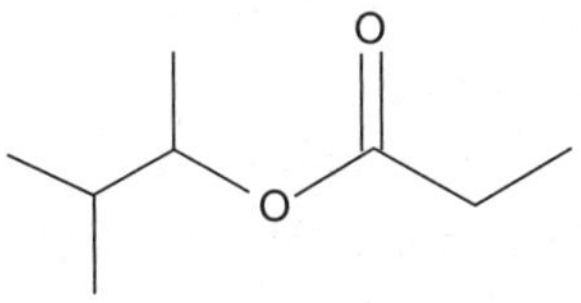

d. OH O

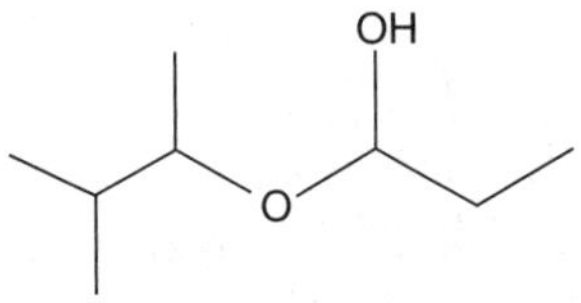

31. What is the IUPAC name for the following molecule?

O H

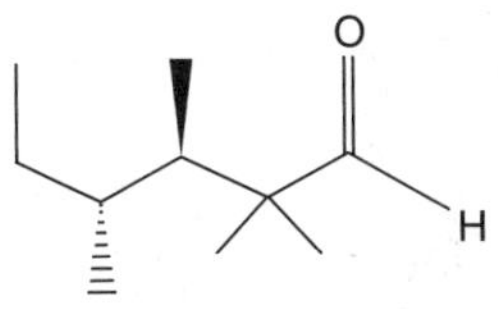

a. (3R, 4R)-2,2,3,4-tetramethylhexenal
b. (3R, 4R)-2,2,3,4-tetramethylhexanal
c. (3R, 4S)-2,2,3,4-tetramethylhexanal
d. (3R, 4S)-2,2,3,4-tetramethylhexanone

32. Rank the following molecules in order of acidity, from least acidic to most acidic.

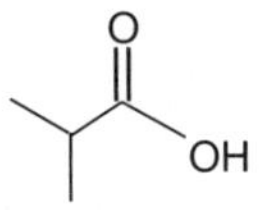

O OH
I

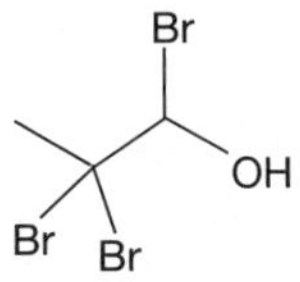

Br OH Br Br
II

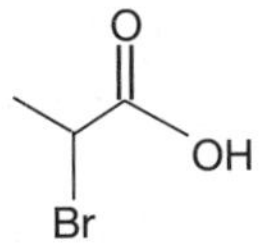

O OH Br
III

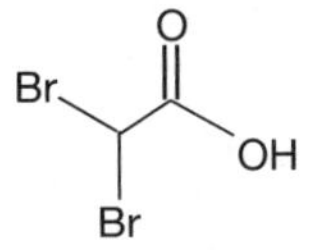

O Br OH Br
IV

a. IV, III, I, II
b. II, I, III, IV
c. I, III, IV, II
d. I, III, II, IV

33. Which of the following substrates is the most reactive in an S_N1 reaction?
a. bromopentane
b. 2-bromopentane
c. 2-bromo–2-methylpentane
d. bromobenzene

34. What is the major S_N1 product from the following reaction?

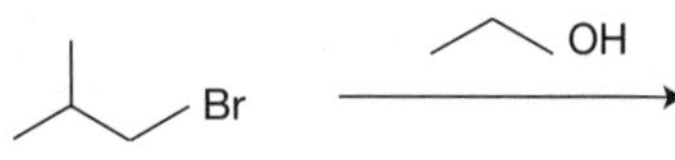

a. 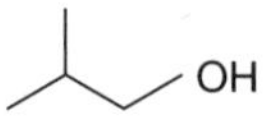 OH

b. 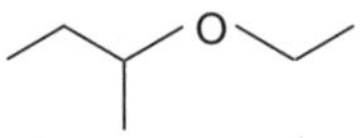 O

c. 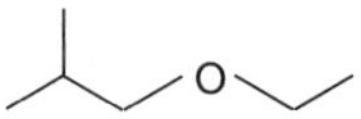 O

d. 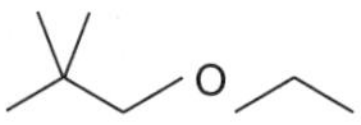 O

35. What is the product of the reaction between hydrogen bromide and 2-methylpentene?

a. 2-bromo–2-methylpentane
b. 1,2-dibromo–2-methyl-pentane
c. 1-bromo–2-methylpentane
d. 2-bromo–2-methylpentene

36. What is the major product produced by the following reaction?

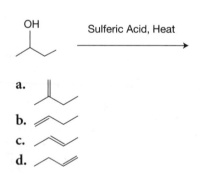

OH Sulferic Acid, Heat

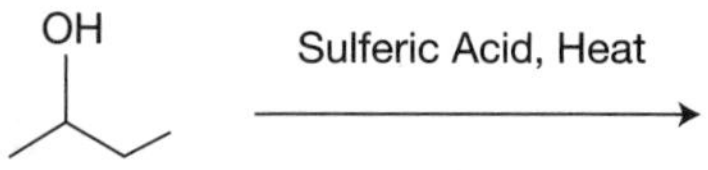

a.

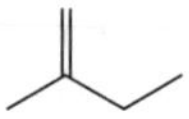

b.

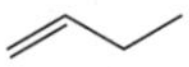

c.

d.

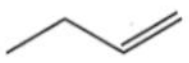

37. Which of following compounds CANNOT be oxidized by chromic acid?

a. cyclohexanol
b. 3-heptanol
c. 2-methyl-hexanal
d. 2-ethyl–2-pentanol

38. What is the product of the following reaction sequence?

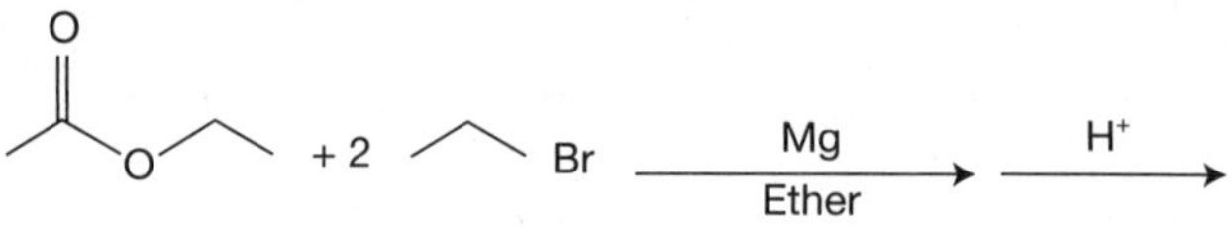

O O + 2 Br Mg Ether H^+

a. primary alcohol
b. secondary alcohol
c. tertiary alcohol
d. ether

39. When a carboxylic acid undergoes dehydration at standard conditions, which CANNOT occur?

a. formation of a ketal
b. synthesis of an acid anhydride
c. intramolecular nucleophilic attack
d. acid catalysis

40. If 4-ethyl cyclohexanol is first treated with an oxidizing agent, disodium chromate, and the product of this reaction is then treated with acetic acid, what is the final product?

a. 4-ethyl cyclohexanoic acid
b. 4-ethyl cyclohexanal
c. 4-ethyl cyclohexanone
d. 4-ethyl cyclohexyl acetate

41. What is NOT true for an acyl chloride?

a. An acyl chloride, also known as an acid chloride, is a very versatile functional group.
b. An acid anhydride is more reactive than an ester, and less reactive than an acyl chloride.
c. The chloride anion is a more stable leaving group than the hydroxide anion of a carboxylic acid.
d. An ester is more reactive toward nucleophilic attack, for it has been more strongly oxidized.

42. Toluene is treated with potassium permanganate, a strong oxidizing agent. It is then treated with water. What is the final product?

a. benzaldehyde
b. benzoic acid
c. phenol
d. benzyl benzoate

43. In the presence of iron(III) chloride, benzene is treated with diatomic chlorine. The major product(s) is/are

a. chlorobenzene.
b. ortho-dichlorobenzene.
c. para-dichlorobenzene.
d. meta-dichlorobenzene.

44. Iodobenzene is treated with fuming nitric acid in the presence of sulfuric acid. What is/are the final product(s)?

a. 1-nitro–3-iodobenzene
b. 1-nitro–3-iodobenzene and 1-nitro–4-iodobenzene
c. 1-nitro–2-iodobenzene and 1-nitro–4-iodobenzene
d. 1-nitro–2-iodobenzene and 1-nitro–3-iodobenzene

45. The electrostatic effects of substituents on aromatic rings play an important role in electrophilic aromatic substitution. Which of the following is NOT correct?

a. Ethers withdraw electron density from the aromatic ring. They serve as meta directors.
b. Activators release electron density into the aromatic ring. They serve as ortho and para directors.
c. Halogens withdraw electron density from the aromatic ring, yet are activators.
d. Nitrates deactivate the aromatic ring by withdrawing electron density. They serve as meta directors.

46. Fluorobenzene is treated with sulfite in sulfuric acid. What is/are the major product(s)?

a. meta sulfonated fluorobenzene
b. ortho and para sulfonated fluorobenzene
c. sulfonated benzene
d. trisulfonated fluorobenzene

47. Benzyl propanone is treated with Zn(Hg) amalgam. It is then acidified in the presence of heat. The final product is

a. benzyl propane.
b. benzyl propanoate.
c. benzyl propanol.
d. benzyl propanal.

48. Benzyl iodide reacts with 1 mole of a diethyl copper lithium alklylation agent. The major product (named via correct IUPAC nomenclature) (named via correct IUPAC nomenclature) is

a. 1-ethyl benzene and 4-ethyl-benzene.
b. 1,4-diethyl benzene.
c. 1,3-diethyl benzene.
d. ethylbenzene.

Section 5: Writing

1 Essay Prompt
Time: 30 minutes

Essay 2

Prompt: Discuss solutions to the issue of the loss of privacy in today's high-technology society.

Section 6: Reading Comprehension

48 Questions
Time: 50 minutes (for the entire Reading Comprehension section)
Directions: Read each passage. Answer the questions that follow by choosing the best answer from the choices given.

Passage 1

(1) The history of microbiology begins with a Dutch haberdasher named Antoni van Leeuwenhoek, a man of no formal scientific education. In the late 1600s, Leeuwenhoek, inspired by the magnifying lenses used by drapers to examine cloth, assembled some of the first microscopes. He developed a technique for grinding and polishing tiny, convex lenses, some of which could magnify an object up to 270 times. After scraping some plaque from between his teeth and examining it under a lens, Leeuwenhoek found tiny squirming creatures, which he called *animalcules*.

(2) His observations, which he reported to the Royal Society of London, are among the first descriptions of living bacteria. Leeuwenhoek discovered an entire universe invisible to the naked eye. He found more animalcules—protozoa and bacteria—in samples of pond water, rainwater, and human saliva. He gave the first description of red *corpuscles*, and he observed plant tissue, examined muscle, and investigated the life cycle of insects.

(3) Nearly two hundred years later, Leeuwenhoek's discovery of microbes aided French chemist and biologist Louis Pasteur to develop his germ theory of disease. This concept suggested that disease derives from tiny organisms attacking and weakening the body. The germ theory later helped doctors to fight infectious diseases, including anthrax, diphtheria, polio, smallpox, tetanus, and typhoid.

(4) Leeuwenhoek did not foresee this legacy. In a 1716 letter, he described his contribution to science this way: "My work, which I've done for a long time, was not pursued in order to gain the praise I now enjoy, but chiefly from a craving after knowledge, which I notice resides in me more than in most other men. And therewithal, whenever I found out anything remarkable, I have thought it my duty to put down my discovery on paper, so that all ingenious people might be informed thereof."

Passage 1 Questions

1. The word *corpuscles* in the second paragraph means
a. blood cells.
b. microbes.
c. bacteria.
d. viruses.

2. According to the passage, Leeuwenhoek's work led to all of the following EXCEPT
a. descriptions of bacteria.
b. effective ways to fight infectious diseases.
c. the germ theory of disease.
d. therapies for cancer.

3. Since it was not mentioned in the passage, which of the following can you assume is NOT an infectious disease?
a. diphtheria
b. smallpox
c. diabetes
d. tetanus

4. The author indicates that Leeuwenhoek
a. sought fame and fortune.
b. was not searching for discoveries.
c. wanted to share information.
d. wanted to be a full-time scientist.

5. The tone of the passage is
a. matter-of-fact.
b. cynical.
c. negative.
d. scientific.

6. The author's attitude toward Leeuwenhoek's contribution to science is
a. neutral.
b. admiring.
c. opposed.
d. disbelieving.

7. Leeuwenhoek is best described as
a. a doctor.
b. a tailor.
c. the first microbiologist.
d. an amateur scientist.

8. The word *animalcules* at the end of the first paragraph means
a. small animals.
b. small plants.
c. microorganisms.
d. microscopes.

Passage 2

(1) Elizabeth Blackwell was the first woman to receive a medical degree in the United States. By establishing the New York Infirmary in 1857, she offered a practical solution for women who were rejected from internships elsewhere but determined to expand their skills as physicians. She also published several important books on the issue of women in medicine.

(2) She was born in Bristol, England, in 1821. Her family moved to America when she was 11. Her father, who was an *abolitionist*, died when she was 17, though she and her siblings continued to campaign against slavery in addition to working for women's rights.

(3) In her book *Pioneer Work in Opening the Medical Profession to Women*, Dr. Blackwell wrote that initially she "hated everything connected with the body, and could not bear the sight of a medical book. . . . My favorite studies were history and metaphysics, and the very thought of dwelling on the physical structure of the body and its various ailments filled me with disgust." Instead she became a teacher, a profession considered more suitable for a woman. She turned to medicine after a terminally ill close friend suggested she would have been spared her worst suffering if her physician had been a woman.

(4) Blackwell consulted with several physicians she knew. They said medical school was a good idea, but told her she was unlikely to be admitted. Attracted by the challenge, she convinced two physician friends to let her read medicine with them for a year, and then she applied to medical schools in New York and throughout the Northeast. She was accepted by Geneva Medical College in 1847. The faculty, assuming that the all-male student body would never agree to a woman joining their ranks, let the students vote on her admission. As a joke, they voted "yes," and she matriculated.

(5) Two years later, in 1849, she received her degree. She worked in clinics in London and Paris for two years, and studied midwifery at La Maternité, where she contracted purulent ophthalmia from a patient. Having lost sight in one eye, she returned to New York, giving up her dream of becoming a surgeon.

(6) Dr. Blackwell established a practice in New York City, but had few patients and few opportunities for intellectual exchange with other physicians and therefore did not have "the means of increasing medical knowledge, which dispensary practice affords." She applied for a job as physician at the women's department of a large city dispensary, but was refused. In 1853, with the help of friends, she opened her own dispensary in a single rented room, seeing patients three afternoons a week. Eventually, she opened the New York Infirmary for Women and Children, which included a medical college for women and provided care for the poor.

Passage 2 Questions

9. The main idea of this passage is best described as
- **a.** the perseverance of one woman and its long-term impact on others.
- **b.** the effects of adversity in shaping Dr. Blackwell's life.
- **c.** the story of the first woman in the United States to attend medical school.
- **d.** one woman's stubbornness in the face of adversity.

10. The word *abolitionist* in paragraph 2 means
- **a.** pro-women's rights.
- **b.** against women going to medical school.
- **c.** antidemocracy.
- **d.** antislavery.

11. Elizabeth Blackwell became a doctor for all but which of the following reasons?
- **a.** A dying friend said she would have liked a woman doctor.
- **b.** She was not afraid of a challenge.
- **c.** She was accepted to medical school.
- **d.** She wanted to cure her sick friend.

12. According to the passage, the other students at Geneva Medical College
- **a.** welcomed Elizabeth Blackwell with open arms.
- **b.** doubted her abilities.
- **c.** voted to admit her.
- **d.** supported the faculty's lack of confidence in her.

13. From the passage, *dispensary practice* most closely means
- **a.** being a sole practitioner.
- **b.** being part of a group practice.
- **c.** working in a hospital.
- **d.** practicing medicine.

14. Elizabeth Blackwell's efforts are best described as
- **a.** selfish.
- **b.** selfless.
- **c.** pioneering.
- **d.** dangerous.

15. According to the passage, Blackwell's dream was to become
- **a.** a teacher.
- **b.** a surgeon.
- **c.** a doctor.
- **d.** a historian.

16. Based on the passage, the author's attitude toward women becoming doctors can best be described as
- **a.** neutral.
- **b.** negative.
- **c.** positive.
- **d.** indifferent.

Passage 3

(1) The U.S. population is going gray. Aging Baby Boomers and increased longevity have made adults 65 and older the fastest-growing segment of today's population. In 30 years, this segment of the population is expected to double to 70 million people over 65. The number of "oldest old"—85 and older—is 34 times greater than in 1900 and likely to expand fivefold by 2050.

(2) This unprecedented "elder boom" will have a profound effect on American society, particularly the field of healthcare. Is our system equipped to deal with the demands of an aging population? Although we have adequate physicians and nurses, many of them are not trained to handle the multiple needs of older patients. Today we have about 9,000 geriatricians. Some studies estimate a need for 36,000 geriatricians by 2030.

(3) Many doctors treat a patient of 75 the same way they would treat a 40-year-old. However, although seniors are healthier than ever, physical challenges often increase with age. By age 75, adults often have two to three medical conditions. Diagnosing multiple health problems, and knowing how they interact, is crucial for effectively treating older patients. Healthcare professionals—often pressed for time—must be *diligent* about asking questions and collecting evidence from their elderly patients. Finding out about a patient's over-the-counter medications or living conditions could reveal an underlying problem.

(4) Lack of training in geriatric issues can result in healthcare providers overlooking illnesses or conditions that may lead to illness. Inadequate nutrition is a common, often unrecognized, problem among frail seniors. An elderly patient who has difficulty preparing meals at home may become vulnerable to malnutrition or other medical conditions. Healthcare providers with training in aging issues may be able to address this problem without the costly solution of admitting a patient to a nursing home.

(5) Depression, a treatable condition that affects nearly five million seniors, often goes undetected. Some healthcare professionals view depression as just part of getting old. Untreated, it can have serious, even fatal consequences. According to the National Institute of Mental Health, older Americans account for a disproportionate share of suicide deaths, making up 18% of them in 2000. Healthcare providers could play a vital role in preventing this outcome—several studies have shown that up to 75% of seniors who die by suicide visited a primary care physician within a month of their death.

(6) Healthcare providers who work with the elderly must understand and address the physical, mental, emotional, and social changes of the aging process. They need to be able to distinguish between normal characteristics associated with aging and treatable conditions. They should look beyond symptoms and consider methods to help seniors maintain and improve quality of life.

Passage 3 Questions

17. The tone of the passage is primarily

a. neutral reporting.
b. argument backed up with facts.
c. anger.
d. frustration.

18. The author implies that when doctors treat all patients the same regardless of their age, they are
a. providing effective care to all patients.
b. may make treatment mistakes in younger patients.
c. doing a disservice to their older patients.
d. mistreating patients.

19. In the passage, the use of the example of untreated depression in the elderly helps the author
a. illustrate specifically why it's important for healthcare providers to have specific training in geriatrics.
b. show that mental illness affects everyone.
c. point to issues faced by the elderly.
d. show the link between mental and physical health.

20. The author implies that doctors should
a. treat only the symptoms older patients report.
b. routinely look beyond obvious symptoms.
c. separate patients by age.
d. provide equal treatment for all patients.

21. The author's attitude toward the current system could best be described as
a. pessimistic.
b. concerned.
c. satisfied.
d. resigned.

22. In paragraph 3, the word *diligent* means
a. careless.
b. accurate.
c. probing.
d. careful.

23. According to the passage, which is NOT true about inadequate nutrition for the elderly?
a. It is a major issue for older people.
b. It may lead to nursing home admissions.
c. It may be due to an inability to cook at home.
d. It can be solved by home delivery of meals.

24. What can you infer is the author's opinion regarding the elderly and medication use?
a. Medication use is necessary, but must be carefully managed by the patient.
b. Medications are overused.
c. Medication use is necessary, but must be carefully managed by the patient and doctor.
d. The elderly should avoid over-the-counter medications.

Passage 4

(1) Although debate about cigarette smoking and health has been around for centuries, it wasn't until a dramatic increase in cigarette smoking in the United States in the twentieth century occurred that the antismoking movement was born. Reformers argued that smoking brought about general *malaise*, physiological malfunction, and declines in mental and physical health. Evidence of the ill effects of smoking was accumulated during the 1930s, 1940s, and 1950s.

(2) Epidemiologists found direct links between the increase in lung cancer mortality and smoking. Scientists confirmed the statistical relationship between smoking and lung cancer, bronchitis, emphysema, and coronary heart disease. Smoking, not air pollution, asbestos contamination, or radioactive materials, was the chief cause of the epidemic rise of lung cancer. In June 1957, U.S. Surgeon General Leroy E. Burney said the official position of the U.S. Public Health

Service was that evidence showed a causal relationship between smoking and lung cancer.

(3) It was an alliance of prominent private health organizations that pushed for an official report on smoking and health. In June 1961, the American Cancer Society, the American Heart Association, the National Tuberculosis Association, and the American Public Health Association wrote to then President John F. Kennedy, calling for a national commission dedicated to "seeking a solution to this health problem that would interfere least with the freedom of industry or the happiness of individuals." In June 1962, the new surgeon general, Luther L. Terry, convened a committee of experts to comb the scientific literature on the smoking question.

(4) Over the next two years, this committee reviewed more than 7,000 scientific articles. The 1964 Surgeon General's Report was front-page news and the lead story on radio and television around the country. It highlighted the deleterious health consequences of tobacco use, and held cigarette smoking responsible for a 70% increase in the mortality rate of smokers over nonsmokers. The report estimated that average smokers had a nine- to tenfold risk of developing lung cancer compared to nonsmokers, and 20-fold for heavy smokers. The risk rose with the duration of smoking and diminished with the cessation of smoking. The report also said smoking was the most important cause of chronic bronchitis and pointed to a correlation between smoking and emphysema, and smoking and heart disease. It noted that smoking during pregnancy reduced the average weight of newborns.

(5) The committee hedged on nicotine addiction, insisting the "tobacco habit should be characterized as an habituation rather than an addiction," in part because the addictive properties of nicotine were not yet fully understood and in part because of differences over the meaning of addiction.

(6) Though the report proclaimed that "cigarette smoking is a health hazard of sufficient importance in the United States to warrant appropriate remedial action," it remained silent on concrete remedies. That challenge fell to politicians. In 1965, Congress required all cigarette packages distributed in the United States to carry a health warning, and cigarette advertising on television and radio was banned in September 1970.

Passage 4 Questions

25. In paragraph 1, the word *malaise* means
a. unhappiness.
b. discomfort.
c. concern.
d. illness.

26. According to the passage, the epidemic rise of lung cancer was due to
a. air pollution.
b. asbestos contamination.
c. radioactivity.
d. smoking.

27. The causal relationship between smoking and lung cancer was scientifically shown in
a. the 1950s.
b. the 1980s.
c. the 1960s.
d. the 1970s.

28. Which of the following diseases is NOT caused by smoking?
a. emphysema
b. lung cancer
c. heart disease
d. tuberculosis

29. The statement in the passage that the 1964 Surgeon General's Report remained silent on concrete remedies implies that it
 a. was leaving those to the legislative branch of government.
 b. did not think action needed to be taken.
 c. was remaining neutral.
 d. could have reinforced remedies it recommended.

30. The tone of the passage is best described as
 a. factual.
 b. informative.
 c. positive.
 d. dispassionate.

31. The author links the following, EXCEPT
 a. statistics and science.
 b. lung cancer and heart disease.
 c. smoking and health.
 d. smoking and growth.

32. The word *hedged* in paragraph 5 means
 a. refused to take a position.
 b. did not discuss.
 c. played down.
 d. addressed the issue directly.

Passage 5

(1) At one time, people wore garlic around their necks to ward off disease. Today, most Americans would scoff at the idea of wearing a necklace of garlic cloves to enhance their well-being. However, many Americans are willing to ingest capsules of pulverized garlic or other herbal supplements in the name of health. Complementary and alternative medicine (CAM), which includes a range of practices outside of conventional medicine such as herbs, homeopathy, massage, yoga, and acupuncture, holds increasing appeal for Americans. According to one estimate, 42% of Americans have used alternative therapies. A Harvard Medical School survey found young adults most likely to use alternative treatments.

(2) The use of unconventional healthcare practices has steadily increased since the 1950s, and the trend is likely to continue. CAM has become a big business, and Americans are willing to dip into their wallets to pay for alternative treatments. A 1997 American Medical Association study estimated that the public spent $21.2 billion for alternative medicine therapies that year, more than half of which were out-of-pocket expenditures not covered by health insurance. By the late 1990s, the total number of visits to alternative medicine providers (about 629 million) exceeded the tally of visits to primary care physicians (386 million).

(3) Still, the public has not abandoned conventional medicine. Most Americans seek alternative therapies *as a complement to* their conventional healthcare, not as a replacement. Why have so many patients turned to alternative therapies? Frustrated by time constraints of managed care and alienated by conventional medicine's focus on technology, some feel that a *holistic* approach better reflects their beliefs and values. Others seek therapies that will relieve symptoms associated with chronic diseases that mainstream medicine cannot control.

(4) As scientific investigation has confirmed their safety and efficacy, some alternative therapies have crossed over into mainstream medicine. For example, today's physicians may prescribe acupuncture for pain management or to control the nausea associated with chemotherapy. Most U.S. medical schools teach courses in alternative therapies, and many health insurance companies offer some benefits for alternative medicine. Yet, despite their gaining acceptance,

the majority of alternative therapies have not been researched in controlled studies. New research efforts aim to test alternative methods and provide the public with information about which are safe and effective and which are a waste of money, or possibly dangerous.

(5) So what about those who swear by the health benefits of the so-called smelly rose, garlic? Observational studies that track disease incidence in different populations suggest that garlic use in the diet may act as a cancer-fighting agent, particularly for prostate and stomach cancer. However, these findings have not been confirmed in clinical studies. And yes, reported side effects include garlic odor.

Passage 5 Questions

33. According to the passage, alternative medicine
- **a.** is proven to work.
- **b.** is unproven.
- **c.** seems to work.
- **d.** is useless.

34. The word *holistic* in paragraph 3 means
- **a.** single-focused.
- **b.** multiple-disease.
- **c.** overall.
- **d.** piecemeal.

35. The author's primary purpose in the passage is to
- **a.** describe why people have turned to alternative medicine even when it is unproven.
- **b.** confirm the safety and effectiveness of alternative treatments.
- **c.** deny the safety and efficacy of alternative treatments.
- **d.** criticize alternative medicine.

36. Which of the following is not an alternative medicine treatment?
- **a.** herbs
- **b.** chiropractic
- **c.** acupuncture
- **d.** vitamins

37. Which of the following best describes the approach of this passage?
- **a.** matter-of-fact narration
- **b.** sarcasm
- **c.** historical reporting
- **d.** facts with a sense of humor

38. The use of the example of the money spent on alternative therapies illustrates that
- **a.** Americans spend too much money on alternative treatments.
- **b.** alternative treatments work.
- **c.** Americans are willing to pay for extra treatments out of their own pockets.
- **d.** alternative treatments should be covered by insurance.

39. The phrase *as a complement to* in paragraph 3 means
- **a.** as a positive statement about.
- **b.** in addition to.
- **c.** instead of.
- **d.** after.

40. The author's attitude about research on alternative therapies can best be described as which of the following?
- **a.** It is a waste of time.
- **b.** It should be done.
- **c.** It will cost too much money.
- **d.** It is not worthwhile.

Passage 6

(1) Obesity rates have soared since the 1980s. The U.S. Centers for Disease Control and Prevention report that the number of obese adults has doubled in the past 20 years. The number of obese children and teenagers has almost tripled, increasing 120% among African-American and Latino children and 50% among white children. The risk for type 2 diabetes, associated with obesity, has increased dramatically, too. Disturbingly, the disease now affects 25% to 30% of children, compared with 3% to 5% two decades ago.

(2) What is behind this trend? Supersized portions, cheap fast food, and soft drinks combined with a sedentary lifestyle of TV watching or Internet surfing have contributed to the rapid rise of obesity. Yet, there may be more to it: Is it a coincidence that obesity rates increased during the same time period in which a low-fat dietary doctrine has reigned?

(3) Before the 1980s, conventional wisdom was that fat and protein created a feeling of *satiation*, so that overeating would be less likely. Carbohydrates were regarded as a recipe for stoutness. This perception began to change after World War II when coronary heart disease reached near-epidemic proportions among middle-aged men. A theory that dietary fat might increase cholesterol levels and, in turn, increase the risk of heart disease emerged in the 1950s and had gained increasing acceptance by the late 1970s. In 1979, the focus of the food guidelines promoted by the United States Department of Agriculture (USDA) began to shift away from getting enough nutrients to avoiding excess fat, saturated fat, cholesterol, and sodium—the components believed to be linked to heart disease. The antifat credo was born.

(4) To date, the studies that have tried to link dietary fat to increased risk of coronary heart disease have remained ambiguous. Studies have shown that cholesterol-lowering drugs help reduce the risk of heart disease, but whether a diet low in cholesterol can do the same is still questionable. While nutrition experts are debating whether a low-fat, carbohydrate-based diet is the healthiest diet for Americans, nearly all agree that the antifat message of the past 20 years has been oversimplified. Some fats and oils like those found in olive oil and nuts are beneficial to the heart and may deserve a larger proportion in the American diet. Likewise, some carbohydrates like the refined carbohydrates contained in white bread, pasta, and white rice are metabolized in the body much the same way as sweets.

(5) So what about those high-fat protein diets that restrict carbohydrates, like the popular Atkins diet and others? A small group of nutrition experts within the medical establishment find it hard to ignore the anecdotal evidence that many lose weight successfully on these diets. They are arguing that those diets should not be dismissed out of hand, but researched and tested more closely. Still others fear that Americans, hungry to find a weight-loss regimen, may embrace a diet that has no long-term data about whether it works or is safe. What is clear is that Americans are awaiting answers, and in the meantime we need to eat something.

Passage 6 Questions

41. The author uses statistics in the first paragraph to illustrate
- **a.** the alarming increase in obesity among adults.
- **b.** the alarming increase in obesity among Americans of all ages.
- **c.** that obesity rates have grown slowly since the 1980s.
- **d.** that obesity rates have stabilized.

42. The author links a rise in obesity rates to all EXCEPT which one of the following?
- **a.** sedentary lifestyle
- **b.** too many carbohydrates
- **c.** the Internet
- **d.** healthy eating

43. The author worries that Americans are
- **a.** looking for fast ways to lose weight.
- **b.** not concerned about fat and carbohydrate intake.
- **c.** concerned only about fat and carbohydrate intake.
- **d.** confused about what types of diets are healthiest.

44. The primary purpose of the passage is to
- **a.** make clear that dieting is not as simple as low fat.
- **b.** debunk the myths about dieting and weight loss.
- **c.** criticize the science behind dieting.
- **d.** advocate for high-fat diets.

45. The tone of the last sentence is
- **a.** pessimism.
- **b.** irony.
- **c.** concern.
- **d.** indulgence.

46. The word *satiation* in paragraph 3 means
- **a.** appetite.
- **b.** fullness.
- **c.** hunger.
- **d.** nausea.

47. According to the author, studies on dietary fat and heart disease are
- **a.** clear-cut.
- **b.** obvious.
- **c.** inconclusive.
- **d.** conclusive.

48. The author uses the word *epidemic* to describe heart disease among middle-aged men after World War II in order to
- **a.** inform.
- **b.** scare.
- **c.** show the seriousness of the issue.
- **d.** detail the diseases of obesity.

Section 7: Quantitative Ability

48 Questions
Time: 40 minutes (for the entire Quantitative Ability section)
Directions: Choose the best answer to each of the following questions.

1. Which of the following would be classified as an integer?
- **a.** 0.04
- **b.** -3
- **c.** $-\frac{1}{2}$
- **d.** all of the above

2. What mathematical property is demonstrated by the following statement?

$4 + (2 + 6) + 8 = 4 + 2 + (6 + 8)$

a. associative property of addition
b. commutative property of addition
c. identity property of addition
d. distributive property

3. Solve:

$25 \div (3 + 2) \times 6 + (10 - 4) =$

a. $\frac{41}{6}$
b. 60
c. $\frac{204}{3}$
d. 36

4. What is $7\frac{3}{14} + 8\frac{2}{7}$? Simplify your answer.
a. $15\frac{7}{14}$
b. $15\frac{5}{21}$
c. $5\frac{3}{14}$
d. $15\frac{1}{2}$

5. Express $\frac{125}{473}$ as a decimal rounded to the thousandths place.
a. 3.78
b. .2642706131
c. 3.784
d. 0.264

6. Divide 3.14×10^6 by 1.25×10^2.
a. 2.512×10^4
b. 3.86×10^{-4}
c. 3.98×10^{-7}
d. 2.512×10^{-8}

7. Divide $x^4 + 3x^3 - 4x^2 + 8x - 5$ by $x - 3$.
a. $x^3 + 6x^2 + 12x - 28$ R. 79
b. $x^3 - 3x^2 + 4x - 8$ R. 5
c. $x^3 - 4x - 4$ R. -17
d. $x^3 + 6x^2 + 14x + 50$ R. 145

8. Solve for x.

$6x^2 + 11x = -3$

a. $x = -\frac{3}{2}, -\frac{1}{3}$
b. $x = -\frac{3}{4}, -2$
c. $x = -\frac{1}{2}, -\frac{4}{3}$
d. $x = \frac{1}{2}, \frac{1}{3}$

9. Solve the following equation.

$8x + 3 = 4x - 5$

a. 4
b. $\frac{1}{2}$
c. 2
d. -2

10. The female-to-male ratio in a second grade class is 3:5. If there are 15 boys in the class, how many girls are there?
a. 9
b. 25
c. 1
d. 13

11. Matt deposits his paycheck worth $527 into his existing bank account, bringing the total of his account's balance to $1,439. What was the percent increase of Matt's bank account during this transaction? Round to the nearest whole percent.
a. 63%
b. 58%
c. 41%
d. 37%

12. Solve the equation using the quadratic formula. Round to the nearest hundredth.

$6x^2 + 7x - 1 = -3$

a. 8.55, –50.55
b. 50.55, –8.55
c. –0.5, –0.67
d. 0.24, –1.40

13. Solve for x and y.

$4x - 7y = 3$
$2x - y = 4$

a. $x = 3.1, y = 2.2$
b. $x = -3.1, y = -10.2$
c. $x = 2.5, y = 1$
d. $x = -2.5, y = -6$

14. Solve the inequality.

$-3x + 4 \leq 13$

a. $x \leq 3$
b. $x \geq 3$
c. $x \leq -3$
d. $x \geq -3$

15. Solve the logarithm for x.

Log(base 3)(x) = 4

a. 64
b. 81
c. 12
d. 7

16. Given the set of numbers {1, 3, 4, 5, 7, 10}, calculate the mean.

a. 30
b. 5
c. 6
d. 4.5

17. If two six-sided dice are rolled, what is the probability, as a percentage, that both numbers will be odd?

a. 11.1%
b. 50%
c. 33.3%
d. 25%

18. Given the set of numbers {1, 5, 5, 5, 8, 12}, calculate the median.

a. 5.5
b. 6
c. 5
d. 12

19. If two quarters are flipped simultaneously, what is the probability, as a percentage, that only one will land heads up?

a. 50%
b. 75%
c. 25%
d. 100%

20. Given the set of numbers {–3, –1, 4, 4, 10, 12}, calculate the range.

a. 12
b. 26
c. 15
d. –3

21. There are 30 balls in a bag; 12 are green, 8 are black, and 10 are red. What is the probability, as a percentage, that a ball drawn at random will be green? What is the probability of the ball being red?

a. 40%, 33.3%
b. 20%, 10%
c. 40%, 10%
d. 20%, 33.3%

22. Given the set of numbers {2, 4, 6, 8, 8, 8, 10}, calculate the mean, median, range, and mode.

a. 8, 8, 2, 8
b. 6.6, 8, 2, 8
c. 6.6, 8, 8, 8
d. 8, 1, 2, 8

23. A poll done before an election states that Joe Brown has a 60% chance of winning in his district, and also shows that Rick Jenkins has a 40% chance of winning in another district. What is the probability, given as a percentage, that both candidates will win? That either candidate will win?

a. 60%, 20%
b. 76%, 24%
c. 20%, 60%
d. 24%, 76%

24. Given the set of numbers {1, 1, 1, 2, 2, 2, 2, 2, 2, 3, 3, 3, 3, 4, 4, 4, 4, 4, 5, 5, 5, 5}, calculate the mode.

a. 4
b. 3
c. 2
d. 3.1

25. For the function $f(x) = 12x + 30$, find $f(2)$.

a. 32
b. 6
c. 54
d. 14

26. What is the order of the following graph?

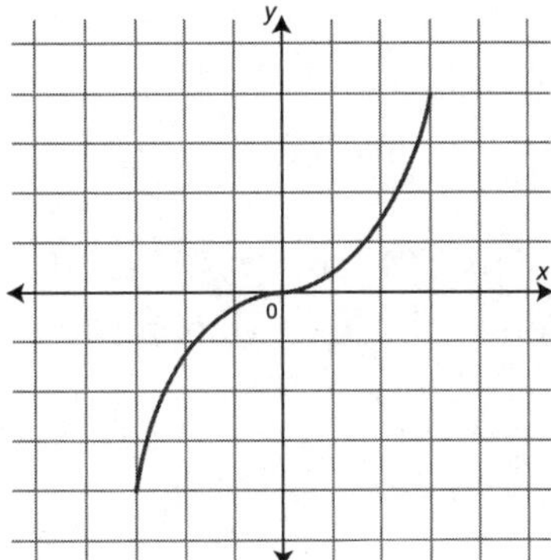

a. first
b. second
c. third
d. fourth

27. For the function $f(x) = x + 2$, what is the solution set for the input set A = {1, 2, 3, 4}?

a. {(1,3), (2,4), (3,5), (4,6)}
b. {(1,–1), (2,0), (3,1), (4,2)}
c. {(3,1), (4,2), (5,3), (6,4)}
d. {(–1,1), (0,2), (5,3), (4,6)}

28. Given $f(x) = 2x + 1$ and $g(x) = x + 4$, find $f[g(3)]$.

a. 9
b. 5
c. 7
d. 15

29. Given the line $y = 4x - 5$, find the slope of a different line that is perpendicular to the one given.

a. $\frac{1}{4}$
b. $-\frac{1}{4}$
c. –4
d. 4

30. What is the slope of the vertical line $x = 2$?

a. 2
b. 1
c. undefined
d. 0

31. Given the points (0,4) and (3,7), find the slope of the line connecting the two points.

a. $\frac{7}{3}$
b. 3
c. $\frac{4}{3}$
d. 1

32. What is the slope of the horizontal line $y = 5$?

a. 0
b. undefined
c. 1
d. 5

33. Which of the following is a line parallel to the line that connects point (4,1) and point (2,7)?

a. $y = 3x + 1$
b. $y = (-\frac{1}{3})x + 5$
c. $y = -3x + 5$
d. $y = (\frac{1}{3})x + 8$

34. The following graph depicts what function?

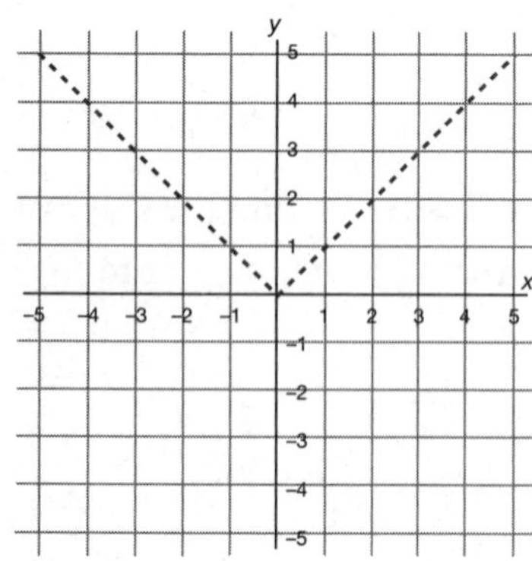

a. $y = x$
b. $y = x^2$
c. $y = \sqrt{x}$
d. $y = \text{abs}(x)$

35. Given $f(x) = x^2 + 2x + 1$ and $g(x) = x + 2$, find $f[g(x)]$.

a. $x^2 + 8x + 8$
b. $x^2 - 2x + 6$
c. $x^2 + 2x + 3$
d. $x^2 + 6x + 9$

36. Determine where the following function crosses the x-axis.

$f(x) = x^2 - 2x - 3$

a. $x = 6, x = 1$
b. $x = 3, x = -1$
c. $x = -3$
d. $x = 1$

37. Find the first derivative of the function $f(x) = x^2 + 4x + 1$.

a. $f'(x) = 2x^3 + 4x^2$
b. $f'(x) = 2x + 4$
c. $f'(x) = {}^{x}3_{3} + 2x^2 + x$
d. $f'(x) = x + 4$

38. Find the slope of the line tangent to the curve $y = x^2 + 6x + 8$ at the point (0,2).

a. 10
b. 0
c. 6
d. 8

39. Find the second derivative of the function $f(x) = 3x^4 - 5x^3 + 2x^2 + 3$.

a. $12x^3 - 15^2 + 4x$
b. $4x^3 - 3x^2 + 2x$
c. $x^3 + 3x^2 + 4x$
d. $36x^2 - 30x + 4$

40. Find the point(s) where the function $f(x) = 12x + 5$ decreases.

a. The function decreases when x is less than 0.

b. The function decreases when x is less than $-\frac{5}{12}$

c. The function never decreases.

d. The function decreases for all values of x.

41. Find the second derivative of the function $f(x) = x^4 + 3x^3 + 6x^2 + 7x + 5$.

a. $4x^3 + 9x^2 + 12x + 7$

b. $12x^2 + 18x + 12$

c. $7x^2 + 11x + 12$

d. $4x^2 + 9x + 12$

42. Find where the graph of the function $f(x) = x^3 + 4x^2 + 3x + 1$ is concave up.

a. The graph is concave up where x is greater than $-\frac{4}{3}$.

b. The graph is concave up where x is greater than zero.

c. The graph is never concave up.

d. The graph is always concave up.

43. Find the local extrema (minima or maxima) for $f(x) = 3x^2 + 2x + 1$.

a. maximum at $x = 6$

b. minimum at $x = 2$

c. minimum at $x = \frac{-1}{3}$

d. maximum at $x = \frac{-1}{3}$

44. Find the antiderivative of the function $f(x) = x^2$.

a. $2x$

b. x^3

c. $\frac{x^3}{2}$

d. $\frac{x^3}{3}$

45. Find the antiderivative of the function $f(x) = 4x^3 + 9x^2 + 12x + 7$.

a. $12x^2 + 18x$

b. $x^4 + 3x^3 + 6x^2 + 7x$

c. $x + 3x^3 + 6x^2 + 7x$

d. $x^2 + 12x$

46. Evaluate the indefinite integral.

$\int x^3 + 3x^2 + x + 2dx$

a. $3x^2 + 6x + 1$

b. $\frac{x^4}{4} + x^3 + \frac{x^2}{2} + 2x$

c. $x^4 + x^3 + x^2 + 2x + C$

d. $\frac{x^4}{4} + x^3 + \frac{x^2}{2} + 2x + C$

47. Evaluate the integral for the interval [0,5].

$\int 3x^2 + 2x + 4dx$

a. 32

b. 55

c. –170

d. 170

48. Find the area under the curve $y = x^2$ for the interval [0,2].

a. $\frac{8}{3}$

b. $-\frac{8}{3}$

c. 4

d. 8

Answers and Explanations

Section 1: Writing

Essay 1

Good Response

The challenge of keeping the U.S. food supply safe has never been greater given that food is being produced on farms both large and small, and increasing amounts of food come to the United States from overseas. The Department of Agriculture and the Food and Drug Administration (FDA) share the responsibility of regulating what is available for Americans to eat, though in recent years the FDA has focused mostly on medications and medication safety. While that continues to be part of its mandate, outbreaks of food-borne disease caused by spinach, eggs, and peanut butter in 2008, 2009, and 2010 have shown that more needs to be done.

Stronger government oversight, including current efforts to strengthen the FDA so it can act on safety issues before outbreaks occur, instead of investigating them afterward, could be helpful. This could include giving the FDA more power to inspect the food supply as well as allowing it to demand accountability from food companies. If the FDA and the Department of Agriculture combined forces, they would be able to regulate more effectively the food supply produced by large and small providers, which is necessary since some of the recent food recalls have been from smaller enterprises.

In addition to increasing inspections at food processing plants, the FDA and others need to expand quality control and the inspection of food that is imported into the United States. This is particularly pertinent since many imports have proliferated dramatically without specific rules and regulations in place about how to ensure that the imported foods are safe for Americans to eat. As of 2010, the FDA inspects a very small fraction of imported foods, and this must change.

Some say the free market should be left to control food safety. However, that seems inadequate based on the increasing number of outbreaks of food-borne disease in this country, the large increase in uninspected and unregulated imported food, and the likelihood that without regulated inspections some food manufacturers and growers will cut corners to decrease costs and increase profits. It is up to the federal government to ensure that all foods, whether processed, natural, or a combination of both, do not make Americans sick.

Since problems at one facility or farm may end up affecting people all over the country, it is vital for the federal government to have the power to move quickly. Government agencies must be able to do whatever is possible to ensure that the food supply is safe so there are fewer instances of sudden recalls after patients show up at emergency rooms all over the country with signs of food poisoning. In other words, we must keep the FDA and the Department of Agriculture strong so our food supply is safe.

Analysis

This is a strong answer not only because the writer seems to know something about the subject, but also because it is well-constructed. There is a lead paragraph, two paragraphs about the proposed solution, a paragraph discussing a counterargument, and a concluding paragraph. There are no spelling or grammatical errors in the response, and there is some use of sophisticated sentence construction.

Weak Response

It is important for us to keep the food supply safe. Otherwise people will get sick from eating bad food. Right now that happens too often.

The way we can keep the food supply safe is to make sure food is inspectid more often. It is the government that we can rely on to do this, they have to make sure they are looking at the food supply more often and they need to inspect farms and manufactureing plants to do this.

There should be laws so that the food supply is inpectid on a regular basis. These laws should be passed by Congress so the whole country's food supply will be safer.

Analysis

This answer is vague and it is short. The argument is not strongly constructed, and there are spelling and grammatical mistakes. In particular, the second sentence of paragraph 2 is a run-on sentence, and should have been split into two or even three separate sentences.

Even if you don't know much about the subject presented, it's possible to write a good essay if you remember the construction—a lead paragraph restating the problem and providing an overview of your solution, two or three paragraphs backing up your solution, a counterexample if you can think of one, and a concluding paragraph. Solutions to the problems that tend to be presented often involve changing behavior through government intervention or regulation, education, and awareness building. While it is certainly the case that the more you know about a subject, the stronger your argument will be, these three elements may help you if you find you are not able to provide specific details based on your own personal knowledge.

Section 2: Verbal Ability

Analogies

1. b. This is an analogy of word degree, going from a lesser degree to a greater one. A shower is a brief rainfall, while a deluge is a heavy downpour. A sentence bridging the two words could be: A shower is lighter or smaller than a deluge, and a pebble is lighter or smaller than a *boulder* (choice **b**). None of the other three answers fit. While you may find a pebble in a *pond* (choice **c**) or on a *walkway* (choice **a**), the given word pair does not have the relationship of finding a shower in a deluge. Choice **d**, *sand*, does not bear a lesser/greater relationship to a pebble.

2. d. The elongated part of the face of certain animals, the part containing the nose, jaws, and possibly other features, is the snout. By starting the bridge sentence with the second word (i.e., A dog has a snout), you are searching for another animal that has a feature similar to a snout, in this case, a beak. *Dolphin* (choice **d**) is the correct answer. An *anteater* (choice **a**) has a snout, not a beak; and, as you well know, a *human* (choice **c**) has a nose. Choice **b**, *rostrum*, is incorrect as it is a synonym for beak or snout, and this is not an analogy based on synonyms. A dog has a snout and a dolphin has a beak.

3. b. This is both a part-to-whole analogy and an analogy of function. The relationship sentence could be: Lungs perform vital roles in/are major parts of the respiratory system just as bones perform vital roles in/are major parts of the skeletal system. Choice **c**, *muscular system*, is the wrong system. Choice **d** is wrong because *musculoskeletal* is not considered a system in basic anatomy. In addition, *musculoskeletal* is an adjective, and the answer must be a noun. Remember, the parts of speech for the first word pair must have the same as for the second word pair; that is, words one and three must be the same part of speech, and words two and four must have the same part of speech. Although bones make up part of the human body, choice **a**, *anatomy*, is not the best answer.

4. a. A calendar is divided into months just as a book is divided into *chapters*. This is a part-to-whole analogy in reverse. Perhaps you were thinking the answer is choice **b**, *pages*, especially if you came up with a sentence like: A calendar contains months just as a book contains *pages*. Remember, you are to select the *best* answer. If the given word pair were CALENDAR : DAYS :: BOOK :, then *pages* would be the correct answer. However, the analogy presents the calendar divided on a larger scale, months, so book, too, must be divided on a scale larger than pages. Choices **c**, *titles*, and **d**, *index*, do not fit the analogy.

5. c. This is an analogy where the first words of the pairs are types of the second words of the pairs. A trapezoid is a type of quadrilateral and an octagon is a type of *polygon*. None of the remaining three answer choices fit.

6. b. This is an analogy of function. A bridge sentence could read: An eraser gets rid of mistakes and detergent gets rid of *grime*. With this word relationship, no other answer choices make sense.

7. d. This is an analogy of synonyms. Paucity is a synonym for dearth just as duplicity is a synonym for *guile*. Both paucity and dearth mean scarcity, and both are nouns. Duplicity and *guile* can be defined as cunning, or deceit; and, as the parts of speech of the word pairs must mirror one another, duplicity and *guile* are nouns.

8. a. This analogy is about an employee and the workplace. An usher works in a theater and a provost works in a *university*. These are the most common places where such workers would be.

9. d. This analogy is one of degree, where the second word in each pair is the first word to an extreme. If people are extremely warm, they can become overheated. If people are extremely anxious, they can become *petrified*. You can construct a sentence starting with the second word as well: To be overheated is to be extremely warm. To be *petrified* is to be extremely anxious. If you tried to plug in the other three answers, you would see *petrified* is the only logical choice, but you must know the meaning of the other words to be sure. *Placated* (choice **a**) means appeased; *disparaged* (choice **b**) means belittled; and *attenuated* (choice **c**) can be defined as thinned, or weakened.

10. b. This is a gender/animal analogy. A female sheep is a ewe, and a female pig is a *sow*.

11. a. This analogy focuses on how an object—in this case, food—is presented. Sugar can be offered in the form of a cube, as butter can be offered in the form of a *pat* (a cube of sugar, a *pat* of butter). Furthermore, this is how such items can be offered individually or in restaurants. Given the word relationship, pat is a noun here, not a verb.

12. d. This analogy contains synonyms. Furtive and surreptitious both mean sly and stealthy. Inchoate, which means incipient, or just beginning, is synonymous with *nascent*. Choice **a**, *quiescent*, means quiet or inactive, so it is incorrect; choice **b**, *plenary*, which can mean absolute, or full, is an antonym for inchoate; and choice **c**, *insidious*, is incorrect as it is a word related to the first word pair, and can be defined as treacherous, or in a stealthy manner.

13. c. This is a cause-and-effect analogy. Glare can cause one to squint, and dust can cause one to *cough*. None of the remaining answer choices could even be considered, unless you struggled with vocabulary, particularly with choice **d**, *descry*, which means to catch sight of; and choice **a**, *squelch*, means to crush, or silence.

14. c. The relationship sentence for this analogy could read: To be ambiguous is to lack clarity; to be obdurate is to lack compassion. Obdurate means hardened against feelings or persistent in wrongdoing. *Compassion* (choice **c**) is the best answer. One may argue that an obdurate person may lack *flexibility* (choice **a**) or *intelligence* (choice **b**), but these would be a real stretch. The analogy calls for the lack of something directly related to the definition of the word, not interpretations. Choice **d**, *pragmatism*, also is incorrect, as being obdurate does not directly indicate lacking practicality.

15. a. This is an analogy of antonyms. Haughty, which means condescendingly proud, is the opposite of modest. Sedulous, which means persevering, diligent, is the opposite of *inactive*. Choice **b**, *impudent*, is an antonym for modest, not sedulous; and neither *honest* (choice **c**) nor *sagacious* (choice **d**) are antonyms for sedulous. *Sagacious* means shrewd.

16. b. This analogy focuses on action and result. The first word is a verb, and the second word is a noun, or the result of the verb's action. A bridge sentence could read: They instigate a conflict; they foster *talent*. The test taker must know the meaning of both verbs to arrive at the correct answer. To instigate is to goad, provoke, which has a negative connotation. On the other hand, to foster is to nurture, cultivate, which has a positive connotation. It would not make sense, then, to foster something negative, such as *controversy* (choice **c**) or *disdain* (choice **d**). *Disdain* means scorn, or a feeling of contempt. In addition, to foster *volatility* (choice **a**) makes little sense.

17. c. This analogy is all about synonyms. In the given word pair, dogged and intransigent both mean uncompromising. Plaintive, which means sad or melancholy, must be paired with a similarly defined word, which leads to *doleful*. Choice **a** is incorrect because *magnanimous* means generous, noble. Choice **b**, *buoyant*, means cheerful, so it is an antonym for plaintive, and is incorrect. *Austere* (choice **d**) means severe, or strict, so it has no relation to plaintive, and is incorrect.

18. a. The second word in this analogy's given pair describes a likely attribute of the first word. A relationship sentence could be: A misanthrope is cynical, whereas a philanthropist is *altruistic.* A misanthrope is someone who loathes humankind, society. Therefore, this type of person is likely to be cynical, or distrustful of people and their motives. A philanthropist wants to see the well-being of humankind increase, and helps by charity or donations. Therefore, this type of person is likely to be altruistic, or selfless with regard to the welfare of others. As such, a philanthropist would not be *egoistic* (choice **b**) or *skeptical* (choice **d**). Also, it would not make much sense to choose **c**, *equivocal*, which means ambiguous.

19. d. This analogy is one of degree. The second word in the first word pair, blubber, means to sob noisily. Therefore, the answer must be a word that means to state something with more gusto, in this case, loudly, or emphatically. Essentially, the second word must exaggerate the first word. *Exclaim*, which means to speak loudly and suddenly, is the correct answer. Choice **a**, *whisper*, would fit only if the analogy called for the second word to diminish the volume of the first word. Choice **b**, *express*, is a synonym for state, so it is incorrect. *Depict* (choice **c**) has no relation to any word in this analogy, and also is incorrect. This analogy also tests your recognition of parts of speech. At first glance, blubber could be a noun, as could state. If you thought this were the case, perhaps trying to construct a sentence with this analogy would be complicated, and a stretch. Scanning the answer choices should indicate that all the words in the analogy are verbs.

20. b. This analogy has to do with two types of chemical reactions. The second word is an example of the type of chemical reaction that is the first word. A relationship sentence could be: An exothermic chemical reaction may include combustion. An endothermic chemical reaction may include *photosynthesis.* It may be easier to grasp the word pair relationship by constructing a sentence starting with the second word of the given pair: Combustion is an example of an exothermic reaction, and *photosynthesis* is an example of an endothermic reaction. While choice **a**, *temperature*, has an impact on both types of reactions, it does not fit into the word relationship. An educated guess would tell you that choice **c**, *explosion*, is too close to combustion to make sense as an endothermic reaction; and choice **d**, *molecules*, makes no sense in this analogy.

21. d. The key to this analogy is recognizing that the tools in the first word pair perform the same action. Both the hacksaw and the knife are used for cutting things, albeit generally different kinds of things. Therefore, the word that goes with caliper needs to perform the same action as does a caliper, which is to measure. *Protractor* is the only tool or device among the answer choices that is used for measuring. Perhaps the bridge sentence could be: A hacksaw and knife are used for cutting things, and a caliper and *protractor* are used for measuring things.

22. a. This analogy has the second word describing the nature of the first. For example, an insult can be described as contemptuous. A stench can be described as *noisome*. Contemptuous can be a synonym for insulting, so it aptly describes an insult. *Noisome*, which can mean offensive to the senses, particularly to the sense of smell, aptly describes a stench. Notice the first word of each word pair is a noun, while the second words are adjectives. Therefore, choice **b**, *offend*, does not work because it is a verb. If it were in its adjectival form, offensive, it would work. The other two choices, **c**, *pleasing*, and **d**, *nosy*, have no place in this analogy, and could throw off the test taker who does not know the meaning of contemptuous or *noisome*.

23. c. You have to dig into your geography knowledge for this one, or make an educated guess. The Caspian Sea is considered the world's largest lake and Lake Superior is considered the largest lake in the United States. Angel Falls is considered the world's tallest waterfall, so you are looking for the tallest waterfall in the United States, which is considered to be *Yosemite Falls*. If choosing the answer is difficult because you are not familiar with these places, it is easier to eliminate the incorrect choices. Choices **b**, *Lake Tahoe*, and **d**, *Baltic Sea*, do not fit, as they are not falls, and even if you do not know about Angel Falls, you can tell from the name that Angel Falls is not a lake or a sea. The only other answer a test taker may consider is choice **a**, *Niagara*, but the answer does not read *Niagara Falls*, and, even if it did, Niagara Falls would also be incorrect. Niagara Falls is one of the most popular waterfalls, but nowhere near the tallest.

24. b. This analogy focuses on tools and what they measure. In chemistry, a hydrometer measures the density of liquids. A *seismograph* measures movements in the ground, such as tremors or earthquakes.

25. d. This analogy is a bit tricky because though the words are synonyms, the second word has a different sense. In the given pair, the second word, abscond, not only means to leave, but to leave secretly and hide. Therefore the answer must not only mean to calm, but to calm in a different sense. The answer, *placate*, means to calm or appease, especially by making concessions. Both words in the given pair are verbs in the present tense, so the second pair must also be verbs in the present tense (or is an adjective). This knocks out choice **a**, *sated*, which is in the past tense. Sate means to satisfy fully, or to excess. Neither choice **b**, *negotiate*, nor choice **c**, *remain*, are logical answers.

26. c. This is an analogy of synonyms. Phlegmatic and stolid mean unemotional. The answer must be a synonym for bilious, which means ill-tempered, as does choice **c**, *cantankerous*. Choice **a**, *fervid*, means zealous, or burning, which is an antonym for the words in the first word pair, and is incorrect. Choice **b**, *apathetic*, which means indifferent, is related to the first word pair, and also is incorrect. *Laconic* (choice **d**) bears no relation to any of the given words, as it means terse or concise. If you did not know the meaning of phlegmatic, you could probably guess it had to do with something sluggish or apathetic, because of phlegm. Bilious has its root in bile, considered to be linked with irritability.

27. b. The first word in this analogy is a type of the second word. Quadratic is a type of equation (in math), while labor is a type of law. Choice **a**, *toil*, and choice **c**, *equalization*, do not fit the relationship. *Holiday* (choice **d**) may be a tempting selection at first, but Labor Day is a type of holiday, not just *labor*, which renders *law* the best answer.

28. a. This analogy takes traits commonly known to particular animals, but uses a lesser-known synonym for these traits. A lion is known for its valor (courage, bravery) and a dog is known for its *steadfastness* (loyalty). Choice **b**, *dogmatism*, which means an arrogant assertion of opinion, does not fit, and choice **c**, *fickleness*, is incorrect. A clever skill or trickery defines *artifice*, so choice **d** is incorrect. Dogs certainly learn tricks, but *artifice* implies a level of ingenuity or cleverness in such tricks. While *artifice* may apply to some dogs, it is not a common trait, leaving *steadfastness* as the best answer.

29. d. This is an analogy of antonyms. Capitulate is the opposite of resist, as blandish is the opposite of *intimidate*. Capitulate means to acquiesce or yield. Blandish means to cajole or coax by flattery. Therefore, none of the other choices fit.

Sentence Completions

30. b. Clue words in this sentence are *even though*, at the beginning of the sentence, and *instead*, at the end of the sentence. Choice **a** is incorrect because it is the opposite of the word that best fits the blank. While it is possible they *faulted* their better judgment, choice **c** is far from the best answer that choice **b**, *ignored*, provides. Choice **d** also is incorrect, as *targeted* makes no sense.

31. d. The sense of the sentence steers you toward choosing a word that would fit with *bounteous* and *finest*. The word may not be a direct synonym, but it will not be an antonym, either. Choice **d**, *richest*, is the only logical fit. Choice **a**, *craven*, means cowardly, which does not fit; choice **b**, *dullest*, makes no sense; and neither does choice **c**, *loquacious*, which means highly talkative.

32. d. This is the only logical choice. Perhaps if you first tried to fill in the blanks with your own words, you came up with *teach* for the first blank. Then, when you looked at the answer choices, there was no such word. However, in looking for something close to *teach*, you probably focused on choices **c** and **d**. Upon further inspection, you would notice that choice **c** does not fit well because the sentence talks about the aim of a science, and to *infer* would be shaky ground for such science. When you plugged in *anatomy* for the second blank, you also would see the phrase *order of anatomy* is not very logical, particularly when the word set in choice **d** fits so logically. In addition, there is a helpful hint, and it appears toward the beginning of the sentence, *general*. If you were plugging in the second words of choices **a**, **b**, and **c**, *general* should have signaled that these choices were all too specific given the sense of the sentence. Moreover, even if you thought they fit, when you plugged in the first words of choices **a**, **b**, and **c**, you would see all three of these word sets did not work.

33. a. This word set is the only one in which both words make sense. While the first word of choice **c** might work, the second does not. Neither word in choice **d** makes sense, given the context, so choice **d** can be eliminated immediately. For choice **b**, *scarcely* could work only if the second word were the opposite of *scarcity*. The sentence does give you clues. In the first sentence, you learn families often are large. *This means* begins the second sentence, letting you know to focus on the ramifications of a large family. Before you even plug in possible answers, you learn that a condition in many of these large families is one that precedes children being *old enough to work*, and thus old enough to bring money into the household. At first glance, the second words in both choices **a** and **b** could fit, but, again, the first word in choice **b** is illogical.

34. b. This sentence is mainly a straight vocabulary test. The sentence lets you know the man is desperate and pacing. Therefore, choice **b** is the only logical choice. Choice **a**, *felicity*, means happiness, which makes no sense. Choice **c**, *efficacy*, is also illogical, and choice **d**, *languish*, is not only the wrong meaning for the blank (*languish* can mean to become weak or feeble), but the wrong part of speech. *Languish* is a verb, and the answer must be a noun.

35. c. The clue to the correct answer, *vacillated*, is in the second part of the sentence. There you learn the woman is generally swayed by the people with whom she speaks. While the other three choices are not ridiculous, they do not fit with the sense of the sentence.

36. b. This is another vocabulary test, and the goal here is to come up with synonyms or related words for *hyperbolize*, but in a different part of speech. If you know the meanings of all the words, then choice **b**, *romanticized . . . exalted* will be the obvious selection. If not, you can take a stab at eliminating choice **a**, because the suffix *-less* in *guileless* lets you know the word means without something, in this case, without deceit, without cunning. An educated guess could help eliminate words likely to be unrelated to *hyperbolize*, or to speak in an exaggerated manner. A word that means lacking something probably does not relate to *hyperbolize*. The other word paired with *guileless* is *innocuous*, which means harmless. The same argument can be made for choice **c**, *dispassionate*, as the prefix *-dis* means not—in this case, not passionate; devoid of emotion. Again, an educated guess could let you know this word might not fit well with *hyperbolize*. The word paired with *dispassionate* is *insipid*, which means tasteless, or dull, another word that does not relate to *hyperbolize*. Choice **d** is incorrect because *elongated* means made longer, or extended; and *mollified* means appeased, soothed.

37. a. The blank in this sentence needs a word similar to *distinguished*. The clue that this is so comes in the second sentence, with *further*. The definitions of choices **b**, **c**, and **d** point to choice **a**, *characterized*, as the clear choice. *Confounded* (choice **b**) means confused; *obviated* (choice **c**) means made unnecessary; and *tempered* (choice **d**) can be defined as moderated.

38. c. The sentence offers a double clue, with *but* coming after *not done in the work of a day*. This provides a hint as to the type of word needed in the blank before *process*, and the sentence implies it is work that takes longer than a day. If you did not know that *prodigal* means lavish or wastefully extravagant, you might have considered choice **d**, which is incorrect. Choice **a** is wrong because *quick* is the opposite of the meaning implied in the rest of the sentence. In addition, *chicanery* means trickery, which does not work in the second blank. Though a stretch, one could argue that *wretched* (**b**) might fit, but the second word, *ropes*, makes little sense, particularly when comparing the process to other great accomplishments, many of which likely did not require *ropes*. Remember, when one word clearly is not a match, eliminate that answer choice. This leaves choice **c**, *gradual . . . experiments*, as the best answer.

39. d. If you were thinking of words on your own, before looking at the answer choices, you might have considered *serious* for the first blank, and *ample*, or *enough*, for the second blank. If you did, you were correct in your thinking, though you had to look for synonyms among the answers. When you skim the choices, you do see *ample*, in choice **b**, but the first word, *limited*, makes no sense, as it has nothing to do with *serious*. Therefore, you can eliminate choice **b**. You also eliminate choice **a** because, while *copious* can serve as a word related to ample (*copious* means plentiful or abundant), the first word does not make sense, as *trivial* is the opposite of serious. In choice **c**, *suitable* functions well in the second blank, but the first word, *neutral*, does not work in the first blank. This leaves choice **d**, *grave . . . sufficient*, as the correct answer.

40. c. This is a vocabulary test once again. If no one had been to the store in a week, the owner likely would be excited to see customers, so the answer must have something to do with being excited, happy, and, overall, in a positive state of mind. Choice **c**, *jubilantly*, is the clear answer, as it means in a joyous manner. There is not even a close second choice. Choice **a**, *sullenly*, means in a sluggish or gloomy manner; choice **b**, *pusillanimously*, means with a lack of courage; and choice **d**, *demurely*, means in a reserved or modest manner. If you did not immediately latch onto *jubilantly*, given the sense of the first part of the sentence, another clue comes at the end of the sentence: *talked incessantly*.

41. b. The answer must contain antonyms for the two words at the end of the sentence: *easy* and *inexpensive*. Choice **a** is incorrect because *hapless* means unfortunate, which has nothing to do with the opposite of *easy*. Moreover, *cheap* is a synonym, not an antonym, for *inexpensive*. While the second word in choice **c**, *exorbitant*, is an antonym for *inexpensive* and completes the second blank correctly, the first word, *facile*, is a synonym, not an antonym, for *easy*, so **c** is incorrect. The reverse is the case with choice **d**, as the first word, *burdensome*, does fit as an antonym for *easy*, yet the second word, *reasonable*, is similar to *inexpensive*, and, thus, incorrect. This leaves choice **b**, *onerous . . . costly*, as the correct answer.

42. **d.** If you came up with your own word prior to looking at the answer choices, it may be that none of the choices was close to yours. It is okay to come up with a few words to describe what will ultimately be one word when thinking what may work in the blank, and then look among the answer choices for a word that describes the few you used. The tone of the sentence is straightforward and factual, so the answer will not be one that makes colorful use of the language; for example, giving the piano the ability to render humanlike actions. Therefore, choice **b**, *renounced*, is incorrect. A piano would not *renounce* the other instruments. *Renounce* means to give up, especially by formal declaration, or to reject. Choice **c**, *subsidized*, makes no sense, as a piano would not financially assist the spinet and harpsichord; and choice **a**, *conceded*, does not work, either. The piano could have *superseded* (choice **d**), or replaced or displaced, the other two instruments. Choice **d** is correct.

43. **a.** If you thought of your own word before reviewing the answer choices, perhaps you came up with *mainly* or *primarily*, both of which fit the sense of the sentence. When you scanned the answers, you saw that choice **a**, *principally*, was the closest match, and the correct answer. Choice **b**, *arbitrarily*, meaning in a random manner, does not work. Choice **c** is not a suitable fit, as *fervently* means ardently, with great zeal; and choice **d** is illogical, as *allegorically* can be defined as characterized by symbolic representation.

44. **c.** To select the correct answer is to connect the first part of the sentence with the second, and to deduce that a name was given to the state because of the great quantity of wild thyme. Thyme is an *herb*, and it makes sense that the explorers would have found thyme growing in great abundance, or *profusion*. If you thought thyme grew in the form of *shrubs*, you could still eliminate choice **b** because *meagerness* is the opposite of great quantity. Choice **a** is illogical, as thyme could not be considered *sustenance*, and even if it grew in great *colors*, the answer as a whole is not the best fit. Choice **d** appears to make sense if one disregards the first part of the sentence, but, because thyme is the theme throughout the sentence, *economy* and *strides* do not make sense.

45. **d.** You may have had an easier time thinking of a word for the first blank than for the second. If you did come up with *conclusion*, or a similar word, you probably saw that *consequence* fit the second blank most logically. If you missed this, one clue in the sentence is the verb preceding the first blank: *to form*. While one may form an *opinion* (choice **a**), the second word, *reconciliation*, or reestablishment of relations, makes no sense. Choice **b** does not work because one generally does not form a *consideration*. Plus, *consideration* is too weak a word for the context. In addition, the second word of choice **b**, *precursor*, is the opposite of the word that fits, *consequence*. Choice **c** is incorrect because *permutation* means transformation, or major change, which makes no sense here, and *conjecture*, or guess, is not something that logically follows *from observation and experiment*.

46. b. This is a vocabulary test that can be tricky. Not only should you know the meanings of the answer choices, but know the difference between two words spelled so similarly that there is only one vowel separating them. One of these words, choice **b**, *ingenious*, is correct. *Ingenious* means clever, inventive, while the word that looks similar, choice **c**, *ingenuous*, means something entirely different: artless, without cunning, straightforward. Thus, choice **c** is incorrect. *Derisive* means mocking, so choice **a** is wrong; and *inept* means incompetent or not fitting, so choice **d** is incorrect. Apart from vocabulary, the sense of the sentence is that the man assumed that shell games, which he considered old-fashioned, were still around and thriving and conning people. Thus, he would have thought such games had long since been abandoned in favor of more inventive, or clever, or *ingenious* games.

47. c. The first sentence sets up what kind of words are needed in the next sentence's two blanks. You should have focused on the pressure not being lowered by ordinary fatigue, which implies something greater than ordinary fatigue is needed to lower the pressure. The only logical choice, then, is choice **c**, *exhaustion . . . decreased*. Choice **b** is incorrect as both words are the opposite of the words in choice **c**. Choice **a** is also incorrect as extreme states of *exercise* would not lower pressure. The second word in choice **a**, *mitigated*, means alleviated or relieved. In choice **d**, your vocabulary knowledge is tested with *turpitude*, which means depravity, the state of moral corruption, so choice **d** makes no sense.

48. a. Not only does this test vocabulary, but it also tests your knowledge of a word's various meanings. Because *Miss Polly did not usually make hurried movements*, then it makes sense to think of a word such as *calmness* for the blank. Given *calmness* is not among the answer choices, you look for a synonym, which you have in choice **a**, *repose*. You may know the meaning of *repose* as the state of being at rest, which somewhat fits, but *repose* has a related definition that even better fits the sentence: calmness or tranquility. However, even the first definition of *repose* works better in the sentence than the other choices, so if at least you know *repose* has to do with rest, you can make an educated guess. Choice **b**, *verbosity*, is wrong, as it means wordiness; choice **c**, *petulance*, is incorrect as it means impatience, or irritability; and choice **d** makes no sense, as *agitation* is the opposite of *repose*.

Section 3: Biology

1. **b.** Divergent evolution is when homologous structures with a common evolutionary origin evolve in different ways such that they develop different traits for the same structure. Choice **a** is incorrect: Micro-evolution refers to a change in the gene frequency within a given population of organisms in a particular area that happens over one or several generations. Choice **c** is incorrect: Convergent evolution is when a biological trait or function is similar in two groups of organisms, but it was not inherited from a common ancestor. The trait or function is an environmental adaptation that both species converged upon despite having different heredity. Thus it is an analogous trait, rather than homologous trait. Choice **d** is incorrect: Parallel evolution is when two species have a common ancestor and a common environment but are geographically separated and independently evolve analogous traits.
2. **d.** Commensalism is a symbiotic relationship in which one organism benefits and the other is unaffected by the relationship. Choice **a** is incorrect: Pleiotropy is when a single gene affects a number of expressed traits. The word *pleiotropy* is derived from the Greek words for many (*pleio*) and changes (*tropo*). This can cause significant disruptions in certain genetic disorders. If a mutation occurs, at least two and possibly many different phenotypic traits will be affected. Choice **b** is incorrect: Parasitic relationships are a type of symbiosis in which one organism benefits while the other sustains harm. Choice **c** is incorrect: Mutualistic relationships are symbiotic relationships that benefit both organisms.
3. **c.** Gene flow refers to the migration of individuals from one population to another taking their contribution to the gene pool with them. Emigration away from a population can diminish genetic variation, potentially harming the vitality of the remaining population, just as immigration into a population can enhance genetic variation, potentially increasing the vitality of the gene pool. Choice **a** is incorrect: Genetic drift refers to random sampling and chance. The alleles that are found in offspring are a result of random sampling. An allele can be eliminated, particularly in a small population, by chance alone. Choice **b** is incorrect: Natural selection refers to the propensity for better-suited individuals to survive and thus reproduce. A particular set of genes is passed on because the reproducing individual has adapted to survive and pass on those traits. Through this process, characteristics become either more prevalent or less frequent in a population. Choice **d** is incorrect: Adaptations are new inheritable traits that increase fitness so that individuals will survive and reproduce. They can be morphological and anatomical, biochemical and physiological, or behavioral.
4. **b.** The correct order of the taxa in the classification system is: domain, kingdom, phylum, class, order, family, genus, and species.

5. b. Archaeabacteria are unicellular prokaryotes. Most of their cell walls contain no peptidoglycan. They can be autotrophs or heterotrophs and most live in extreme environments. Choice **a** is incorrect: Members of the Fungi kingdom are either unicellular or (mainly) multicellular eukaryotic heterotrophs. Their cell walls are made of chitin. Choice **c** is incorrect: Eubacteria are unicellular prokaryotes that have cell walls that contain peptidoglycan. They can be autotrophs or heterotrophs. Choice **d** is incorrect: Protista are mainly unicellular eukaryotes that either have no cell wall (protozoa) or have cell walls composed of only cellulose or cellulose combined with other substances (algae). The water and slime molds are not true molds of the Fungi kingdom because they have no chitin in their cell walls. Both also contain cellulose in their cell walls. Protists can be either autotrophs or heterotrophs.

6. c. Autotrophs are organisms that can make their own food using photosynthesis. They do not consume other organisms. Choice **a** is incorrect: Decomposers are heterotrophs (bacteria and fungi), which begin digestion externally using enzymes. They then absorb the partially broken-down materials from dead plants and animals and the waste of other organisms. Choice **b** is incorrect: Detritivores are animal heterotrophs that ingest dead or decaying organisms (mostly plants) and fecal material. Detrivores directly ingest dead and decomposing organic matter, while decomposers secrete enzymes to digest organic matter and then absorb the molecules. Choice **d** is incorrect: Heterotrophs are organisms that obtain their food energy from consuming other organisms.

7. a. Members of the Fungi kingdom are either unicellular or (mainly) multicellular eukaryotic heterotrophs. Their cell walls are made of chitin. Choice **b** is incorrect: Archaeabacteria are unicellular prokaryotes. Most of their cell walls contain no peptidoglycan. They can be autotrophs or heterotrophs, and most live in extreme environments. Choice **c** is incorrect: Eubacteria are unicellular prokaryotes that have cell walls that contain peptidoglycan. They can be autotrophs or heterotrophs. Choice **d** is incorrect: Protista are mainly unicellular eukaryotes that either have no cell wall (protozoa) or have cell walls composed of only cellulose or cellulose combined with other substances (algae). The water and slime molds in the kingdom Protista are not true molds of the Fungi kingdom because they have no chitin in their cell walls. Both also contain cellulose in their cell walls. Protists can be either autotrophs or heterotrophs.

8. d. A paraphyletic taxon is a group of organisms that includes the most recent common ancestor of all of the organisms, but does not include all the descendants of the most recent common ancestor. Choice **a** is incorrect: A monophyletic taxon, also called a natural group or clade, is a group of organisms that includes the most recent common ancestor of all of those organisms and all of the descendants of the most recent common ancestor. Choice **b** is incorrect: A polyphyletic taxon is a group of organisms in which the most recent common ancestor of all of the organisms is not included. It is not an evolutionarily valid grouping. This type of group usually has a biological trait or function in common that was not inherited from the most recent common ancestor. Choice **c** is incorrect: A natural group is the same as a monophyletic taxon. It is a group that includes the most recent common ancestor of all of the organisms in the group and all of the descendants of the most recent common ancestor.

9. c. The nucleoid is the nonmembrane-bound single circular chromosome, or circular DNA molecule of prokaryotic cells. It contains the genes that code for the proteins needed by the cell. Choice **a** is incorrect: Flagella are organelles made of the protein flagellin that allow some prokaryotes to accomplish movement. Choice **b** is incorrect: Ribosomes are organelles composed of RNA and proteins that serve as the site of protein synthesis. Choice **d** is incorrect: The cell wall is a rigid structure that protects prokaryotic cells from their watery environments and gives them strength, structure, and shape.

10. b. Receptor proteins are the adhesion and communication proteins. They bind specific molecules such as hormones and cytokines. The specificity of receptor proteins allow the cell to respond to the outside environment in many different ways. When a molecule binds to the cell at a receptor protein, it initiates signal transduction. Choice **a** is incorrect: Channel proteins form pores for the facilitated transport of small molecules and ions across the cell membrane. Choice **c** is incorrect: Recognition proteins identify a particular cell type. They also function in self versus foreign identification. Most cell-recognition proteins are glycoproteins. The carbohydrate chains are different in different species. Different types of cells in a single organism also have different carbohydrate chains. Choice **d** is incorrect: Carrier proteins transport attached molecules and ions via facilitated diffusion and active transport.

11. a. The Golgi complex is composed of flat disks called cisternae that are stacked in piles and surrounded by a complex network of tubules and vesicles. The Golgi complex is the packaging center for storage, distribution, and excretion. Many Golgi apparatuses are found in kidney cells. They are responsible for sorting and modifying proteins and lipids received from the rough endoplasmic reticulum (RER) and the smooth ER (SER) and for folding polypeptides to create proteins. These molecules are sorted and packaged into vacuoles and vesicles for storage, for transport to other parts of the cell, or for secretion. Choice **b** is incorrect: The ER is a series of internal channels formed by invaginations of the cell membrane to connect the nuclear membrane with the pores in the plasma membrane. The smooth ER (SER) provides a surface area for lipid synthesis, particularly phospholipids and steroids. It also metabolizes carbohydrates and steroids and controls calcium concentration. The rough ER (RER) has ribosomes attached to its outer surface. It produces and modifies newly formed proteins, manufactures new membrane, and performs roles in the transport of these proteins and membrane to other locations within the cell. Choice **c** is incorrect: Lysosomes are a type of membrane-bound vesicle referred to as a suicide sac or destruction vacuole because they contain digestive enzymes to break down macromolecules. They are synthesized by the endoplasmic reticulum and the Golgi complex and can break down nucleic acids, proteins, and polysaccharides. They take in and break down older nonfunctioning or sick cells and organelles so that the products can be reused to make new organelles. Choice **d** is incorrect: Centrioles are cylindrical structures located near the nucleus in eukaryotic animal cells consisting of a ring of nine evenly spaced bundles of three microtubules. Centrioles play a role in the formation of cilia and flagella. A pair of centrioles forms a centrosome, also called the microtubule organizing center (MTOC). During animal cell division, the mitotic spindle forms between centrioles. They produce the microtubules that form the spindle fibers, which separate the chromosomes during cell division.

12. d. Mitochondria are double membrane-bound, rod-shaped organelles in the cytoplasm that have their own DNA and ribosomes and can replicate to create new mitochondria. Mitochondria function during cellular respiration to produce ATP, the energy supply molecule for life processes. This is why they are often referred to as the powerhouses of the cell. Choice **a** is incorrect: Vesicles are small single phospholipid membrane-bound storage and transport organelles that are numerous in the cell. They function to organize cellular substances to keep the cell environment safe. They are also involved in metabolism and can function as enzyme storage compartments and as chemical reaction chambers. Choice **b** is incorrect: The cytoskeleton is composed of microfilaments, intermediate filaments, and microtubules that provide cellular support and flexibility to perform tasks associated with movement. Eukaryotic animal cells, which do not have a rigid cell wall, require the support of the cytoskeleton to stabilize their shape. Cell movements—for example, the crawling movement of white blood cells and amoebas or the contraction of muscle cells—depend on cytoskeletal filaments. In both mitosis and meiosis, the cytoskeleton organizes and controls the movement of the chromosomes during cell division. It also functions in the constriction of animal cells during cytokinesis. Choice **c** is incorrect: Peroxisomes are also membrane-bound organelles. They also contain enzymes that catalyze a variety of metabolic reactions. Examples include the detoxification of harmful substances such as alcohol and hydrogen peroxide. In cellular respiration, the final acceptor in the electron transport chain is an oxygen atom. Oxygen readily accepts the electrons, which then combine with protons (H^+) to form water. Occasionally, oxygen reacts with other substances in the electron transport chain and only one electron is transferred, creating the reduced O_2^- called superoxide. This must be converted to hydrogen peroxide (by the enzyme superoxide dismutase), and then the H_2O_2 must be converted to water (by the enzyme catalase). Both O_2^- and H_2O_2 can react with DNA or proteins to disrupt cell functions and cause cell death.

13. c. The cytoskeleton of eukaryotic animal cells is composed of microfilaments, intermediate filaments, and microtubules. Microtubules are composed of the globular protein tubulin. They form hollow tubes, which provide structural support for the cell and are also flexible and function in movement tasks such as cell and organelle movement and cell division. Flagella and cilia in eukaryotes are both composed of tubulin. Choice **a** is incorrect: Microfilaments are made of the protein actin. The cytoskeleton of eukaryotic animal cells is composed of microfilaments, intermediate filaments, and microtubules. The solid rodlike construction of microfilaments provides cellular support and their flexibility enables them to form structures that can perform tasks such as engulfing material in the extracellular environment and cell division. Choice **b** is incorrect: The sister chromatids are attached in the center at the centromere. Cohesin is the binding protein in the centromere. Choice **d** is incorrect: Flagellin is the protein that comprises prokaryotic flagella. The flagellin forms a hollow tube with a hook at the end. The N and C termini of the protein form the inside of the helical tube and allow it to polymerize into a filament.

14. c. Gap or communication junctions form regions in the cell membranes of animal cells where intracell communication takes place. Cells on opposite sides of the junction deposit special proteins in the plasma membrane that form channels to transport both nutrient molecules and electrical currents between the connected cells. They allow for the rapid movement of both materials and messages between cells; for example, in cardiac cells they can be used to send signals for contraction. They are not found in plant cells, because the cell membranes do not come into close contact due to the cell wall. Choice **a** is incorrect: Tight or occluding junctions form bands around a cell where they are joined in localized spots to adjacent cells. The bands form a complex that increases in efficiency with each additional band. No chemicals can be transferred at these points—for example, the blood-brain barrier. None of the spaces are wide enough to allow passage. They form a leakproof barrier. Choice **b** is incorrect: Spot desmosomes or anchoring junctions are extensions of the cytoskeleton that hold cells together like a button and anchor the internal intermediate filaments. They are not leakproof and are found in cells that need to stretch, such as the skin and bladder. Choice **d** is incorrect: Plasmodesmata are similar to gap junctions. They are delicate strands of cytoplasm that extend through the cell membrane and the cell wall to interconnect plant cells to form a transportation system. Plants need to rapidly move the glucose made in the leaves to the rest of the plant. They must also move water quickly. Osmosis would be much too slow. These extensions form the transportation system for plant cells.

15. d. Carrier proteins transport attached molecules and ions via facilitated diffusion and active transport. Choice **a** is incorrect: Channel proteins form pores for the facilitated transport of small molecules and ions across the cell membrane. Choice **b** is incorrect: Receptor proteins are the adhesion and communication proteins. They bind specific molecules such as hormones and cytokines. The specificity of receptor proteins allow the cell to respond to the outside environment in many different ways. When a molecule binds to the cell at a receptor protein, it initiates signal transduction. Choice **c** is incorrect: Recognition proteins identify a particular cell type. They also function in self versus foreign identification. Most cell-recognition proteins are glycoproteins. The carbohydrate chains are different in different species. Different types of cells in a single organism also have different carbohydrate chains.

16. a. Microfilaments are made of the protein actin. The cytoskeleton of eukaryotic animal cells is composed of microfilaments, intermediate filaments, and microtubules. The solid rodlike construction of microfilaments provides cellular support and their flexibility enables them to form structures that can perform tasks such as engulfing material in the extracellular environment and cell division. Choice **b** is incorrect: The sister chromatids are attached in the center at the centromere. Cohesin is the binding protein in the centromere. Choice **c** is incorrect: The cytoskeleton of eukaryotic animal cells is composed of microfilaments, intermediate filaments, and microtubules. Microtubules are composed of the globular protein tubulin. They form hollow tubes, which provide structural support for the cell and are also flexible and function in movement tasks such as cell and organelle movement and cell division. Flagella and cilia in eukaryotes are both composed of tubulin. Choice **d** is incorrect: Flagellin is the protein that comprises prokaryotic flagella. The flagellin forms a hollow tube with a hook at the end. The N and C termini of the protein form the inside of the helical tube and allow it to polymerize into a filament.

17. c. Gametogenesis is the production of the haploid gametes in a mature organism. The production of sperm is spermatogenesis and the production of eggs is oogenesis. Choice **a** is incorrect: Gastrulation is the process that occurs after implantation, when the blastula sphere invaginates such that the single layer of blastula cells becomes a three-layer ball of cells that is indented to form a cavity in the center. This structure is called the gastrula. Choice **b** is incorrect: Spermiogenesis is the process of differentiation that spermatids undergo to become sperm. Choice **d** is incorrect: Blastulation is the process by which the morula differentiates, developing an interior space that becomes filled with fluid called the blastocoel. The hollow ball of cells is called a blastula or blastocyst, and this is what will implant in the uterine wall.

18. d. The mesoderm is the middle layer of the gastrula and is the germ cell layer from which all connective tissue is derived. This includes bone, blood, cartilage, extracellular matrix, collagen, and muscles, including the heart muscle. The excretory system, gonads, and parts of the liver, pancreas, thyroid gland, and lining of the bladder also arise from the mesoderm. Choice **a** is incorrect: The endoderm, which is the inner layer of the gastrula, is the germ layer responsible for the epithelial tissue that lines the digestive and respiratory tracts. Parts of the pancreas, liver, lining of the bladder, and thyroid gland also arise from the endoderm. Choice **b** is incorrect: Nervous tissue and many tissues of the integumentary system derive from the ectoderm, which is the outer germ cell layer of the gastrula. This includes the epidermis, hair, and nails, as well as the epithelial tissue of the mouth, nose, and anal canal. The lens and retina also arise from the ectoderm. Choice **c** is incorrect: The archenteron is the cavity or pouch at the center of the gastrula, where the blastula invaginated after implantation in the uterine wall. It is also called the primitive gut. The opening into the archenteron is the blastopore.

19. b. The allantois develops from the posterior of the gastrointestinal (GI) tract of the embryo and forms a sac. It functions in gas exchange, (O_2 and CO_2), water and salt exchange, and nitrogenous waste removal. Choice **a** is incorrect: The chorion is the outer membrane that protects the embryo in all reptiles, birds, and mammals. Its function is gas exchange. Choice **c** is incorrect: The amnion contains the amniotic fluid, which functions as a protective cushion for the embryo. The amnion membrane develops the amniotic sac in reptiles, birds, and mammals. Choice **d** is incorrect: The yolk sac encloses the yolk, which nourishes the egg. A network of blood vessels supplies the embryo with food. Oviparous amniotes have a large external yolk sac that contains nutritional stores. In bony fishes, sharks, reptiles, birds, and lower mammals, the yolk sac is attached to the embryo. In humans, the yolk sac performs all of the roles of the circulatory system before the embryonic circulatory system is functioning.

20. c. Bacilli are rods that can have flagella. Choice **a** is incorrect: Spirilla are spirals that can have flagella. Choice **b** is incorrect: Cocci a re spherical shaped and rarely have flagella. Choice **d** is incorrect: Vibrio are a type of spirilla that is an incomplete spiral or half-moon shape.

21. **d.** Mesophiles thrive in moderate temperatures. Their optimum growth temperatures are between 25°C and 45°C. Most bacteria are mesophilic, including soil bacteria and bacteria that live in and on the body. Choice **a** is incorrect: Psychrophiles are cold-loving bacteria with optimum growth temperatures between –5°C and 15°C. They are found in Arctic and Antarctic regions and streams fed by glaciers. Choice **b** is incorrect: Hyperthermophiles are extreme heat-loving organisms. Their optimum growth temperatures are between 70°C and 110°C. They are usually members of Archaea and grow near hydrothermal vents at great depths in the ocean, in hot springs such as those in Yellowstone National Park, and in solfataric fields. Choice **c** is incorrect: Thermophiles are heat-loving organisms. Their optimum growth temperatures are between 45°C and 70°C. They are found in hot springs and compost heaps.

22. **a.** Apocrine sweat glands are located in the armpits and axillary region and are not present at birth. They develop at puberty and release their product into an associated hair follicle. They do not function in thermoregulation. Apocrine sweat glands release pheromones, which are used in communication. The odor is a signal for sexual availability and other messages. Apocrine sweat glands use the merocrine mechanism, exocytosis. Choice **b** is incorrect: The ceruminous glands produce cerumen (ear wax) and are a modified apocrine sweat gland. Mammary glands are also modified apocrine sweat glands. Choice **c** is incorrect: Sudoriferous glands are another name for sweat glands. They open on epithelial tissue but are located in the connective tissue of the dermis. Apocrine and eccrine sweat glands are types of sudoriferous glands. There are 2.5 million sweat glands, but none on the lip margins, nipple, and portions of the external genitalia. Otherwise, they are everywhere else on the skin. Choice **d** is incorrect: Eccrine sweat glands are most numerous on the hands, feet, and forehead. They release their product via the merocrine mechanism, exocytosis. They open via a duct to the cell surface.

23. **b.** Diarthroses are freely movable joints. Choice **a** is incorrect: Synarthroses are immovable joints. Choice **c** is incorrect: Synostoses are fused bony joints such as when the sutures in the skull become bony and completely fused when the epiphyseal plate is gone after growth is complete. Choice **d** is incorrect: Amphiarthroses are slightly movable joints.

24. b. The adrenal medulla, inner nervous tissue of the adrenal glands, produces two hormones: epinephrine and norepinephrine. These hormones are part of the sympathetic nervous system and the fight-or-flight response. Their release is stimulated by preganglionic fibers of the sympathetic nervous system in reaction to stress, and their effects mimic sympathetic nervous system activation. Choice **a** is incorrect: Cortisol is one of the glucocorticoids released from the zona fasciculata, which is the middle part of the adrenal cortex. Cortisol is stimulated by ACTH from the anterior pituitary gland and targets the body cells to make more glucose through gluconeogenesis, the creation of glucose from nonglucose sources (fats and proteins). Choice **c** is incorrect: Aldosterone is the main mineral corticoid and is released from the zona glomerulosa, which is the outer region of the adrenal cortex. Its release is stimulated by a high concentration of K+ in the bloodstream or a low concentration of Na+, by adrenocorticotropic hormone (ACTH) from the anterior pituitary under stress conditions, or by renin, a protein released from the kidney when the blood pressure is low, which causes an enzyme cascade to form angiotensin II. Choice **d** is incorrect: The gonadocorticoids; mainly androgens, are released from the zona reticularis, which is the innermost part of the adrenal cortex. They are converted to estrogen and testosterone after their release and are thought to be responsible for the onset of puberty, for jump-starting the ovaries and testes, for the female sex drive, and for postmenopausal estrogen production.

25. c. Gomphoses are specialized fibrous joint between the teeth and the mandible and maxilla. These are peg-in-socket joints secured with the periodontal ligament. They are immobile, synarthroses joints. Choice **a** is incorrect: Syndesmoses are fibrous joints that are held together by ligaments. These joints mostly have only some give to them. They are synarthroses (immovable) though they are sometimes referred to as amphiarthroses, or slightly movable. Choice **b** is incorrect: Synchondroses are cartilaginous joints in which a bar or plate of hyaline cartilage unites the bones. Almost all are immovable synarthroses. Examples include the temporary joint between the epiphyseal plate and the diaphysis and the costal cartilage of the first rib to the manubrium of the sternum. Choice **d** is incorrect: Sutures are fibrous joints found only in the skull. The bones interdigitate or have a double-zigzag holding them together. These are synarthroses, or immovable joints.

26. b. Plantar flexion and dorsiflexion describe the up-and-down movements of the foot. In plantar flexion, the toes point, like a ballet dancer, downward or away from the body. In plantar dorsiflexion, the toes point up toward the knee. Choice **a** is incorrect: Flexion decreases the angle of the joint. It is a bending movement that brings the articulating bones closer together. Extension increases the angle of the joint, for example, straightening a flexed neck, body trunk, elbow, or knee. At the shoulder and hip, extension carries the limb to a point posterior to the joint. Choice **c** is incorrect: Inversion and eversion describe the movements of the foot from the ankles. Inversion is when the sole of the foot turns medially (inward). Eversion is when the sole of the foot turns laterally (outward). Choice **d** is incorrect: In regard to the foot, pronation refers to the combined motion of the foot in a normal gait when the outer edge of the heel hits the ground and the foot rolls inward and flattens out, and supination refers to the heel lifting off the ground as the front of the foot and toes push the body forward. Pronation and supination also refer to the palms up and palms down movements of the hand.

27. d. The Volkmann's canals run at right angles, perforating out from the Haversian canals. They connect the blood and nerve supply of the periosteum to the central Haversian canals and to the medullary cavity. Choice **a** is incorrect: Lacunae are little hollow cavities in which osteocytes, mature bone cells, are housed. Choice **b** is incorrect: Haversian or central canals are the channels through the core of each osteon that run along the bone axis and contain blood and lymph vessels and nerves. Choice **c** is incorrect: Lamellae are the series of layers that make up osteons, the structural unit of compact bone. This is why compact bone is often referred to as lamellar bone.

28. a. Crenation occurs when the environment is hypertonic to the cell. Water must leave the cell in order for equilibrium to be established on either side of the membrane. The cell shrinks, taking on a scallop-edged shape. Choice **b** is incorrect: When the environment is hypotonic to eukaryotic animal cells, water enters, causing the cells to swell until they lyse or burst in the process called osmotic lysis or cytolysis. Choice **c** is incorrect: When the environment is hypotonic to eukaryotic plant cells, water enters, causing the cells to become turgid, or swollen and distended, but they do not lyse. Choice **d** is incorrect: When the environment is hypotonic to the cell, water enters the cell from the exterior, where there are fewer solutes relative to water.

29. c. Melatonin is released from the pineal gland. It is released cyclically with higher levels in the evening. It is involved in sleep/wake cycles, the regulation of the biological clock, and possibly the onset of puberty. Choice **a** is incorrect: Thyroxine (T4) and triiodothyronine (T3) are released from the thyroid gland, causing increased metabolic activity, which produces body heat. They are also involved in maintaining blood pressure and in the normal growth and development of the reproductive, skeletal, and nervous systems. Calcitonin, which lowers the concentration of Ca2+ in the bloodstream, is also released from the thyroid gland. Choice **b** is incorrect: The hormones released from the anterior pituitary gland are growth hormone (GH), prolactin, and four tropic hormones: thyroid-stimulating hormone (TSH or thyrophin), luteinizing hormone (LH), follicle-stimulating hormone (FSH), and adrenocorticotropic hormone (ACTH). Choice **d** is incorrect: The two hormones released from the thymus are thymosin and thymopoietin, both of which are involved in the immune response, specifically in stimulating the maturation of T-cells.

30. c. The stationary period lasts for 24 to 48 hours and there is an equal rate of growth and death so that overall bacterial numbers stay the same. Choice **a** is incorrect: The decline or death period lasts for 48 to 96 hours and is when rapid cell death by cell lysis occurs. The colony has reached its maximum capacity given the environmental conditions. Cell lysis is now outpacing binary fission. Spore production commences in spore-forming bacteria. Choice **b** is incorrect: The logarithmic period of growth lasts for 12 to 24 hours and is when active doubling, or active reproduction occurs. Choice **d** is incorrect: Lag time lasts for 20 to 30 minutes and constitutes the generation time (GT). It is when a new colony is establishing and beginning to reproduce.

31. c. Each fascicle, or bundle of muscle fibers, is covered by a connective tissue layer called the perimysium. Choice **a** is incorrect: The periosteum is the outer fibrous layer of dense, irregular connective tissue on the outside of bone. Choice **b** is incorrect: The endomysium is the connective tissue layer in which each muscle fiber is wrapped. Choice **d** is incorrect: The epimysium is the connective tissue layer on top of a muscle.

32. b. Penicillin and its derivatives are ineffective against *Mycoplasma* because the latter do not have a cell wall. Penicillins and cephalosporins kill the cell wall by stopping the formation of peptidoglycan (PG). However, they kill only Gram-positive bacteria with their thick layer of PG and are of no use on *Mycoplasma*, which has no cell wall. Choice **a** is incorrect: Bacteria in the genus *Mycoplasma* are not classified as either Gram negative or Gram positive, because they lack a cell wall. Choice **c** is incorrect: Capsules aid bacteria by preventing phagocytosis by neutrophils that cannot attach to their slimy surface, by helping bacteria to attach to cells, by helping to prevent dehydration of bacteria that thrive in deserts, and because they can store sugars. They perform no function in blocking antibiotics from entering the cell. Choice **d** is incorrect: The name *Mycoplasma* comes from the Greek words for fungus, *mykes*, and formed, *plasma*. The name arose in the nineteenth century due to its fungus-like characteristics; however, it is not a fungus. Mycoplasma infections are generally treated with tetracycline or doxycycline, in contrast to most pneumonias, which are treated with penicillin.

33. a. *Cryptococcus neoformus* yeast is found in soil contaminated with certain types of bird droppings, particularly pigeons. Humans inhale the dust containing *C. neoformus* and develop flulike symptoms, which can progress to pneumonia and eventually lung scarring. Healthy people with strong immune systems may remain asymptomatic. In compromised patients with HIV infections, people with Hodgkin's disease, chemotherapy patients, or people taking high doses of corticosteroids, it can spread through the circulatory system to the meninges and the brain, becoming a cryptococcal meningoencephalitis. Choice **b** is incorrect: Coccidioidomycosis is caused by the systemic mold *Coccidioides immitis*. Humans inhale spores in the dry dusty air of semiarid desertlike environments, and in the body the mold takes on the nonmycelial form and is seen as endosporulating spherules. It causes a chronic, long-term tuberculosis (TB)-like illness. Choice **c** is incorrect: Blastomycosis is caused by the systemic mold *Blastomyces dermatitidis*. In the body, the mold is found in the yeast form with a characteristic thick cell wall. Blastomycosis is thought to become a problem when soil is disturbed such that the vegetative hyphae and spores are elevated above the soil surface. Both humans and animals breathe in the spores, which germinate in the lungs to the nonmycelial form. It is seen more often in dogs than in humans but can infect compromised patients and spread to the skin, central nervous system, and bones. Lung infections produce symptoms similar to histoplasmosis and coccidioidomycosis. Choice **d** is incorrect: Histoplasmosis is caused by the systemic mold *Histoplasma capsulatum* and is generally found in the soil in moist climates, primarily in the Eastern United States, Great Lakes, and Mississippi and Ohio River valleys. The mold form grows best in soil contaminated with bird droppings or bat droppings, referred to as guano. Humans inhale the spores from the contaminated soil and the spores germinate in the lungs where the fungus grows as a budding encapsulated yeast. They develop a flulike illness, which can become chronic, causing lung scarring.

34. b. The tertiary consumers are carnivores, which are depicted at the top of the pyramid of energy supported by all of the higher-energy levels below. At each level, energy is absorbed, consumed, and lost as heat and to the death of organisms. Only 10% to 15% of the absorbed energy is transferred up to the next level. The least amount of energy is available to the top-level consumers. Choice **a** is incorrect: The pyramid of energy starts at the wide base where the most energy is stored in the photosynthetic green plants. Choices **c** and **d** are incorrect: The primary consumers are the animals that eat green plants, the herbivores. They are the second energy level up from the bottom of the pyramid where the most energy is stored in the photosynthetic green plants.

35. b. The myocardium is the bulk of heart. It is contractile muscle tissue. The left ventricle is much thicker than the right because it must sustain higher pressure. It must pump blood to the body. However, there are always equal amounts of blood on each side even though the size and thicknesses differ. Choice **a** is incorrect: The epicardium is the innermost outer covering of the heart. It is also called the visceral layer of serous pericardium and is part of the heart wall. Choice **c** is incorrect: The interventricular sulci are grooves on the outside of the heart that mark the location of the interventricular septum, which separates the right and left ventricles. Choice **d** is incorrect: The endocardium is the innermost part of the heart. It lines the chambers of the heart, covers the valves, and is continuous with the blood vessels. It is composed of epithelial and connective tissue.

36. d. The three vessels of the right atrium are the superior vena cava, the inferior vena cava, and the coronary sinus. The superior vena cava delivers blood from everything in the systemic circuit superior to the diaphragm to the right atrium. The inferior vena cava delivers blood from everything inferior to the diaphragm to the right atrium. The coronary sinus collects blood from the myocardium and is part of the coronary circuit that supplies the heart with blood. Choice **a** is incorrect: The three vessels of the right atrium are the superior vena cava, the inferior vena cava, and the coronary sinus. The right pulmonary vein enters the left atrium, as do all four of the pulmonary veins. There are four vessels of the left atrium; all are pulmonary veins, two left pulmonary veins and two right pulmonary veins. Choice **b** is incorrect: The three vessels of the right atrium are the superior vena cava, the inferior vena cava, and the coronary sinus. The brachiocephalic artery is one of the three branches off the aortic arch. It supplies blood to the head and brain. Choice **c** is incorrect: The coronary sinus and the superior vena cava along with the inferior vena cava enter the right atrium. All four pulmonary veins enter the left atrium.

37. a. Late erythroblasts accumulate hemoglobin and become normoblasts. Normoblasts eject the nucleus to become reticulocytes. It is the reticulocytes that are released by the red bone marrow. The count tells how well the bone marrow is producing new RBCs. The reticulocytes persist for two days in the bloodstream and become erythrocytes. Choice **b** is incorrect: Normoblasts are the last erythroblast stage after hemoglobin has been accumulated by the immature erythrocyte. The normoblast ejects the nucleus to become a reticulocyte, which is released by the red bone marrow and is an indicator of how well erythropoiesis is occurring. Choice **c** is incorrect: Hemocytoblasts are RBC stem cells. They also give rise to the white blood cells (WBCs) and platelets depending on pathway. Once a hemocytoblast becomes a proerythroblast, it is a committed cell and must become an RBC. Choice **d** is incorrect: Proerythroblasts are the next stage after the RBC stem cells, the hemocytoblasts, which can also develop into WBCs and platelets. Once a hemocytoblast becomes a proerythroblast, it is a committed cell and must become an RBC.

38. d. *Chlamydia* and *Rickettsia* are obligate intracellular parasites. They must grow inside the living cells of their host. They cannot be grown in the laboratory on any medium. *Rickettsia* generally prefer to grow inside cells that line the blood vessels, the endothelial cells. A number of diseases are caused by *Rickettsia*, including typhus, Rocky Mountain spotted fever, and Brill-Zinzer disease, a delayed relapse of typhus. *Chlamydia* are smaller than most bacteria, and have very little peptidoglycan in their cell walls. They cause a number of important infections, including trachoma, psittacosis, lymphogranuloma venereum, and genitourinary infections. Choice **a** is incorrect: *Mycoplasma* are smaller than most bacteria, generally 0.15 to 0.3 μm long, and their distinguishing characteristic is that they do not have a cell wall. Since they lack rigidity, they are pleomorphic, taking on many different shapes. They are the smallest microorganisms to grow on agar plates, and this growth is very slow, taking up to one week; but they do grow on laboratory media, unlike the obligate parasites, which must grow inside the living cells of their hosts and cannot be grown in the laboratory on any medium. *Rickettsia* are obligate intracellular parasites. They must grow inside the living cells of their hosts and cannot be grown in the laboratory on any medium. Choice **b** is incorrect: The genera *Bacillus* and *Clostridium* are the primary producers of endospores. *Bacillus* are Gram-positive, aerobic, spore-forming bacteria. The rod-shaped cell produces one spore within the cell. *Clostridium* are Gram-positive, anaerobic spore formers. The much smaller rod, which is sausage- or cigar-shaped, produces a tennis racket–shaped cell due to the endospore at one end. Choice **c** is incorrect: *Chlamydia* are obligate intracellular parasites, which must grow inside living cells. They cannot be grown in the lab. They cause a number of important infections, including trachoma, psittacosis, lymphogranuloma venereum, and genitourinary infections. *Mycoplasma* are smaller than most bacteria, and their distinguishing characteristic is that they do not have a cell wall. Since they lack rigidity, they are pleomorphic, taking on many different shapes. They are the smallest microorganisms to grow on agar plates, and this growth is very slow, taking up to one week; but they do grow on laboratory media, unlike the obligate parasites, which must grow inside the living cells of their hosts and cannot be grown in the laboratory on any medium.

39. c. Basophils are granulocytes with dark-staining, purplish-black granules and an S- or U-shaped nucleus. They are the least abundant WBCs, comprising 0.5% to 1% of the WBC population. They release histamine, a chemical used in the inflammatory response that stimulates vasodilation, an increase in blood vessel diameter. They also attract more WBCs to infected areas to help remove infection. Choice **a** is incorrect: Neutrophils are the most abundant WBC type, comprising 50% to 70% of the WBC population. They are granulocytes and stain purple/lilac, have a multilobed nucleus, and phagocytize bacteria. They are short-lived, because they are constantly encountering bacteria to phagocytize and this process causes death. Choice **b** is incorrect: Eosinophils are non-phagocytic granulocytes with a bilobed nucleus. Their granules stain red and they attack parasitic worms by releasing a substance from the granules that contains digestive enzymes. They also respond to allergic reactions by destroying some of the inflammatory chemicals released during an allergy attack and helping to eliminate antigen/antibody complexes formed during an allergy attack. Choice **d** is incorrect: Monocytes are agranulocytes that comprise 3% to 8% of the WBC population. They are very large cells and are easy to identify due to their purple color and U-shaped nucleus. When they leave the bloodstream, they become macrophages, which attack virus-infected cells and some bacteria. They are important in chronic illnesses such as TB. If the monocyte count is elevated, it could indicate some type of chronic, long-term infection.

40. a. The chlorophyll and other photosynthetic pigments as well as electron transport chains are on the thylakoid membrane. The light-dependent reactions of photosynthesis occur on the thylakoid membrane. Choice **b** is incorrect: The thylakoid membrane encloses the fluid-filled thylakoid interior space, called the thylakoid compartment or thylakoid lumen. During photophosphorylation, protons are pumped across the thylakoid membrane into the lumen, creating a proton gradient. The energy stored in this gradient is captured by the enzyme ATP synthase complex. The ATP synthase is activated by the ion flow down the concentration gradient and catalyzes the formation of ATP from ADP + Pi. Choice **c** is incorrect: The light-independent (dark) reactions of photosynthesis occur in the stroma, where photosynthetic enzymes are stored. The stroma, a fluid-filled region inside the inner membrane of the chloroplast, contains the necessary enzymes for the light-independent reactions. Choice **d** is incorrect: The thylakoids are disklike sacs formed by the infoldings of the thylakoid membrane. Sometimes the thylakoids form a stack called a granum.

41. c. Sickle-cell anemia is an example of pleiotropy and incomplete dominance. One amino acid in a β chain that comprises the globin protein in the hemoglobin molecule is mutated, causing the shape of the red blood cell to sickle or become a half-moon shape. This in turn causes problems with multiple organ systems in the body. Homozygous recessive individuals inherit the full-blown disease. Heterozygous individuals carry the sickle cell trait and have controllable symptoms. Only homozygous dominant individuals are normal. Sickle-cell anemia is a point mutation. Glutamic acid is produced instead of valine because histidine (CAC) is produced rather than tyrosine (UAC). Choice **a** is incorrect: Tay-Sachs disease is an autosomal recessive trait. The HEXA gene codes for a protein that is used to manufacture the enzyme β-hexosaminidase A. Lysosomes carry β-hexosaminidase A to break down a lipid substance called GM2 ganglioside. When the two alleles of the mutated gene are inherited, GM2 ganglioside accumulates and becomes toxic to neurons in the brain and spinal cord. Choice **b** is incorrect: Marfan syndrome is an example of pleiotropy and autosomal dominance. A mutation in the FBN-1 gene that codes for the protein fibrillin-1 causes multiple symptoms in the aorta, eye, skin, and bones. Fibrillin-1 is an integral part of elastic cartilage tissue. The FBN-1 gene is autosomal dominant, so individuals who inherit one mutated allele exhibit the symptoms of the disease. Choice **d** is incorrect: Huntington's disease is an autosomal dominant trait caused by trinucleotide repeats (cytosine-adenine-guanine repeats on chromosome 4). The good gene that does not contain the repeats is recessive. Individuals who have one of these alleles on chromosome 4 will display the disease at some point in their lives.

42. d. Epistasis is when one or more genes inhibit the expression of another gene. The inhibiting gene and the effected gene are on different loci on the genome, although they may be tightly linked. The effect can be either genotypic or phenotypic. One example is albinism. The gene that causes albinism masks the gene that codes for eye color and hair color. Albinism is autosomal recessive. Choice **a** is incorrect: Hypostasis is when the expression of a gene is masked by an epistatic gene. In epistasis, when one or more genes inhibit the expression of another gene, the phenotype that is expressed is epistatic and the phenotype that is inhibited or masked is hypostatic. Choice **b** is incorrect: Polygenic inheritance is when many genes are involved in the expression of a particular trait. The phenotype is expressed due to the relationships and interactions between a number of genes. Skin color, height, and body shape are all the result of multiple genes interacting. Choice **c** is incorrect: Pleiotropy is when a single gene affects a number of expressed traits. It can cause significant disruptions in certain genetic disorders. If a mutation occurs, at least two and possibly many different phenotypic traits are affected.

43. c. In codominance, two different alleles for a gene are both expressed phenotypically. Blood type is an example. Capital I indicates the dominant alleles (A or B), while lowercase i denotes the recessive O allele. If a heterozygous type A female is crossed with a heterozygous type B male, the probability is that 25% of their offspring will be type AB, the codominant blood type in which both the A and B antigens are present on the red blood cells and neither the A nor the B antibodies are present. Another 25% will likely be homozygous recessive type O; 25% each will be heterozygous type A and heterozygous type B.

		Female	
		I^A	i
Male	I^B	I^AI^B	I^Bi
	i	I^Ai	ii

44. **a.** Anthrax is caused by *Bacillus anthracis*, a Gram-positive aerobic spore former. The spores are naturally found in deep anaerobic soil. When humans open up the soil in some manner, most commonly via overfarming and erosion, we bring them to the surface. The spores attach to animal fur, hair, and skin or can be inhaled in dry, dusty, blowing soil particles. The spores germinate and the bacteria produce necrotizing toxins. On the skin, this causes blisters and sores from the dead tissue. In the lungs, sores and hemorrhaging result. Pulmonary anthrax has a very high death rate of between 20% and 50%. Choice **b** is incorrect: Lymphogranuloma venereum (LGV) is a sexually transmitted disease (STD) caused by the atypical bacterium *Chlamydia*, which is an obligate intracellular parasite. When it infects the lymph nodes in the groin, hard, swollen, black lumps, or granulomas, develop. It used to be called black syphilis because it resembles syphilis. Choice **c** is incorrect: Giardiasis is caused by the anaerobic, flagellated protozoan *Giardia intestinalis. Giardia* belongs to a group of flagellates referred to as the diplomonads, which have two nuclei in a double cell structure that each have four flagella. The disease's mode of transmission is ingestion of water or food contaminated with the cysts. The cysts can be ingested due to improper hygiene (fecal-oral transmission), because there are many asymptomatic carriers of the parasite. *Giardia* trophozoites colonize the small intestine. The symptoms of giardiasis are explosive diarrhea, lethargy, flatulence that can be so severe that it induces vomiting, nausea, bloating, and resultant weight loss. Compromised patients can suffer extended infections. This includes those with immunodeficiency disorders and disorders of the digestive system that result in diminished gastric acid production. Choice **d** is incorrect: Trachoma is a type of conjunctivitis considered to be the world's leading cause of blindness. It is caused by the atypical bacteria *Chlamydia*, which are an obligate intracellular parasite. It is spread when water that is contaminated with human or animal waste gets into the eye.

45. **b.** Plasma is the fluid component of blood. It constitutes about 55% of whole blood. It is the least dense and therefore the top layer upon centrifugation. Choice **a** is incorrect: RBCs or erythrocytes comprise approximately 45% of whole blood. When centrifuged, the bottom layer is the erythrocytes because they are the densest. This constitutes the hematocrit or packed cell volume in a complete blood count. Choices **c** and **d** are incorrect: The next layer up from the densest erythrocyte layer at the bottom of the centrifuge is the buffy coat consisting of WBCs and platelets. It constitutes approximately 1% of whole blood.

46. d. The complementary base pairs that form rungs of the DNA ladder are held together by hydrogen bonds. Hydrogen bonds form on molecules that have polar covalent bonds such that one atom carries a partial positive charge and one carries a partial negative charge. When one charged part of the molecule forms an electrostatic interaction with an oppositely charged part of another molecule, these weak bonds can easily and rapidly form, break, and reform. However, in a molecule such as DNA, even though a hydrogen bond individually is far weaker than a covalent bond or an ionic bond, when there are millions of hydrogen bonds, molecular stability is significantly enhanced. Choice **a** is incorrect: A phosphodiester bond is formed between a phosphate group and two adjacent carbons via ester linkages. This covalent bond forms between the phosphate group on the 5′ carbon of one deoxyribonucleotide and the hydroxyl (OH) group on the 3′ carbon of the deoxyribose of another to form the sugar-phosphate backbone of the DNA. Choice **b** is incorrect: Carbon-hydrogen bonds are the covalent bond essential to life. Chemical energy is found in food, macromolecules with carbon-hydrogen bonds, where energy is stored in cells. Carbon-hydrogen bonds are potential energy and matter. Anabolism is a reduction reaction in which carbon-hydrogen bonds are built or synthesized. Energy is stored in the larger molecules that are built in an endergonic reaction. Choice **c** is incorrect: adenosine triphosphate (ATP) is held together by high-energy phosphate bonds. These are covalent bonds, but they are highly unstable and thus easily broken. The instability is caused by the oxygen molecules, which add negative polarity to the molecules. This is why ATP carries the energy for the cell.

47. a. Mutations are changes in the sequence of nitrogen bases on a DNA strand. They can be caused by errors when the nitrogen base sequence is copied during cell division and by exposure to radiation, chemicals, or viruses. Point mutations or single substitutions are when a single nucleotide is changed to another. Sickle-cell anemia is a point mutation on the hemoglobin beta gene (HBB) found on chromosome 11. Glutamic acid is produced instead of valine because histidine (CAC) is produced rather than tyrosine (UAC). Frame-shift mutations are when the deletion or insertion of a nucleotide causes the reading frame for the mRNA to change. When there are more or less nucleotides, all of the codons on the mRNA are changed from the point of insertion or deletion onward. If a nucleotide is added or deleted, it can cause an entirely different protein to be made. If the deletion or insertion occurs late in the sequence, it may result in a functioning protein, but it may not. Usually if the mistake is early in the sequence, the protein will be badly damaged or nonfunctional.

48. b. Glycolysis produces two pyruvate molecules and two molecules of ATP. All cells can perform glycolysis in the cytosol. It is a multistep metabolic pathway that involves the partial oxidation of glucose ($C_6H_{12}O_6$). No oxygen is required. After a glucose molecule is broken down into 2 PGAL (3-phosphoglyceraldehyde) molecules fueled by the input of two ATP molecules, a series of reactions results in two pyruvate molecules, a net gain of two ATP molecules and two NADH molecules. In short, PGAL → pyruvate (pyruvic acid). The complete reaction is:

$C_6H_{12}O_6 + 2\ NAD^+ + 2\ ADP + 2\ P_i \rightarrow 2\ NADH + 2\ Pyruvate + 2\ ATP + 2\ H_2O + 2\ H^+$

The products of glycolysis can be used in either anaerobic respiration or aerobic respiration. In anaerobic respiration, the next pathway is a series of reactions collectively called fermentation. In aerobic respiration, the products of glycolysis are sent to the citric acid, or Krebs cycle. Choice **a** is incorrect: These are the products of the cellular respiration reaction. The overall cellular respiration equation is:

$C_6H_{12}O_6 + 6O_2 \rightarrow 6CO_2 + 6H_2O + 36\text{–}38\ ATP$

Choice **c** is incorrect: The transition reaction produces two acetyl CoA molecules and two molecules of CO_2. The transition reaction in aerobic respiration is also referred to as the oxidation of pyruvate. The two molecules of pyruvate from glycolysis enter the matrix of the mitochondria, where they are converted to two molecules of acetyl CoA, a two-carbon molecule. This oxidative decarboxylation reaction will continue as long as there is oxygen supplied to the mitochondria. If not, the pyruvate will be shuttled to the fermentation reactions. The enzyme that catalyzes the reaction is pyruvate dehydrogenase. Two NAD^+ molecules are reduced. Each gains two electrons to yield two NADH and two H^+. Pyruvate is catabolized in the process, resulting in the release of two molecules of CO_2. The other product of the breakdown, acetyl, instantly bonds with coenzyme A to form acetyl CoA. The acetyl CoA then enters the Krebs cycle. The complete reaction is:

$2\ Pyruvate + 2\ NAD^+ + 2\ Coenzyme\ A \rightarrow 2\ Acetyl\ CoA + 2\ NADH + 2\ H^+ + 2\ CO_2$

Choice **d** is incorrect: Two lactate molecules and two molecules of ATP are produced in lactic acid fermentation. Fermentation refers to the conversion of pyruvate to acetic acid, alcohol, or a number of other organic compounds. Lactic acid (lactate) fermentation occurs in certain fungi, prokaryotes, and animal cells. The summary reaction is:

$C_6H_{12}O_6 \rightarrow Pyruvate \rightarrow 2\ Lactate + NAD^+ + 2\ ATP$

The two pyruvic acids are broken down into lactic acid + NAD^+. Pyruvate is reduced and NADH is oxidized. Lactic acid fermentation occurs in muscle cells, where an accumulation causes cramps.

Section 4: Chemistry

General Chemistry

1. a. The specific heat capacity of a substance can help us relate its changes in heat to its changes in temperature by using the calorimetric equation $Q = m\ C_p\ \Delta T$ (where Q is the change in heat/enthalpy, m is the mass of the substance, C_p is the heat capacity, and ΔT is the change in temperature). In this question, the scientist knows the amount of heat applied, the mass, and the change in temperature; these values can be used to calculate the heat capacity. The heat of fusion (choice **b**) measures the change in enthalpy when a solid melts or a liquid freezes, while the heat of vaporization (choice **c**) measures the change in enthalpy when a liquid vaporizes or a gas condenses. Heat conductivity (choice **d**) cannot be measured using simple calorimetry and requires a separate measurement.

2. b. Before answering this question, it may help to draw a potential energy diagram for an exothermic reaction:

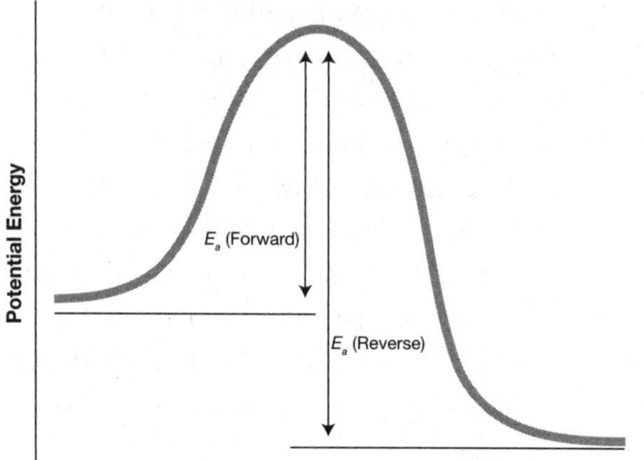

If the reaction is exothermic (and, consequently, releases energy—meaning that the starting energy on the y-axis is higher for starting materials than for products), we can see that the products must be storing less potential energy than the reactants. Exothermic reactions give off heat (energy), which explains the energy difference between the starting materials and the products: The products must be lower down on the diagram than the reactants. The activation energy is equal to the difference between the initial potential energy and the maximum potential energy (which could be either an intermediate or, more likely, a transition state). Therefore, we can see that the activation energy is greater for the reverse reaction, which is endothermic (requiring a net surplus of energy for the reverse reaction to proceed). Assuming no catalysts or other variables, a simple exothermic reaction will have a lower activation energy than its corresponding endothermic reverse reaction.

3. b. The first step is to balance this equation. Sulfur trioxide (SO_3) has three oxygen atoms, while an oxygen molecule (O_2) has only two oxygen atoms. Since the oxygen molecule cannot simply be split for the reaction, the balanced reaction must use three oxygen molecules and form two sulfur trioxide molecules. Here is the unbalanced reaction as well as the balanced reaction:

$$S + O_2 \longrightarrow SO_3$$
$$2S + 3O_2 \longrightarrow 2SO_3$$

In the balanced reaction, three moles of oxygen are consumed for every two moles of sulfur; consequently, 1.5 moles of oxygen are consumed for every mole of sulfur.

4. b. The first atomic energy level contains only a single *s*-orbital, which can hold a total of two electrons. The smallest atom to fill this energy level would, therefore, require two electrons. Of the stable neutral elements, only helium has the two electrons necessary to fill this outer (valence) shell. This is behavior shown by all other noble gases (argon, xenon, etc.), although helium is smallest in size. The loss or gain of electrons from atoms is a major driving force in chemical reactions, due to the extra stability associated with having a filled valence shell.

5. c. While all four choices listed are on the heavier side of the Periodic Table, xenon and krypton will have relatively low densities because they exist as gases at room temperature and standard pressure. Iodine and bromine have similar chemical properties, but density increases as we move down the Periodic Table within the same family. While the atomic radius of atoms increases as you go down a column in the periodic table (meaning that fewer molecules can be packed into a given space, which would lead to a lighter density), each atom in turn has more mass due to its increased number of protons and neutrons. Iodine (density = 4.94 g/ml) is in fact more dense than bromide (3.12 g/ml).

6. c. A general rule: As a chemical bond becomes stronger, it also becomes shorter. Triple bonds are generally stronger than single bonds or double bonds because they involve more shared electron pairs. Consequently, a C≡C bond will generally be shorter than a C=C bond or a C–C bond.

7. a. Alkali metals have only one electron in their valence shell, so they carry a +1 oxidation state in virtually all of their compounds. All of the other choices can carry a variety of different positive charges in different types of reactions.

8. b. The electrons on the left side of this reaction are used to oxidize the chromium ion in $Cr_2O_7^{2-}$. In order to determine the number of electrons involved, we must first calculate the oxidation state of this chromium ion. Oxygen nearly always carries a –2 charge, so the total charge from the O_7 is equal to –14. In order to form a complex with a net charge of –2, the two chromium ions must carry a total charge of +12; each individual chromium ion, therefore, has an oxidation state of +6 on the left side of the equation. The chromium ion on the right side of the equation has an oxidation state of +2, so we can see that four electrons are required to produce one of these ions. Alternatively, you can balance the equation using standard techniques to arrive at the result: $Cr_2O_7^{2-} + 14H^+ + ?e^- \rightarrow 2Cr^{2+} + 7H_2O$. In order to complete the balanced equations, the charges must balance; there is a net charge of +12 on the left side of the reaction arrow, and +4 on the product side of the reaction arrow. Therefore, a total of eight electrons (carrying a –1 charge each) completes the balanced equation, which produces two Cr^{2+}. Since the equation asks how many electrons are needed to produce just one Cr^{2+}, the correct answer is ($\frac{8}{2}$), or four electrons: choice **b**.

9. c. A reagent is considered to be a reducing agent if it donates electrons, thereby reducing one of the other reagents. An atom is most likely to lose an electron if it has a valence shell with only one electron within it, as the most stable configurations are those in which the valence shell (outermost shell) is completely filled. Choice **c** (potassium) has a single valence electron, so it can achieve a stable configuration if it donates that electron. Choice **d** (calcium) is also more likely to donate electrons, but it is not as powerful a reducing agent because its full 4s orbital makes it more stable than potassium. Choices **a** (sulfur) and **b** (chlorine) have valence shells that are nearly full, so they are much more likely to accept electrons in order to fill their outer shells.

10. c. In β^- decay, a neutron is converted to a proton, while a negatively charged β particle (an electron) as well as an electron neutrino are emitted into the environment. This is common in isotopes that have too many neutrons and not enough protons; the net effect is an increase in the atomic number with no change in the atomic mass, since protons and neutrons have similar atomic mass values. Conversely, β^+ decay involves the conversion of a proton to a neutron along with the emission of a positively charged β particle (a positron) along with an electron neutrino. This decreases the atomic number. α decay is defined by the emission of a helium nucleus (two protons and two neutrons), which leads to a decrease in the atomic number and the atomic mass. γ decay simply involves the release of energy with no change in atomic number or atomic mass.

11. c. A catalyst increases the rate of a reaction by lowering the activation energy, thereby allowing the reaction to achieve the activation energy more rapidly. In a multistep reaction, the most effective use of a catalyst would be to increase the rate of the slow step, which is also known as the rate-determining step; a change in the rate of the fast step will not have a significant effect on the rate of the reaction. It is also important to note that the addition of a catalyst will have no impact on the net change in enthalpy or the equilibrium constant of the reaction.

12. a. When in solution, many of the transition metals produce a strong characteristic color. Electrons in the *d*-orbital are able to transition between different energy states, causing the ion to absorb light energy. The color of the light depends on the amount of energy that is absorbed in any given transition, but copper is known to produce blue and green solutions with different anions. In this question, some of the copper has reacted with hydrochloric acid to produce hydrogen gas and copper (II) chloride, which appears green in solution. The other three answer choices are not transition metals and, consequently, are less likely to form a colored solution.

13. c. In order to solve a problem like this, it is best to first convert all quantities into moles. The question can be divided into a few steps: We need to calculate (1) the number of moles of NaOH, (2) the number of moles of HCl, (3) the number of moles of the product formed, and (4) the concentration of the product formed.

1. (4 g NaOH) (1 mol/40 g NaOH) = 0.1 mol NaOH
2. (0.1 mol/L HCl) (100 mL solution) (1 L/1,000 mL) = 0.01 mol HCl
3. $NaOH + HCl \rightarrow NaCl + H_2O$. Since there is 10 times more NaOH than HCl, HCl acts as a limiting reagent and 0.01 moles of NaCl are produced.
4. $\frac{0.01 \text{ moles NaCl}}{0.1 \text{ L of solution}} = 0.1$ M NaCl solution. Note that we still have a large amount of NaOH floating around in solution, but without more HCl with which to react, it does not contribute to a higher concentration of NaCl.

14. a. While most of the acid halides are considered strong acids, HF is a weak acid. The K_a, or the acid dissociation constant, quantifies a compound's level of acidity by measuring how much of it will dissociate in solution. Strong acids dissociate completely, so they generally have very high K_a values, while weak acids dissociate in smaller quanitities and have much smaller K_a values. For this list of acids, the acids increase in strength in the order HF, HCl, HBr, and HI. HI is the strongest acid on this list, with a pK_A ($-\log[H^+]$) of approximately –11. This is 14 orders of magnitude stronger than the acidity of HF. HF is the weakest acid on the list, so the correct answer is choice **a**.

15. d. The ideal gas law, $PV = nRT$, provides an accurate estimate of gas behavior in most cases. More precise calculations can be made using van der Waals's equation, which also considers the value of the attractive forces between particles (the strongest of which is the van der Waals force) and, to a lesser extent, the total atomic/molecular volume taken up by individual particles. Several other factors are also involved in the function of real gases, but the most significant factor not considered by the ideal gas law is the intermolecular force. Choice **a** is incorrect because potential energy is a relative calculation, and there is no such thing as a "total potential energy" stored by a particle. Choice **b** is incorrect because kinetic energy of a gas molecule is a direct function of its temperature, and has therefore already been considered in the ideal gas law. Choice **c** is incorrect because a particle's volume has more of an impact than its mass, and neither is as important as the intermolecular forces.

16. c. At the triple point, a substance can coexist as solid, liquid, and gas. The substance will generally be most likely to evaporate into a gas if the temperature is increased or the pressure is decreased. The temperature of water's triple point is 273°K, or about 0°C; since this is the temperature at which water coexists as solid and liquid at 1 atm, we know that the pressure must be far lower than 1 atm for water to approach the gas phase.

17. a. Electronegativity increases as we move toward the top right of the Periodic Table, with the exception of the noble gases. It may be easier to remember this trend if you just remember that fluorine is the most electronegative element on the table.

18. b. Like most other compounds, liquid water generally expands when heated, thereby decreasing its density. However, while most compounds are densest in their solid form, water is an exception due to its unique crystal lattice structure; this is why ice floats in liquid water. Water is most dense at temperatures that are slightly above the freezing point.

19. b. This diagram depicts the two resonance structures of a thiocyanate ion. Thiocyanate shares its negative charge between its sulfur atom and its nitrogen atom, either of which is capable of forming an ionic bond with a cation. In order for the negative charge to be shared in this manner, the central carbon atom (which can form four total bonds because it has four valence electrons to share) can form bonds to create either of the resonance structures in the diagram.

20. d. Aluminum generally forms compounds with an oxidation state of +3, while a carbonate ion carries a –2 charge. In order for aluminum to form an ionic bond with carbonate, the net charge must add up to zero; for this to happen, the final compound must have two aluminum atoms and three carbonate ions.

21. c. Ionic bonds form between a cation and an anion, while covalent bonds form between various atoms regardless of their ionic properties. Generally, bonds between metals and nonmetals are ionic and bonds between nonmetals (especially carbon) are covalent. In choices **a**, **b**, and **d**, oxygen is bonded to a metal; meanwhile, in choice **c** (formaldehyde), the central atom is carbon and all of its bonds are covalent.

22. b. In a CH_4 molecule, the carbon is surrounded by four electron pairs, each of which is shared with a hydrogen atom. When there are four electron pairs around a central atom, they arrange in the form of a tetrahedron, a three-dimensional figure with four vertices at approximately equal angles.

23. c. Assuming no heat lost to the environment, the amount of heat transferred in a process can be related to the temperature change in each substance involved by the formula $Q = mC_p\Delta T$, where Q is the total amount of heat transferred, m is the mass of the substance, C_p is the specific heat, and ΔT is the change in temperature. The value for Q will be the same for both liquids, since the amount of heat lost by the warm liquid will be equal to the amount of heat gained by the cold liquid. In this example, ΔT is also the same for both liquids, so the only two variables are the mass and the specific heat; therefore, we can say that mC_p for the unknown liquid is equal to mC_p for the water sample. Since the specific heat of water is exactly twice that of the unknown liquid, the mass of water must be half of the unknown liquid, or 50 g.

24. a. According to Planck's law, the energy of light is directly proportional to its frequency. In the visible spectrum, red light carries the least energy and violet light carries the most. Infrared radiation carries slightly less energy than red light, while ultraviolet radiation carries slightly more energy than violet light. Microwave radiation and radio waves, meanwhile, carry less energy than infrared light.

25. a. The bridge in a galvanic cell is also called a "salt bridge." A salt is generally composed of a metallic cation and a nonmetal anion; a common example is copper sulfate, or $CuSO_4$. By contrast, Cu (copper) is a metal, Br_2 (bromine) is a diatomic molecule, and CH_2O (formaldehyde) is an aldehyde.

26. d. The *g* subshell does not exist in any known elements, but its properties are easily predictable based on the properties of the other subshells. The *s* subshell holds one electron pair, the *p* subshell holds three pairs, the *d* subshell holds five pairs, and the *f* subshell holds seven pairs. Since each increasing subshell gains two extra pairs, we can conclude that a *g* subshell would hold nine pairs, or 18 total electrons.

27. b. A pi bond is a bond that is generally formed between electrons from *p*-orbitals. By contrast, a sigma bond is formed between electrons from *s*-orbitals. A single bond is made from one sigma bond, a double bond contains one sigma bond and one pi bond, and a triple bond contains one sigma bond and two pi bonds.

28. c. The K_a of a weak acid is approximately equal to the product of the concentrations of the products divided by the concentration of the acid itself. Chlorous acid dissociates into ClO_2^- and H^+ in equal concentrations, so the K_a is equal to $[ClO_2^-][H^+]/[HClO_2]$. The percent dissociation will be constant regardless of the concentration of the acid, so we can set the concentration equal to 1 for simplicity; also, since the concentration of ClO_2^- is equal to the concentration of H^+, we can replace $[ClO_2^-][H^+]$ with simply x^2. This allows us to determine the concentration of H^+ with the equation $x^2 = K_a = 10^{-2}$, and $x = 10^{-1} = 0.1 = [H^+]$. The percent dissociation is $[H^+]/[HClO_2] = 0.1/1 = 10\%$. For any monoprotic weak acid, there is a shortcut to this calculation: The percent dissociation will always be equal to the square root of the K_a.

Organic Chemistry

29. c. The structures are not completely different compounds, because each structure has the same number of carbons, hydrogens, and oxygens. The structures are stereoisomers, as they possess the same sequence of bonds and atoms. The structures are in fact exactly identical because the two stereocenters present in the molecule have identical configurations when compared to each other. To determine the relationship between the two structures, label each stereocenter as either *R* or *S*. Both stereocenters in the structure on the left are in *S* configurations. Both stereocenters in the structure on the right are also in *S* configurations. Remember that in Fischer projections, bonds drawn going left/right are envisioned as coming "out of the page," and bonds going north/south are envisioned as going "into the page." A plastic model kit or free chemistry software such as ISISDraw may help to convince you of this fact. Since each stereocenter retained the same configuration, the structures are exactly identical.

30. c. This is an example of a Fischer esterification. In a Fischer esterification, a carboxylic acid and an alcohol combine (in the presence of an acid catalyst) to produce an ester. During this reaction, water is produced as a by-product, forming from the loss of a proton from the alcohol and a hydroxyl group from the carboxylic acid. The *R* groups (the alkyl groups attached to the alcohol and to the acid) remain unchanged in this reaction. The equation is simplified, in that this reaction is an equilibrium process, and therefore both reactants and products will be present after the reaction occurs. Choices **a**, **b**, and **d** are incorrect because the structures are not esters, and this is a Fischer esterification whose product is always an ester. The structure in choice **c** is an ester, with the expected unchanged *R* groups.

31. **b.** The molecule shown is an aldehyde because of the –COH group on the molecule. Aldehydes are named based on the name of the parent molecule. To name an aldehyde, replace the *-e* at the end of the name of the parent hydrocarbon with an *-al*. For example, a five-carbon aldehyde would be named pentanal, after pentane, the parent five-carbon alkane. The molecule drawn here has six carbons in the longest chain; therefore, the parent molecule is hexane, and the molecule is a hexanal. The carbon with the aldehyde group has the highest priority for purposes of nomenclature, and is labeled as carbon #1. The substituents are as follows: two methyl groups on carbon #2, one methyl group on carbon #3, and one methyl group on carbon #4. Thus the molecule is 2,2,3,4-tetramethylhexanal. Carbon #3 and carbon #4 are both chiral, and the configuration must be determined and designated (i.e., *R* or *S*). The substituents of the third carbon have the following priorities: $C(CH_3)_2COH$ has priority 1, $CH(CH_3)CH_2CH_3$ has priority 2, the methyl group has priority 3, and the hydrogen has priority 4. Therefore, the carbon #3 is in the *R* configuration. The substituents of the fourth carbon have the following priorities: $CH(CH_3)C(CH_3)_2COH$ has priority 1, CH_2CH_3 has priority 2, the methyl has priority 3, and the hydrogen has priority 4. Therefore, carbon #4 is in the *R* configuration. The correct name is (3*R*, 4*R*)-2,2,3, 4-tetramethylhexanal. Choice **a** is incorrect because the molecule is not an alkene; it does not contain any carbon-carbon double bonds. Choice **c** is incorrect because the listed stereochemistry is incorrect. Choice **d** is incorrect because the molecule is not a ketone.

32. b. Carboxylic acids are more acidic than alcohols, as the resultant anion (upon losing the proton) can be resonance stabilized over the carboxylate group. Therefore, molecule II is the least acidic, as it is the only nonacid in the group. Halogen substituents on a molecule increase the acidity due to electron-withdrawing effects; the resulting anion (from loss of a proton) can be stabilized if it is close to an electronegative atom such as a halogen. This has the net effect of making halogen-containing molecules more acidic. Among the carboxylic acids, molecule I is the least acidic, as it contains no halogens. Molecule III has the next highest acidity, with one halogen present. Molecule IV has the most halogens, and is also a carboxylic acid. It is therefore the most acidic.

33. c. An S_N1 reaction is a two-step reaction with a carbocation intermediate formed during the first, rate-determining step. The carbocation is formed when the leaving group leaves with the two electrons from the covalent bond; this is the slow step of the mechanism. In each of the structures listed, the leaving group is bromine. The loss of bromine from structure **a** produces a primary carbocation, which is very unstable due to a lack of alkyl substitutents to help stabilize the positive charge through inductive effects. This translates to a very, very slow loss of bromine from structure **a**. The loss of bromine from structure **b** produces a secondary carbocation, which is more stable than a primary carbocation, but still not completely ideal. Structure **d** does not undergo an S_N1 reaction, because the carbons on the ring are not sp^3 hybridized; bromobenzenes can undergo substitution reactions, but not via an S_N1 mechanism. The loss of bromine from structure **c** produces a tertiary carbocation. Since carbocation stability increases with increasing substitution, tertiary carbocations are the most stable carbocations. The substrate with a tertiary carbocation intermediate is therefore the most reactive in an S_N1 reaction. The correct answer is **c**, 2-bromo–2-methylpentane.

34. d. An S_N1 reaction is a two-step reaction with a carbocation intermediate formed during the first, rate-determining step. The second step of an S_N1 reaction is a fast, nucleophilic attack by the nucleophile. The nucleophile in this example is the oxygen on the alcohol, as it has an abundance of electron density with which to attack an electrophile such as a carbocation. In this example, loss of the leaving group (bromine) produces a primary carbocation. Since primary carbocations are not very stable, the molecule quickly rearranges via a hydride shift to produce a more stable tertiary carbocation. A methyl shift would also be possible, but this would result in a (less favorable) secondary carbocation, and therefore the hydride shift is preferred. The next step is attack by the nucleophile (the alcohol). The final step is the loss of the proton from the oxygen. The final product of this reaction is an ether. Choice **a** is an alcohol, and is not product formed by this reaction. Choice **b** would be the product formed by the methyl shift (via the secondary carbocation intermediate), but it is not a significant product of this reaction due to the much more favorable hydride shift, which results in a tertiary carbocation. Choice **c** is a minor product formed from the primary carbocation that is initially formed, if that carbocation were attacked by the nucleophile before the rearrangement occurred. Choice **d** is the major product formed, and is produced by the nucleophilic attack on the rearranged, tertiary carbocation.

35. a. The reaction between hydrogen bromide and 2-methylpentene proceeds via a carbocation intermediate. In the first step, the double bond acts as a nucleophile and attacks the proton of hydrogen bromide. Markovnikov's rule is followed, in that the intermediate formed is as stable as possible; tertiary is preferred over secondary, which is preferred over primary. In this case, the carbocation is formed on carbon #2, giving a stable tertiary carbocation. Resultant attack of the bromide nucleophile (left over from the original hydrogen bromide reactant) completes the reaction, yielding 2-bromo–2-methylpentane.

36. c. This reaction represents the dehydration of an alcohol, which proceeds via an E_1 elimination. The first step of this reaction is protonation of the hydroxyl group by a proton from sulfuric acid. In the next (rate-determining) step, this protonated alcohol leaves as a water molecule, which produces a secondary carbocation. The final step is abstraction of a proton from a neighboring carbon to the carbocation by the hydrogen sulfate anion (which is left over from the sulfuric acid reagent, having already given up one of its protons). The electrons that were in the bond between the carbon and the proton flow over to the carbocation and form a double bond. The major product of this reaction is the alkene that has the most highly substituted double bond, as double bonds increase in stability as they gain substituents. Lower-energy (more stable) products are generally the preferred products in chemical reactions. Choice **a** has one more carbon than the reactant, and is not a possible product from this reaction. Choices **b** and **d** are the same monosubstituted product, drawn in a different orientation. Choice **c** is the only disubstituted product that can be formed from this reaction, and is the most stable.

37. d. Chromic acid is an oxidizing agent. Chromic acid oxidizes primary alcohols to carboxylic acids, secondary alcohols to ketones, and aldehydes to carboxylic acids. Chromic acid is unable to oxidize tertiary alcohols, because tertiary alcohols lack hydrogens on the carbon attached to the hydroxyl group; attempts to oxidize a tertiary alcohol would result in a five-bonded carbon atom, which breaks the rules of valence. Choices **a** and **b** are secondary alcohols, and can be oxidized by chromic acid. Choice **c** is an aldehyde, and can be oxidized by chromic acid. Choice **d** is a tertiary alcohol, and cannot be oxidized by chromic acid.

38. c. This reaction is a Grignard reaction. The bromoethane reacts with Mg in the presence of an ether solvent to produce a Grignard reagent, where the magnesium metal inserts into the carbon-bromine bond to form ethyl magnesium bromide. This reverses the normal chemical behavior of ethyl bromide (electrophilic), as magnesium is more electropositive than carbon, and therefore there is a buildup of electron density on the carbon atom attached to the magnesium. The Grignard reagent therefore functions as a carbanion/nucleophile, and attacks the carbonyl carbon present in the ester. The first nucleophilic attack adds an ethyl group to the carbonyl carbon; since carbon can support only four covalent bonds, the ethoxy group has to leave as a leaving group (ethoxide). The resulting molecule is a ketone, which still has a carbonyl carbon that is electrophilic and open to nucleophilic attack. A second equivalent of ethyl magnesium bromide can then perform another nucleophilic attack on the carbonyl carbon (which has a buildup of positive charge character, due to its proximity to the electronegative oxygen carbonyl atom). This produces a tertiary alcohol. Therefore, the correct answer is choice **c**.

39. a. When a carboxylic acid dehydrates, an acid anhydride can form. Intramolecular nucleophilic attack is also possible, particularly when five- or six-membered rings can be formed. Acid catalysis is often necessary in dehydration reactions. A ketal would never form from the dehydration of a carboxylic acid.

40. c. The alcohol is oxidized to the ketone. The chromate anion is a strong oxidizing agent.

41. d. An ester is less reactive than an acyl chloride. The alcohol group is not as good as a leaving group as the chloride anion.
42. b. Potassium permanganate is a strong oxidizing agent. When it reacts with toluene and then is treated with water, benzoic acid forms.
43. a. The iron(III) chloride is a Lewis acid catalyst. In electrophilic aromatic substitution, hydrogen can be replaced with chlorine under the proper conditions. These conditions require the Lewis acid catalyst and diatomic chlorine.
44. c. The ortho and para products form. The iodine anion is an ortho/para director. The nitro group adds to the ortho and para sites on the benzene ring.
45. a. Ethers donate electron density to the aromatic ring. They activate the aromatic ring toward electrophilic aromatic substitution.
46. b. The fluorine anion is an ortho/para director.
47. a. This is a Clemmensen reduction, with Zn(Hg) amalgam as the reducing agent. The ketone is reduced to an alkane.
48. d. One mole of benzyl ethane forms as this aklylating agent adds one mole of the ethyl group to the benzyl iodide.

Section 5: Writing

Essay 2

Good Response

While there are some people, like Facebook founder Mark Zuckerberg, who believe that the age of privacy in our society is over, there are others who think that privacy is something we should attempt to preserve. In an age of social media overload and increased use of the Internet to conduct personal and work-related business transactions, is it possible, or even desirable, to fight for privacy? From parents who want to protect their children to individuals and businesses that want to avoid cyberfraud and stolen identities, the answer is definitely yes. But how?

If you are a parent, you probably have rules about how much television your children may watch and what programs are acceptable for them. Applying similar rules about the Internet may help protect your child's privacy. For example, if you decide to allow your young teenager to have a Facebook page or Twitter account, discuss the rules and expectations with your child in advance. Then monitor the page frequently to make sure your child is following the agreed-upon rules. Such parameters may be about the amount of time spent on the Internet as well as specifics regarding the types of comments he or she is allowed to make and updates he or she is allowed to post. You will probably want to make rules regarding photos as well.

For yourself, you should be wary of providing information like your Social Security number to any website or online business, even if it's a bank. While stolen credit card numbers are a risk when purchasing online, the theft of your Social Security number is more damaging. Keep your number as private as possible, since sharing your Social Security number can enable someone to steal your identity, open new cards in your name, and commit other types of fraud that can be very difficult to undo.

You should also set an example for your children by sharing with them the way you use the Internet and the information that you choose to share. Family photos from the holidays may be fine to post, but beware of photos and language demonstrating negative behaviors you wouldn't want your boss to see. These days, potential employers can find significant information about job applicants online, and no one should lose out on a job because of an embarrassing photograph on Facebook.

In closing, while certain types of privacy have disappeared in today's world, some level of privacy can still be preserved if people choose to be careful about what information they and their families share online. Everyone should think about the implications of any information shared on the Internet getting into the hands of anyone a person might want to impress now or in the future. Children will need their parents to guide them on this, since most children learn from the good examples set them.

Analysis

This is a strong response because it is well written and it approaches the privacy issue from more than one angle—discussing what adults can do, what they can do to help their children be careful about the information they share on the Internet, and how they can set good examples for their children.

At the end of the first paragraph it uses the rhetorical device of asking a question that the next paragraph will answer. While this doesn't work in all cases, in this instance it sets up the solutions nicely.

Weak Response

The loss of privacy is a serious concern for American citizens today. It is a major problem for all of us. We need ways to solve it.

One way would be for people to spend less time on the Internet, where they often give too much information out about themselves in emails and in social media. Other people might use that information in bad ways, and if it's not out there, it can't be used.

Another way is to not buy things online, so you don't give your credit card information out online. That makes it harder for someone to steal your credit card and charge things on it. Instead people can shop online for what they like and go buy it in stores. It's not as convenient, but it might help with privacy.

A third way is to control the way your children use the Internet. If you limit the time they can be online, and keep them off of certain websites, they are less likely to write or post things that could effect their privacy or your's.

Another way is to remember that anything you write online, in an email or on Facebook, is there forever, so think before you post.

If all of us did these things and were a little more careful, we'd have more privacy.

Analysis

While this essay is not a bad one in terms of answering the question, it is a very simple argument that lacks the sophistication of the good response. The paragraphs are short, it appears to be more of a list than an argument, and there are grammatical and spelling errors at the end of the fourth paragraph. The correct word in the second sentence should be *affect*, as in have an impact on, not *effect*, which implies cause and effect. In addition, an apostrophe does not belong in the word *yours.*

This essay response is just adequate. Compare it to the good response, read the explanations, and you will be able to see what you have to do to write a good essay.

Section 6: Reading Comprehension

Passage 1

1. a. While Leeuwenhoek saw microbes and bacteria (viruses are too small to see under the kind of microscope he had), the word *corpuscles* refers specifically to blood cells.

2. d. Leeuwenhoek's work led to the germ theory of disease, which led to descriptions of disease-causing agents like bacteria, which led to effective ways to fight infectious disease. His work did not lead to cancer therapies.

3. c. Diabetes is the only one of the choices not in the passage, and it is a chronic disease, not an infectious disease.

4. c. His discoveries were almost accidental, and he was not searching for fame and fortune. In the quote from him, he talks about sharing information and knowledge.

5. a. The author is telling the story in a straightforward manner, so the tone is neither cynical nor negative. While there is scientific information in the passage, it is focused more on the history of Leeuwenhoek's life than on scientific details.

6. b. The author admires the early work Leeuwenhoek did, particularly since he was an amateur.

7. d. Although he was a tailor and he ended up being the father of microbiology, the best description of Leeuwenhoek from this passage is an amateur scientist.

8. c. In the passage, the word *animalcules* refers to all of the microorganisms Leeuwenhoek saw through his microscope.

Passage 2

9. a. While Dr. Blackwell did face adversity, and she was the first woman in the United States to go to medical school, and she might be considered to have been stubborn, the main idea of the passage was that her perseverance had a long-term impact on many other women.

10. d. The word *abolitionist* is associated with the antislavery movement in the United States prior to the Civil War.

11. d. As her friend's illness was terminal—not curable—she was not able to help her survive, though her friend was Blackwell's inspiration.

12. c. While it is likely that the other students at Geneva Medical College doubted Elizabeth Blackwell's ability and probably didn't have much confidence in her, the passage directly states that they voted to admit her; therefore, choice **c** is the correct answer. All of the other statements are inferences, not facts.

13. b. The context of the use of the words *dispensary practice* indicates it involves doctors working in groups, and makes it clear that Dr. Blackwell was looking for collaborators and partners as opposed to being a sole practitioner.

14. c. While Dr. Blackwell was often selfless, and may have chosen a path that was dangerous at the time, the best description of her efforts, according to the passage, is that they were pioneering.

15. b. While the passage refers to Blackwell becoming a teacher, and is about her becoming a doctor later, there is specific reference to her dream of becoming a surgeon in paragraph 5 of the passage.

16. a. Because the tone of this passage is very factual, although it describes a first for women, it does not take a position about whether women should be in medicine, so the best answer is choice **a**. Even though you might infer that the author wouldn't write about the subject otherwise, you can't know that for sure; you can only base the answer on the passage in front of you.

Passage 3

17. b. The author has a clear point of view, so choice **a**, neutral reporting, is not the correct answer. And while the author may be angry (choice **c**) and frustrated (choice **d**), the passage itself includes arguments and facts, so choice **b** is the best answer.

18. c. The author states that treating patients of all ages the same way is not the most effective way to meet their needs. While the author certainly believes that doctors should provide effective care to all patients, the theme of the passage is focused on elderly patients, so choice **c** is the best answer.

19. **a.** In the passage, the use of depression as an example is to discuss a specific issue that elderly patients face in high proportion and use it to illustrate the need for specialized training. While all other choices are true statements, choice **a** is the one that reflects the ideas from the passage.

20. **b.** Choices **c** and **d** may be true statements, but the author of this passage thinks doctors should routinely look beyond the obvious symptoms when dealing with older patients.

21. **b.** The author's attitude, based on the passage, is one of concern with the current system. Pessimistic (choice **a**) is too strong, resigned (choice **d**) is not accurate because there are implied suggestions for improvement, and satisfied (choice **c**) is the opposite of the author's attitude.

22. **c.** The use of the word *diligent* in this context means probing, in other words continuing to ask questions. Careless (choice **a**) is the opposite, and the other two choices are not as accurate as choice **c**.

23. **d.** While choice **d** may be true, it is the only choice not mentioned in the passage. Therefore it is the correct answer choice.

24. **c.** While choice **a** looks like the correct answer, it leaves the doctor out of the equation, and the author clearly states that patients and doctors must work together to manage medications. While the author might agree that elderly patients should avoid over-the-counter medications, this is not stated in the passage and therefore is not the best answer choice.

Passage 4

25. **b.** The word *malaise* most closely means discomfort and unease, so choice **b** is the correct answer.

26. **d.** The passage clearly states that the epidemic rise of lung cancer in the twentieth century was due to smoking and not the other choices.

27. **c.** The causal relationship between smoking and lung cancer was shown scientifically in the 1960s when the committee reviewed thousands of scientific articles and experiments and compiled the results.

28. **d.** While tuberculosis is a respiratory disease, it is caused by a bacterium. The other three diseases may be caused all or in part by smoking.

29. **a.** According to the passage, the 1964 Surgeon General's Report defined the issue more specifically than it had been defined before, and showed significant research evidence to back up its statements, but it left the concrete remedies to the legislative branch of government. The report clearly indicated that action was needed and it was not neutral. While the report might have suggested remedies, the Surgeon General's office would have no power to carry them out unless they were made into laws by the legislature.

30. **b.** The tone of the passage is best described as informative. Factual isn't broad enough, and the author clearly cares about the subject, so the tone is not dispassionate.

31. **d.** Although there is reference to low-birth-weight babies, there is no direct reference to smoking and growth. All of the other choices are directly stated in the passage.

32. **c.** In the passage the word *hedged* most closely means that the report played down the direct association between nicotine and addiction. While it is implied that the committee thought nicotine was addictive, they chose to make a much softer statement in the report.

Passage 5

33. c. Choice **c** is the best answer because, although alternative medicine has not been proven to work, according to the passage, many people feel it does help them.

34. c. In the context of the passage, the word *holistic* refers to overall treatment that would include standard medical therapy and alternative medicine. Piecemeal (choice **d**) and single-focused (choice **a**) are opposites, and holistic in this context refers to patients, not diseases (choice **b**).

35. a. The primary purpose of the passage is closest to choice **a**. The passage does not confirm or deny the safety and effectiveness of alternative treatments, and it is not critical of them.

36. d. The first three choices are considered alternative medicine. Vitamins, although their value is sometimes debated, are considered part of mainstream medicine.

37. d. Although the author of the passage provides useful information about the subject, the beginning and end of the piece set a tone of facts with a sense of humor. There is no sarcasm, and the passage does not focus on history.

38. c. The author uses the amount of money spent on alternative treatments to illustrate that Americans are willing to pay for alternative treatments even though they are usually not covered by insurance and they may not work. The author does not make a judgment about how much Americans spend (answer choice **a**), whether alternative treatments should be covered (choice **d**), or whether they work (choice **b**).

39. b. In this context, the phrase *as a complement to* means in addition to/along with. Choice **a**, as a positive statement about, could be true only if the word were spelled *compliment.* The other choices, instead of (choice **c**) and after (choice **d**), do not fit the context.

40. b. The author implies that research on alternative therapies to show whether they work would be valuable and should be done. The author does not discuss the cost of such research or say it would be useless or not worthwhile.

Passage 6

41. b. While the first sentence talks about adults, the rest of the paragraph expands to discuss children and different ethnic groups, so although choice **c** is true, choice **b** is the best answer.

42. d. The author links the rise in obesity rates to choices **a**, **b**, and **c**. Healthy eating is not mentioned as a cause, so choice **d** is the correct answer.

43. d. The author discusses the confusion about different types of diets and the medical evidence to support them, so the best answer is that people are confused about what is healthy and what diet is best. While people are looking for fast ways to lose weight (choice **a**), that is not the focus of the passage. People are concerned about fat and carbohydrate intake, among other things, so choices **b** and **c** are not correct.

44. a. The author's purpose is to include confusing and contradictory information in the passage to show that dieting and eating properly are not as simple as low fat. The author does not address myths about dieting and weight loss (choice **b**), criticize the science behind dieting (choice **c**), or advocate for high-fat diets (choice **d**).

45. b. The tone of the last sentence is ironic. After a passage about what we should and shouldn't eat, you might expect an answer or conclusion at the end. Instead the author does the opposite, and says that we're all hungry so we have to eat something, though after reading the passage we don't know what we should eat.

46. b. Satiation and satiety refer to the feeling of fullness. Even if you don't know the meaning of the word, the context in this case should help to make it clear that the author is discussing feeling full.

47. c. The author states clearly that studies linking dietary fat and heart disease are inconclusive.

48. c. Although the word *epidemic* implies something scary, in this case, the author uses the word to show the reader how serious the issue of heart disease among middle-aged men was after World War II. Choice **c** is the best answer.

Section 7: Quantitative Ability

1. b. An integer is defined as any number with no fractional or decimal parts, including negative whole numbers and zero.

2. a. The associative property of addition allows you to group different numbers together, still resulting in the same solution.

3. d. The order of operations follows the saying Please Excuse My Dear Aunt Sally: parentheses, exponents, multiplication and division (from left to right), then addition and subtraction (from left to right).

4. d. To add mixed numbers, first create common denominators in the fractional parts. Add the two whole numbers together ($7 + 8 = 15$), then add the fractions ($\frac{3}{14} + \frac{4}{14} = \frac{7}{14}$). Simplify the fractional part to get 15 and $\frac{1}{2}$.

5. d. To convert a fraction to a decimal, divide the denominator by the numerator. When you divide 473 by 125 you get 0.2642706131. However, the question asks you to round the decimal to the thousandths place, or the third digit after the decimal point, giving you 0.264.

6. a. Divide the coefficients, $3.14 \div 1.25$, which gives you 2.512. Then subtract the exponents, $6 - 2$, which equals 4. The result is 2.512×10^4.

7. d. Use long division to solve this problem. The goal for each step is to eliminate the first term of the dividend. First you multiply the divisor by x^3, which gives you $x^4 - 3x^3$. Subtract this expression from the dividend, canceling out the x^4, and bring down what's left of the dividend after cancellation and subtraction. Place what you multiplied the divisor by on top of the division sign over the term of the same power. Repeat this until you have only a constant left over after subtraction. This constant is your remainder. If the constant is zero, you have no remainder.

$$
\begin{array}{rl}
 & x^3 + 6x^2 + 14x + 50 \quad \text{R. } 145 \\
x - 3 \,\big) & x^4 + 3x^3 - 4x^2 + 8x - 5 \\
 & -x^4 - 3x^3 \\
 & \qquad 6x^3 - 4x^2 \\
 & \qquad -6x^3 - 18x^2 \\
 & \qquad\qquad 14x^2 + 8x \\
 & \qquad\qquad -14x^2 - 42x \\
 & \qquad\qquad\qquad 50x - 5 \\
 & \qquad\qquad\qquad -50x - 150 \\
 & \qquad\qquad\qquad\qquad 145
\end{array}
$$

8. a. Add 3 to both sides first; then there are two ways this problem could be solved. The first and simplest way is by factoring into $(2x + 3)(3x + 1)$. Set the two factors equal to zero and solve for x. The other way is to plug the coefficients into the quadratic formula.

9. d. Subtract 3 from both sides; then subtract $4x$ from each side. Divide both sides by 4 to find out what x is.

10. a. Set up equivalent ratios, using any variable as the unknown amount of females. We are given the female-to-male ratio 3:5 and a quantity of 15 boys. The ratio containing the unknown should mirror the order of girls and boys in the given ratio. Cross multiply to solve for the variable in your ratio, which tells how many females are in the class.

11. b. Subtract $527 from $1,439 to find how much money was in Matt's account before the deposit: $912. Divide $527 by $912, the amount of increase divided by the original value.

12. c. Add 3 to both sides in order to have the polynomial set equal to zero, resulting in $6x^2 + 7x + 2$. Let $a = 6$, $b = 7$, and $c = 2$. Plug these values into the quadratic equation:

$$x = \frac{-b \pm \sqrt{b^2 - 4ac}}{2a}$$

$$x = \frac{-7 \pm \sqrt{7^2 - (4 \cdot 6 \cdot 2)}}{2 \cdot 6}$$

$$x = \frac{-7 \pm \sqrt{49 - 48}}{12}$$

$$x = \frac{-7 \pm \sqrt{1}}{12}$$

$$x = \frac{-6}{12},\ x = \frac{-8}{12}$$

$$x = \frac{-1}{2},\ x = \frac{-2}{3}$$

$$x = -0.5,\ x = -0.67$$

13. c. First solve for one variable. In this case, y is the easiest to solve for in the second equation. After solving for y, you get $y = 2x - 4$. Substitute this for y in the first equation to solve for x.

14. d. Solve the inequality just as you would an equation with an equal sign. First subtract 4 from both sides. Then divide each side by negative 3. Whenever you multiply or divide an inequality by a negative number, you must change the sign to the opposite operation. In this case, $\leq$ becomes $\geq$.

15. b. For any log(base b)(x) = a, $b^a = x$. For this particular logarithm, 3 to the fourth power is 81.

16. b. To calculate the mean, or average, of a set of numbers, add the numbers together and divide the total by the number of numbers in the set. For this example there are six numbers in the set, so: $1 + 3 + 4 + 5 + 7 + 10 = 30$. $\frac{30}{6} = 5$.

17. d. To determine the probability of two separate events happening simultaneously, find the probability of each event happening individually and multiply the probabilities together. The probability of an odd number being rolled on a die is $\frac{1}{2}$. Thus, multiplying $\frac{1}{2}$ by $\frac{1}{2}$ becomes $\frac{1}{4}$, or 0.25. Multiply by 100 to get the percentage, 25%.

18. c. To calculate the median of a set of numbers, find the center value(s). The center values are 5 and 5, so the median is 5.

19. a. In the case of two coins flipped simultaneously, there are four possible outcomes: HH, TT, HT, and TH. Out of the four possible outcomes, two outcomes satisfy the problem statement and contain one coin that lands heads up. Thus, two out of four, or $\frac{2}{4}$ (50%), outcomes satisfy the problem.

20. c. To determine the range of a set of numbers, subtract the lower limit from the upper limit. Thus, $12 - (-3) = 15$.

21. a. To determine the probability of a single event, divide the chances of the specific event occurring by the chances of any event occurring. Thus, divide the number of green balls by the number of total balls: $\frac{12}{30} = 0.4$ or 40%. Do the same for the red balls: $\frac{10}{30} = 0.333$ or 33.3%.

22. c. To calculate the mean of a set of numbers, add the numbers together and divide the total by the number of numbers in the set. For this example there are seven numbers in the set, so: $2 + 4 + 6 + 8 + 8 + 8 + 10 = 46$; $\frac{46}{7} = 6.6$. To calculate the median, determine the total number of values, which is seven. The fourth (middle) value, 8, is the median. To determine the range, subtract the lower limit from the upper limit. Thus, $10 - 2 = 8$. To calculate the mode, determine which number appears in the set most frequently. The number 8 appears the most times, so the mode is 8.

23. d. To determine the probability of two separate events happening simultaneously, find the probability of each event happening individually and multiply the probabilities together. Thus, you get $\frac{4}{10}$ multiplied by $\frac{6}{10}$, which is $\frac{24}{100}$ or 0.24, or 24%. To find the probability of either of these events happening, add the probabilities together and subtract the probability that both events will occur: $\frac{4}{10} + \frac{6}{10} - \frac{24}{100} = \frac{76}{100}$ or 76%.

24. c. To calculate the mode, determine which value in the set of numbers occurs the most frequently. The number 2 occurs six times, more than any other number, so it is the mode.

25. c. Substitute 2 for x and calculate $12(2) + 30 = 54$.

26. c. The order of a function is the highest exponent in the function. Determine the function that produces the graph, $f(x) = x^3$, and find the highest exponent, 3. Thus, this graph (and function) is a third-order function.

27. a. Substitute the input numbers into the function. Your answers should be in the form of ordered pairs.

28. d. Plug 3 in for x in $g(x)$, which gives you 7. Then substitute 7 for x in $f(x)$ and solve. The answer is 15.

29. b. The slopes of any two perpendicular lines are multiplicative and additive inverses of each other. You need to change the sign *and* flip the number ($\frac{4}{1} \rightarrow \frac{1}{4}$). The result is $-\frac{1}{4}$.

30. c. The slope of any vertical line is undefined.

31. d. To find the slope given two points, look at the rise over run, or the change in y over the change in x. In this case, subtract 4 from 7 and divide the result by the difference between 3 and zero: $(7 - 4) \div (3 - 0) = 1$.

32. a. The slope of any horizontal line is zero.

33. c. Find the slope by computing the rise over run. Then find the equation of the line with the same slope. Parallel lines always have the same slope. Slope $= (7 - 1) \div (2 - 4) = 6 \div 2 = -3$.

34. d. If you don't know what function this graph depicts by looking at it, you can make an input/output table to find the pattern.

35. d. Substitute $g(x)$ everywhere you see an x in $f(x)$. Then simplify as far as possible.

36. b. Where the graph crosses the x-axis, y will equal zero. Set $f(x)$ equal to zero and solve for x by factoring: $(x - 3)(x + 1)$.

37. b. Given $f(x) = x^n, f'(x) = nx^{n-1}$. Take the derivative of each term individually by bringing the exponent out front and subtracting 1 from the exponent. $f'(x) = 2x + 4$.

38. c. Find the first derivative and find $f'(0)$;
$f'(x) = 2x + 6, f'(0) = 6$.

39. d. Take the first derivative by deriving each term individually. Then do the same again to obtain the second derivative.

$f'(x) = 12x^3 - 15x^2 + 4x$

$f''(x) = 36x^2 - 30x + 4$

40. c. A function is decreasing wherever its derivative is less than zero. Take the derivative of the function, which is 12. Twelve is always positive; therefore, it is *never* less than zero, so it *never* decreases; $f'(x) = 12$.

41. b. Take the first derivative by deriving each term individually. Then do the same again to obtain the second derivative.

$f'(x) = 4x^3 + 9x^2 + 12x + 7$

$f''(x) = 12x^2 + 18x + 12$

42. a. Find the second derivative and set it greater than zero. Then solve for x.

$f'(x) = 3x^2 + 8x + 3$

$f''(x) = 6x + 8$

$6x + 8 > 0$

$6x > -8$

$x > -\frac{8}{6}$

$x > -\frac{4}{3}$

43. c. Find where the first derivative equals zero to identify where the local extrema (maxima or minima) are. Then find the second derivative at that point (plug the point into the second derivative) to determine whether the extreme point is a minimum or a maximum. The point is a minimum if your answer after plugging it into the second derivative is positive, and a maximum if your answer after plugging it into the second derivative is negative.

$f'(x) = 6x + 2$

$f''(x) = 6$

$6x + 2 = 0$

$6x = -2$

$x = -\frac{2}{6}$

$x = -\frac{1}{3}$

44. d. Antiderivative is synonymous with integral. Given $f(x) = x^n$, the integral of $f(x)$ equals x^{n+1} divided by $(n + 1)$. Add 1 to the exponent and divide by the new exponent.

45. b. Antiderivative is synonymous with integral. Given $f(x) = x^n$, the integral of $f(x)$ equals x^{n+1} divided by $(n + 1)$. Add 1 to the exponent and divide by the new exponent. Follow this process for each term.

46. d. Integrate each term individually using the same method described in the previous problem.

47. d. Integrate each term individually then substitute 5 for x in the result. Substitute zero for x in the result and find the difference between the two resulting numbers.

$\int 3x^2 + 2x + 4dx = x^3 + x^2 + 4x$

$f(5) = 5^3 + 5^2 + 4 \times 5 =$

$125 + 25 + 20 = 170$

$f(0) = 0$

$170 - 0 = 170$

48. a. Integrals can be used to find area. Integrate the function. Substitute 2 for x and subtract the result by the result of zero substituted for x.

$\int x^2\,dx = \frac{x^3}{3}$

$f(2) = \frac{2^3}{3} = \frac{8}{3}$

$f(0) = 0$

$\frac{8}{3} - 0 = \frac{8}{3}$

ADDITIONAL ONLINE PRACTICE

Whether you need help building basic skills or preparing for an exam, visit the LearningExpress Practice Center! Using the code below, you'll be able to access additional PCAT online practice. This online practice will also provide you with:

Immediate Scoring
Detailed answer explanations
Personalized recommendations for further practice and study

Log in to the LearningExpress Practice Center by using the URL: **www.learnatest.com/practice**

This is your Access Code: **7878**

Follow the steps online to redeem your access code. After you've used your access code to register with the site, you will be prompted to create a username and password. For easy reference, record them here:

Username: ______________________ **Password:** ______________________

With your username and password, you can log in and access your additional practice materials. If you have any questions or problems, please contact LearningExpress customer service at 1-800-295-9556 ext. 2, or e-mail us at **customerservice@learningexpressllc.com**

NOTES

NOTES